OXFORD MEDICAL PUBLICATIONS

Oxford Handbook of
Paediatrics

Published and forthcoming Oxford Handbooks

Oxford Handbook for the Foundation Programme 3e
Oxford Handbook of Acute Medicine 3e
Oxford Handbook of Anaesthesia 3e
Oxford Handbook of Applied Dental Sciences
Oxford Handbook of Cardiology 2e
Oxford Handbook of Clinical and Laboratory Investigation 3e
Oxford Handbook of Clinical Dentistry 5e
Oxford Handbook of Clinical Diagnosis 2e
Oxford Handbook of Clinical Examination and Practical Skills
Oxford Handbook of Clinical Haematology 3e
Oxford Handbook of Clinical Immunology and Allergy 3e
Oxford Handbook of Clinical Medicine – Mini Edition 8e
Oxford Handbook of Clinical Medicine 8e
Oxford Handbook of Clinical Pathology
Oxford Handbook of Clinical Pharmacy 2e
Oxford Handbook of Clinical Rehabilitation 2e
Oxford Handbook of Clinical Specialties 9e
Oxford Handbook of Clinical Surgery 4e
Oxford Handbook of Complementary Medicine
Oxford Handbook of Critical Care 3e
Oxford Handbook of Dental Patient Care 2e
Oxford Handbook of Dialysis 3e
Oxford Handbook of Emergency Medicine 4e
Oxford Handbook of Endocrinology and Diabetes 2e
Oxford Handbook of ENT and Head and Neck Surgery
Oxford Handbook of Epidemiology for Clinicians
Oxford Handbook of Expedition and Wilderness Medicine
Oxford Handbook of Gastroenterology & Hepatology 2e
Oxford Handbook of General Practice 3e
Oxford Handbook of Genetics
Oxford Handbook of Genitourinary Medicine, HIV and AIDS 2e
Oxford Handbook of Geriatric Medicine
Oxford Handbook of Infectious Diseases and Microbiology
Oxford Handbook of Key Clinical Evidence
Oxford Handbook of Medical Dermatology
Oxford Handbook of Medical Imaging
Oxford Handbook of Medical Sciences 2e
Oxford Handbook of Medical Statistics
Oxford Handbook of Nephrology and Hypertension
Oxford Handbook of Neurology
Oxford Handbook of Nutrition and Dietetics 2e
Oxford Handbook of Obstetrics and Gynaecology 2e
Oxford Handbook of Occupational Health 2e
Oxford Handbook of Oncology 3e
Oxford Handbook of Ophthalmology 2e
Oxford Handbook of Oral and Maxillofacial Surgery
Oxford Handbook of Paediatrics 2e
Oxford Handbook of Pain Management
Oxford Handbook of Palliative Care 2e
Oxford Handbook of Practical Drug Therapy 2e
Oxford Handbook of Pre-Hospital Care
Oxford Handbook of Psychiatry 3e
Oxford Handbook of Public Health Practice 2e
Oxford Handbook of Reproductive Medicine & Family Planning
Oxford Handbook of Respiratory Medicine 2e
Oxford Handbook of Rheumatology 3e
Oxford Handbook of Sport and Exercise Medicine
Oxford Handbook of Tropical Medicine 3e
Oxford Handbook of Urology 3e

Oxford Handbook of
Paediatrics

Second Edition

Edited by

Robert C. Tasker

Professor of Neurology and Anaesthesia (Pediatrics),
Harvard Medical School; Chair in Neurocritical Care,
Children's Hospital, Boston, USA

Robert J. McClure

Neonatologist, Paediatrician and Anatomical Pathologist
Queen Elizabeth Medical Centre, Nedlands,
Perth, Western Australia

Carlo L. Acerini

University Senior Lecturer,
Cambridge University Clinical School,
Cambridge, UK

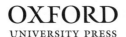

OXFORD
UNIVERSITY PRESS

OXFORD
UNIVERSITY PRESS

Great Clarendon Street, Oxford, OX2 6DP,
United Kingdom

Oxford University Press is a department of the University of Oxford.
It furthers the University's objective of excellence in research, scholarship,
and education by publishing worldwide. Oxford is a registered trade mark of
Oxford University Press in the UK and in certain other countries

First edition published 2008
Second edition published 2013 , Reprinted 2014 , 2015 , 2016 , 2017 , 2018 , 2019

Impression: 11

British Library Cataloguing in Publication Data
Data available

ISBN 978–0–19–960830–0 (flexicover: alk.paper)

Printed in China by
C&C Offset Printing Co. Ltd.

Foreword to the first edition

Textbooks have been the mainstay of medical education for centuries. Clearly, the development of the information superhighway via the Internet has changed how we learn, find information, and communicate. What does yet another paediatric textbook add to the current long list of titles?

Drs Tasker, McClure, and Acerini have conceived of and edited a new book. It is a handbook of paediatrics that joins a stable of similar publications from Oxford University Press. There are 23 contributing editors. Using a well-tested format for presentation, the handbook consists of 31 chapters, ranging from sections on epidemiology, evidence, and practice, through the more traditional topics, such as nephrology and neurology, and concluding with international health and travel, and paediatrics, ethics, and the law. Each chapter follows the same format, 5–40 sections, followed by bulleted points. Both signs and symptoms of illness, as well as specific diseases are covered. Virtually all topics are limited to 1–2 pages of important information. Tables are carefully inserted, and complement the text. Doses of important drugs are included in the text and/or the tables. There are a limited number of figures, but like the tables, they supplement the text and have been carefully chosen to add clarity.

The *Oxford Handbook of Paediatrics* is a worthy addition to your library. It will be particularly appealing to medical students and younger physicians, who have learned to digest a great deal of information quickly and in an abbreviated format. Its availability on a CD-ROM is an added and necessary benefit. Drs Tasker, McClure, and Acerini have done a wonderful job in ensuring consistency, clarity, and completeness.

Professor Howard Bauchner,
Boston University School of Medicine/Boston Medical Center,
Vice-Chair, Academic Affairs,
Editor in Chief, Archives of Disease in Childhood,
January 2008

Preface

The first 'boke' of paediatrics printed in English was written by Thomas Phaire (1510–1560), a man from East Anglia who studied medicine at Oxford University. The book had 56 pages, measured 3 7/8 inches (9.8cm) by 2 5/8 inches (6.7cm), and covered '… innumerable passions & diseases, wherunto the bodye of man is subiecte, and as well moste commonly the tender age of chyldren is chefely vexed and greued with these diseases folowyng. Apostume of the brayne, swellyng of the head …'.[1] In 1553, the 'innumerable passions & diseases' came to 39 presenting clinical problems. As clinicians, we first met and worked in the heart of East Anglia (Cambridge University) and have now collaborated with Oxford University Press in this venture, a new handbook of paediatrics. Our similarity with Thomas Phaire has not escaped us, particularly as we see the importance of basing a text on common presenting clinical problems.

Our principal aim is to provide a compact source of information and clinical thinking that can be used in the clinic or hospital ward, at a time when the child is being seen. The challenge, therefore, was to distil the content of information found in several textbooks into a conveniently sized handbook without the loss of important information. We easily reached the limit in pages given to us, and so we have had to be strict in sifting out key facts crucial to clinical practice. Our intention is that the handbook be used from the start of one's education in paediatrics all the way through to higher general training in the field.

We have kept with the tradition of providing content and text that often exceeds that required by the generalist—we believe it important for learners and readers to see the full landscape. There are spaces where more notes can be added from lectures, other reading, and personal experience. This is intended. It means that the handbook can be made personal, develop with you, and be used in whatever your chosen practice— hospitalist, generalist, or community and family practice. Above all, we hope that the handbook will give you confidence to manage paediatric clinical problems effectively and safely.

RCT
RJM
CLA
April 2012

Reference

1 Phaire T (1553). *The boke of chyldren*. [Reprint edited by Neale AV, Wallis HRE (1965). Edinburgh: E&S Livingstone Ltd, Edinburgh.

Authors' disclaimer

All reasonable efforts have been undertaken in order to ensure the accuracy of drug doses in this book. UK readers are advised to also consult the British National Formulary for children (2012; see http://www.bnf.org/bnf/index.htm)). Other readers should refer to their own regional or national guidelines. The authors cannot be held responsible for any errors here in.

Acknowledgements

We would like to extend our thanks and gratitude to all the contributors. We would also like to thank our colleagues who reviewed and advised on the content of our chapters, in particular Dr Robert Ross-Russell, Dr Roddy O'Donnell, Jenny Pool, Amy Stewart, Clare Bradley Stevenson, and Liesje Cornwell for their helpful comments. We are also indebted to Dr Stephan Sanders for his comments and criticisms of our draft manuscript. We would also like to thank Drs Kim Jones and Tony Jaffa, Profs Deirdre Kelly and Brett McDermott, and Ms Julia Smith, Kelly Lamour, and Lynne Radbone for their contribution to the last edition. We are especially grateful to Beth Womack and Elizabeth Reeve at OUP for their help and assistance, and for their patience with us. Finally, but not least, a special thanks goes to our respective families for their encouragement, support, and understanding throughout the preparation of this book.

Robert C. Tasker
Robert J. McClure
Carlo L. Acerini

RJM is indebted to Marge, Hannah, and Thomas, for their endless love, support, and sacrifice.

Contributors

Mr David Albert
Consultant Otolaryngologist,
Great Ormond Street Hospital for
Children NHS Foundation Trust,
London

Miss Louise Allen
Consultant Paediatric
Ophthalmologist
Cambridge University Hospitals
NHS Foundation Trust,
Cambridge, and
Associate Lecturer, University of
Cambridge, UK

Dr R Mark Beattie
Consultant Paediatric
Gastroenterologist
University Hospital Southampton
Southampton, UK

Mr Yogesh Bajaj
Consultant Paediatric
Otolaryngologist
Barts, and the London Children's
Hospital, London

Dr Ian Balfour-Lynn
Consultant in Respiratory
Paediatrics
Royal Brompton Hospital, London

Dr Detlef Bockenhauer
Honorary Consultant
Renal Unit, Great Ormond Street
Hospital NHS Trust;
HEFCE Clinical Senior Lecturer,
UCL Institute of Child Health,
London, UK

Dr Tony Caccetta
Dermatology Registrar
Princess Margaret Hospital, Perth,
Western Australia

Professor Imti Choonara
Professor in Child Health,
Academic Division of Child
Health, University of Nottingham,
Derbyshire Children's Hospital
Derby, UK

Dr David Coghill
Ninewells Hospital and
Medical School,
Dundee, UK

Mr David Crabbe
Consultant Paediatric Surgeon
Leeds Teaching Hospitals NHS
Trust and Bradford Teaching
Hospitals NHS Foundation Trust,
UK

Dr Saul N Faust
Reader in Paediatric Immunology
and Infectious Diseases and
Director, NIHR Wellcome
Trust Clinical Research Facility,
University of Southampton, UK

Dr Rob Freeman
Consultant Orthopaedic Surgeon,
Robert Jones and Agnes
Hunt Orthopaedic Hospital NHS
Trust, Shropshire, UK

Dr Georgina Hall
Consultant, Paediatric
Haematology/Oncology Unit, John
Radcliffe Hospital, Oxford, UK

Dr Peter Heinz
Consultant Paediatrician
Cambridge University Hospitals
NHS Foundation Trust,
Cambridge, UK

Dr Ewen D Johnston

Consultant Neonatologist
Simpson Centre for Reproductive
Health, Royal Infirmary of
Edinburgh,
UK

Dr Samir Latifi

Consultant in Paediatric Intensive
Care, Akron Children's Hospital
Akron, Ohio, USA

Dr Elaine Lewis

Consultant Community
Paediatrician, Cambridge
University Hospitals NHS
Foundation Trust,
Cambridge, UK

Dr James C Nicholson

Consultant Paediatric Oncologist
Cambridge University Hospitals
NHS Foundation Trust,
Cambridge, UK

Dr Roddy O'Donnell

Consultant in Paediatric Intensive
Care, Cambridge University
Hospitals NHS Foundation Trust,
Cambridge, UK

Dr Alasdair Parker

Consultant Paediatric Neurologist,
Cambridge University Hospitals
NHS Foundation Trust,
Cambridge, UK

Dr Willie Reardon

Consultant Clinical Geneticist,
Our Lady's Hospital for Sick
Children, Dublin, Ireland

Dr Lesley Rees

Consultant Paediatric
Nephrologist
Great Ormond Street Hospital for
Children Foundation Trust,
London

**Professor Benjamin J
Stenson**

Consultant Neonatologist
Simpson Centre for Reproductive
Health, Royal Infirmary of
Edinburgh, UK

Dr Robert M R Tulloh

Consultant in Paediatric
Cardiology, Bristol Royal Hospital
for Children and Bristol Royal
Infirmary, UK

Contents

Detailed contents

6   Neonatology

7   Practical procedures   201

10   Gastroenterology and nutrition   297

13   Growth and puberty   455

14   Neurology   495

Symbols and abbreviations

☛	controversial topic
↑	increased
↓	decreased
↔	normal
→	leading to
1°	primary
2°	secondary
♂	male
♀	female
+/–	with or without
+ve	positive
–ve	negative
AABR	Automatic auditory brainstem response
ABC	airway, breathing, circulation
ABCD	airway, breathing, circulation, disability
ABPM	ambulatory blood pressure monitoring
ACE	angiotensin converting enzyme
ACh	acetylcholine
ACL	anterior cruciate ligament
ACTH	adrenocorticotrophin
AD	autosomal dominant
ADEM	acute disseminated encephalomyelitis
ADH	antidiuretic hormone
ADHD	attention deficit hyperactivity disorder
ADP	adenosine 5-diphosphate
ADPKD	Autosomal dominant polycystic kidney disease
ADR	adverse drug reaction
A&E	accident and emergency (department)
AFP	alpha-foetoprotein
AG	anion gap
AIDS	acquired immune deficiency syndrome
AIS	androgen insensitivity syndrome
AKI	acute kidney injury
ALA	aminolevulinic acid
ALCL	anaplastic large cell lymphoma
ALD	adrenoleucodystrophy

ALL	acute lymphoblastic leukaemia
ALP	alkaline phosphatase
ALS	advanced life support
ALT	alanine transferase
AML	acute myeloid leukaemia
AN	anorexia nervosa
ANA	anti-nuclear antigen
ANC	antenatal care
ANCA	anti-neutrophil cytoplasmic antibodies
ANLL	acute non-lymphoblastic leukaemia
AP	antero-posterior
APC	activated protein C
APD	automated peritoneal dialysis
APH	antepartum haemorrhage
APRT	adenine phosphoribosyltransferase
APTT	activated partial thromboplastin time
AR	autosomal recessive
ARA	acute rheumatoid arthritis
ARDS	acute respiratory distress syndrome
ARF	acute renal failure
ARM	artificial rupture of membranes
ARPKD	autosomal recessive polycystic kidney disease
ARR	absolute risk reduction
AS	Angelman syndrome
ASA	5-aminosalicylic acid
ASCA	anti-Saccharomyces cerevisiae antibodies
ASD	atrial septal defect
ASIS	anterior superior iliac spine
ASOT	anti-streptolysin O titre
AST	aspartate transaminase
AT	ataxia telangiectasia
ATP	adenosine triphosphate
AV	arteriovenous
AVP	arginine vasopressin
AVSD	atrioventricular septal defect
AXR	abdominal X-ray
AZA	azathioprine
BA	bone age
BAL	British anti-Lewisite

BBS	Bardet-Biedl syndrome
BCG	Bacille Calmette–Guérin
bd	twice a day
BiPD	bipolar disorder
BLCL	diffuse large B cell
BLS	basic life support
BM	bone marrow
BMD	Becker muscular dystrophy
BMI	body mass index
BMT	bone marrow transplantation
BP	blood pressure
BPD	bronchopulmonary dysplasia
BSS	Bernard–Soulier syndrome
BWS	Beckwith–Wiedemann syndrome
BXO	balanitis xerotica obliterans
CA	choanal atresia
CACT	carnitine–acylcarnitine translocase
CAD	coronary artery disease
CaSR	calcium-sensing receptor
CAH	congenital adrenal hyperplasia
CAM	cystic adenomatoid malformation
CAMHS	child and adolescent mental health services
CBT	cognitive behaviour therapy
CCNU	Lomustine
CD	Crohn's disease
CDD	conduct disorder
CDGP	constitutional delay in growth and puberty
CDH	congenital diaphragmatic hernia
CDS	congenital dyserthropoietic anaemia
CeO	cerebral oedema
CER	control event rate
CF	cystic fibrosis
CFAM	cerebral function analysis monitoring
CFRD	cystic fibrosis related diabetes
CFS	chronic fatigue syndrome
CFTR	cystic fibrosis transmembrane receptor
CGA	corrected gestational age
CGM	continuous glucose monitoring
CGMS	continuous glucose monitoring system
CH	cystic hygroma

CHARGE	coloboma, heart defects, choanal atresia, retarded growth, genital anomalies, ear abnormalities
CHC	choriocarcinoma
CHD	congenital heart disease
CHEOPS	Children's Hospital of Eastern Ontario Pain Scale
CHO	carbohydrate
CI	confidence interval
CIE	congenital ichthyosiform erythroderma
CJD	Creutzfeldt–Jakob disease
CK	creatine kinase
CLD	chronic lung disease
CLE	congenital lobar emphysema
CMG	congenital Myasthenia gravis
CML	chronic myeloid leukaemia
CMV	cytomegalovirus
CNS	central nervous system
CO	carbon monoxide
CoA	coarctation of aorta
CONS	coagulase-negative staphylococci
CoRF	corticotrophin-releasing factor
CP	cerebral palsy
CPAP	continuous positive airway pressure
CPR	cardiopulmonary resuscitation
CPS	carbamyl phosphate synthetase deficiency
CRF	chronic renal failure
CRIES	Crying, Requires oxygen for saturation >95%, Increased vital signs, Expression, Sleepless
CRMO	chronic recurrent multifocal osteomyelitis
CRP	C-reactive protein
CRT	capillary refill time
CS	Caesarean section
CSF	cerebrospinal fluid
CSII	continuous subcutaneous insulin infusion
CStE	convulsive status epilepticus
CT	computerized tomography
CTG	cardiotocogram
CVP	central venous pressure
CVS	cardiovascular system
CXR	chest X-ray
CYP	cytochrome P450

DALY	disability-adjusted life year
DCD	developmental coordination disorder
DCT	direct Coombs' test
DDAVP	deamino-8-d-arginine vasopressin (desmopressin)
DDH	developmental dysplasia of the hip
DEND	developmental delay, epilepsy, and neonatal diabetes
DEXA	dual-energy X-ray absorptiometry
DHAP	dihydroxyacetone phosphate
DHEAS	dehydroepiandrosterone sulphate
DI	diabetes insipidus
DIC	disseminated intravascular coagulation
DIP	distal interphalangeal (joint)
DJF	duodenojejunal flexure
DKA	diabetic ketoacidosis
DMARD	disease-modifying antirheumatic drug
DMD	Duchenne muscular dystrophy
DMSA	dimercaptosuccinic acid
DPG	diphosphoglycerate
DPT	diphtheria, pertussis, tetanus
DSM	*Diagnostic and statistical manual*
DTPA	diethylenetriamine pentaacetic acid
DVM	delayed visual maturation
DVT	deep vein thrombosis
EAR	estimated average (nutritional) requirement
EBM	expressed breast milk
EBV	Epstein–Barr virus
EC	embryonal carcinoma
ECG	electrocardiogram
ECLS	Extracorporeal life support
ECMO	extracorporeal membrane oxygenation
EDS	Ehlers-Danlos syndrome
EEG	electroencephalogram
EER	experimental event rate
EHEC	enterohaemorrhagic E. coli
ELBW	extremely low birth weight
ELISA	enzyme-linked immunosorbent assay
EM	electron microscopy
EMDR	eye movement desensitization and reprocessing
EMG	electromyogram
EMU	early morning urine

EMV	electromagentic valve
ENT	ear, nose and throat
EPO	emergency protection order
ERCP	endoscopic retrograde cholangiopancreatography
ES	Ewing's sarcoma
ESR	erythrocyte sedimentation rate
ESRF	end-stage renal failure
ET	essential thrombocytheaemia
ETT	endotracheal tube
FA	Fanconi's anaemia
FB	foreign body
FBC	full blood count
FDG	18F-fludeoxyglucose
FDP	fibrin/fibrinogen degradation products
FEL	familial erythrophagocytic lymphohistiocytosis
FEV1	forced expiratory volume in 1 second
FFP	fresh frozen plasma
FH	familial hypercholesterolaemia
FHL	familial haemophagocytic lymphohistiocytosis
FiO_2	fractional inspired oxygen
FISH	fluorescence in situ hybridization
FIX	factor IX
FLAG	fludarabine, ara-C, and G-CSF (regime)
FRAXA	fragile X syndrome
FRC	functional residual capacity
FSGS	focal segmental glomerulosclerosis
FSH	follicle-stimulating hormone
FTT	failure to thrive
FVC	forced vital capacity
FVL	factor V Leiden
GA	general anaesthetic
GAD	generalized anxiety disorder
GBS	group B streptococcus
G-BS	Guillain–Barré syndrome
GCS	Glasgow coma scale
G-CSF	granulocyte colony-stimulating factor
GCT	germ cell tumour
GDAP	ganglioside-induced differentiation-associated protein
GFR	glomerular filtration rate
GH	growth hormone

GHIS	growth hormone insensitivity syndrome
GHRH	growth hormone-releasing hormone
GI	gastrointestinal
GluA	glutaric aciduria
GluAD	glutamic acid decarboxylase
GN	glomerular nephritis
GnRH	gonadotrophin-releasing hormone
GOR	gastro-oesophageal reflux
GORD	gastro-oesophageal reflux disease
GP	general practitioner
GPI	glycosylphosphatidylinositol
G6PD	glucose-6-phosphate dehydrogenase
GSD	glycogen storage disease
GU	genitourinary
GVHD	graft versus host disease
HAV	hepatitis A virus
Hb	haemoglobin
HBeAg	hepatitis B virus e antigen
HBL	hepatoblastoma
HBsAg	hepatitis B surface antigen
HBV	hepatitis B virus
HCC	hepatocellular carcinoma
hCG	human chorionic gonadotrophin
Hct	haematocrit
HCV	hepatitis C virus
HD	haemodialysis or
HE	hereditary elliptocytosis
HELLP	haemolytic anaemia–elevated liver enzymes–low platelet count
HFOV	high frequency oscillatory ventilation
HH	hypogonadotrophic hypogonadism
HHV6	human herpes virus 6
HIDA	hepato-iminodiacetic acid
HIE	hypoxic–ischaemic encephalopathy
HIH	hiatus hernia
HIT	heparin-induced thrombocytopenia
HIV	human immunodeficiency virus
HL	Hodgkin's lymphoma
HLA	human leukocyte antigen
HLH	haemophagocytic lymphohistiocytosis

HLHS	hypoplastic left heart syndrome
HMG-CO	3-hydroxy-3-methyl-CoA
HOCM	hypertrophic obstructive cardiomopathy
HPA	human platelet antigen
HPLC	haemoglobin electrophoresis
HPRT	hypoxanthine–guanine phosphoribosyltransferase
HR	heart rate
HRCT	high resolution computerized tomography
HS	hereditary spherocytosis
HSD	Hirschsprung's disease
HSP	Henoch–Schönlein purpura
HSV	herpes simplex virus
HUS	haemolytic–uraemic syndrome
HVA	homovanillic acid
IAA	insulin auto-antibody
IAP	intrapartum antibiotic prophylaxis
IBD	inflammatory bowel disease
IBS	irritable bowel syndrome
ICA	islet cell antibody
ICD	International Classification of Diseases
ICP	intracranial pressure
IDM	infant of diabetic mother
IDDM	insulin-dependent diabetes mellitus
I:E	ratio of inspiratory time to expiratory time
iem	inborn error of metabolism
IEM	inborn errors of metabolism
IGF	insulin-like growth factor
Igs	immunoglobulins
IGT	impaired glucose tolerance
IHPS	idiopathic hypertrophic pyloric stenosis
IIH	idiopathic intracranial hypertension
ILAR	International League of Associations for Rheumatology
IO	intraosseous
IM	intramuscular
IMD	inherited metabolic disease
INR	international normalized ratio
IPPV	intermittent positive pressure ventilation
IRT	immunoreactive trypsinogen
IT	intrathecal
ITP	idiopathic thrombocytopenic purpura

ITT	insulin tolerance test
ITU	intensive therapy unit
IU	international units
IUGR	intrauterine growth restriction
IUT	intrauterine blood transfusion
IV	intravenous
IVC	inferior vena cava
IVGT	intravenous glucose tolerance test
IVH	intraventricular haemorrhage
IVI	intravenous infusion
IVIG	intravenous immunoglobulin
JCA	juvenile chronic arthritis
JDM	juvenile dermatomyositis
JIA	juvenile idiopathic arthritis
JRA	juvenile rheumatoid arthritis
JVP	jugular venous pressure
KS	Kallmann syndrome
LBW	low birth weight
LCH	Langerhan's cell histiocytosis
LDH	lactate dehydrogenase
LDL	low density lipoprotein
LFT	liver function test
LGA	large for gestational age
LH	luteinizing hormone
LHRH	luteinizing hormone-releasing hormone
LI	lamellar ichthyosis
LIP	lymphoid interstitial pneumonitis
LKM	liver/kidney microsomal (antibodies)
LKS	Landau-Kleffner syndrome
LMW	X-linked lymphoproliferative
LOC	level of consciousness
LOS	lower oesophageal sphincter
LP	lumbar puncture
LR	likelihood ratio
LRD	living related donor
LRTI	lower respiratory tract infection
LS	linear scleroderma
LSCS	lower segment Caesarean section
LSE	left sternal edge
M4Eo	acute myelomonocytic leukaemia with eosinophilia

MA	microalbuminuria
MAG-3	mercaptoacetyltriglycine
MAHA	microangiopathic haemolytic anaemia
MAOI	monoamine oxidase inhibitor
MAP	mean airway pressure
MAS	meconium aspiration syndrome
MCAD	medium chain acyl-CoA dehydrogenase deficiency
McAS	McCune–Albright syndrome
MCD	minimal change disease
MCDK	multicystic dysplastic kidneys
MCH	mean cell haemoglobin
MCHC	mean corpuscular haemoglobin concentration
MCP	metacarpal phalangeal (joint)
M,C&S	microscopy, culture, and sensitivity
MCTD	mixed connective tissue disease
MCUG	micturating cystourethrography
MCV	mean cell volume
MD	Meckel's diverticulum
MDI	metered dose inhaler
MDP	myeloproliferative disorder
MDS	myelodysplastic syndrome
MeA	mesenteric adentitis
MELAS	mitochondrial encephalopathy–lactic acidosis and stroke-like episodes (syndrome)
MEN	multiple endocrine neoplasia
MFS	Marfan syndrome
MGN	membranous glomerulonephritis
MIBG	meta-iodo-benzylguanidine
MLD	metachromatic leucodystrophy
MMA	methylmalonic acidaemia
MMF	mycophenolate mofetil
MMR	measles, mumps, rubella (vaccination)
MODY	maturity onset diabetes of young
MPGN	membranoproliferative glomerulonephritis
MPH	mid-parental height
MPS	mucopolysaccharidosis
MRD	minimal residual disease
MRI	magnetic resonance imaging
MSbP	Munchausen syndrome by proxy
MSH	melanocyte-stimulating hormone

MSU	midstream urine
MTHFR	methyltetrahydrofolate reductase
MTP	metatarsal phalangeal (joint)
MTX	methotrexate
NAGS	N-acetylglutamate synthetase deficiency
NAHI	non-accidental head injury
NAI	non-accidental injury
NAIT	neonatal alloimmune thrombocytopenia
NC	nasal cannula
NCStE	convulsive status epilepticus
NEC	necrotizing enterocolitis
NF	neurofibromatosis (NF1, NF2)
NFCS	neonatal facial coding scale
NG	nasogastric
NGT	nasogastric tube
NHL	non-Hodgkin's lymphoma
NIMH-MTS	National Institute of Mental Health-Multimodal Treatment Study
NIPS	Neonatal and Infant Pain Scale
NMJ	neuromuscular junction
NNT	number (of patients) needed to treat
NNU	neonatal unit
NS	Noonan syndrome
NSAID	non-steroidal anti-inflammatory drug
NSE	neuron-specific enolase
nvCJD	new variant Creutzfeldt–Jakob disease
OA	oesophageal atresia
OAE	otoacoustic emission
OCD	obsessive–compulsive disorder
od	once daily
OD	observed difference
ODD	oppositional defiant disorder
OFC	occipitofrontal circumference
OGTT	oral glucose tolerance test
OI	osteogenesis imperfecta
OMIN	Online Mendelian Inheritance in Man (database)
OS	osteosarcoma
OSA	obstructive sleep apnoea
OSAS	obstructive sleep apnoea syndrome
OTC	ornithine transcarbamylase deficiency

$PaCO_2$	arterial carbon dioxide tension
p-ANCA	perinuclear antineutrophil cytoplasmic antibody
PANDAS	paediatric autoimmune neuropsychiatric disorder associated with *Streptococcus*
PaO_2	arterial oxygen tension
PBSCT	peripheral blood stem cell transplants
PCA	patient-controlled analgesia
PCH	paroxysmal cold haemoglobinuria
PCKD	polycystic kidney disease
PCOS	Polycystic ovarian syndrome
PCP	pneumocystis pneumonia
PCR	polymerase chain reaction
PCV	packed cell volume
PD	peritoneal dialysis
PDA	patent ductus arteriosus
PDD	pervasive developmental disorder
PDPE	psychologically determined paroxysmal events
PE	pulmonary embolism
PEEP	positive end-expiratory pressure
PEFR	peak expiratory flow rate
PEG	polyethylene glycol
PET	positron emission tomography
PFA	platelet function assay
PGE1	prostaglandin E1
PHP	pseudohypoparathyroidism
PHVD	post-haemorrhagic ventricular dilatation
PICU	paediatric intensive care unit
PIE	pulmonary interstitial emphysema
PIP	peak/positive/proximal inspiratory pressure
PIPP	Premature Infant Pain Profile
PK	pyruvate kinase
PKU	phenylketonuria
PMDI	propellant metered dose inhaler
PML	promyelocytic leukaemia
PN	parenteral nutrition
PNDM	Permanent neonatal diabetes mellitus
PNET	primitive neuroectodermal tumour
PNH	paroxysmal nocturnal haemoglobinuria
PO	orally/by mouth
PP	precocious puberty

PPHN	persistent pulmonary hypertension of newborn
PPI	proton pump inhibitor
PPROM	preterm prolonged rupture of membranes
PR	rectally, per rectum
PResp	parental responsibility
PrIP	proximal interphalangeal (joint)
PROM	prolonged rupture of membranes
PSS	progressive systemic sclerosis
PT	prothrombin time
PTH	parathyroid hormone
PTHrP	PTH-related peptide
PTSD	post-traumatic stress disorder
PTT	partial thromboplastin time
PTV	patient-triggered ventilation
PUJ	pelviureteric junction
PUV	posterior urethral valve
PV	vaginally, per vagina
PVH	periventricular haemorrhage
PVL	periventricular leucomalacia
PWS	Prader-Willi syndrome
qds	four times a day
RA	rheumatoid arthritis
RAS	reflex anoxic seizures
RAST	radioallergosorbent test
RBC	red blood cell
RCC	red cell count
RCM	red blood cell mass
RCT	randomized, controlled trial
RDS	respiratory distress syndrome
RF	rheumatoid factor
rhGH	recombinant human growth hormone
RIF	right iliac fossa
RMS	rhabdomyosarcoma
RNP	ribonucleoprotein
ROM	range of movement
ROP	retinopathy of prematurity
RP	retinitis pigmentosa
RR	respiration rate
RRR	relative risk reduction
RSV	respiratory syncytial virus

RTA	renal tubular acidosis
RV	residual volume
SAA	severe aplastic anaemia
SAD	separation anxiety disorder
SaO_2	arterial oxygen saturation
SBR	serum bilirubin
SC	subcutaneous
SCD	sickle cell disease
SCID	severe combined immunodeficiency
SCII	SC insulin infusion
SCL	subcortical leucomalacia
SDH	subdural haemorrhage
SE	standard error
SENCO	special educational needs co-ordinator
SGA	small for gestational age
SHBG	sex hormone-binding globulin
SIADH	syndrome of inappropriate antidiuretic hormone
SIDS	sudden infant death syndrome
SIMV	synchronized intermittent mandatory ventilation
SIPPV	synchronized intermittent positive pressure ventilation
SLE	systemic lupus erythematosus
SM	sternomastoid muscle
SMA	spinal muscular atrophy or superior mesenteric artery
SMN	survival motor neuron
SN	sensorineural
SOB	shortness of breath
SOS	self-referral of symptoms
SPA	suprapubic aspiration
SpO_2	pulse oximetry measurement of oxyhaemoglobin saturation
SR	steroid-resistant
SS	steroid-sensitive
SSC	systemic sclerosis
SSPE	subacute sclerosing panencephalitis
SSRI	selective serotonin reuptake inhibitors
StE	status epilepticus
STI	sexually transmitted infection
subE	subependymal
SUDI	sudden unexpected death in an infant
SUFE	slipped upper femoral epiphysis

SVC	superior vena cava
SVT	supraventricular tachycardia
T1DM	type 1 diabetes mellitus
T2DM	type 2 diabetes mellitus
T3	triiodothyronine
T4	thyroxine
TA	tricuspid atresia
TaGVHD	transfusion-associated graft versus host disease
TAPVD	total anomalous pulmonary venous drainage
TAR	thrombocytopenia–absent radius (syndrome)
TAT	transanamastic tube
TB	tuberculosis
TBI	total body irradiation
TBM	tuberculous meningitis
$TcCO_2$	transcutaneous carbon dioxide pressure
TcO_2	transcutaneous oxygen pressure
TCPL	time-cycled, pressure limited
TDC	thyroglossal duct cysts
TDD	total digitalizing dose (for digoxin)
tds	three times a day
TdT	terminal deoxynucleotidyl transferase
TE	expiratory time
TEC	transient erythroblastopenia of childhood
TEG	thromboelastogram
TEWL	transepidermal water loss chapter 6
TFT	thyroid function test
TH	therapeutic hypothermia
Ti	inspiratory time
TIBC	total iron binding capacity
TLC	total lung capacity
TNDM	Transient neonatal diabetes mellitus
TNF	tumour necrosis factor
TOF	tracheo-oesophageal fistula
TORCH	toxoplasmosis, others, rubella, cytomegalovirus, herpes virus II
TPA	tissue plasminogen activator
TPN	total parenteral nutrition
TPPPS	Toddler—Preschooler Postoperative Pain Scale
TRAB	TSH receptor antibody
TRALI	transfusion-related acute lung injury

TSC	tuberous sclerosis complex
TSH	thyroid-stimulating hormone
TSS	toxic shock syndrome
TT	thrombin time
TTG	tissue transglutaminase IgA antibody
TTN	transient tachypnoea of newborn
TTP	thrombotic thrombocytopenic purpura
UAC	umbilical arterial catheter
UC	ulcerative colitis
U&E	urea and electrolytes
UNC	urine net charge
UNHS	universal newborn hearing screening
UP:UCr	urinary protein to urinary creatinine (ratio)
URTI	upper respiratory tract infection
US	ultrasound
USS	ultrasound scan
UTI	urinary tract infection
UV	umbilical vein
UVC	umbilical venous catheter
VACTERL	vertebral anomalies, anal atresia, cardiac malformations, tracheo-oesophageal fistula, renal and limb anomalies
VEGF	vascular endothelial growth factor
VDDR	vitamin D-dependent rickets
VDRL	Venereal Disease Research Laboratory (test)
VF	ventricular fibrillation
VHL	von Hippel–Lindau (disease)
VIP	vasoactive intestinal polypeptide
VLBW	very low birth weight
VLDL	very low density lipoprotein
VMA	vanillylmandelic acid
VOD	vaso-occlusive
VSAA	very severe aplastic anaemia
VSD	ventricular septal defect
VT	ventricular tachycardia
V/Q	ventilation–perfusion ratio
VUJ	vesicoureteric junction
VUR	vesicoureteric reflux
vWD	von Willebrand's disease
vWF	von Willebrand's factor
VZV	varicella zoster virus

WAGR	Wilms, aniridia, gonadal dysplasia, retardation
WBC	white blood cell
WCC	white cell count
WG	Wegener's granulomatosis
WS	Williams syndrome
XLP	X-linked lymphoproliferative
YST	yolk sac tumour
ZIG	zoster immunoglobulin

Chapter 1

Practising paediatrics

Reading and learning paediatrics

Welcome to paediatrics and child health! You will find this area of medicine challenging, rewarding, and above all fun. We have written this handbook to help you develop as a practitioner—whether it's in the emergency department, inpatient wards, outpatient clinic, or family health surgery.

Six basic goals in your learning

If you are a novice in the field, you will find that every day requires new skills, and sometimes this can seem daunting. Take heart. We hope that this experience will provide an education in the aspects of general paediatrics that are important for all medical practitioners. Your curriculum goals should be the following.

- *Acquire basic knowledge of growth and development:* learn about physical, physiological, and psychosocial change from birth through to adolescence and see how this applies to clinical practice.
- *Develop communication skills:* this will help you to speak to children, adolescents, and their families.
- *Become competent in physical examination* of babies, infants, toddlers, children, and adolescents.
- *Learn enough core knowledge* so that you can make a diagnosis and start treatment of common acute and chronic paediatric illnesses.
- Improve your clinical problem-solving skills.
- *Take a broader perspective* and understand more about the upbringing and health of children in modern society, and in our different communities.

As you scan through the handbook you will see that all of the chapters cover some aspect of these points. We hope that you will take time to annotate particularly helpful guides and record what you have learnt. Perhaps, with time, things will not appear quite so daunting.

What next after this foundation?

For those who are using this handbook to progress in their postgraduate level of learning we have been more prescriptive in the next sections. We have itemized certain objectives that are deemed essential for professional conduct, attitudes, skills, and knowledge. Use these as a checklist and monitor your progress as you work through the handbook. Again, most chapters cover aspects of the material that you will need.

Professional conduct and attitudes

- *Have you learnt to adapt your clinical approach to patients of all ages?* Can you communicate with the child or adolescent and family in the clinic? What about dealing with confidentiality and privacy? (see 📖 p.1038).
- *Can you communicate clearly and sensitively?* How do you break bad news to new parents, or to the newly-diagnosed adolescent with chronic illness or disability? (see 📖 p.794).
- *Do you work well in a team?* Do you treat each member of the team with courtesy and recognize the contributions of each?
- Are you aware of cultural, ethnic, and socio-economic factors in your practice?
- *Do you have a foundation in basic ethical principles?* Do you appreciate the ethical challenges specific to paediatrics and child health? (see 📖 pp.1032, 1038).

Professional skills

Interviewing (📖 Chapter 3)

- *Can you obtain a complete medical history?* The history of the perinatal period, immunizations, development, diet, family and social history, and systems review is unique to paediatrics. Can you collect this information in a timely manner—40min in a complex case history. You should also be able to modify the medical history depending on the age of the child, with particular attention to the following age groups—neonate; infant, toddler, school age, and adolescence.
- *Can you obtain a focused medical history?* In an emergency you will need to know what are the important questions to ask—what is going to help you now with your treatment.

Physical examination (📖 Chapter 3)

- *Can you complete a full physical examination of an infant, child, and adolescent, including the observation and documentation of normal physical findings?* You should be able to do this 'long case' examination in less than 10min.
- *Can you carry out a problem-orientated examination?* For example, in the child with a limp: what are the important positive and negative clinical findings?
- *Are you a good observer?* Do you take time to look first?
- *Can you assess behaviour, neurodevelopment, and pubertal staging?*

Communication

- *Can you establish rapport with the patient and family?* Are you able to identify the main concerns of the patient and family? Can you communicate information to both the patient and parent, making sure both understand the diagnosis and treatment plan, and do you give them the opportunity to ask questions?
- *Can you write a discharge letter for the family doctor?*
- *Can you write a full medical summary for the medical notes?*
- *Can you present to colleagues a well-organized summary of your patient?* Can you communicate effectively with other health care workers, including nurses and social workers, and explain the thought process that led to your diagnosis and treatment?

Clinical problem solving

- *Can you compile a problem list and differential diagnosis for each of the common clinical presentations?* Can you use your knowledge of key signs and symptoms, and the frequency and prevalence of diseases at different ages to develop a likely differential diagnosis?
- *Can you make a management plan of investigations?* Can you interpret the results of commonly ordered laboratory tests, such as the full blood count, urinalysis, and serum electrolytes, and recognize that the normal values of some tests may vary with the age of the patient?

- Can you use the medical paediatric literature to research the diagnosis and management of clinical problems? Can you critically appraise a topic (i.e. patient, intervention, outcome—see 📖 Chapter 2, p.16) and decide on best evidence for treatment?

Practical procedures (📖 Chapter 7)

- Do you know when certain procedures are needed (e.g. lumbar puncture, intravenous (IV) line, nasogastric (NG) tube, etc.)?
- Can you explain these procedures to parents and children?
- Specialist trainees in paediatrics should be able to perform the procedures in the Boxes 1.1 and 1.2.

Box 1.1 Diagnostic procedures

- Venepuncture and venous cannulation for blood sampling (📖 p.203)
- Collection of blood from central lines and umbilical arterial lines (📖 pp.204–209)
- Capillary blood sampling (📖 p.202)
- Electrocardiogram (ECG)
- Lumbar puncture (LP, 📖 p.220)
- Suprapubic aspiration of urine (📖 p.219)
- Non-invasive blood pressure (BP) measurement
- Urethral catheterization (📖 p.218)
- Urine analysis using standard bedside tests
- Blood sugar measurement using standard point-of-care glucometers

Diagnostic procedures with supervision

- Peripheral arterial cannulation (📖 p.205)
- Needle thoracentesis of pleural effusion for microbiology and cytology

---

Box 1.2 Therapeutic procedures

- Bag, valve, and mask ventilation (📖 p.211)
- Placement of an oral airway (📖 p.210)
- External chest compression
- Tracheal intubation of term newborn babies (📖 p.212)
- Removal and replacement of a blocked tracheotomy tube
- Percutaneous long-line insertion (📖 p.209)
- Placement of NG tube

Therapeutic procedures with supervision

- *Injections:* intradermal, subcutaneous (SC), intramuscular (IM), and IV
- Insertion of an intraosseous (IO) needle
- Administer surfactant
- Tracheal intubation of preterm and older child
- Chest drain insertion for pneumothorax

Knowledge

During your reading you should consider these questions as a starting point to the knowledge that would be expected of a junior paediatrician.

Growth (📖 Chapter 13)

- *What are the intrauterine factors that affect growth of the foetus?*
- *Can you explain how growth charts are used in the longitudinal evaluation of height, weight, and head circumference?*

In particular, consider the following.

- Can you recognize abnormalities of growth that warrant further evaluation?
- What is the significance of crossing centiles on a growth chart?
- What is the significance of discrepancies between height, weight, and head circumference?
- What are: short stature; constitutional delay; failure to thrive; obesity; microcephaly; and macrocephaly?

Development (📖 Chapters 15, 24, and 27)

Why is following development important in clinical paediatrics?

- What are the normal changes in reflexes, tone, and posture in the infant?
- What is the normal progression in motor milestones in the first year?
- What are the signs of cerebral palsy?

Behaviour (📖 Chapters 15, 16, and 21)

What are the typical presentations of common behavioural problems at various developmental levels and ages?

- What are temper tantrums?
- How may somatic complaints represent psychosocial problems?
- In what types of situations does pathology in the family contribute to childhood behaviour problems?

Nutrition (📖 Chapter 10)

- *What factors contribute to the development of failure to thrive in infancy?*
- *What factors contribute to the development of child obesity?*
- *What are the special dietary needs of children with chronic illness?*
- *What caloric intake is needed for normal growth in infants and small children?*

Also consider the following.

- What are the major differences between human milk and commonly available formulas?
- What are the advantages of breastfeeding?

Newborns (📖 Chapter 6)
- What diseases are detected by neonatal blood screening?
- What important historical information, physical examination findings, and laboratory data are needed for the differential diagnosis of the following problems:
  - jitteriness or seizures;
  - jaundice;
  - lethargy or poor feeding;
  - respiratory distress;
  - cyanosis;
  - bilious vomiting;
  - non-bilious vomiting;
  - hypoglycaemia;
  - sepsis?

Genetics and congenital malformations (📖 Chapters 23 and 25)
- What are the effects of teratogenic agents such as alcohol and phenytoin?
- What are the findings and implications of the common chromosomal abnormalities:
  - trisomy 21;
  - sex chromosome abnormalities (e.g. Turner's syndrome, fragile X syndrome);
  - other genetic disorders (cystic fibrosis, sickle cell disease)?

Common paediatric illnesses
For each of the common 'presentations' and 'conditions' in this handbook can you review:
- cause;
- pathophysiology;
- natural history;
- presenting signs and symptoms;
- initial laboratory test and/or imaging needed for diagnosis;
- plan for initial management?

Epidemiology, evidence, and practice

Introduction

The aim of this chapter is to provide the epidemiological information that we find useful in supporting our every-day clinical practice. You may have read an article and need a quick reference. Alternatively, you may want to examine some data published in a report and apply it to your work. Asking questions is a skill that you, the clinician, should develop. It is important to ask questions that fall into two main categories:

- *Those that define the burden of disease:* i.e. what, who, where, and when questions.
- Those that understand or search for the cause of childhood disease: i.e. why, and how questions.

The answers to these questions will require the use of numerical reasoning and statistics. In your professional development you should seek an understanding of:

- *Quantifying* disease in populations.
- *Research design*, methodology, and implementation.
- *Basic statistical tests* and their interpretation.
- *Clinical guidelines*, systematic reviews and meta-analyses.
- *Critical appraisal* of the literature.

This chapter will highlight some of these areas. Other texts should be read for a fuller account of statistics and evidence-based medicine.

Descriptions in populations

Measurements

- *Prevalence:* the proportion of a study population who have a disease at one instant, or period in time. This number includes both new and old cases.
- *Incidence:* the proportion of people in a study population who develop a new condition or diagnosis.

Mortality rates

- *Still birth:* an infant born after the 24th week of pregnancy who does not, at any time after being born, breathe or show any other sign of life.
- *Perinatal mortality:* still births plus deaths in first week of life.
- *Infant mortality:* deaths from birth to 1yr.
- *Post-neonatal mortality:* deaths from 4wks of age to 1yr.
- *Under 5-yr-old mortality:* deaths from birth to under 5yrs.

Summary of study designs

Here are the common types of clinical study that you will read about.

Experimental study

- *Randomized controlled trial (RCT):* this is the gold-standard of clinical intervention studies. These studies assign subjects to receive treatment or no treatment. The RCT provides the best evidence for causation
- *Quasi-experimental:* other studies with an intervention and measurement of an outcome

Observational study

In populations

These are descriptive studies and can, at best, provide an ecological correlation

In individuals

These studies can be descriptive, as in case series; or they can be analytical, as in case-control, cohort, and cross-sectional studies.

- *Case-series (retrospective) review:* these studies are essentially reviews of practice or uncontrolled treatment in a defined patient group.
- *Case-control (retrospective) study:* these studies have cases that are defined by their disease, and controls that do not have disease. Typically, cases are compared with controls, but there is considerable potential for bias. This type of evidence for causation is weak.
- *Cohort (prospective) study:* these studies observe, over time, the effect of exposure to a risk factor or disease in a study cohort and a suitable control group not exposed to the factor or disease. Population studies can be used to define incidence and they provide stronger evidence of causation.
- *Cross-sectional study:* these studies examine, at the same time, an outcome or disease, and the presence of a risk factor. Cross-sectional studies can be used to define prevalence.

Levels of evidence

Evidence-based medicine is a method used for guiding clinical decision-making based on critically analysed information. There are now standard texts for this discipline. These approaches, however, are now common-place and the clinician should be aware of the types of information that are available:

Systematic reviews

A systematic review is a summary of the medical literature that uses a standardized methodology for searching databases, appraising the content of individual studies, and synthesizing all the data in a coherent and statistically rigorous manner. When this process involves quantitative data then it could be called a 'meta-analysis'.

Guidelines

A clinical guideline is a series of systematically developed statements that are used to assist clinical decisions. Guidelines should provide a summary of the evidence (quality and level) on which the statements are based, and an instruction on applying the evidence in practice.

Expert opinions

In areas where there is little in the way of systematic or high-quality data, one may have to resort to the advice of a panel of experts. The approach can be systematized with a technique called the 'Delphi' approach. In this iterative process one brings together a panel of experts who each assign a score (0–9) to statements about practice, management or care. The process continues with changes to statements until consensus is achieved. Each step, for acceptance or rejection, has strict criteria.

The GRADE (GRades of recommendation, Assessment, Development, and Evaluation) system for presenting 'Quality of Evidence' (Table 2.1):

Table 2.1 The GRADE system for presenting 'Quality of Evidence'

Quality rating	Underlying methodology
High	Randomized controlled trials (RCT) yielding consistent and directly applicable results, or well-done observational studies yielding large effects
Moderate	RCT with important limitations, or well-done observational studies with yielding large effects
Low	Well-done observational studies, or RCTs with serious limitations
Very low	Poorly controlled observational studies and unsystematic clinical observations such as case series, or case reports

Basics of statistics

In the following section we describe the terms and tests that we often refer to when assessing as study.

Commonly used term

- *Significance (α) level of a statistical test:* often set at 5% (0.05), this is the probability of finding a statistical association by chance alone when there really is no association.
- *Power (1-β) of a statistical test:* often 80% (0.80), the probability of finding a statistical association when there is one.
- *Sample size:* the number of subjects needed in a clinical study to achieve a sufficiently high power and low α, in order to obtain a result that is of value clinically.
- *P-value:* this value quantifies the probability of a finding by chance alone. If the *P*-value is less than the preset α, then the finding is considered not due to chance.
- *Confidence interval (CI):* often set at 95% probability: the interval where there is 95% chance of finding the true value.
- *Relative risk:* this value is the ratio of incidence of disease among people with a risk factor to the incidence of disease among people without the risk factor.
- *Odds ratio:* in case-control studies, the ratio of odds of having the risk factor in people with disease to odds of having the risk factor in people without the disease.

The hypothesis test for the difference between two proportions

There will be instances where you want to re-analyse some data that have been presented (see Table 2.2)

Table 2.2 Frequency table to display data

Feature	Group 1	Group 2	Total
Present	A	B	A+B
Absent	C	D	C+D
Total patients	A+C = n_1	B+D = n_2	A+B+C+D= $n_1 + n_2$

When a comparison is being made, you need:
- *An estimate of the 95% CI in each group:* in small series ($n \leq 100$) you should consult standard tables. When the proportion is zero (i.e. 0/n), where $n \leq 100$, use the 'rule-of-3' to calculate the upper limit of the 95% CI, i.e. upper limit = 3/n.
- Then draw a 2 x 2 frequency table to display the data (see Table 2.2).
- *The observed difference (OD)* in the proportions with the feature, between groups 1 and 2: OD = A/n_1 – B/n_2.
- The proportion (p) in both groups combined: p = (A + B)/(n_1 + n_2).
- *The standard error (SE) of the difference* between the two proportions is: SE = $\sqrt{p(1-p)\,(1/n_1 + 1/n_2)}$.

- Difference in sample proportions will be normally distributed with mean 0.
- To calculate the observed difference in SE units away from hypothesized difference of zero: OD/SE.
- Exact level of significance can be read from the table of the normal distribution.

Assessing the validity of an RCT

Calculate the number of patients that you need to treat (NNT) with the experimental therapy in order to prevent one additional bad outcome, as follows:

- *Relative risk reduction (RRR):* RRR = (CER − EER)/CER, where CER is the control event rate, and EER is the experimental event rate.
- *Absolute risk reduction (ARR):* ARR = CER − EER.
- *Number needed to treat:* NNT = 1/ARR
- *The 95% CI on a NNT − 1/limits on the CI of its ARR:* ± 1.96/CER × $(1 - CER)/n_1$ + EER × $(1 - EER)/n_2$ where n_1 is the number of controls and n_2 the number treated.

Measurements for evaluating a clinical test

When you want to know whether a test will affect management, assess the importance of the study in diagnostic terms (see Table 2.3).

Table 2.3 Assessing the importance of a study in diagnostic terms

	Disease status	
Test result	Positive	Negative
Positive	A (true positive)	B (false positive)
Negative	C (false negative)	D (true negative)

- *Sensitivity:* the proportion of all diseased who have positive (+ve) test (use Table 2.3) = A/(A + C).
- *Specificity:* proportion of all non-diseased who have a negative (−ve) test = D/(B + D).
- *Positive predictive value:* proportion of all those with +ve tests who truly have disease = A/(A + B).
- *Negative predictive value:* proportion of all those with −ve tests who truly do not have disease = D/(C + D).
- *Likelihood ratio (LR) positive:* ability of a +ve test result to confirm disease status = Sensitivity/(1-specificity).
- *LR negative:* ability of a −ve test result to confirm non-diseased status = Specificity/(1-sensitivity).
- *Pre-test probability* or prevalence = (A + C)/(A + B + C + D).
- *Pre-test-odds* = prevalence/(1-prevalence).
- *Post-test odds* = Pre-test odds × LR.
- *Post-test probability* = Post-test odds/(Post-test odds + 1).

Having analysed the data, ask 'Will the change from pre-test probability (prevalence) to post-test probability make a difference?'

Training and special knowledge skills

During clinical practice, as a postgraduate trainee or an undergraduate medical student, there are many opportunities to demonstrate your ability and skills at approaching common questions at the core of paediatrics and child health. We suggest that writing a report will often help to clarify your thoughts. The format should follow this sequence:

• Identify the problem you want to address.
• Define a structured question.
• Find the best evidence using original primary studies or evidence summaries.
• Ask yourself 'how valid is the evidence?'
• Summarize the results.
• Then ask, 'how should I apply the results to patient care?'

The following format for critically appraising a topic can be used as a guide—the word lengths are approximate:

Clinical setting (~150 words)

Give a description of the clinical setting that gave rise to your question for critical appraisal (e.g. where you saw the patient, what interested you?).

A structured question (a sentence)

Your question should demonstrate that you have thought about specific knowledge which relates to managing patients. It will have four essential components:

• A [patient] or [problem].
• An [intervention].
• A comparison [*intervention*] if relevant.
• A clinical [*outcome*].

For example, in a wheezing child, admitted to hospital with bronchiolitis [*patient*], treatment with nebulized salbutamol [*intervention*] reduces the duration of oxygen therapy and hospital admission [*outcomes*].

A brief report of search methods (3 sentences)

List in order the sources of information you have used:

• Secondary sources.
• Systematic reviews (Cochrane Library see 📖 p.18).
• Primary research (PubMed query using MeSH 'subject headings').
• *Search results:* have you identified any papers as being relevant to your question.

A structured summary of search results (use a table)

Using the information you have gained from reading the papers you identified construct a table listing:

- The citation.
- The type of study.
- The outcome or endpoint of the study.
- The key result.
- Your personal comments.

Commentary on the papers listed in your table (300 words)

Write two paragraphs that draw together your knowledge and insights on the subject.

Your clinical message or bottom line (50 words)

Have an answer to your question and what you will do in your practice. Also, set a review date when you we review this topic.

References

Incorporate a list of all of the references.

The final length of your written report should be 500–600 words. Some medical journals will accept these items for publication.

Practice point

You will find it helpful to present the results of your appraised topic to your colleagues. We suggest that you do this with no more than 10 presentation slides (see Table 2.4).

Table 2.4 Suggested presentation slides

Slide	Content
1	The clinical setting
2	Your structured question
3	The search strategy
4, 5, and 6	Your findings and results
7	A summary
8 and 9	How this evidence applies to your patient or problem
10	The clinical bottom line

Useful websites and resources

Useful synopses and syntheses of the medical literature:
- *Cochrane Database of Systematic Reviews:* covers a broad range of disciplines examining therapy and prevention. Available at: ♪ http://www.cochrane.org/index.htm
- *Database of Abstracts of Reviews of Effects (DARE):* covers all disciplines and concentrates on therapy and prevention. Available at: ♪ http://www.york.ac.uk/inst/crd/crddatabases.htm
- *Bandolier:* useful for primary care. Available at: ♪ http://www.medicine.ox.ac.uk/bandolier

Primary sources of the medical literature that give access to reports of studies:
- MEDLINE has lots of primary studies across all disciplines and areas of research which is free through PubMed. Available at: ♪ http://www.ncbi.nlm.nih.gov/pubmed
- *GOOGLE Scholar:* when all else fails—you can't remember the right search term to use or the type of study—the fastest way to find high-impact studies that have recently made the headlines. Available at: ♪ http://scholar.google.com

References

Guyatt G, Rennie D. (2002). Users guide to the medical literature: a manual for evidence-based clinical practice. Chicago: American Medical Association.

Sackett, DL, Straus, SE, Richardson, WS, et al. (2000). Evidence-based medicine. How to practice and teach EBM, 2nd edn. Edinburgh: Churchill Livingstone.

Clinical assessment

Communication skills

Skill at communication is central to paediatric medical practice. In time you will develop the following abilities and traits.

Personal

- *Courtesy* to families, colleagues, and members of the multidisciplinary team.
- *Patience and sensitivity* in your communication with children and their families.
- *Empathy* with children, young people, and their families experiencing difficulty and distress.
- *Insight* into personal limitations and when help should be sought in managing sensitive and complex situations.

Professional

See also 📖 pp.575–576, 794, 1005, 1034–1035.

- Understand how to manage consultations with babies, young children, adolescents, and their families effectively.
- Learn how to listen to children and young people, i.e. hear their needs, respect their views, and respond in an age-appropriate manner where the child is feeling vulnerable.
- Develop an effective way of communicating information about a diagnosis, prognosis, or emotional issue to children, young people, families.
- Know when and what assistance is required when communicating with children and families who unable to speak or understand English.
- Learn what information is appropriate to share with children based on their physical and mental maturity.

Taking a paediatric history: introduction

This section provides a system for reviewing the full paediatric medical history and examination. With experience, there are short-cuts, but it is wise for newcomers to the field to be thorough. As you become more adept, develop your own style and process—the key point is *do not miss important information*. When you write-up notes, record the important +ve and −ve findings and observations. Remember, these are a form of communication—between you and your colleagues, or for you at a later date—they should be legible, clear, and logical, and written in black ink.

Practice point

Always record:
• Date and time when you undertook the consultation
• Who was present
• Who gave the history

The presenting complaint

There are over 100 ways in which the human body can respond to illness or disease. To the clinician, the presenting complaint may be a symptom, a sign, a finding, or a laboratory abnormality. If it is not clear to you what the problem is then ask yourself or the patient/carer 'Why has this child, and their family, sought medical attention now?' Record the patient or parent's description of the problem.

Box 3.1 lists, in alphabetical order, a selection of common paediatric symptoms and problems. A more detailed account of these complaints can be found in the chapters indexed, and the reader should refer to these sections (see Box 3.1).

Box 3.1 Common paediatric symptoms and problems

- Abdominal mass and abdominal pain, 📖 pp.310, 351, 668, 845
- Anaemia, 📖 pp.192, 610–629
- Anaphylaxis, 📖 p.64
- Antisocial behaviour, 📖 p.598
- Apnoea, 📖 p.48
- Ataxia, 📖 p.524
- Attention deficit and hyperkinesis, 📖 p.600
- Bleeding, bruising, or purpura, 📖 p.632
- Breathlessness, 📖 p.258
- Coma and head injury, 📖 pp.72–79
- Constipation, 📖 pp.304, 306
- Cough (acute, chronic), 📖 p.257
- Cyanosis, 📖 pp.60–63, 226
- Dehydration, 📖 p.90
- Developmental delay, 📖 p.564
- Diarrhoea (acute, chronic), 📖 pp.302–305
- Ear pain or discharge, 📖 p.900–901
- Electrolyte disturbance, 📖 p.89–93
- Failure to thrive, 📖 p.308
- Fatigue (chronic), 📖 p.990
- Fever and febrile neutropenia, 📖 pp.682–683, 696–702
- Headache, 📖 pp.516–518
- Hypotonia, 📖 pp.136, 538
- Joint pain, limp, 📖 pp.734–737
- Lymphadenopathy, 📖 p.654
- Oedema, 📖 pp.138, 226
- Polyuria and urinary frequency, 📖 p.350
- Rash, 📖 p.806
- Red eye, 📖 p.890
- School performance (poor), 📖 pp.986, 991
- Seizures and status epilepticus, 📖 pp.80, 134, 505
- Shock, 📖 pp.54–58, 65
- Sleep disturbance, 📖 p.279
- Sore throat, 📖 p.282
- Stature (short, tall), 📖 pp.466, 474
- Stridor, 📖 p.256
- Vomiting, 📖 p.300
- Walking (delayed), 📖 p.564
- Wheeze, 📖 p.255
- White blood cell count (abnormal), 📖 **pp.**608, 626, 656–659, 724

History of present illness

Once you have established the presenting problem you will need to answer the following questions:

- When did the current problem start. What was it like?
- Has the problem changed at all? If so, when and in what way?
- Has the patient sought medical attention before now? If so, what investigations have been done so far? What treatments have been tried?
- Ask specifically about current state: eating, drinking, passing urine, stool, acting their normal self, and vomiting.

Past health history

On reviewing the child's past health history there are five areas that should be covered by your questioning. It is important to consider and record at least those that relate to the current health problem.

Prenatal history

- How many pregnancies has mother had; what were the outcomes?
- What was the length of the pregnancy with this child?
- Were there any complications during the pregnancy, such as abnormal bleeding, illness, or infection?
- Did the mother take any medication during pregnancy?

Birth history

- What was this child's gestation at birth and what was the weight?
- How long was labour?
- Was there maternal fever or premature rupture of membranes?
- Was any intervention required at delivery?

Neonatal period

- Did the child have any neonatal problems, e.g. jaundice, cyanosis, or respiratory distress?
- Was vitamin K given?
- Was the baby treated on the special care baby unit?
- When did the baby and mother go home?

Child development

- When did the baby achieve key developmental milestones, e.g. smiling, rolling over, sitting unaided, standing, speaking, and toileting skills?
- How well has the child grown in weight and length/height?
- Have there been any concerns about development, vision, hearing?

Immunization

What immunizations has the child had? Start from birth and review the date when each was given, as well as what was given. If any immunizations have been missed or omitted, identify any reasons, e.g. was the child unwell?

Past medical history

In this part of the history you will need to find out about past visits to the doctor and any admissions to hospital that the child has had.

- *Childhood illness and infections:* What infections and illnesses has the child had? Does the child have asthma, diabetes, epilepsy?
- *Is the child on any medication?* Why? Are there any allergies? Which?
- *Surgical procedures and investigations:* What, if anything, has been done in the past?
- *Is the child seeing another clinician?* What for?

Symptom review

If you haven't done so already, you need to find out about the child's general condition. Do they feel unwell, tired, or fatigued? The following list of questions can be used for further review, although it is not exhaustive. Some of these questions will have been covered in your assessment of the presenting problem, so there is no point repeating them. However, it is important that you tailor this part of the history to issues you think relevant to the child's condition—particularly when you suspect multisystem disease.

Head
Is there a history of injury, headaches, or infection?

Eyes
- How good is visual acuity—are glasses needed?
- Is there a history of infection, injury, or surgery?

Ear, nose, and throat
- Is there a problem with hearing or balance?
- Is there a history of ear infection or discharge?
- Is there any difficulty with breathing?
- Is there a history of nasal discharge, snoring, or bleeding?
- Are there any enlarged lumps or glands?
- Is there a history of sore throat, dental problems, or mouth ulcers?

Chest
- Is there any limitation to exercise?
- Is there a history of cough, wheeze, chest pain, or haemoptysis?
- Has there been any exposure to tuberculosis?
- Has the child ever had a chest X-ray (CXR)?
- Are there any smokers in the family?
- Are there any smoke-free zones in the family accommodation?

Heart
- Is there a history of heart murmur or rheumatic fever in the patient or family?
- Is there a history of dyspnoea, orthopnoea, chest pain, or cyanosis?

Gastrointestinal
- How good is the child's appetite?
- Have there been any recent changes in weight, food tolerance, or bowel movements?
- Has there been any rectal bleeding?

Genitourinary

- Is there a history of infection?
- How frequent is urination?
- Is there any dysuria, or haematuria, or discharge?
- Is there a history of bedwetting?
- What was the age of menarche?

Joints, limbs, and tissue

- Is there any pain?
- Is there swelling or limitation in movement?
- Is there muscle weakness?
- Is there any difficulty walking or a limp?

Nervous system

- Is there a history of fits, faints, or funny turns?
- Is there a history of febrile seizures?
- Are there any abnormal involuntary movements or tremors?
- How has the child being doing at school—has there been a recent change that has concerned the teachers or the family?
- Is there a history of hyperactivity?

Skin

- Is there a rash?
- Are there any birthmarks or unusual marks on the skin?

Family history

In paediatrics, the family history is one of the most important components of the history:

- *Ages of parents and siblings*: you will need to be able to draw the family tree. Include the whole extended family with ages.
- *Illness in the family*: does anyone have a history of seizures, asthma, cancer, heart disease, tuberculosis, or any other medical condition? What was the age of onset and the medical advice so far?
- *Death in the family*: have there been any deaths in the family? What was the cause and age at death? Were any in infancy or childhood?
- *Social history*: where and how does the family live? What are the occupations of the family members? Are there any pets?

Practice point

Draw a family tree to assist your note-taking, and identification of key family and social history information

Examining a child: introduction

The physical examination of a child is one of the hardest parts of the doctor–patient interaction. You will need to have gained the confidence of the family and the child if you are to get the information that you require. How you approach the family (and how you communicate with them) throughout the interaction will be picked up by the child. In fact, a child may decide very early into the interview whether you've gained their confidence, and whether or not they will let you examine them. No amount of coercing will improve the situation—the parent will often be your advocate and do the convincing for you. It is therefore very worthwhile investing in the art of communication—how to talk with toddlers to teenagers and how to speak effectively with parents of sick children.

The following description is not meant to be prescriptive. There is much overlap between the different systems and you will have to decide on when, and in what order, you do things. For example, the tongue is assessed in the respiratory, cardiovascular, and GI systems—just look at it once!

General condition

- *State of health:* make a note of the child's general appearance. Is there any evidence of chronic illness? Make an assessment of their mental state: is their behaviour appropriate. Does the child interact with the parents? Is the child alert, tired, lethargic, or uncomfortable?
- *Height, weight, and head circumference:* these measurements are often made before you see the child. Acquaint yourself with how they are done in the clinic or on the paediatric ward. Certain measurements, e.g. the head occipitofrontal circumference (OFC), you will want to do yourself. In a growth clinic, length or height measurements are best done by the auxologist.
- *Hydration:* capillary refill, mucous membranes, anterior fontanelle, sunken eyes, skin turgor, and pulse.

Practice point

- In those under 2yrs old, obtain a length measurement using a table stadiometer. In older children, height can be measured standing
- Weigh the child unclothed
- Measure the head OFC at the maximum point of the occipital protuberance posteriorly and at the mid-forehead anteriorly
- Each of these measurements should be plotted on standard charts and the centiles recorded with the raw data

Vital signs

See also 📖 p.37. See Tables 3.1 and 3.2 for normal values of respiratory rate, heart rate (HR), and BP at different ages.

- *Temperature*: there are various ways in which the body temperature can be measured. Different units use different methods:
  - an electronic thermometer in the axilla;
  - a chemical dot thermometer in the axilla; *or*
  - an infrared tympanic thermometer 📖 p.696.
- A sick child could have a high, or abnormally low, temperature.
- *Pulse rate*: the pulse rate should be assessed from the radial pulse. (In the younger child you may find it easier to use brachial pulse.) Assess the rate, character, and rhythm at the radial pulse.
- *Respiratory rate*: in the older child you can observe the chest and count the number of breaths/min. Breaks or pauses in breathing that last longer than 15s are abnormal. In the infant, count abdominal movements over 1min, if you find it is easier to see diaphragmatic, rather than chest wall movement.
- *BP*: measurement is commonly performed using an automated method with BP displayed on-screen. It is important that the size and width of the cuff is appropriate for the size of limb in which pressure is being measured. It should cover 50–75% of the upper arm or thigh. A single measurement is required in most cases, but if heart disease is suspected, 4-limb measurements are needed. If considering hypertension, a standard technique is required; plot observations on BP centile charts.

Table 3.1 Normal values of respiratory rate and heart rate at different ages

Age	Respiratory rate (breaths/min)	Heart rate (beats/min)
0–6mths	30–50	120–140
6–12mths	20–40	95–120
1–5yrs	20–30	90–110
6–10yrs	18–25	80–100
>10yrs	12–25	60–100

Table 3.2 Normal values of blood pressure at different ages

Age	BP, mean (mmHg)	BP range, 90% (mmHg)
0–6yrs	95/65	80/50–115/80
10yrs	110/70	90/55–130/85
15yrs	120/75	110/60–145/90

Respiratory system

See also 📖 p.254.

- *Lips and buccal mucosa:* what is the colour of the mucous membranes and lips? Is the tongue in good condition? What is its colour? Are there any plaques, white patches, or spots?
- *Oropharynx:* what is the colour and size of the tonsils? Is there an exudate? What is the shape of the palate, uvula, and posterior pharynx?
- *Chest:* what is the shape of the chest? Are there scars or deformity? What is the position of the trachea? What is the chest like on percussion? (hyperresonant or dull? Where?)
- *Breathing:* are there any signs of respiratory distress. Is there nasal flaring, intercostals, subcostal, and sternal recession, use of accessory muscles, forced expiration, grunting, or tracheal tug? Is there an audible noise during inspiration or expiration?
- *Auscultation of the lungs:* listen for breath sounds in all regions of the chest. Evaluate inspiration and expiration. In the crying child you will still be able to listen during inspiration. Are there any fine crackles, rhonchi, or wheezes? Is there a pleural friction rub?
- *Ears:* the child will need to be positioned correctly for this part of the examination. It is often easier to have the child sitting on the mother's lap; one of her arms should be held around the upper body, and with the other arm she should place her hand against the side of the child's head so that it is held firm against her. Is there evidence of otitis externa? Is there a rash in the post-auricular area (a feature of dermatitis, measles, and rubella)? On otoscopy, check the state of the tympanic membrane. What is its colour and degree of lucency? Is it perforated, or is there a myringotomy tube present?
- *Nose:* is there discharge? Can the child breathe through each nostril?

Practice point

You should also consider the following as additional features essential to the respiratory examination:
- Sputum pot contents
- Peak flow rate measurement and assessment in relation to height
- Inhaler technique in those using such devices
- Evidence of previous tracheotomy or use of current one

You should be able to recognize the following patterns of abnormal signs:
- Consolidation
- Collapse or removal of a lung
- Pleural effusion
- Pneumothorax
- Airflow obstruction
- Bronchiectasis

Cardiovascular system

- *Colour and cyanosis* (see 📖 respiratory system, pp.55, 60, 254): examine the colour of the sclerae and conjunctivae.
- *Teeth:* assess the number and condition of the teeth.
- *Clubbing:* assess fingers and toes. Is there any peripheral oedema?
- *Pulses and rhythm:* compare the strength of the femoral and right brachial pulse. Pulse rate varies with the phase of respiration. It increases with inspiration and decreases with expiration.
- *Chest:* identify the position of the apex beat and consider whether it is displaced. In young children (<7yrs) it will be in the 4th intercostal space, to the left of the mid-clavicular line, on the left. In the child older than 7yrs, it will be in the 5th to 6th intercostal spaces. If it is not palpable, check the right side to exclude dextrocardia. Can you feel any other pulsations, heaves, or vibrations in the chest wall?
- *Murmurs:* auscultate the heart with the child in the sitting and supine positions. Listen over the whole precordium—the apex, the 2nd intercostal space to the left of the sternum (pulmonary valve area), the 2nd intercostal space to the right of the sternum (aortic valve area), and the 4th intercostal space over the sternum (tricuspid valve area). Listen to the heart sounds in each of these areas. Are the sounds muffled and suggestive of pericardial fluid? In the pulmonary valve area, is the second heart sound split during inspiration? (Fixed splitting is found with atrial septal defect.) At the apex, is a third heart sound present, indicating mitral valve prolapse or atrial septal defect? Is there a gallop rhythm of congestive heart failure?

Murmurs (see 📖 pp.228–231)

Now listen for added noises during the cardiac cycle. If there is one, then it should be described according to:
- *Loudness:* grade I to VI
- *Timing in the cardiac cycle:*
  - diastolic or systolic
  - early, mid, or late
- *Pitch:* high or low
- *Quality:* blowing, musical, or rough
- *Location where best heard:* apex, pulmonary, aortic, or left sternal
- *Radiation:* where, if anywhere, does the noise transmit across the chest? Listen to the back

Gastrointestinal system

For hands, mouth, tongue, and eyes see respiratory and cardiovascular systems (pp.50, 254). Assess whether the child is jaundiced.

Abdomen

The child needs to be relaxed and positioned supine, with the knees bent and hands by the sides.

- *Look at the shape of the abdomen:* is it distended? Is the umbilicus everted?
- *Does the abdominal wall move?* Is the child in pain? Is peristalsis visible?
- *Let the child know that you are going to touch the abdomen:* they should be free to tell you if it hurts. *Do not hurt the child.* First auscultate for bowel sounds, and then percuss in your assessment of hepatomegaly and ascites. In the right mid-clavicular line an enlarged liver extends more than 2cm below the costal margin. The normal span of the liver—between its upper and lower margins—is shown in Table 3.3.
- *Palpate the abdomen and check for any tenderness before assessing rebound:* palpate for masses during inspiration and deep expiration. Can you feel an abnormal spleen, liver, or kidney?
- *Watch the child feeding.*

Rectum and anus

In most instances you will only need to observe the patency of the anus and to look for fissures and rectal prolapse. However, if the child has abdominal symptoms, a digital examination may be required to check for sphincter tone, masses, and tenderness.

- This examination should only be done once and you will need to decide whether this test should be performed by a senior colleague, or by the surgeon should the child have an acute abdomen.
- Never perform a rectal examination as a senior house officer.

Table 3.3 Normal span of liver (between its upper and lower margins)

Age	Normal span of liver
At 6mths	2cm below costal margin
At 3yrs	4cm span
At 10yrs	6cm span
In adults	10cm span

Genitourinary system

See also 📖 p.484, 868. For hands, mouth, tongue, abdomen, and eyes see 📖 Respiratory system, Cardiovascular system, and Gastrointestinal system. The external genitalia are examined for any evidence of ambiguity, congenital abnormality, and size. For this examination you should have a chaperone present for both sexes. In the older child you must ensure privacy and preserve the child's dignity with the appropriate use of covers and gowns. Examine once only.

• *In boys:* development of the penis, testes, scrotum, and pubic hair can be staged using a standardized system (Tanner scale). Look at the state of the foreskin. Is there evidence of infection or discharge. Locate the position of the penile meatus. Have both testes descended?

• *In girls:* Tanner stage the pubic hair. Is there evidence of fused labia, enlarged clitoris, or infection with discharge or bleeding?

Musculoskeletal system

See also 📖 p.732.

• *Congenital anomalies:* examine the fingers, toes, hands and feet, legs and arms. Look at the shape of the bones.

• *Deformities:* are there deformities due to fracture? Are the lower limbs of equal length? What is the range of motion of each joint? Are the skin folds in the upper thigh normal? In the infant under 6mths check for congenital hip dislocation. Inspect the full length of the spine looking for tufts of hair, dimples, masses, or cysts at the base. Check for torticollis in the neck. Observe for any abnormal curvature or posture with the child standing and bending over touching their toes.

• *Gait:* watch the child walk and describe it in light of your other findings.

Practice point See also 📖 **pp.496–499, 557**

You should be able to recognize the gaits associated with:
• Myopathy (waddling)
• Hemiplegia
• Spastic diplegia
• Cerebellar ataxia
• Painful limb (antalgic gait)
• Foot drop
• Trendelenburg gait

Resuscitation

Cardiopulmonary arrest

Cardiopulmonary arrest in children often develops as a progression of respiratory failure and shock. The outcome of out-of-hospital arrest is poor, but respiratory arrest alone is associated with a rate of survival of 80%.

In hospital, even though unexpected cardiac arrest is now a rare event (1 per 5000 paediatric admissions), it is important that events or signs that may lead to arrest are recognized early. Children with any of the features in Table 4.1 warrant urgent medical review (see 📖 p.30 for normal values of vital signs).

Rapid cardiopulmonary assessment

The rapid cardiopulmonary assessment should take less than 1min.

Airway
Is it patent?

Breathing
- What are the effort and work of breathing? Is there recession, nasal flaring, grunting, use of accessory muscles, stridor, or wheeze?
- What is the air entry like in the chest?
- What is the respiratory rate: is it fast or slow?
- What is the skin colour?

Circulation
- What is the heart rate?
- What is the systemic perfusion? Check pulse volume, capillary refill, skin temperature, level of consciousness, and urine output.
- What is the BP?

Disability
- What is the level of consciousness?
- What are the pupils like: size and reaction?

Table 4.1 Warning signs for acute deterioration

Threatened airway obstruction Tachypnoea

Age	Action respiratory rate (breaths/min)
Term to 3mths	>60
4–12mths	>50
1–4yrs	>40
5–12yrs	>30
>12yrs	>30

Bradycardia or tachycardia

Age	Bradycardia (beats/min)	Tachycardia (beats/min)
Term to 3mths	<100	>180
4–12mths	<100	>180
1–4yrs	<90	>160
5–12yrs	<80	>140
>12yrs	<60	>130

Hypotension

Age	Action systolic pressure (mmHg)
Term to 3mths	<60
4–12mths	<65
1–4yrs	<70
5–12yrs	<80
>12yrs	<90

Altered mental state or convulsion

Low pulse oximetry values: <90% in any supplemental oxygen (<60% if cyanotic heart disease)

Paediatric basic life support

Cardiopulmonary arrest in children usually results from hypoxia due to respiratory or neurological failure or shock. If it occurs, irrespective of the cause, basic life support (BLS) must be started immediately.

Paediatric basic life support algorithm

1 First things
- Assess the safety of the situation.
- Stimulate the child and check responsiveness.

2 Shout for help

3 Open the airway
Give head tilt and chin lift, or jaw thrust

4 Assess breathing
Look, listen, and feel

5 If no breathing: rescue breaths
- *Child*: 5 breaths mouth to mouth
- *Infant*: 5 breaths mouth to mouth and nose

6 Assess the pulse
- *Child*: at the carotid artery
- *Infant*: at the brachial or femoral artery

7 If HR <60/min and poor perfusion: chest compressions
- *Child >8yrs*: use two-handed method for rate of 100/min and ratio of 15 compressions to 2 breaths
- *Child 1–8yrs*: use heel of hand on the lower third of the sternum for rate of 100/min and ratio of 15 compressions to 2 breaths
- *Infant*: use two fingers or the encircling chest technique if you have help at rate of 100/min and ratio of 15 compressions to 2 breaths

8 Provide 1min of life support

9 Contact emergency medical services

Choking children

The algorithm for emergency management of choking children using the Resuscitation Council (UK) protocol is as follows (Fig. 4.1):

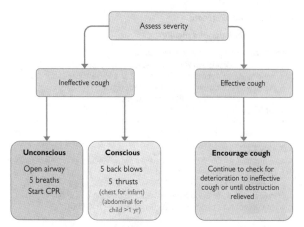

Fig. 4.1 Resuscitation Council Guidelines, Paediatric FBAO treatment algorithm 2010. Reproduced with permission.

Paediatric advanced life support

Paediatric advanced life support (ALS) algorithm

1 Basic life support

2 Ventilate and oxygenate

3 Attach defibrillator and monitor

4 Assess cardiac rhythm and check pulse
- *If ventricular fibrillation (VF) or pulseless tachycardia (VT):*
  - defibrillate as necessary: 4J/kg for initial and all subsequent shocks
  - *then* give cardiopulmonary resuscitation (CPR) for 2min
  - *then* reassess rhythm and pulse and respond
- *If not VF or VT:* asystole or pulseless electrical activity:
  - give CPR for 4min
  - then reassess rhythm and pulse, and respond

5 During CPR
- *Attempt and verify:*
  - tracheal intubation
  - IV or IO access
- *Check:* electrode or paddle placement: the position and contact.
- *Give:* epinephrine every 3–5min (0.1mL/kg IV (1:10,000))
- *Consider:*
  - giving anti-arrhythmics and alkalizing agents
  - potentially reversible causes—hypoxia; hypovolaemia; hypokalaemia; hyperkalaemia; hypocalcaemia; tension pneumothorax; cardiac tamponade; toxins; thromboemboli

6 Are there difficulties in ventilation?
Rule out the following potential problems
- Is the endotracheal tube *displaced*?
- Is there an *obstruction*?
- Does the child have a *pneumothorax*?
- Is there *equipment* failure?
- Is there air in the *stomach* causing diaphragmatic splinting?

Useful formulae in children

- *Estimation of weight*
  - *0–12 months*—Weight (kg) = (0.5 × Age (mths)) + 4
  - *1–5yrs*—Weight (kg) = (2 × Age (yrs)) + 8
  - *6–12yrs*—Weight (kg) = (3 × Age (yrs)) + 7
- *Endotracheal tube*
  - *Size* = (Age (yrs)/4 + 4)
  - *Length for oral tube* = (Age (yrs)/2 + 12) cm
  - *Length if nasal tube* = (Age (yrs)/2 + 15) cm

The algorithm for ALS using the Resuscitation Council (UK) protocol is shown in Fig. 4.2.

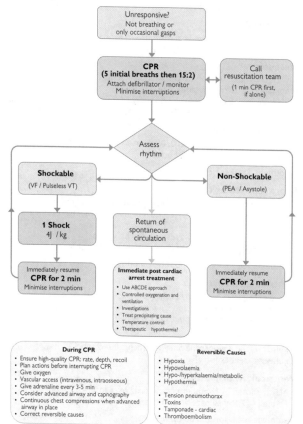

Fig. 4.2 Resuscitation council guidelines 2010. Paediatric Advanced Life Support algorithm. Reproduced with permission.

Rhythm disturbances

See 📖 pp.55–57, 250–251.

Bradycardia
- Bradycardia is often the final response to hypoxia.
- A preterminal rhythm leading to asystole.

Treatment
- Oxygen, with attention to airway and inflation.
- Epinephrine 10 micrograms/kg IV
- May require atropine 20 micrograms/kg IV (minimum 100 micrograms; maximum 1mg) if triggered by vagal stimulation.

Sinus tachycardia
- Heart rate can be as high as 220/min in an infant, but not higher.
- Caused by fever, pain, and shock.

Treatment Treat the cause.

Supraventricular tachycardia
- The most common primary arrhythmia in infancy and childhood.
- Onset sudden. Heart rate: >220/min in infants; >180/min in children over 3yrs.
- Rhythm is regular and P waves may not be visible.
- Infants may present with shock, sweatiness, and poor feeding.

Treatment See algorithms opposite, 📖 pp.57, 250.

Ventricular tachycardia
- Rare in children; caused by primary cardiac problem or overdose.
- Heart rate: between 120 and 250/min.
- Rhythm is almost regular, but QRS is wide (>2 small squares).

Treatment
- *Pulse present:* amiodarone 5mg/kg; synchronized shock.
- *Pulseless:* treat as for VF.

Ventricular fibrillation
- Mainly caused by hypothermia and drug overdose.
- Found in 27% of all paediatric in-hospital arrests.

Treatment See algorithm on 📖 p.41.

Asystole
- Mainly caused by hypoxia and acidosis.
- 60% of all paediatric arrests.

Treatment See algorithm on 📖 p.41.

Pulseless electrical activity
See algorithm on 📖 p.41.

Treating supraventricular tachycardia

Attach cardiac monitor and check BP.

Algorithm for treating patient with supraventricular tachycardia, but not in shock

1 Trial of vagal manoeuvres

2 Adenosine
- 50–100microgram/kg given as a rapid IV push into the most central IV access available followed by fast IV flush
- If no response, then 100–200microgram/kg
- If no response, then increase at increments of 50–100microgram/kg to a maximum single dose of 500microgram/kg

3 Consider
- Synchronous DC shock
- Amiodarone (IV bolus over 10min) 5mg/kg
- Procainamide (IV loading dose of 15mg/kg over 30–60min). Stop infusion if QRS widens or hypotension occurs
- Flecainide (IV 2mg/kg bolus over 20min)
- Seek advice

Algorithm for treating patient with SVT who is in shock

1a Attempt vagal manoeuvres but do not delay progress to step 2

1b If IV access is available give adenosine (see preceding algorithm) but do not delay progress to step 2

2 Synchronous DC shock
- 1J/kg
- If no response, then 2J/kg
- If no response, then 2J/kg

3 Consider using anti-arrhythmics (amiodarone)

4 Synchronous DC shock
- Return to step 2 in the algorithm at 2J/kg

Following unsuccessful resuscitation

The death of a child is distressing. The family should be spoken to sympathetically and in private. Most parents will want to see and hold their dead child and they should be offered this opportunity.

Report to the coroner (UK)

- Unexpected deaths (see 📖 Sudden unexpected death in an infant (SUDI)).
- Infants brought in dead to the emergency department or who die soon after arrival.
- Deaths where there has been recent surgery or an accident.
- Deaths where there are suspicious circumstances.

Sudden unexpected death in an infant (SUDI)

Parents or carers

- Take and record a detailed clinical history.
- Explain that a referral has been made to the coroner. Explain the role of the police and warn the family that they may visit the house.

Child

After failed resuscitation the endotracheal tube and IO needle can be removed, but venous access should be retained. Retain the child's clothing/bedding and nappy for the police. Take the following samples:

- *Nasopharyngeal aspirate*: virology and bacteriology.
- *Urine*: biochemistry and freeze immediately.
- *Blood*: toxicology, cultures, metabolic and coagulation screen.
- *Lumbar puncture* (cerebrospinal fluid (CSF) for virology and culture): if indicated.

Other professionals

Inform the following:

- Senior clinical staff: in the UK a designated SUDI team will investigate these deaths and a home visit will be made by the paediatrician and police within 24hr.
- Family general practitioner.
- Health visitor (or community midwife).
- Neonatologist (if a neonate).

Follow-up

- Arrangements should be made for the family to discuss the results of the coroner's post-mortem.
- Genetic counselling may be needed.
- Bereavement counselling should be offered: this may be provided by the family practitioner, the paediatric team, or from other agencies (e.g. Foundation for the Study of Infant Deaths, Child Death Helpline, and CRUSE).

Emergency and high dependency care

The ABC of high dependency

Emergency and high-dependency care is about providing the right care and support in a timely manner. Practising paediatrics under these conditions means that you will need to anticipate what could happen next, which can be very difficult. Therefore, we shall start with an emphasis on patient safety—the ABC—the assessment of Airway, Breathing, and Circulation. Then, we shall cover most of what is needed next for acute care—knowledge, assessments, and treatments.

A—establish an airway

Provide oxygen

Use fractional inspired oxygen (FiO_2) 100%; use the optimum method for patient size and monitor.
- *Neonates, infants:* head-box oxygen with *in situ* FiO_2 monitor.
- *Infants, toddlers:* nasal cannulae (NC). The ideal estimate of FiO_2 from tidal volume (7mL/kg) and NC flow rate is shown in the following example.

Consider a 6kg infant on 0.25L/min NC oxygen (tidal volume = 42mL; NC flow = 250mL/min, 4mL/s; inspiratory time = 1s).
FiO_2 value is: 4mL × 1.0 = 4mL oxygen, plus 38mL × 0.21 = 8mL oxygen. FiO_2 = (4 + 8)/42 = 0.29.

- *Toddler, pre-school:* NC, face mask.
- *School-age child:* non-rebreathing mask.

Maintain airway and air movement
- *Support airway when needed with jaw lift:* suction nasopharynx and mouth as needed. Provide oral or nasopharyngeal airway.
- *Maintain patient in upright position:* do not force a distressed patient to lie down. Minimize discomfort.

B—use respiratory support for breathing
- *Identify the level of respiratory involvement:* treat specific problems appropriately (e.g. bronchodilators).
- *Assist work of breathing with non-invasive support:* this can be achieved with nasopharyngeal continuous +ve airway pressure (see bronchiolitis, 📖 p.288), or −ve pressure ventilation.
- *Intubation and mechanical ventilation.*

C—assess circulation; establish IV access
- Start *pulse oximetry* and *cardiac monitoring.*
- *Provide IV fluids:* when the circulation is good it is advisable to limit fluid intake to an amount ranging from restricted to just below maintenance.

Respiratory distress

Respiratory distress is defined as increased work of breathing that causes a sense of altered well-being. The hallmarks are use of accessory muscles and tachypnoea. Distress can be caused by disorders of gas exchange (O_2 absorption, or CO_2 elimination), respiratory drive, neuromuscular disease, and infection (see Box 5.1).

Box 5.1 Differential diagnosis of respiratory distress

Nasopharynx
- *Nose:* choanal atresia, stenosis
- *Oropharynx:* tonsillar hypertrophy
- *Tongue:* glossomegaly
- *Pharynx:* peritonsillar abscess, retropharyngeal abscess, diphtheria

Upper airway obstruction
- *Larynx:* vocal cord dysfunction, laryngomalacia, papilloma, haemangioma, croup
- *Epiglottis:* epiglottitis, foreign body

Lower airway disorder
- *Trachea:* tracheitis, tracheobronchomalacia, foreign body, pulmonary artery sling
- *Bronchi:* bronchitis, bronchomalacia
- *Bronchioles:* asthma, bronchiolitis, pertussis

Disordered gas exchange
- *Haemoglobin:* carbon monoxide poisoning, methaemoglobinaemia, acidosis
- *Shunt:* pulmonary oedema, haemorrhage, atelectasis, or embolism
- *Dead space ventilation:* asthma, bronchiolitis, pulmonary hypertension
- *Other:* sickle chest syndrome, pneumonia, pneumothorax

Respiratory drive
- *Hyperventilation:* psychogenic, brainstem tumour
- *Hypoventilation:* apnoea, drugs

Neuromuscular
- *Respiratory muscle weakness:* Duchenne muscular dystrophy, spinal muscle atrophy, central nervous system (CNS) depression

Other
- *Pleural:* pneumothorax, chylothorax, haemothorax, pleural effusion, empyema
- *Chest wall:* flail chest, rib fractures

Definitions

Broadly, we can define the two major causes of respiratory distress as follows.

Respiratory failure

- *Hypoxaemia despite high FiO₂:* arterial oxygen tension (PaO$_2$) <8kPa in previously well child.
- *Acidosis:* pH <7.25; no specific arterial carbon dioxide tension (PaCO$_2$) since the child may have a chronic 'compensated' problem.
- *Increasing fatigue, or absence of improvement with therapy:* based on your observations on child's breathing and mental state.

Neuromuscular weakness

- *Clinical:* bulbar dysfunction with poor or absent cough, gag, swallow, *or* chest wall weakness of neurological or muscular origin.
- *Physiological:* use spirometry to assess vital capacity <12mL/kg, or manometry to assess maximum inspiratory force <−20mmHg.

Respiratory distress: management

Clinical assessment

Assess the patient for the following:
- *Colour:* pallor or cyanosis.
- *Respiratory drive:* pattern and timing of breathing may reflect a central or brainstem cause.
- *Inspiration and expiration of air at the mouth and nose:* upper airway obstruction produces stridor; lower airway obstruction leads to cough, wheeze, and a prolonged expiratory phase.
- *Chest wall movement:* chest and abdominal wall dynamics may indicate flail-chest, diaphragmatic palsy, pneumothorax, or foreign body inhalation.
- *Position and level of agitation.*
- *Mental state.*
- *Heart rate and perfusion:* these may reflect impending arrest.

Investigations

- *Non-invasive:* pulse oximetry measurement of oxyhaemoglobin saturation, pulse oximetry measurement of oxyhaemoglobin saturation (SpO_2).
- *Arterial blood gas:* assessment of acid–base, PaO_2, $PaCO_2$. A capillary blood sample is a good alternative (for pH, PCO_2) if the extremity is warm and the blood flows freely.
- *Blood tests:* full blood count (FBC), electrolytes, glucose, and cultures.
- *CXR:* for diagnosis (e.g. severe pneumonia); for assessment of complications (e.g. pulmonary oedema, pneumothorax).

Monitoring

- Pulse oximetry.
- Continuous ECG.
- BP.
- Temperature.
- Fluid balance.
- Conscious level.

Therapy

There are specific therapies for each condition listed in the 'Differential diagnoses' on 🕮 p.48 (see individual sections). With regard to fluid therapy, we generally restrict total volume to 80% maintenance for the following reasons.
- *Distress with retraction:* high –ve intrathoracic pressure will pull fluid out of capillaries into the interstitial space and will aggravate breathing with pulmonary oedema.
- *Syndrome of inappropriate antidiuretic hormone (SIADH):* this is a common problem in moderate to severe respiratory distress.
- *Diuresis is limited:* in the hydrated patient consider using furosemide (0.5–1mg/kg, IV). It may help the patient with extra-interstitial water without overt oedema.

Foreign-body inhalation

Foreign-body (FB) aspiration is more common in toddlers and infants, who tend to put objects in their mouths. FBs can be inhaled into the airway, or they may get caught in the oesophagus and compress the trachea.

Symptoms

The symptoms of a FB in the aerodigestive tract range from no symptoms to complete airway obstruction.
- *Larynx:* usually causes hoarseness, cough, dysphonia, haemoptysis, stridor, wheezing, dyspnoea, cyanosis, or apnoea due to complete obstruction.
- *Trachea and bronchus:* can cause chest pain. After initial symptoms, there may be an asymptomatic period followed by features of pneumonia (see 📖 p.290).
- *Oesophagus:* will produce drooling, dysphagia, or vomiting and, if the trachea is compressed, may produce dyspnoea, stridor, respiratory failure, or apnoea (see 📖 pp.256, 258).

Aetiology

Inhaled FB should be considered in all patients with a history of choking or gagging.

Diagnosis

- A monophonic *wheeze or absent breath sounds* on one side of the chest may be noted on examination.
- Chest and neck *radiographs*, with lateral views, may be helpful in identifying the location of an object. Inspiratory and expiratory films may show an area of hyperinflation.
- *Arterial blood gas* analysis is indicated when the patient is in severe distress.

Initial treatment

Follow a standard protocol.
- *ABC.*
- *FB removal:* if the child is calm with good air exchange, removal of the FB should take place under controlled circumstances; manipulation may change the position of the object, inducing more severe obstruction. If the child is in distress, but maintaining good air exchange, back blows and chest thrusts may be performed as per the standard technique for paediatric advanced life support (ALS).
- An unconscious child with poor air entry should be given oxygen (FiO$_2$ 100%) via a face mask until rigid bronchoscopy and object removal can be performed.

Drowning

Drowning is caused by submersion in water. When water has been aspirated into the lungs it is usually a small amount (<22mL/kg). In ≤10% there has been laryngospasm without aspiration of water. The location—sea, freshwater, brackish water—is of little consequence. However, the temperature of the water is important, and the incident is classified as warm, cold, and very cold when the water temperature is 20°C, 6–19°C, and ≤5°C, respectively.

Symptoms

Respiratory acidosis occurs with inadequate ventilation.
- If there has been a hypoxic–ischaemic insult, brain swelling, and raised intracranial pressure (ICP) may develop.
- Hypoxaemia and inadequate perfusion will cause acidosis, arrhythmia, and shock.

Aetiology

Children under 3yrs old and teenagers are most at risk. Young children may have accidents in pools and bathtubs if left unattended. Assess the duration of submersion, water temperature, and presence of cyanosis or apnoea. Emergency staff should provide details of resuscitation and the time taken to establish a pulse and cardiac output. Consider:
- head and neck injuries from diving;
- pre-existing cardiac arrhythmia;
- pre-existing seizure disorder;
- drug and alcohol abuse.

Initial treatment

Follow a standard protocol.
- *AB:* the neck may be injured and the airway may be obstructed by material from the water. Clear the mouth and immobilize the neck. If there is no gagging, hypoxaemia, or apnoea, then endotracheal intubation is needed. At the time of intubation use in-line traction.
- *C:* poor perfusion occurs in children with severe hypoxic–ischaemic injury or pulmonary oedema.
- *Temperature:* remove all wet clothing in order to avoid cooling. Warm the child to achieve a core temperature >35°C (use a heating blanket). In profound hypothermia, more invasive methods of warming may be used on the intensive care unit (e.g. heart–lung bypass or internal bladder and gastric lavage).

After resuscitation

- *Assess:* vital signs, chest, heart, and the central nervous system.
- *Start:* pulse oximetry and cardiac monitoring.
- ECG.
- *Look closely for signs of lower respiratory tract involvement:* use of accessory respiratory muscles, nasal flaring, tachypnoea, cough, wheeze, and crackles.

Circulation: cardiovascular difficulty

Shock

The failure to deliver adequate oxygen to the tissues:
- *Heart rate disturbance:* bradycardia, dysrhythmias.
- *Decreased stroke volume:* hypovolaemia; vasodilatation; poor contractility.

Congestive heart failure

Cardiac fatigue due to:
- *Excess volume load:* from left-to-right cardiac lesions (ventricular septal defect (VSD), patent ductus arteriosus (PDA), atreriovenous (AV) canal), AV fistula, severe anaemia, hypervolaemia.
- *Excess pressure load:* from systemic vascular system (aortic stenosis, coarctation of the aorta, or hypertension) or pulmonary vascular system (pulmonary stenosis, pulmonary hypertension, chronic hypoventilation, or severe upper airway obstruction).
- *Myocardial problems:* including cardiomyopathy, myocarditis, myocardial ischaemia (anomalous coronary artery, cardiac thrombosis in Kawasaki), metabolic disorders (📖 p.962).
- *Excess myocardial demand:* due to fever, thyrotoxicosis.

Dysrhythmia

See also 📖 pp.42–43, 55–57, 250; uncommon, but consider:
- *Supraventricular tachycardia.*
- *Congenital heart block.*

Hypertension

See also 📖 pp.55, 390; causes of hypertension are:
- *Renal:* glomerulonephritis; haemolytic–uraemic syndrome; pyelonephritis; obstructive nephropathy; vascular disease.
- *Cardiac:* coartation of the aorta.
- *Neurological:* infection; drugs; tumour; cerebral oedema.
- *Endocrine:* phaeochromocytoma; Cushing's syndrome; corticosteroids; hyperthyroidism.
- *Toxins and poisons.*
- *Primary essential hypertension.*

Anaphylactic shock

See also 📖 p.64; main causes are food, medication, and insect bites. Life-threatening problems are:
- *Respiratory:* airway narrowing of upper and lower airway.
- *CVS:* shock, vasodilatation, and increased vascular permeability.

Pericarditis See 📖 p.246 The causes include infection, rheumatological disorders, trauma, malignancy, and post-pericardiotomy syndrome.

Congenital heart disease See 📖 pp.232–241

Cardiovascular system difficulty: assessment

See also 📖 pp.226–231.

Shock

In early shock, findings can be subtle. Hypotension is a late sign, so look for a decreased stroke volume (decreased pulse amplitude) and increased systemic vascular resistance (perfusion changes to skin and muscle). In classic shock there are features of decompensation. Late shock is a pre-arrest phenomenon.

Shock

Early shock
- *Pulse*: tachycardia
- *BP*: normal but postural drop
- *Breathing*: tachypnoea
- *Limbs*: cool and mottled
- *CNS*: agitated
- *Laboratory*: mild metabolic acidosis

Classic shock
- *Pulse*: tachycardia and weak pulses
- *BP*: hypotension
- *Breathing*: tachypnoea and grunting
- *Limbs*: cool, clammy, and pale or blue
- *CNS*: depressed level of consciousness
- *Laboratory*: metabolic acidosis

Late shock
- *Pulse*: tachycardia and thready pulses; bradycardia is pre-arrest
- *BP*: profound hypotension
- *Breathing*: tachypnoea; bradypnoea signifies pre-arrest
- *Limbs*: cold (blue to white)
- *CNS*: coma
- *Laboratory*: metabolic acidosis, multisystem derangement

Congestive heart failure

The patient may have: sweating on exertion or feeding; malaise and irritability; decreased appetite. The physical findings include:
- *Tachycardia*: ± gallop rhythm on auscultation.
- *Tachypnoea*: ± wheeze and crackles on auscultation.
- *Raised jugular venous pressure*: ± hepatosplenomegaly and oedema.
- *Pale or mottled and cool extremities.*
- *Hypotension.*
- *Features of the underlying cause*: e.g. murmur in VSD or pallor in anaemia.

- *CXR:* showing cardiomegaly, and pulmonary vascular congestion to pulmonary oedema.

Arrhythmias

A 12-lead ECG and BP are needed for diagnosis.

Bradycardia

If there is haemodynamic instability (i.e. hypotension or poor perfusion), significant bradycardia is present if the HR is:
- <80/min in neonates.
- <50/min in infants.
- <40/min in older children.

Tachydysrhythmia

These may be:
- *Narrow complex:* QRS duration <0.1s in children or <0.12s in adolescents (e.g. supraventricular tachycardia (SVT) and atrial flutter). There are no P waves in SVT;
- *ventricular:* prolonged QRS.

Hypertension

To diagnose hypertension strict criteria should be followed: three measurements in non-stressful circumstances with values >2 standard deviations above mean for age and sex. Standard charts should be consulted (📖 p.391–392), but, by age, the upper limits of normal BP are:
- *<2yrs:* systolic BP, 110mmHg; diastolic BP, 65mmHg;
- *3–6yrs:* systolic BP, 120mmHg; diastolic BP, 70mmHg;
- *7–10yrs:* systolic BP, 130mmHg; diastolic BP, 75mmHg;
- *11–15yrs:* systolic BP, 140mmHg; diastolic BP, 80mmHg.

Pericarditis

There may be chest pain or features of the underlying cause. Look for:
- Congestive heart failure.
- Friction rub.
- Pulsus paradoxus (>10mmHg).

When cardiac tamponade is present there are classic signs:
- Shock.
- Distended jugular veins.
- Heart sounds appear distant.
- *ECG:* decreased voltage, elevated ST segments, T-wave inversion.
- *CXR:* the heart will look enlarged if an effusion is present.

Congenital heart disease

In cyanotic babies the history and examination can be used to exclude respiratory causes of cyanosis. The assessment also includes the hyperoxia test (measurement of PaO_2 in FiO_2 100%).
- *PaO_2 < 13.3kPa (100mmHg):* possible cyanotic heart disease.
- *PaO_2 13.3–26.7kPa (100–200mmHg):* possible heart disease with complete mixing and increased pulmonary blood flow.
- *PaO_2 > 33.3 kPa (>250mmHg):* cyanotic heart disease unlikely.

Cardiovascular system difficulty: therapy—1

Shock

Initial therapy includes the following.

- *Oxygen:* provide supplemental oxygen, FiO_2 100%. Intubate if required.
- *Position:* in shock, elevate the legs to improve venous return. In congestive heart failure elevate the head.
- *IV access:* central access may be required, particularly when using inotropes.
- *Temperature:* control fever with antipyretics (paracetamol 15mg/kg).
- *Metabolic state:* correct hypoglycaemia and hypocalcaemia. Acidosis of respiratory cause should be controlled with ventilation.

Fluid volumes for shock

- *Hypovolaemia:* IV 20mL/kg of normal saline. In severe volume depletion give 40–60mL/kg of normal saline, with additional increments of 10mL/kg to restore volume if small heart size on CXR, and CVP <5–10mmHg.
- *Stop resuscitation with volume:*
  - when clinical improvement is achieved;
  - when clinical signs of improvement fail to appear;
  - if there are signs of volume overload: hepatosplenomegaly, JVP distension, gallop rhythm, wheeze and crackles.

Inotropes for shock

- *Start inotropes:*
  - when circulation remains unsatisfactory and CXR shows large heart, pulmonary vascular congestion, pulmonary oedema, or pleural effusion;
  - when CVP >10–15mmHg; once initiated, titrate dose upward to produce the effect required.
- *Hypotension with tachycardia:*
  - *dopamine*—1–20microgram/kg/min (start at 5microgram/kg/min).
  - *dobutamine*—2–20microgram/kg/min (start at 5microgram/kg/min). Can use peripheral IV.

Dysrhythmias

See also 📖 pp.42–43, 250–251.

Sinus bradycardia and heart block

- Do not treat if haemodynamically stable (i.e. BP and perfusion).
- Consider other treatable causes of bradycardia, such as raised ICP, acidosis, or hypercapnia.
- *Atropine:* 0.02mg/kg IV (min 0.1mg; max 1mg).

Intensive care treatments for shock

Hypotension with normal or low HR

- *Adrenaline:* 0.05–1microgram/kg/min (start at 0.05–0.10 microgram/kg/min)
- *Noradrenaline:* 0.05–1microgram/kg/min (start at 0.05–0.10 microgram/kg/min)
- *Amrinone:* load 0.75mg/kg IV over 3min, then give 5–10microgram/kg/min

Hypotension refractory to volume and single inotrope

- Seek intensive care advice as these patients will usually need intubation and ventilation, and steroids (see 📖 p.714)
- Combinations of inotropes are used in this instance
- Afterload reduction may be required with sodium nitroprusside: 0.5–7micrograms/kg/min (start 0.5microgram/kg/min)

Diuresis for volume overload

- *Start diuretics:* after circulation is restored expected urine volume is 1mL/kg/hr
- If oliguria or anuria use furosemide 0.5–1mg/kg IV or mannitol 0.5–1g/kg IV

Tachydysrhythmia—SVT

Treatment will require consultation with a cardiac specialist. If haemodynamically stable, consider the following:

- *Vagal manoeuvres:* ice bag to face for 15–20s or unilateral carotid massage or Valsalva manoeuvre. Do not compress orbits.
- *Adenosine:* 50–100micrograms/kg initially, as rapid IV push.
- *DC shock:* synchronized countershock 1J/kg should be reserved for the haemodynamically unstable. Intubation and appropriate analgesia and sedation are required.
- *Other drugs:* amiodarone, procainamide, flecainide.

Ventricular tachycardia

If haemodynamically stable and pulse, consider the following after advice from cardiac specialist:

- *If pulse present:* amiodarone 5mg/kg; synchronized shock.
- Pulseless (see 📖 Chapter 41, p.41).

Cardiovascular system difficulty: therapy—2

Congestive heart failure

Use fluid restriction and inotropic support after cardiological advice.

Digoxin may be used for primary cardiac problem (total digitalizing dose, TDD). By age TDDs are as follows.

- *Neonate:* 30micrograms/kg PO or 20micrograms/kg IV.
- *<2yrs:* 40–50micrograms/kg PO or 30–40micrograms/kg IV.
- *2–10yrs:* 25–35micrograms/kg PO or 20–30micrograms/kg IV.
- *10yrs:* 0.75–1.25mg PO or 0.5–1mg IV.

Digoxin administration

Split the TDD at the following times:
- *Initial:* give 50% of TDD.
- *8hr:* give 25% of TDD.
- *16hr:* give 25% of TDD.

Hypertension

See 📖 pp.390–397. For severe, symptomatic hypertension, the BP should be lowered by 20–25%. Do not aim for normal levels. Patients should be monitored in a high-dependency area. Discuss with nephrologist. Hypertensive encephalopathy is an emergency and too rapid lowering of BP may lead to stroke. Short-acting antihypertensives are the treatment of choice. Consider:

- *Diazoxide:* 1–3mg/kg IV by rapid infusion; repeat after 5–15min.
- *Hydralazine:* 100–500micrograms/kg IV over several minutes (max dose 20mg). May repeat dose in 20–30min.
- *Sodium nitroprusside.*

Congenital heart disease: alprostadil

See also 📖 p.232. In neonates, consider alprostadil (prostaglandin E1 (PGE1) infusion if:

- PaO_2 <4–5.3kPa (30–40mm/kg).
- Oxygen saturation <70% in FiO_2 100%.
- Femoral pulses are diminished or absent with poor perfusion.
- Metabolic acidosis persisting after volume and inotropes.

PGE1 dose

0.01–0.20micrograms/kg/min (start at 0.05micrograms/kg/min, increase in 0.05micrograms/kg/min increments if response is not adequate). Be aware that apnoea may develop.

Cyanosis: assessment

Cyanosis is the result of deoxygenated haemoglobin or abnormal haemoglobin in the blood. Cyanosis is apparent when there is 4g/dL of reduced haemoglobin or 0.5g/dL of methaemoglobin. Anaemic patients may not become cyanotic even in the presence of marked arterial desaturation. In light-skinned patients, cyanosis is usually noted with arterial saturation <85%. In dark-skinned patients, the saturation must be lower. Cyanosis is caused by the following problems.

- *Lung pump:*
  - alveolar hypoventilation;
  - ventilation–perfusion inequality;
  - impairment of oxygen diffusion.
- *Cardiovascular pump:* right-to-left shunting.
- *Haematological:* decreased affinity of haemoglobin for oxygen.

Differential diagnosis for cyanosis

Alveolar hypoventilation
- *CNS:* seizures; cerebral oedema; haemorrhage; infection; hypoxia–ischaemia; drugs
- *Hypothermia*

Ventilation–perfusion inequality
- *Lung:* bronchiolitis; pneumonia, pneumothorax; pleural effusion; respiratory muscle dysfunction (muscular dystrophy, myasthenia gravis, Guillain–Barré); tracheal compression
- *Cardiac:* decreased pulmonary blood flow (tricuspid atresia, pulmonary atresia with intact septum, critical pulmonary stenosis, tetralogy of Fallot); decreased systemic perfusion (coarctation of the aorta, sepsis)

Impairment of oxygen diffusion
- *Lung:* bronchopulmonary dysplasia; hypoplasia; diaphragmatic hernia

Right-to-left shunting
- *Cardiac:* congenital heart defect; Eisenmenger syndrome; AV fistula—pulmonary or systemic
- Decreased *oxygen affinity for haemoglobin*
- *Methaemoglobinaemia:* hereditary; aniline dyes; nitrobenzene; azo compounds and nitrites
- *Carboxyhaemoglobinaemia*

Clinical assessment

Also see 📖 pp.31–32. The key part of the assessment is respiratory and cardiovascular.

Vital and general signs

• Record the temperature.
• Record HR.
• Record BP in all four limbs.
• Is there evidence of failure to thrive?

Clubbing

This sign may be present in the older infant or child. It should be looked for in the fingers and toes. The causes can be:

• hereditary;
• idiopathic;
• congenital heart disease (CHD);
• infective endocarditis;
• pulmonary conditions (e.g. cystic fibrosis);
• GI disease (e.g. Crohn's, ulcerative colitis, cirrhosis).

Respiratory

In the neonate increased respiratory rate (usually <80breaths/min) with no respiratory distress suggests cyanotic heart disease, but with respiratory distress pulmonary disease is suggested. In the older child a full respiratory examination is required—look at all components of the examinations.

Cardiovascular

The absence of a murmur does not exclude congenital heart disease. Is the liver enlarged?

Cyanosis: management

Investigations

Blood tests
- FBC with differential.
- Blood cultures.
- Glucose.
- *Bedside diagnosis of methaemoglobinaemia:* place a drop of blood on a piece of filter paper. After 30s exposure to air, normal blood turns red, while blood taken from a patient with methaemoglobinaemia remains chocolate brown.

Infection
- Lumbar puncture as indicated.
- Urinary culture.

Arterial blood gas
In the older child a single measurement is needed. In the neonate, assess the change in PaO_2 in response to FiO_2 100% for 5–10min (see hyperoxia test, 📖 p.55).

Chest X-ray
See also 📖 p.231. In the neonate the lung fields should be assessed for signs of increased vascularity, pulmonary congestion, or oligaemia. Characteristic radiographic findings are:
- *Egg on a string:* transposition of the great arteries.
- *Boot-shaped heart:* tetralogy of Fallot (Box 5.2), pulmonary atresia, ventriculoseptal defect.
- *Snowman sign:* supracardiac total anomalous pulmonary venous drainage.
- *Wall-to-wall heart:* Ebstein's anomaly.

Electrocardiogram
See also 📖 p.231. Characteristic findings include:
- *Superior left axis:* tricuspid atresia; endocardial cushion defect; primum atrial septal defect.
- *Left axis deviation:* pulmonary atresia ± atrial atresia.
- *Marked right atrial hypertrophy:* Ebstein's anomaly.

Echocardiography
Assessment for specific cardiac lesions.

Monitoring
Standard cardiorespiratory monitoring (see 📖 p.50).

Therapy
Therapies for specific cardiac, respiratory, and poisoning conditions are discussed elsewhere.

Box 5.2 Tetralogy of Fallot ('tet spell') See also 📖 p.235

Patients may have attacks of paroxysmal hyperpnoea and increased cyanosis that occur spontaneously or after early morning feeds, prolonged crying, or defecation

Emergency treatment
- Place the patient in the knee-to-chest position
- Administer oxygen
- Insert IV line and administer phenylephrine, morphine sulphate, and propranolol
- Prolonged attacks require sodium bicarbonate
- Refer to cardiac centre

Anaphylaxis

Anaphylaxis is a life-threatening allergic event. It is the extreme clinical example of an immediate hypersensitivity reaction.

Symptoms

The reaction includes involvement of:
- *Skin*: urticaria and angioedema.
- *Respiratory*: acute airway obstruction with laryngeal oedema and bronchospasm.
- *Gastrointestinal*: severe abdominal cramping and diarrhea.
- *Systemic*: hypotension and shock.

Aetiology

The symptoms of anaphylaxis are abrupt, often within minutes of exposure to an antigen. The causes are:
- *Drugs*: penicillin, aspirin.
- *Injections*: radiographic contrast dyes.
- *Stings*: bites and envenomations.
- *Foods*: shellfish, nuts, peanuts, eggs.

Diagnosis

Take a careful history and aim to determine the time between onset of symptoms and exposure to the potential precipitating cause.

Initial treatment

Follow a standard protocol
- ABC.
- *Epinephrine (adrenaline)*: give SC 0.01mL/kg (1:1000, maximum dose 0.5mL). Repeat every 15min if required.
- *Hypotension*: put the patient head-down at 30° (Trendelenburg position) and give IV normal saline (20mL/kg bolus). IV epinephrine may be given over 2–5min (0.1mL/kg, 1:10,000), while an infusion is being prepared.
- *Salbutamol*: give nebulized salbutamol 0.05–0.15mg/kg in 3mL normal saline. Approximately 2.5mg for child <30kg and 5mg for child >30kg, every 15min if required.
- *Antihistamine*.
- *Steroid*: give IV bolus methylprednisolone (2mg/kg). This dose should be followed by IV methylprednisolone 2mg/kg/day (divided every 6hr), or oral prednisolone 2mg/kg (bolus once a day).

Hypovolaemic shock

Shock is characterized by inadequate systemic perfusion. The most common type, hypovolaemic shock, is related to abnormally low circulating blood volume.

Symptoms
See 📖 p54.

Aetiology
The causes of hypovolaemia are:
- Trauma.
- GI bleeding (📖 pp.312–313).
- Burns (📖 pp.66–68).
- Peritonitis.
- Diarrhoea (📖 pp.302–303).
- Diabetic ketoacidosis. (📖 pp.98–101)

Diagnosis
Perform a rapid clinical examination and direct your initial treatment toward the patient's vital signs.

Initial treatment
Follow a standard protocol
- *Airway, Breathing, Circulation, Disability (ABCD).*
- *Blood:* in patients with significant blood loss, transfusion will be required (about 2mL/kg to increase haemoglobin concentration by 1g/dL). (Patient may need O –ve unmatched blood in an emergency). Monitor the response with laboratory testing.
- *Fluid:* acutely, blood pressure and perfusion need to be restored with crystalloid infusion. IV bolus of normal saline, 20mL/kg, can be given over 15min and repeated if necessary. If more than 60mL/kg is required consider endotracheal intubation and ventilatory support. In the patient who is dehydrated, the water and electrolyte deficit needs to be replaced (see, 📖 pp.90–93).
- *Refractory hypotension:* intubation and intensive care monitoring and therapy are required (see 📖 p.714).

Burns

There are different forms of thermal injury to the body:
- Contact with fire.
- Scalding fluids.
- Chemicals.
- Electricity.
- Inhalation of flame, heated vapour, and toxic fumes.
- Cold: freezing injury.

The severity of a burn to the skin is assessed according to its severity and total surface area.

Severity

Severity of the burn site is categorized according to the degree of involvement of the skin:
- *First degree:* limited to epidermis; painful and erythematous.
- *Second degree:* epidermis and dermis. Superficial is blistered and painful, and deep is white and painless.
- *Third degree:* epidermis and all of the dermis; painless and leathery.

Surface area

The extent of the burn as a proportion of the body surface area (% body surface area) can be calculated by making a sum of the individual areas involved in the injury. Table 5.1 gives the percentage of the body surface area taken up by the individual areas at different ages.

Table 5.1 Contribution of different body parts to total body surface area at different ages

Body part	Body part area/total body surface (%) at ages		
	<1yr	1–11yrs	>11yrs
Head	18	13	9
Trunk (front)	18	18	18
Trunk (back)	18	18	18
Arm	9	9	9
Leg	14	16	18
Genitalia	1	1	1

Symptoms

Features of hypovolaemia, pain, and signs of inhalation injury may be present.

Symptoms of inhalation in the lung
- Tachypnoea.
- Stridor.
- Crackles.
- Wheeze.
- Cough.
- Respiratory distress.
- Black sputum.

Other burn symptoms
Brain
- Confusion.
- Dizziness.
- Headache.
- Restlessness.
- Coma.
- Seizures.

Skin
- Facial burns.
- Nasal burn.
- Cherry-red colour.

Aetiology
You should find out the following about the injury:
- Its mechanism.
- The duration of exposure.
- Environmental factors (closed or open space).
- Loss of consciousness during the accident.

Investigations
Minor burns
There is no need for routine investigations in children with minor burns, i.e. burns that are:
- partial thickness and <5% body surface; *or*
- full thickness and <2cm^2 (unless hands, face, genitals, joints involved).

Major burns
- Arterial blood gas.
- Carboxyhaemoglobin level.
- Blood count and cross-match.
- Blood urea, creatinine, and electrolytes may be tested.

Consider child protection issues!

Burns: treatment

Initial treatment

Follow a standard protocol

- *ABC:* if there is evidence of inhalation then pulmonary toilet with endotracheal intubation may be needed.
- Assume that there is *carbon monoxide poisoning* and measure carboxyhaemoglobin level and PaO_2. Give humidified 100% oxygen until results are available.
- Follow serial arterial blood gases and CXRs.
- Consider *cyanide exposure and poisoning* if the breath smells of almonds, or if the accident is fire-related, or if there is metabolic acidosis with raised anion-gap.
- In infants with burns >10% of body surface area, or children with >15% burns, consider an IV bolus of normal saline (10–20mL/kg). Further fluid resuscitation should be directed toward maintaining a urine output of 0.5–2mL/kg/h. In patients with >25% burns use the Parkland's formula as a guide to fluid therapy Box 5.3.

Box 5.3 Parkland's formula

0–24hr after burn

Crystalloid

- 4mL/kg per 1% burn
- Use 50% of this volume in the first 8hr

24–48hr after burn

Crystalloid + colloid

- Use 50–75% of fluid requirements on day 1
- Add albumin (1g/kg/day) to maintain serum level above 2g/dL

- *Analgesia:* pain must be treated. First ensure that ventilation, oxygenation, and perfusion are adequate. Use IV analgesics if required.
- *Other injuries:* do a secondary survey of associated traumatic injuries. Assess for cardiac and skeletal muscle injury in electrical accidents. In chemical burn, wash and neutralize the chemical.
- Place a *nasogastric tube* (NGT) and *urinary catheter*. Follow outputs.
- *Pulse oximetry* and *cardiac monitoring* are useful, but remember their limitations in carbon monoxide poisoning.
- *Eyes:* examine the eyes for burn or abrasion, and treat with topical antibiotics if required.
- Give tetanus *immunoprophylaxis* if required.

Sepsis

Sepsis is bacterial infection of the bloodstream accompanied by signs of systemic toxicity. In this section we will consider the recognition and specific treatment for sepsis. Shock and respiratory failure are covered elsewhere in the chapter (see 📖 pp.48, 54).

Clinical assessment

Clinically, there may be fever in the older child, but be aware that fever or hypothermia can be the presenting feature in the infant. Perfusion is usually poor and there may be evidence of shock and coagulopathy (i.e. petechiae or purpura).

Investigations

All organ systems may be involved in sepsis so it is important to perform the following tests.

Blood
- FBC with differential.
- Coagulation state.
- Serum electrolytes with urea and creatinine.
- Liver function tests.
- Arterial or capillary blood gas.
- Inflammatory markers (e.g. CRP and erythrocyte sedimentation rate (ESR)).

Urine
Urinalysis.

Imaging
- CXR.
- Abdominal X-ray (AXR).

Sepsis screen
- *Blood culture:* bacteria (aerobic and anaerobic), virus, fungi. (Remember that blood cultures may not be positive, so repeat when there is fever).
- Urine culture.
- Stool swab.
- CSF.
- *Other cultures:* respiratory; wound; and all ports of any indwelling catheters.

Monitoring

Ensure the ABCs. Then, the form and type of monitoring will be dictated by the patient's condition. Start with:
- Continuous pulse oximetry.
- ECG monitoring.
- Intermittent BP monitoring.
- Hourly urine output.

Therapy

Antibiotics

- *When:* do not delay the first dose because of tests, but it is worthwhile trying to get a blood culture first.
- *Should I do a lumbar puncture?* This can wait until you have stabilized the child—you may even have to defer it if there is any coagulopathy.
- *What:* the choice of antibiotics you should use will depend on the patient, as well as your local microbial flora. In general, you can start with a third generation cephalosporin and use the following antibiotics for specific groups of patients.

Age <8 weeks

Consider group B streptococcus—ampicillin.

Indwelling catheter

Consider *Staphylococcus aureus*—anti-staphylococcal cover that is appropriate in your institution.

Intra-abdominal cause

Consider gut anaerobes—metronidazole, gentamicin.

Immunosuppressed or oncological

- *Pseudomonas:* ceftazidime, gentamicin.
- *Fungi:* amphotericin B.
- *Herpes, Varicella:* aciclovir.

Cellulitis or fasciitis

Consider group A streptococcus—penicillin.

Altered level of consciousness

See also 🛲 p.552.

The brain can be injured in many ways. Its responses to injury, however, are uniform and include any combination of:
- Altered level of consciousness (LOC).
- Seizures or dystonia.
- Impaired respiratory function.
- Loss of cardiovascular autoregulation.
- Cerebral swelling.
- SIADH.
- Weakness.

Take a note of:
- When symptoms started, and their progression (gradual versus sudden).
- Possible ingestion or exposure to medication or toxins.
- Possible recent trauma, illness, or exposure to infection.
- *History:* seizures; diabetes; allergies; chronic illness.
- Family history/consanguinity.
- Previous altered LOC.

Aetiology

Infectious causes
- Meningitis, encephalitis (🛲 pp.78–79, 720–721).
- Toxic shock (🛲 p.719).
- Subdural empyema, cerebral abscess.

Autoimmune

Acute disseminated encephalomyelitis (ADEM) 🛲 p.520.

Toxins See poisoning (🛲 pp.82–88).

Neoplastic causes Brain tumours (🛲 pp.662–665).

Trauma
- *Head injury:* concussion or contusion.
- *Haemorrhage:* epidural; subdural; brain.

Vascular causes
- AV malformation.
- Aneurysm, venous thrombosis.

Metabolic causes
- Hypoglycaemia (🛲 p.96).
- Diabetic ketoacidosis (🛲 pp.98–101).
- Electrolyte abnormalities.
- Inborn errors of metabolism (🛲 p.102).
- Hepatic encephalopathy.
- *Hormonal abnormalities:* thyroid; adrenal; pituitary (🛲 pp.424, 449).
- Uraemic encephalopathy.

Other
- Hypothermia.
- Hyperthermia.
- Seizures and post-ictal state (📖 pp.506–507).
- Hypertension (📖 p.396).
- Hydrocephalus (📖 p.535).
- Hypoxia–ischaemia.
- Sepsis (📖 p.714).
- Intussusception (📖 p.860).

Altered level of consciousness: clinical assessment

Initial examination
General examination can provide an explanation for the patient's state.

General
- *Vital signs:* make a note of the adequacy and rate and depth of respiration, the pulse rate and rhythm, BP, and body temperature.
- *Medic-Alert bracelet:* search for a bracelet or tag, or other information that may indicate a longstanding medical problem.
- *Skin:* examine for evidence of trauma, rash, petechiae, jaundice, and needle tracks.
- *Breath:* check for odours of alcohol, ketones, hydrocarbons, or toxins.

Head and neck
- *Head:* if the anterior fontanelle is patent, a tense fontanelle indicates raised ICP, whereas a sunken fontanelle suggests dehydration.
- *Nose and ears:* leakage of blood or CSF; 'raccoon eyes' or Battle sign suggests basal skull fracture.

Pupils
- *Small (2–3mm) reactive pupils:* suggest metabolic cause of coma.
- *Midsize (4–5mm) unreactive, midposition pupils:* suggest midbrain lesion.
- *Pinpoint (1–2mm) pupils:* indicate a pontine disorder, but are also commonly associated with opiates.
- *Unequal pupils with one fixed and dilated:* suggest a brain disorder on the side of the dilated pupil.
- *Bilateral fixed dilated pupils:* imply a poor prognosis, although similar pupils may be produced by mydriatics, barbiturate intoxication, and hypothermia.

Fundi
Examine for evidence of retinal haemorrhages and papilloedema.

After the ABCs, a focused neurological assessment is needed (see Box 5.4). Look for evidence of increased ICP and potential site of intracranial lesion.

Signs of raised ICP
The signs of raised ICP include:
- Abnormal respiratory pattern.
- Unequal or unreactive pupils.
- Impaired or absent oculocephalic or oculovestibular responses.
- Systemic hypertension, bradycardia.
- Tense fontanelle.
- Abnormal body posture or muscle flaccidity.

Box 5.4 Detailed neurological examination

Pattern of respiration
- *Cheyne–Stokes* (alternating apnoea and hyperpnoea) can be seen with metabolic disturbance, bilateral cerebral hemisphere dysfunction, and insipient temporal lobe herniation
- *Central neurogenic hyperventilation* (deep rapid respiration) can occur with hypoxia–ischaemia, hypoglycaemia, or lesion between low midbrain and midpons
- *Ataxic respiration* (irregular depth and rate) can be caused by abnormality of the medulla and impending respiratory arrest
- *Apneustic breathing* (gasping, respiratory arrest in inspiration) indicates pontine involvement

Eye movements
- *Roving eye movements* are seen in light coma without structural brain disease
- *Extra-ocular movements* with coma suggests a metabolic disorder or a supratentorial disorder
- *Absence of movements* suggests infratentorial disorder or drug intoxication
- *Abnormality of lateral gaze:* the eyes are deviated toward the side of a destructive cerebral lesion and away from an irritative cerebral lesion. In a brainstem lesion the eyes are directed away from the side of the lesion
- *Skew deviation* is seen with posterior fossa lesions
- *Ocular bobbing* is seen in pontine lesions

Lateral eye movement reflexes
Lateral eye movements are mediated by brainstem structures and require an intact midbrain and pons. These are assessed clinically by:
- *Oculocephalic reflex (doll's eye):* sudden turning of the head from one side to the other normally causes conjugate deviation of the eyes in the direction opposite to that in which the head is turned.
  - *Do not test when the neck is unstable*
- *Oculovestibular reflex (cold caloric):* cold water irrigated into the ear with the head held 30° above the horizontal normally causes conjugate deviation of the eyes toward the side of the irrigation

Motor function and posture
- *Decorticate rigidity:* the arms are held in flexion and adduction, the legs in extension. This signifies a lesion in the cerebral white matter, internal capsule, or thalamus
- *Decerebrate rigidity:* arms are extended and internally rotated. Legs are extended. Occurs with lesions from midbrain to midpons, and with bilateral anterior cerebral lesions. Can also be seen with metabolic abnormalities, hypoxia–ischaemia, or hypoglycaemia.

Altered level of consciousness: Glasgow coma scale

As a summary of conscious state, the GCS score should be used (Tables 5.2 and 5.3). It is also a useful tool for monitoring changes. The full score is calculated from the sum of E + V + M. A score ≤8 is used as a criterion for endotracheal intubation in the head-injured.

Table 5.2 Glasgow coma scale: scores for older children

Response	Score
Eye opening (E)	
Spontaneous	4
To verbal stimuli	3
To pain	2
None	1
Best verbal (V)	
Orientated	5
Confused speech	4
Inappropriate words	3
Non-specific sounds	2
None	1
Best motor (M)	
Follows commands	6
Localizes pain	5
Withdraws to pain	4
Flexes to pain	3
Extends to pain	2
None	1

Reproduced from Teasdale G, Jennett B. (1974) Assessment of coma and impaired consciousness. A practical scale. *Lancet* Jul 13; 2(7872): 81–4, with kind permission from Elsevier

Table 5.3 Glasgow coma scale: scores for infants

Response	Score
Eye opening (E)	
Spontaneous	4
To speech	3
To pain	2
None	1
Best verbal (V)	
Coos and babbles	5
Irritable cries	4
Cries to pain	3
Moans to pain	2
None	1
Best motor (M)	
Normal	6
Withdraws to touch	5
Withdraws to pain	4
Abnormal flexion	3
Abnormal extension	2
None	1

Reproduced from Teasdale G, Jennett B. (1974) Assessment of coma and impaired consciousness. A practical scale. *Lancet* Jul 13; 2(7872): 81–4, with kind permission from Elsevier

Altered level of consciousness: management

Investigations Consider the following if the cause of the coma is unknown.

Blood
- FBC, clotting, and bleeding time.
- Glucose, electrolytes, urea, liver function tests, ammonia, and lactate.
- Save two extra tubes of clotted blood for storage in the laboratory.

Toxicology
- Urine, blood, gastric aspirate for ingestions.
- Serum lead and free erythrocyte protoporphyrin.

Acid–base Arterial blood gas.

Microbiology Blood and urine cultures.

Imaging
- Cranial CT scan.
- MRI particularly for posterior fossa or white matter lesions. Cranial imaging should only be performed if the child is well enough to leave the emergency department, i.e. a full assessment has been undertaken, and the child is stable, or intubated if GCS<9

Electroencephalography Standard EEG.

Lumbar puncture

Defer LP until a CT scan has been obtained if there are signs of raised ICP or focal neurology, *and* until after intubation if GCS<9. Examine CSF for microscopy, culture, glucose, and protein (see also 📖 pp.720–721).

Meningitis
- 20–20,000 white blood cells (WBC)/mm^3 with a polymorphonuclear neutrophil leucocyte predominance.
- An elevated protein level >100mg/dL.
- Low glucose <2mmol/L (or <50% of plasma level).

Encephalitis
- 20–1000cells/mm^3 with lymphocyte predominance.
- The presence of red blood cells (RBC) up to 500 cells/mm^3 suggests herpes simplex virus (HSV) infection.
- CSF protein can be normal or mildly elevated.
- Glucose is usually normal (770% of plasma level).

Monitoring

The form and type of monitoring will be dictated by the underlying cause of the patient's state. Generally, after initial evaluation, monitor hourly:
- Vital signs, pupil reaction, fluid balance.
- The GCS for neurological review—in those with GCS 9–11 a gastric tube and urinary catheter may be needed.

Treatment
Follow a standard protocol
- *ABC:* the initial priority.
- *Glucose:* whenever the cause of coma is not clearly obvious, 25% glucose (250–500mg/kg) should be given IV after a blood sample has been taken for laboratory blood glucose testing.
- *Specific therapies* should be considered (see Box 5.5).

Box 5.5 Specific therapies See also 📖 p.720

Meningitis
- Immediately begin the appropriate antibiotics (see Antibiotics, p.79)
- Dexamethasone (IV 150micrograms/kg, qds for 4 days) if >3mths

Encephalitis
In the presence of a compatible clinical history, treat for HSV encephalitis with aciclovir (IV 10mg/kg, tds for 10–14 days)

Suspected raised ICP
- GCS ≤8: rapid sequence endotracheal intubation
- Ventilate to achieve normocapnia and normoxia
- Elevate the head of the bed to 30°
- Keep the head in the midline
- Mannitol (IV 0.25–1g/kg) and/or furosemide (IV 1mg/kg)

SIADH secretion
Limit the fluids to 67% maintenance

Antibiotics
Antimicrobial therapy is often given presumptively. The choice will depend on local epidemiology, public health, immunization, and antibiotic policy. In the comatose child, consider the following.
- *Age <4 weeks:* group B streptococcus, Gram –ve bacteria, and *Listeria monocytogenes: Recommend:* ampicillin + aminoglycoside.
- *Infants 1–3 months:* group B streptococcus, Gram-negative bacteria, *Streptococcus pneumoniae, Neisseria meningitides. Recommend:* ampicillin + aminoglycoside/3rd generation cephalosporin.
- *>3 months: Streptococcus pneumoniae, Neisseria meningitides. Recommend:* 3rd generation cephalosporin.

In the comatose older child where no CSF is available, a combination of antimicrobials to cover HSV, *Streptococcus pneumoniae,* and *Mycoplasma pneumoniae* infection is often prescribed.
- Cefotaxime (IV 50mg/kg qds; maximum 12g/day).
- Erythromycin (IV 10mg/kg qds).
- Aciclovir (IV 10mg/kg, tds).

Status epilepticus

Status epilepticus (StE) is a prolonged seizure lasting over 30min or recurrent seizures during which the patient does not fully regain consciousness within a 30min period. However, in practical terms, once a child has been fitting for more than 5min, the chances of the seizure lasting more than 30min are dramatically increased, and therefore the common practice is to start therapy at this point. The success of treatment depends on prompt recognition and treatment (see Box 5.6, also 📖 p.505).

Symptoms
StE is classified as convulsive (C) or non-convulsive (NC). NCStE is diagnosed with electroencephalogram (EEG), and should be considered in the comatosed.

Aetiology
The common causes of childhood StE include:
- A regular occurrence in a child with a known/difficult epilepsy.
- Fever.
- Subtherapeutic anticonvulsant levels.
- Central nervous system (CNS) infections.
- Trauma.
- Poisoning.
- Metabolic abnormalities.

Note: in teenagers diagnosed with convulsive StE in the emergency department, who do not have a pre-existing disability, up to 50% will be having voluntary movements of psychological origin ('pseudoseizures'). So consider whether it is definitely a genuine epileptic seizure.

Investigations
After emergency life-supporting therapies, useful diagnostic tests include:
- Brain imaging: computerized tomography (CT), magnetic resonance imaging (MRI).
- EEG.
- Lumbar puncture* caution, see 📖 pp.720–721;
- *Blood:* magnesium, electrolytes, calcium, glucose, and creatinine levels.
- Arterial blood gas.
- *Toxicology:* blood and urine.
- Anticonvulsant levels in those on anticonvulsants.
- FBC and WBC differential.

Initial treatment
Box 5.6 summarizes the treatments according to time after seizure begins. At any stage, if there is respiratory depression, intubate the trachea and support breathing.

Box 5.6 Anticonvulsants in status epilepticus

0–5min: ABC
- Note time
- Call for help
- Consider whether it is a genuine epileptic seizure
- Check glucose
- Establish IV access
- Monitor vital signs, especially pulse oximetry saturation
- Give 100% oxygen via mask

5–15min: start anticonvulsants
- Use IV lorazepam (50–100micrograms/kg, up to 4mg) *or*
- Rectal diazepam (0.5mg/kg, up to 10mg)

15–20min: anticonvulsants

If there is no response, repeat the dose of lorazepam or diazepam (if no IV access).

Note if the child has been given a benzodiazepine already, e.g. paramedics, give only *one* dose.

15–35min: if seizure persists
- Load with IV phenytoin (18mg/kg, at rate <1mg/kg/min) *or*
- IV phenobarbital (18mg/kg, at rate <1mg/kg/min)

45min: refractory seizure
- If seizures persist intensive care should be initiated
- Intubate the trachea and support breathing
- Intensive care medications include midazolam and thiopentone
- EEG monitoring

Once the seizure has stopped

Whilst the child is convulsing there is a reasonable amount of oxygen perfusing the brain. Hence, the advice to parents that home oxygen is not indicated for the treatment of StE. However, once the convulsion ends, the child may have a respiratory arrest. So this is the critical period for vigilance of ABC. Roll into the recovery position, keep the oxygen running, watch the SpO_2, and other observations carefully. *Do not* transfer the child or perform potentially dangerous procedures, such as LP until the child has a GCS that is both improving and >9.

Poisoning

The peak incidence of childhood accidental poisoning is between the ages of 2 and 3yrs. Most cases occur at home. In older children, accidental self-poisoning should be suspected as a possible suicide gesture.

Aetiology

Parents usually know the name and often have a good idea of the amount of material ingested. Obtain the bottle or container of the ingestant. Get these details in the history.

- *Exact name of the drug* or chemical exposure.
- *Preparation and concentration* of the drug exposure.
- *Probable dose* (by history) of drug ingested in mg/kg, as well as maximum possible dose.
- *Time since ingestion or exposure.*
- *Check the National Toxicology database.*

Symptoms and signs

There are various signs and symptoms produced by poisoning. It is helpful to consider the derangement in body systems and think of potential causes (see Box 5.7). In addition, there are specific odours that may lead to diagnosis.

Odours
- Acetone.
- Alcohol.
- Bitter almonds (cyanide).
- Garlic (heavy metals).
- Oil of wintergreen (methyl salicylates).
- Pears (chloral hydrate).
- Carrots (water hemlock).

Diagnosis

The likely type of poisoning may be indicated by its clinical effect (see Box 5.7). Bedside or laboratory tests should also be performed.

- Urinary dip-tests and toxicology.
- Arterial blood gas.
- Blood glucose.
- Co-oximetry (carboxyhaemoglobin level).
- Serum urea and electrolyte.
- Osmolar gap: [osmolality – $(2 \times Na)$ + urea + glucose].
- Drug levels.
- *ECG:* 12-lead for assessment of rhythm and QT interval.
- *X-rays:* abdomen to detect radio-opaque tablets (e.g. iron).

Box 5.7 Clinical effect and causative drugs or poisons

- *Depressed respiration:* antipsychotics, carbamate pesticides, clonidine, cyclic antidepressants, alcohol, narcotics, nicotine
- *Tachycardia and hypertension:* amphetamines, antihistamines, cocaine
- *Tachycardia and hypotension:* salbutamol, carbon monoxide, tricyclic antidepressants, hydralazine, iron, phenothiazine, theophylline
- *Bradycardia and hypertension:* clonidine ergotamine, ephedrine
- *Bradycardia and hypotension:* calcium-channel blockers, clonidine, digoxin, narcotics, organophosphates, phentolamine, propranolol, sedatives
- *Atrioventricular block:* astemizole, β-adrenergic antagonists, calcium-channel blockers, clonidine, cyclic antidepressants, digoxin
- *Ventricular tachycardia:* amphetamines, anti-arrhythmics (encainamide, flecanide, quinidine, procainamide), carbamazepine, chloral hydrate, chlorinated hydrocarbons, cocaine, tricyclic antidepressants, digoxin, phenothiazine, theophylline
- *Torsade de pointes:* amantadine, antihistamines (astemizole), cyclic antidepressants, lithium, phenothiazine, quinidine, sotalol
- *Coma with miosis:* alcohol, barbiturates, bromide, chloral hydrate, clonidine, ketamine, narcotics, organophosphates, phenothiazines
- *Coma with mydriasis:* atropine, carbon monoxide, cyanide, cyclic antidepressants, glutethimide
- *Hypoglycaemia:* alcohols, insulin, oral hypoglycaemic agents, propranolol, salicylates
- *Seizures:* amphetamines, anticonvulsants (carbamazepine, phenytoin), anticholinergic, antihistamines, camphor, carbon monoxide, chlorinated hydrocarbons, cocaine, cyanide, tricyclic antidepressants, isoniazid, ketamine, lead, lidocaine, meperidine, phenothiazine, phenylpropanolamine, propranolol, theophylline
- *High anion gap ($Na - [Cl + HCO_3]$)) metabolic acidosis:* alcohol, carbon monoxide, cyanide, ethylene glycol, iron, isoniazid, methanol, salicylate, theophylline
- *Low anion gap:* bromide, lithium, hypermagnesaemia, hypercalcaemia

Poisoning: management

Initial treatment

Follow a standard protocol for ABCD and seek advice from your regional or national poisons centre.

Gastrointestinal decontamination

Avoid if airway is unprotected. Otherwise consider the following.

Activated charcoal

- *Oral or nasogastric:* 1g/kg is used for substances that can be adsorbed.
- Do not use when there is *risk of aspiration* (e.g. bowel obstruction, ileus, absent gag reflex).
- Do not use after ingestion of alcohol, iron, boric acid, caustics, lithium, or electrolyte solutions.

Gastric lavage

- May be useful if the patient arrives within 1hr of ingestion (longer if salicylates or iron).
- Do not use if there has been caustic or hydrocarbon ingestion.
- Do not use if co-ingestion of sharp objects.
- The lavage is performed via a large bore gastric tube with normal saline (15mL/kg/cycle, maximum 200mL/cycle) until the gastric contents are clear.

Ipecacuanha

- Useful within 30min of ingestion.
- Use 10mL for infants ≥6mths.
- Use 15mL for children 1–2yrs.
- Use 30mL for child ≥12yrs.
- Do not use when there has been caustic ingestion.
- Do not use if the child has altered LOC or is at risk of seizures.
- After taking ipecacuanha the child should be placed in the prone or lateral position.

Bowel irrigation

- Nasogastric polyethylene glycol solution (GoLYTELY® 25–40mL/kg/h for 4–6hr or until clear effluent) is useful after toxic iron, lithium, or lead ingestion.
- GoLYTELY® may be useful some hours after ingestion of enteric-coated tablets (salicylates, calcium channel blockers, β-blockers).
- Do not use in cases of coma when the airway is not protected.
- Do not use in cases of GI haemorrhage, obstruction, and ileus.

Enhanced elimination
- Urinary alkalinization (pH 7–8) aids elimination of weak acids (salicylates, barbiturates).
- Use IV $NaHCO_3$ (1–2mmol/kg) followed by increased maintenance fluids (1.5–2 times) with added $NaHCO_3$.
- Beware of further electrolyte disturbance.
- Haemodialysis is useful for low molecular weight substances that have low volume of distribution and low binding to plasma proteins (aspirin, theophylline, lithium, phenobarbitone, and alcohols).

Poisoning: antidotes and substrates

Antidotes and substrates are useful in only a minority of poisonings. Poison centres will provide exact advice.

Antidotes and substrates

Paracetamol (acetaminophen)

- Children taking >150mg/kg need assessment
- Take blood 4hr after ingestion and use nomogram. Give N-acetylcysteine if criteria are met. Check liver function tests (LFTs) and International normalized ratio (INR)
- *N-acetylcysteine:* PO or NG loading 140mg/kg, then 70mg/kg/dose qds for 17 doses. IV used if GI bleeding. Repeat blood level at 24hr

Anticholinergics, antihistamines (diphenhydramine), plants (deadly nightshade, jimson weed, henbane), anti-Parkinsonian drugs, dilating eye drops, skeletal muscle relaxants

- *Benzodiazepines:* used for agitation and seizures (avoid phenytoin)
- *Physostigmine:* useful for anticholinergic syndrome. It reverses central effects of agitation and seizures. **Not** for tricyclic antidepressant overdose, asthmatics, GI obstruction, genitourinary (GU) obstruction. Give slow IV 20micrograms/kg/dose (up to 500micrograms) over 5min. Repeat every 5min, but maximum cumulative dose should be below 2mg. Have atropine available for cholinergic symptoms (0.5mg for every mg of physostigmine). Response is rapid

Benzodiazepines: chlodiazepoxide, clonazepam, diazepam, temazepam

- If ABCs are stable there is little need to do more than observe
- *Flumazenil.* Reverses lethargy and coma. **Not** for tricyclic antidepressant or chloral hydrate overdose, or child with seizure disorder on benzodiazepines. Give 10micrograms/kg over 1min (maximum 500micrograms/dose, or 1mg overall). Response is rapid, but resedation may occur. May induce seizures

β-adrenergic antagonists: atenolol, esmolol, labetalol, propranolol

- *Glucagon* is useful for reversing bradycardia and hypotension. Give 0.05–0.1mg/kg bolus, followed by 0.1mg/kg/h infusion
- *Atropine, isoprenaline, and amiodarone* can be used if bradycardia or hypotension persist after glucagon
- Cardiac pacing may be needed. If cardiac arrest occurs, massive doses of adrenaline (*epinephrine*) may be required

Calcium channel blockers: diltiazem, nifedipine, nimodipine, verapamil

- Use *glucagon, amrinone, isoprenaline, atropine, and dopamine* for hypotension unresponsive to fluids and calcium

- Give *calcium chloride* (20mg/kg of 10% solution) or *calcium gluconate* (100mg/kg of 10% solution) for hypotension and bradyarrhythmias
- Consider *cardiac pacing*

Carbon monoxide (CO) fire; exhaust from fuel engines, furnaces, or burners; paint remover with methylene chloride
- Ensure ABCs and give 100% oxygen
- Check COHb level
- Consider hyperbaric oxygen if COHb >40%, or if symptoms persist after 4h despite 100% oxygen
- Also consider cyanide toxicity if smoke inhalation

Cyanide
- There are special kits for rescue that will be in Pharmacy
- *Sodium nitrate 3%:* dose depends on Hb level, but do not give if CO poisoning as well
- *Sodium thiosulphate 25%:* dose depends on Hb level

Digoxin
- Measure serum drug level. Toxicity occurs with level >2ng/mL
- Check electrolytes, magnesium, thyroxine, and calcium
- Correct hypokalaemia (IV 0.5–1mmol/kg/dose as infusion 0.5mmol/kg/h over 2hr)
- If hyperkalaemic (>5mmol/L) give insulin, dextrose, sodium bicarbonate, and Kayexalate®. Do *not* give calcium chloride or calcium gluconate because these potentiate ventricular arrhythmias
- *Digoxin-specific antibody* (FAB fragments). Give for ventricular dysrhythmias, or supraventricular bradyarrhythmias (if resistant to IV atropine 10–20micrograms/kg), hyperkalaemia, hypotension, heart block, and ingestion >4mg. Phenytoin may be used to improve AV conduction. Avoid quinidine, procainamide, isoprenaline, or disopyramide if AV block present

Ethylene glycol, methanol
- *Fomepizole* (loading 15mg/kg, then 10mg/kg bd for 4 doses, then 15mg/kg bd until levels ≤20mg/dL): antidote for methanol and ethylene glycol. Indications: level ≥20mg/dL, or high anion gap metabolic acidosis
- If not available, use *ethanol* (loading dose 0.6g/kg; load over 1hr followed by infusion 100mg/kg/hr)
- Other agent: *pyridoxine* 2mg/kg and *thiamine* 500micrograms/kg. In the case of methanol, also give *folate* (50–100mg over 6hr)

Iron
- Measure serum concentration 2–6hr after ingestion. A level >350micrograms/dL is frequently associated with systemic toxicity. If ingestion <20mg/kg no treatment needed
- *Desferrioxamine*: IV infusion 5–15mg/kg/hr in all cases of serious poisoning (i.e. based on symptoms, AXR, serum level >500micrograms/dL). Continue until symptoms have resolved

Isoniazid

For stopping seizure use *pyridoxine* (vitamin B_6) 3–5g

Lead
- Immediate intervention for blood level ≥70micrograms/dL
- *Oral chelation with dimercaptosuccinic acid (DMSA)*: first 5 days 30mg/kg/day divided every 8hr; next 14 days 20mg/kg/day divided every 12hr
- *Parenteral chelation with British antilewisite (BAL)*: initial dose 75mg/m^2 deep IM; then 4hr later start $CaNa_2EDTA$ (1500mg/m^2/day via continuous IV infusion for 48hr). If there is risk of cerebral oedema, then give IM. BAL is continued simultaneously at 75mg/m^2/dose IM 4-hourly for 48hr
- BAL is suspended in peanut oil, and may cause haemolysis in patients with G6PD deficiency

Methaemoglobinaemia: sulphonamides, quinines, phenacetin, nitrates, aniline dyes, naphthalene
- Measure level and if >30% start treatment
- *Methylene blue 1%*: 1–2mg/kg (0.1–0.2mL/kg) IV over 5min. May repeat dose (maximum total 7mg/kg) if symptoms present after 1hr
- Beware of methylene blue in G6PD deficiency
- Consider hyperbaric oxygen or exchange transfusion if no response

Narcotics: codeine, dextromethorphan, propoxyphene, pentazocine, butorphanol, methadone
- *Naloxone* useful for reversing coma caused by opiates. Give IV, IM, or via ETT 2mg (10micrograms/kg, if < 12yrs inc to 100micrograms/kg). Response is rapid and repeat doses or infusion can be used.

Organophosphates: pesticides
- *Atropine*: initial dose 20micrograms/kg (max 2mg) IV; then additional doses if bronchorrhoea
- *Pralidoxime*: 25–50mg/kg/dose (up to 1g) IV; consider 10–15mg/kg/hr infusion for severe cases

Phenothiazine
- For extrapyramidal syndrome, *diphenhydramine*: 1mg/kg/dose slow IV over 5min.
- Also if life-threatening, IV *benzatropine* 20–50micrograms/kg/dose (1–2 doses per day in children >3yrs)

Fluid and electrolytes

Normal fluid requirements

All children with serious acute illness in hospital are given fluid and electrolyte solutions. It is important to match what you prescribe to what
the child actually needs. There are a number of ways of calculating daily
requirements, but the method we most commonly use is based on patient
weight (see Box 5.8).

Box 5.8 Calculating fluid and electrolyte requirements

24-hr fluid requirements
- *100mL/kg*: for the first 10kg of weight
- *+50mL/kg*: for the second 10kg of weight
- *+20mL/kg*: for the remaining weight above 20kg

24-hr electrolyte requirements
- *Sodium*: 2–4mmol/kg
- *Potassium*: 1–2mmol/kg

Normal fluid therapy is based on the above calculations. In the fasting patient, the type of fluid given should contain dextrose (usually 5%), sodium
chloride, and added potassium chloride. Outside the neonatal period we
use 0.9% or 0.45% saline with dextrose and additives. Do not use plain 5%
dextrose in water or 5% dextrose 0.18% saline. The volume of fluid administered should be increased in dehydration (see 📖 p.91), and restricted to
50–75% of the usual maintenance volume in cases of:
- SIADH (📖 pp.92, 448).
- Fluid overload (📖 p.53).
- Congestive heart failure (📖 p.226).
- Renal failure with oliguria or anuria (📖 pp.362–365).

Fluid and electrolytes: dehydration

Dehydration can lead to shock, severe metabolic acidosis, and death, particularly in infants. Its severity can be assessed using change in weight or the following physical signs.

Mild dehydration (0–5%)

- *Weight loss:* 5% in infants and 3% in children.
- *Skin turgor:* may be decreased.
- *Mucous membranes:* dry.
- *Urine:* may be low.
- *Heart rate:* increased.
- *Blood pressure:* normal.
- *Perfusion:* normal.
- *Skin colour:* pale.
- *Consciousness:* irritable.

Moderate dehydration (5–10%)

- *Weight loss:* 10% in infants and 6% in children.
- *Skin turgor:* decreased.
- *Mucous membranes:* very dry.
- *Urine:* oliguric.
- *Heart rate:* increased.
- *BP:* may be normal.
- *Perfusion:* prolonged capillary refill (capillary refill time (CRT) > 2s).
- *Skin colour:* grey.
- *Consciousness:* lethargic.

Severe dehydration (10–15%)

- *Weight loss:* 15% in infants and 9% in children.
- *Skin turgor:* poor with tenting.
- *Mucous membranes:* parched.
- *Urine:* anuric.
- *Heart rate:* increased.
- *Blood pressure:* decreased.
- *Perfusion:* prolonged CRT.
- *Skin colour:* mottled; blue or white.
- *Consciousness:* comatose.

After you have assessed the degree of dehydration in your patient, two problems need to be addressed—water and electrolyte losses. In practice, our treatment is aimed at correcting both the water and electrolyte losses (Table 5.4).

Table 5.4 Water and electrolyte losses in 10% dehydration

Losses in 10% dehydration			
H2O (mL/kg)	Na (mmol/kg)	K (mmol/kg)	Cl (mmol/kg)
Isotonic dehydration (Na, 130–150mmol/L)			
100–120	8–10	8–10	8–10
Hyponatraemic dehydration (Na < 130mmol/L)			
100–120	10–12	8–1	10–12
Hypernatraemic dehydration (Na > 150mmol/L)			
100–120	2–4	0–4	2–6

Isotonic and hyponatraemic dehydration
- First assess the degree of dehydration (use weight change and signs).
- Calculate the fluid deficit.
- FBC with differential.
- Serum electrolytes (Na, K, Ca) with urea, creatinine, and glucose.

Emergency treatment is directed toward restoring any compromise in the circulation. (See shock, 📖 p.56: use 20mL/kg IV normal saline). Monitoring should include: vital signs, losses (urine output, stool, vomitus, NG), daily weights, and blood tests. After the initial phase, fluid administration should be calculated to correct deficits over 48hr. Overall, take into account the deficit, maintenance requirements, and any ongoing losses:

Hourly rate = (24hr maintenance + deficit − resuscitation fluids)/24

Hypernatraemic dehydration
- Water losses exceed sodium loss.
- Cerebral oedema is a risk during rehydration, so correction of the deficit should be achieved slowly and evenly, over 48hr.
- Emergency treatment of shock is treated with 10–20mL/kg IV saline. Thereafter, calculate the deficit and restore patient's needs.
- Monitor as above, with at least 8-hourly electrolyte studies.
- Use 0.9% saline so that sodium correction occurs slowly.

Seizures and cerebral oedema may complicate the rehydration phase of hypernatraemic dehydration. If these occur, treat symptomatically and refer to an intensive care unit. There may be a number of causes of these problems—your initial role in this emergency is to do the ABCs. Further investigations and CT scan may be needed.

Fluid and electrolytes: abnormalities

Hyponatraemia (<130mmol/L)
Assess the problem. Is the patient hypovolaemic or overloaded?

Sodium depletion
- *Associations:* hypovolaemia and low urine Na (<10mmol/L).
- *Causes:* inadequate Na intake, excessive Na losses.
- *Treatment:* restore circulation, replace water and salt deficits.
- *Symptomatic therapy (<120mmol/L):* if there are seizures, the serum Na level should be acutely raised by 5–10mmol/L in about 1hr. Use 3mmol NaCl/kg IV over 30–60min.

Dilution
- *Associations:* normovolaemia (occasionally overload), paradoxically high urine Na (usually >300mmol/L), and sometimes cerebral oedema.
- *Causes:* impaired water excretion; excess water given.
- *Treatment:* correct the volume overloaded circulation with diuretics (furosemide 0.5–1.0mg/kg IV). Provide oxygen and inotropes if required. Restrict fluids to less than maintenance.
- *SIADH:* There are many causes of SIADH. The features are low urine volume and high urine osmolality in the absence of hypovolaemia, renal disease, and adrenal disease. Urine Na is paradoxically high (20–30mmol/L) in the presence of hyponatraemia 'secondary to volume overload (see 📖 p.448).

Hypernatraemia (>150mmol/L)
Besides hypernatraemic dehydration and salt poisoning, you will see hypernatraemia in diabetes insipidus (DI), where there is excess renal water loss. The urine is 5–10 times usual volume, with low osmolality (50–100mOsm/L), in the absence of glycosuria. So, assess the underlying problem, and restore compromised circulation (see 📖 p.91).

Anti-diuretic hormone (ADH) deficiency
- *Causes:* severe asphyxia, and CNS trauma, surgery, or infection.
- *Treatment:* use two IV solutions—one at 30–40% maintenance for replacement of insensible losses; the other for replacing urine losses. Check urine Na/K and prepare IV replacement solution to match.
- *Hormone replacement:* DI is sometimes transient and so initial fluid therapy is reasonable. However, if this problem is established, hormonal replacement is needed: nasal deamino-8-d-arginine vasopressin (DDAVP) 1–40micrograms/day in 1 or 2 doses; parenteral (IV) DDAVP 2–4micrograms/day in 2 doses. You should see a response within 1hr.

Hypokalaemia (<3mmol/L)

- *ECG changes:* flattened, prolonged, or inverted T waves; prominent U waves; ST segment depression; atrioventricular block.
- *Dysrhythmias, hypotension.*
- *Neuromuscular:* weakness; hypotonia; hyporeflexia; paraesthesiae.
- *GI:* ileus; constipation.

Correction

- *Urgent:* ECG changes, children on digoxin, or serum <2.5mmol/L.
- *Treatment.* use 0.5mmol KCl/kg IV over 1hr via a central line. The bolus should not exceed 20mmol, and should not be more concentrated than 40mmol/L KCl/L. Monitor with continuous ECG and repeat serum K level after 1–2hr.

Hyperkalaemia (>5.5mmol/L)

- *ECG changes:* peaked T waves; widened QRS; depressed ST segments progressing to increasingly aberrant ECG complexes;
- *Dysrhythmias:* bradycardia; VT; VF; cardiac arrest.

Approach

Treatment guided by the level, but first repeat a venous sample in case of haemolysis. Stop all potassium and monitor the ECG, while you wait for the result.

Symptomatic treatment (>8.0mmol/L or ECG changes)

- *Protect the myocardium:* calcium gluconate 10% (100mg/kg/dose IV at maximum rate 100mg/min; 1.5–3.3mL/min, 50mg/mL) and monitor for bradycardia and hypotension.
- *Increase intracellular K uptake:* $NaHCO_3$ (1–2mmol/kg IV over 5–10min); insulin with glucose (0.1unit/kg IV *with* dextrose 25% 0.5g/kg IV over 30min).
- *Induce kaluresis:* salbutamol nebulizer.
- *Decrease total load of K:* Kayexalate® (1g/kg/dose PR 2-hourly with 5mL 20% sorbitol).

Hypocalcaemia (<1.1mmol/L)

See also 📖 p.442. Low ionized values of Ca can result in:
- *ECG changes:* prolonged QT, AV block;
- *Shock.*
- *CNS effects:* seizures, tetany, and weakness.

Symptomatic therapy

- Calcium gluconate 10% for seizures, tetany, hypotension, arrhythmias.
- Monitor HR and BP during treatment.

Refractory hypocalcaemia

- *Check magnesium level and serum albumin:* if low, correct (25–50mg/kg. IV magnesium sulphate over 30min, 6-hourly for 3 doses).
- If these are normal, with *raised phosphate*, decrease phosphate intake and use phosphate binders. Check renal function.

Renal insufficiency

Acute renal failure is the sudden reduction or cessation of renal function to the point where body fluid homeostasis is compromised, leading to accumulation of nitrogenous waste products, with or without reduced urine output. Children in this state need immediate attention and transfer to a specialized renal unit. More commonly, we see patients with a degree of renal insufficiency that is complicating an acute medical illness—it may be present at the time of presentation or it may evolve during hospital admission. The causes of renal insufficiency are discussed on 🕮 p.362.

Clinical assessment

Take a thorough history and do a full examination. Assess whether there is hypertension or hypotension. Check the urine output (oliguria <0.5mL/kg/hr) and if anuric suspect obstruction. The particular points you should consider are the following:

- Whether there has been any preceding throat infection (streptococcus), gastroenteritis (haemolytic-uraemic syndrome (HUS)), or exposure to drugs or toxins.
- Is there any evidence of general illness with pallor, anorexia, oedema, weakness, and fatigue?
- Is there a rash, and is it petechial or purpuric?
- Is there hypertension or signs of heart failure?
- Is there tachynoea, cough, or haemoptysis?
- Is there any nausea, vomiting, bleeding, flank mass, or ascites?
- Is there any evidence of altered consciousness?

Investigations

The following tests are required in acute care:

- *Blood:* FBC with differential.
- *Serum biochemistry:* electrolytes with urea and creatinine, and arterial or capillary blood gas.
- *Urine:* check for any protein, blood, or active sediment (red cell casts, tubular cells, white cell casts, or other evidence of urinary tract infection (UTI)).
- *Imaging:* organize a CXR, AXR, and abdominal and renal ultrasound (US) examination with Doppler studies of renal vessel blood flow.
- *Other tests:* consider taking blood samples for complement levels (C3, C4), serum titres (e.g. anti-streptolysib O (ASO) titres).

Monitoring

The form and type of monitoring will be dictated by the patient's condition. Start with:

- Continuous pulse oximetry.
- ECG monitoring.
- Intermittent BP monitoring.
- Insert a urinary catheter and follow hourly output.

Acute therapy

In the acute setting first assess the ABCs. Then, to assess intravascular volume, come to a decision about whether the patient is hypovolaemic or hypervolaemic.

Hypovolaemia

- Administer 20mL/kg 0.9% normal saline as an IV bolus, and repeat if necessary.
- If the cause of anuria is fluid depletion, fluid resuscitation should restore urine flow within 6hr.
- Give blood if necessary and continue to monitor.
- Acute tubular necrosis is likely if there is no response to the above. Repeat the fluid bolus with furosemide (1–5mg/kg IV), but do not use if obstructive uropathy is suspected—refer to a urologist.
- If the patient produces urine, expect large amounts (which will need to be replaced) as polyuric renal failure may be present.

Hypervolaemia

- Consider a single dose of furosemide (1–5mg/kg IV).
- If the urine output is minimal then treat as acute renal failure.

Acute renal failure and kidney injury

A child in acute renal failure will need to be transferred to a renal unit. Hypertension, hyperkalaemia, hyponatraemia, and seizures will need to be treated. You should continue to monitor volume state, BP, ECG, and electrolytes. Standard treatment includes the following.

BP

- Hypertension is present if BP >95th centile (see 📖 pp.391–392).
- Restrict salt intake.
- Consider antihypertensive drugs.

Fluids

- Continue to correct and replace volume loss with normal saline.
- Thereafter, restrict fluids to urine replacement and insensible losses (300–400mL/m^2/day).

Electrolytes

- Correct hyponatraemia if causing seizures.
- Correct hypocalcaemia if symptomatic—do this before correcting any acidosis.
- Discontinue any potassium administration. (Remember that for every 0.1 fall in pH, potassium will rise by 0.4mmol/L, so you may need to treat acidosis if pH <7.2 and bicarbonate <10mmol/L.)

Diet

Limit protein to 0.5–1.0g/kg/day.

Glucose: hypoglycaemia

In infants and children this emergency is defined as a blood value <2.2–2.6mmol/L (see also 📖 pp.132, 412, 967).

Aetiology

Hypoglycaemia is a sign of an underlying disease process that interferes with carbohydrate intake or absorption, gluconeogenesis, or glycogenolysis. These conditions are discussed in detail in Chapter 26 (see 📖 p.967). Outside the neonatal period, in the acute setting, the causes of hypoglycaemia can be grouped as follows.

Endocrine
- Hyperinsulinism.
- Hypopituitarism.
- Growth hormone deficiency.
- Hypothyroidism.
- Congenital adrenal hyperplasia.

Metabolic
- Glycogen storage disease.
- Galactosaemia.
- Organic acidaemia.
- Ketotic hypoglycaemia.
- Carnitine deficiency.
- Acyl CoA dehydrogenase deficiency.

Toxic
- Salicylates.
- Alcohol.
- Insulin.
- Valproate.

Hepatic
- Hepatitis.
- Cirrhosis.
- Reye syndrome.

Systemic
- Starvation.
- Malnutrition.
- Sepsis.
- Malabsorption.

Clinical assessment

Take a thorough history and identify the timing of hypoglycaemia in relation to feeding and medication. On examination assess for:
- Short stature (📖 p.466).
- Failure to thrive (📖 p.308).
- Hepatomegaly (📖 p.960).
- Features of any generalized metabolic disorder (📖 p.954).

Investigation

If possible, during an acute episode you should try to:
- Save blood and urine for metabolic and endocrine testing.
- Check blood glucose in the laboratory.
- Blood electrolytes, urea, liver function, and osmolality.
- Blood gas.
- Toxicology screen.

Monitoring

Ensure ABCs. Then start with continuous pulse oximetry and ECG monitoring, and intermittent BP monitoring.

Treatment

Asymptomatic child

Oral glucose drink or gel.

Symptomatic child

- *Glucose:* 10% 5–10mL/kg IV, or 25% 2–4mL/kg IV.
- *Followed by:* continuous infusion of salt solution with 5–10% glucose (6–8mg/kg/min), e.g. 0.45% saline and 5% glucose.
- If *hypoglycaemia persists* increase the glucose to 10–12mg/kg/min.
- If there is *no response* consider glucagon, hydrocortisone, or diazoxide. These patients will need advice from a specialist.

Diabetic ketoacidosis

See also 📖 p.413.
Diabetic ketoacidosis (DKA) is a diabetic emergency and such patients can die from hypovolaemic shock, cerebral oedema, hypokalaemia, or aspiration pneumonia. DKA is defined as:
- Hyperglycaemia (>11mmol/L).
- pH < 7.3.
- Bicarbonate <15mmol/L.
- Urinary ketones.

Patients who meet the above criteria, who are more than 5% dehydrated, or who have altered level of consciousness require careful supervision and treatment. Some patients may need referral to an intensive care unit (e.g. pH < 7.1, severe dehydration with shock, <2yrs of age).

Clinical assessment
- Degree of dehydration (📖 p.90).
- Level of consciousness (📖 pp.74–77).
- Full examination for evidence of cerebral oedema, infection, and ileus.
- Weight.

Investigations
The key tests are as follows.

Blood
- FBC with differential.
- Serum electrolytes with urea and creatinine.
- Glucose.
- LFTs (transaminases).
- Arterial or capillary blood gas.
- Lactate level.
- Ketone level.

Urine
- Urinalysis.
- Ketones.
- Reducing substances.
- Organic and amino acids.
- Drug screen.

Monitoring
- *Ensure the ABCs:* after that the form and type of monitoring will be dictated by the patient's condition.
- *CNS:* follow the neurological state. If there is headache or altered consciousness, treat as though raised ICP has developed.
- *Continuous pulse oximetry and ECG monitoring:* T-wave changes should alert you to hypokalaemia or hyperkalaemia.
- *Intermittent BP monitoring.*
- *Hourly urine output:* test for ketones.

Diabetic ketoacidosis: treatment

Fluid therapy

We have already discussed the management of dehydration (📖 pp.90–93). Our therapy is similar in DKA, with the following caveats.

Resuscitation fluid

- Use 0.9% saline for resuscitation of the circulation.
- This alone will bring down the glucose level.
- Remember to include the initial resuscitation volume in your calculation of total fluid replacement to be given in the 48hr.

Calculation of deficit

- Never use more than 10% dehydration in the calculations.
- Restore deficit over 48hr.

Type of fluid

- Use normal saline initially.
- When glucose has fallen to 14mmol/L add glucose to the fluid. If this fall occurs within 6hr, the child may still be sodium depleted. In this instance add glucose to 0.9% saline. Usually the fall in glucose occurs after 6hr and it is safe to change the fluid type to 0.45% saline with 5% glucose.
- Potassium should be started with the rehydration fluids after the first 500mL provided the patient is passing urine. Add 40mmol KCl/L (i.e. 20mmol KCl to each 500mL bag).

Bicarbonate and phosphate

- There is no evidence for using bicarbonate/phosphate in DKA.[1]
- However, under extreme conditions and in critical illness these are sometimes considered.

Electrolytes

Check these 2-hourly after resuscitation, and then 4-hourly.

Oral fluids

- Initially nil by mouth ± NGT.
- Juices and rehydration solutions should only be given after substantial clinical improvement.
- These fluids should be added to the overall calculation of fluid intake.

Insulin therapy

Once the rehydration fluids and potassium have been started insulin should be used to switch off ketogenesis and reverse DKA. There is no need for an initial bolus dose; continuous low-dose IV insulin is the preferred method of administration.

Insulin treatment in diabetic ketoacidosis

Insulin infusion
- Make up a solution of 1U/mL of human soluble insulin (50U in 50mL of 0.9% saline)
- Attach this to a second IV line or 'piggy-back' to one line with the replacement fluids
- Give 0.1U/kg/h (i.e. 0.1mL/kg/hr)

Glucose fall
- If the rate of blood glucose fall exceeds 5mmol/L/hr, or falls to around 14–17mmol/L, then add glucose (equivalent to 5–10%) to the IV fluids
- Insulin dose needs to be maintained at 0.1U/kg/hr in order to switch off ketogenesis—*do not stop it*. If the blood glucose falls below 4mmol/L, give a bolus of 2mL/kg of 10% glucose and increase the glucose concentration of the infusion

Recovery
- Once the pH is >7.3, the blood glucose <14mmol/L, and a glucose-containing fluid has been started, consider reducing the insulin infusion rate, but to no less than 0.05U/kg/hr
- Once the child is drinking well and able to tolerate food, IV fluids and insulin can be discontinued
- Start SC insulin in the newly-diagnosed diabetic, according to local protocol. Resume usual insulin regimen in known diabetics
- Discontinue the insulin infusion 60min after the first SC injection

Treatment failure
If blood glucose is uncontrolled, or the pH worsens after 4–6hr, check IV lines, dose of insulin, and consider possible sepsis

Complications
The most concerning complication of DKA is cerebral oedema. The warning signs include:
- Headache, behavioural change with restlessness, drowsiness.
- Body posturing, cranial nerve palsy, seizures.
- Slowing of HR, haemodynamic instability.
- Respiratory arrest.

Once identified:
- Start ABCs.
- Emergency mannitol (1.0g/kg) IV.
- Transfer to the intensive care unit.

Reference
1 Dunger DB, Sperling MA, Acerini CL, et al. (2004). ESPE/LWPES consensus statement on diabetic ketoacidosis in children and adolescents. *Arch Dis Child* **89**: 188–94.

Inborn error of metabolism

Inborn errors of metabolism are rare. If such conditions are suspected during the neonatal period, then there is a specific course of action that should be followed (see 📖 p.187, and Chapter 26). Very occasionally, however, infants or children present outside the neonatal period with a catabolic state induced by an intercurrent illness such as viral infection, or fasting. The differential diagnosis at this time is broad and includes:

- *Infection:* generalized sepsis; CNS infection.
- *Gastrointestinal:* pyloric stenosis; gastroenteritis.
- *Cardiac:* duct-dependent CHD.

Clinical assessment

History

- A thorough history is important.
- Assess whether there is any consanguinity, or death of siblings from unknown or metabolic diseases.
- Identify specifically developmental progress.
- Has there been intermittent vomiting, sleepiness, or seizures.

Examination

- A full examination is needed here.
- Think about abnormal odours.
- Check on growth, failure to thrive.
- *Skin:* dermatitis or alopecia.
- *Eyes:* cataracts.
- *Breathing pattern:* Kussmaul or central hyperventilation.

Investigations

Until you know the diagnosis, the key tests are as follows.

Blood

- FBC with differential.
- Serum electrolytes with urea and creatinine.
- Glucose, LFTs (transaminases).
- Arterial or capillary blood gas.
- Lactate, pyruvate, ketones.
- Plasma amino acids.
- Ammonia.
- Carnitine.
- Drug screen.

Urine

- Urinalysis.
- Ketones.
- Reducing substances.
- Organic acids.
- Amino acids.
- Drug screen.

Monitoring

Ensure the ABCs. Then, the form and type of monitoring will be dictated by the patient's condition. Start with continuous pulse oximetry and ECG monitoring, and intermittent BP monitoring. Follow hourly output.

Therapy

In the acute setting, prior to transfer (if needed), treatment will be supportive, and directed towards any complicating metabolic acidosis or hypoglycaemia. All protein intake and oral feeds should be discontinued until the diagnosis is confirmed. In order to avoid catabolism give continuous glucose infusion (10–15%) during illness or periods of fasting.

Supportive care

• The underlying or precipitating illness needs to be treated.
• Later on, as a means of prevention against infection, ensure that immunizations are up to date.

Acidosis

• Correct and optimize ventilation and circulation.
• After this, bicarbonate replacement may be needed.
• For more persistent problems, treat in specialist centres.

Hypoglycaemia

Use glucose 25% (2–4mL/kg/dose IV).

Other acid–base problems

Since respiratory derangements in acid–base have already been discussed, we will restrict this section to metabolic acidosis (see 📖 p.958). An acidotic pH (<7.30), with low bicarbonate (<20mmol/L), suggests a primary metabolic acidosis. In an emergency, an alkalotic pH (>7.50) with raised bicarbonate (>30mmol/L) is most usually seen when supportive ventilation has been started in a patient with chronic hypercapnia.

Differential diagnosis of metabolic acidosis

Calculate the anion gap (AG)

$$AG = [Na] - ([HCO_3] + [Cl])$$

Normal AG = 10–12mmol/L

Increased anion gap metabolic acidosis

This is due to the production of exogenous acid. As an *aide-mémoire*, think of 'a mudpile'
- Alcohol or aspirin
- Methanol
- Uraemia
- DKA
- Paraldehyde
- Ingestion or inborn error
- Lactate
- Ethylene glycol

Normal anion gap metabolic acidosis

This is commonly due to loss of bicarbonate from the gut or kidney, or impaired acid secretion by the kidney
- *Diarrhoea*
- *Type I (distal) renal tubular acidosis (RTA):* inability to excrete hydrogen ion; urine pH always high (>6.5); caused by a variety of medications or inherited; often associated with hypokalaemia and hypercalciuria
- *Type (proximal) II RTA:* impaired reabsorption of bicarbonate from proximal tubule: usually associated with other proximal tubular dysfunction such as phosphaturia or glycosuria (Fanconi syndrome)
- *Type IV (hyperkalaemic) RTA*—inadequate aldosterone production or inability to respond to it: seen in acute pyelonephritis or obstructive uropathy

Clinical assessment

History

A thorough history is important. You will need to identify any symptoms of fever, flank pain, and vomiting (pyelonephritis), lethargy, or altered mental state (metabolic disease or poisoning). Then ask specific questions about the gastrointestinal and renal tracts, and growth. Last there may be a significant family history of renal disease, kidney stones, or early infant death.

Examination

A full examination is needed. Assess:
- Hydration.
- Growth.
- Respiratory state (compensation for metabolic acidosis).
- Abdomen.
- CNS.

Investigations

Until you know the diagnosis, the key tests are as follows.
- *Blood.* FBC with differential, serum electrolytes with urea and creatinine, glucose, LFTs (transaminases), arterial or capillary blood gas, lactate, pyruvate, ketone, plasma amino acids, ammonia, carnitine, and drug screen.
- *Urine:* urinalysis, ketones, reducing substances, organic and amino acids, and drug screen.
- *Imaging:* renal US scan looking for nephrocalcinosis (type I RTA).

Monitoring

Ensure the ABCs. Then, the form and type of monitoring will be dictated by the patient's condition. Start with continuous pulse oximetry and ECG monitoring, and intermittent BP monitoring. Follow hourly output.

Therapy

If the patient is dehydrated then this problem should be treated with oral or IV replacement. This alone may improve serum bicarbonate. However, for the specific metabolic disorders:
- *Increased AG:* identify cause and treat;
- *Distal or proximal RTA:* bicarbonate supplementation (see also 📖 pp.382–385);
- *Hyperkalaemic RTA:* correct serum bicarbonate and increase fluids to improve sodium delivery to the distal tubule (this will enhance potassium secretion).

Bicarbonate treatment

If you are using bicarbonate then:
- Estimate the deficit = $(20 - [HCO_3]) \times$ weight (kg) $\times 0.5$mmol;
- Replace over 24–48hr with oral supplements.

Further reading

BSPED-recommended DKA Management Guidelines (2009). Available at: ℘ www.bsped.org.uk/professional/guidelines/docs/DKAGuideline.pdf

Wolfsdorf J, Craig ME, Daneman D, et al. (2007) ISPAD Clinical Practice Consensus Guidelines 2006–2007. *Pediat Diabet* **8**: 28–43. For the evidence base to the DKA management guidelines, see the 2007 ISPAD guidelines. Available at: ℘ http://www.ispad.org/FileCenter/10-Wolfsdorf_Ped_Diab_2007,8.28–43.pdf

Neonatology

Newborn life support

All who attend deliveries should be proficient in newborn resuscitation, ideally taught on a recognized course (newborn life support (NLS) or equivalent). The algorithm on 📖 p.109 demonstrates a general approach to resuscitation (see Fig. 6.1). Preterm infants require special consideration (📖 p.114).

Before birth
- Check equipment.
- Ask about: Gestation? Foetal distress? Meconium?

At birth
- For uncompromised babies, a delay in cord clamping of at least one minute is recommended.
- There is insufficient evidence to recommend a delay in babies who require resuscitation.

Meconium
- Vigorous infants born through meconium stained liquor do NOT require airway suctioning either on the perineum or the resuscitaire.
- Pale, floppy, poor respiration, or bradycardia? Inspect oropharynx and perform suction if required.
- If appropriate expertise is available, tracheal intubation and suction may be useful in non-vigorous babies. If expertise not available, or if attempted intubation is prolonged or unsuccessful, start mask ventilation, particularly if there is persistent bradycardia.

Lung inflation
- Inflation breaths are given initially, use air (21% O_2).
- 3s each breath, 7 30cmH$_2$0 (term infants)—give in sets of 5.
- Once the chest is moving, ventilation breaths (shorter and gentler) are given at a rate of 30–40/min if required.

Airway manoeuvres
- Jaw thrust (2 person technique very useful).
- Direct inspection of oropharynx and airway suction.
- Guedel airway.
- Intubation (if competent).

Chest compressions
- Rate ~100/min, using two thumbs technique.
- 3 chest compressions per lung inflation (3:1 ratio).
- Re-assess infant after each 30secs (15 cycles).

Drugs
- Give through umbilical venous catheter (UVC) or IO (high dose endotracheal tube (ETT) adrenaline can be considered).
- Remember, drugs are B.A.D. (Bicarbonate/Adrenaline/Dextrose 10%).

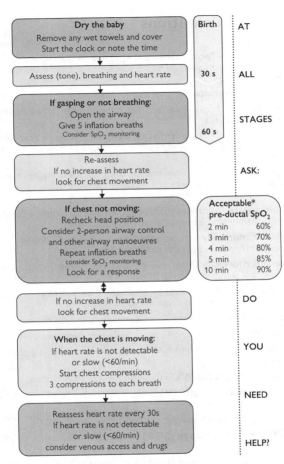

Fig. 6.1 Newborn life support. SpO₂ values are 25th centile for term infants. Reproduced with kind permission of Resuscitation Council (UK) 2010.

Perinatal definitions

See also 📖 p.10.

Gestational age (post-menstrual age) Age measured from the first day of the last menstrual period before conception and expressed in complete weeks or days.

Chronological/postnatal age Time elapsed from birth.

Corrected age Chronological age minus the number of weeks born before 40wks gestation.

Spontaneous abortion (miscarriage) A conceptus born after spontaneous labour without any signs of life before 24 completed weeks gestation.

Live birth A baby that displays any sign of life (i.e. breathing, heart beat, cord pulsation, or voluntary movement) after complete delivery from the mother, irrespective of gestation.

Stillbirth (late foetal death) Foetal death prior to complete delivery from the mother after 24 completed weeks gestation.

Perinatal mortality Includes all stillbirths and neonatal deaths in the first week. UK rate ~7–8 per thousand total births.

Neonatal mortality Death amongst live births before 28 days of age (whatever the gestation at birth). UK rate ~3 per thousand live births.

Neonatal period From birth to 28 postnatal days in term infants. If preterm, from birth to 44wks post-menstrual age.

Preterm Birth before 37 completed weeks gestation. ~8% of births.

Term birth Between 37 and 42 completed weeks gestation.

Post-term (post-mature) Birth after 42 completed weeks gestation. <5% of births.

Low birth weight (LBW) Birth weight <2500g. 7% of births.

Very low birth weight (VLBW) Birth weight <1500g. 1.2% of births.

Extremely low birth weight (ELBW) Birth weight <1000g.

Small for gestational age (SGA) Birth weight <10th centile for gestational age.

Large for gestational age (LGA) Birth weight >90th centile for gestational age.

Small for gestational age

SGA is birth weight <10th centile for gestational age. Intrauterine growth restriction (IUGR) is failure of growth *in-utero* that may or may not result in SGA.

- *Symmetric (proportional) SGA:* all growth parameters symmetrically small; suggests foetus affected from early pregnancy, e.g. chromosomal disorder or constitutional.
- *Asymmetric (disproportional) SGA:* weight centile < length and head circumference. Usually because of IUGR due to insult in late pregnancy, e.g. pre-eclampsia. Asymmetric SGA infants at risk of complications.

Causes

- Constitutional, i.e. small parents (commonest).
- Restricted foetal O_2 or glucose supply, e.g. placental dysfunction, maternal hypertension, multiple pregnancy, maternal illness.
- Foetal abnormality, e.g. chromosomal disorders, congenital anomalies and syndromes, congenital infection.
- Maternal substance exposure, e.g. alcohol, smoking, therapeutic or other drugs.

Complications

- ↑ Risk of foetal death and asphyxia (SGA indicates foetal compromise).
- May have congenital infection, toxoplasmosis, others, rubella, cytomegalovirus, herpes virus II (TORCH) or malformation (📖 p.182).
- Hypoglycaemia (due to decreased glycogen stores; 📖 p.187).
- Hypothermia.
- Polycythaemia (secondary to chronic intrauterine hypoxia; 📖 p.192).
- Necrotizing enterocolitis and/or intolerance of feeds (chronic foetal bowel hypoxia; 📖 p.178).
- Thrombocytopenia/neutropenia/coagulopathy (bone marrow/hepatic compromise; 📖 p.193).
- Meconium aspiration syndrome (2° to foetal hypoxia; 📖 p.152).

Management

Ideally manage on a postnatal ward with increased ratio of midwives.

- Routine postnatal care.
- Evaluate clinically for features suggestive of underlying cause.
- Particular attention to thermal care and blood glucose monitoring.
- Observe temperature, pulse, and respiration for at least the first 48hr.
- Admit to neonatal unit if birth weight <1800g.
- Well infants can be discharged when: they are sucking all feeds 3–4-hourly; weight gain is satisfactory (20–30g/day); body temperature is maintained at room temperature; mother is capable of caring for infant.

Prognosis

See also 📖 p.117. Neurodevelopmental impairments more common in SGA infants. Symmetric SGA infants often stay small. The Barker hypothesis suggests IUGR infants with a small placenta are at risk in later life of coronary disease, stroke, obesity, and hypertension.

Large for gestational age

Defined as birth weight >90th centile for gestational age.

Causes
- Most frequently constitutional, i.e. large parents.
- Infant of a mother with diabetes mellitus.
- Foetal hyperinsulinism, pancreatic islet cell hyperplasia.
- Hydrops foetalis (📖 p.138).
- Beckwith–Wiedemann syndrome (BWS; 📖 p.949).

Complications
- Perinatal asphyxia, nerve palsies, shoulder dystocia, fractures.
- Hypoglycaemia, especially if due to maternal diabetes or in BWS.
- Problems associated with the underlying cause LGA.

Management
- Careful obstetric management to prevent obstetric complications.
- Examine for associated features, e.g. BWS or signs of birth injury.
- Prevent hypoglycaemia (📖 p.132).

Prognosis Generally excellent (unless hydrops foetalis) if managed well.

Infant of a mother with diabetes mellitus
Pathophysiology
Maternal hyperglycaemia → ↑ foetal glucose → ↑ foetal insulin secretion (antenatally has growth hormone function) → macrosomia, organomegaly, and polycythaemia. Rarely, maternal vascular disease results in foetal IUGR.

Associated complications
- *2–4 × risk of congenital abnormalities:* caudal regression syndrome (sacral and femoral agenesis or hypoplasia); transient hypertrophic cardiomyopathy; small left colon syndrome; neural tube defects.
- *Obstetric complications* (see 📖 Complications): increased risk of spontaneous miscarriage, intrauterine foetal death, and prematurity.
- *Hypoglycaemia:* generally resolves as serum insulin level falls.
- *Respiratory disease:* respiratory distress.
- *Polycythaemia.* Risk of secondary thrombosis (e.g. renal vein).
- Exaggerated physiological jaundice.
- Hypocalcaemia and hypomagnesaemia.

Management
Optimize maternal glycaemic control during pregnancy (↓ risk of complications except for congenital abnormalities; see 📖 p.120).

Prognosis
- Normoglycaemia occurs within 48hr in vast majority.
- 7 × increased risk of diabetes mellitus in later life.
- Increased risk of later obesity and, possibly, poor development.

Prematurity

Birth before 37 completed weeks gestation. 8% of all births. Most problems seen in with infants born <32 completed weeks (~2% of all births).

Predisposing factors
- Idiopathic (40%).
- Previous preterm birth.
- Multiple pregnancy.
- Maternal illness, e.g. chorioamnionitis, polyhydramnios, pre-eclampsia, diabetes mellitus.
- Premature rupture of membranes.
- Uterine malformation or cervical incompetence.
- Placental disease, e.g. dysfunction, antepartum haemorrhage.
- Poor maternal health or socio-economic status.

Associated problems
- Respiratory: surfactant deficiency causing respiratory distress syndrome (RDS; 📖 p.150), apnoea of prematurity (📖 p.154), chronic lung disease/bronchopulmonary dysplasia (CLD/BPD) (📖 p.166).
- *CNS*: intraventricular haemorrhage, periventricular leucomalacia; retinopathy of prematurity (📖 p.188).
- *GI*: necrotizing enterocolitis (📖 p.178); inability to suck; and poor milk tolerance.
- Hypothermia.
- Immuno-compromise resulting in ↑ risk and severity of infection.
- Impaired fluid/electrolyte homeostasis (↑ transepidermal skin water loss, poor renal function).
- Patent ductus arteriosus (📖 p.169).
- Anaemia of prematurity (📖 p.192).
- Jaundice (liver enzyme immaturity; 📖 p.130).
- Birth trauma (📖 p.126).
- Perinatal hypoxia (📖 p.120).
- *Later*: increased risk of adverse neurodevelopmental outcome, behavioural problems, sudden infant death syndrome (SIDS), non-accidental injury (NAI), and/or parental marriage break up (due to impaired infant–maternal bonding, stress of long-term complications, etc.).

General management—antenatal
- Delivery should be planned in a centre capable of caring for preterm infants.
- If a woman has threatened preterm labour in a centre unable to care for the baby, possible *in-utero* transfer should involve discussion between neonatology and obstetrics teams preferably at consultant level. Consider foetal fibronectin screening to aid diagnosis and tocolysis to delay birth to allow for transfer.
- Give mother IM corticosteroids, 2 doses, 12–24hr apart, of either beta- or dexamethasone, if <34wks gestation. Steroids ↓ mortality by up to 40% (↓ severity of RDS, periventricular haemorrhage, and necrotizing enterocolitis) provided they are given >24hr before birth. Benefit persists for at least 7 days. Effect of repeated doses remains unclear—may have adverse impact on later growth.

General management—postnatal

- Most preterm infants require stabilization and support in transition– *not* resuscitation.
- Senior paediatrician should be present at birth if very preterm, e.g. <28wks.
- Delay cord clamping for 1min if infant not compromised.
- Immediately after birth, place in food grade plastic bag and under radiant heater.
- Provide respiratory support as required:
  - use positive end-expiratory pressure (PEEP) (5cmH$_2$O);
  - start with lower peak inspiratory pressure or proximal (PIP) (20cmH$_2$O);
  - consider elective intubation and ETT surfactant if <27/40;
  - may be possible to stabilize with PEEP/nasal continuous positive airway pressure (CPAP) only.
- Monitor oxygen saturation levels if available (right wrist = pre-ductal), and target oxygen therapy appropriately:
  - must be familiar with normal values;
  - approx 10% well preterm infants will have SpO$_2$ <70% at 5min;
  - ☞ 'correct' starting dose of O$_2$ unclear, therefore, can start in air;
  - easy to hyperoxygenate if start in high FiO$_2$.
- Once stable, well infants >1800g, and >35/40 may be transferred to a suitable postnatal ward if midwifery staffing and expertise exists for the required additional care. Otherwise admit to a neonatal unit.
- Measure weight and temperature on admission and monitor closely:
  - <1000g 37–37.5C;
  - >1000g 36.5–37C;
  - nurse in 80% humidity for first 7 days if <30/40.
- Monitor and maintain blood glucose with enteral feeds (expressed breast milk), total parenteral nutrition (TPN) or 10% glucose as appropriate. Encourage ALL mothers to express breast milk from day 1.
- Start broad spectrum antibiotics if any possibility of infection, e.g. benzylpenicillin, and gentamicin.
- Start specific treatment for associated diseases and complications of prematurity, e.g. surfactant for RDS.
- Aim for minimal handling of infant with appropriate levels of noise and cycled lighting in the nursery.
- Support parents.

Birth at the limit of viability

WHO defines the perinatal period as starting at 22wks gestation, which is realistically the earliest gestation of viability. In the UK threshold viability is generally accepted to be when birth is between 22 and 25 completed weeks gestation, typically 500–1000g birth weight.

Management before birth

As gestation falls, the likelihood of mortality and serious long-term disability increases. When preterm birth at threshold viability is threatened there should be close collaboration between paediatrician, obstetrician, midwife, and family.

Unless delivery is precipitate a senior paediatrician should meet parents before birth to assess and do the following:
- Ascertain whether estimate of gestation is likely to be reliable.
- Give relevant information.
- Outline potential problems.
- Outline possible management (including option of not resuscitating).
- Describe relevant survival and disability rates.
- Parents should fully participate in any decision about the appropriateness of any later attempted resuscitation.

Management at birth

- *<22wks gestation:* rarely suitable for resuscitation, but it may still be beneficial for a senior paediatrician to attend birth to reassure parents and support staff in provision of comfort care.
- *22–25wks gestation:* a senior obstetrician and paediatrician should be present to assess size, maturity, and condition of the newborn and then manage appropriately. If an infant appears viable, respiratory support should be given. External cardiac massage or resuscitation drugs are not generally considered appropriate. If junior doctors are present alone at such a delivery full resuscitation should be started and continued until a senior paediatrician arrives and makes an assessment. If parents do not wish life-sustaining care in an infant born before 25wks their view should be respected and taken into account. However, if the infant appears unexpectedly vigorous or more mature, full treatment should be started.

If resuscitation is withheld on a delivery ward the infant should be kept warm and comfortable, as well as offered to parents to cuddle. For management after death see 📖 p.198.

Management after birth

Clinical progress after the initial resuscitation and further discussion with the parents will dictate whether it is appropriate to continue or withdraw life-sustaining treatment. Where doctors and parents, or parents themselves, cannot agree as to the best or most appropriate management it is almost always best to continue as the situation will become clearer with time and agreement is usually then reached.

Outcome following prematurity

Risk of complications and associated morbidity/mortality steadily lessen as gestation advances. Infants who are well in the first 24hr and are >32wks gestation are at low risk of suffering adverse outcomes. The EPICure and EPICure2 studies give the best available guide to likely outcome in UK for infants born at less than 26wks gestation (Table 6.1).[1]

Table 6.1 Likely outcomes in UK for infants born at <26wks gestation

	Weeks of gestation		
Survival to discharge (%)	22–23	24	25
1995	19	35	54
2006	26	47	67
Statistically significant increase?	No	Yes+	Yes++
Overall survival of live births free of disability at age 6yrs (%)*EPICure 1*	<0.5	9	20

Disabled survivors in EPICure were categorized as approximately; 1/3 Severe, 1/3 Moderate, 1/3 Mild. The overall rate of severe IVH (13–15%) or chronic lung disease (74–75%) was unchanged between 1995 and 2006.

Typical disabilities were;
• Cerebral palsy, most commonly spastic (diplegia > quadriplegia > hemiplegia).
• Squint (strabismus).
• Blindness.
• Hearing loss.
• Epilepsy.
• Cognitive impairment and behavioural disorders, e.g. attention deficit hyperactivity disorder.

Generally smaller, more immature infants will have a poorer outcome than larger, mature babies.

Knowledge of your own unit's outcome is important. However, the numbers will be small, and national figures (where available) should be used. Note that many things influence outcome, e.g. a singleton infant, born spontaneously at 25wks gestation after an otherwise uncomplicated pregnancy in a mother treated with 48hr of steroids, has a better prognosis than a triplet born suddenly at 26wks after the mother developed severe chorioamnionitis.

Reference

1 Marlow, N., Wolke, D., Bracewell, et al. (2005). Neurologic and developmental disability at six years of age after extremely preterm birth. *N Engl J Med* 352: 71–2.

Basic obstetrics

The aim of obstetrics is to monitor and promote foetal and maternal well-being during pregnancy and labour, and to identify and manage high risk pregnancies or complications. In the UK most women choose to deliver in hospital, although planned home deliveries are on the increase. Depending on local provision women may also choose to deliver in a birthing centre, community midwifery unit, or midwife-led unit attached to an obstetric centre.

All 'high-risk' deliveries should be in a consultant-led obstetric unit, and clear protocols should be in place for the transfer in of women from outlying centres if problems arise during labour.

Routine antenatal care of the low risk pregnancy

In the UK, care is usually shared among GP, community midwife, and obstetrician.
- First antenatal ('booking') visit usually occurs at 10–12wks gestation when significant risk factors should be identified.
- Foetal US is usually performed to determine gestational age.

Women are assessed every few weeks to monitor:
- general health;
- haemoglobin (Hb);
- BP, urine glucose and albumin;
- foetal growth, movements, HR, and lie (liquor volume).

Routine prenatal screening

Maternal testing is offered for:
- Blood group and antibodies (iso-immune haemolytic disease);
- Serology for syphilis, rubella, hepatitis B, and human immunodeficiency virus (HIV);
- Urine for protein, glucose, and bacteria.

Blood tests are also offered at 17–18wks to screen for chromosomal disorders and structural anomalies. Controversy exists as to what is most cost-effective and they may include:
- α-fetoprotein (AFP);
- Human chorionic gonadotrophin (hCG);
- Oestriol (combined with above 2 tests = 'triple test');
- Triple test plus inhibin ('quadruple test');
- Quadruple test plus pregnancy-associated protein-A (PrAP-A) ± US nuchal thickness.

A detailed foetal US looking for abnormalities is usually done at ~18wks.

Chorionic villus biopsy (>10wks gestation) or amniocentesis (usually at 15–16wks) is offered for chromosomal, enzymatic, or gene probe analysis, if screening tests show high risk of serious problems (also if maternal age >35yrs, previously abnormal baby, +ve family history). Both diagnostic tests carry a risk of miscarriage (~1%, slightly higher with cardiovascular system (CVS)).

Induction of labour
Indicated when delivery is safer for either mother or baby than to remain *in utero*. Method: use prostaglandin (PO or vaginally, per vagina (PV)) or amniotomy.

Normal labour
Occurs >37wks and should result in delivery within 24hr of starting.
- *1st stage:* from the onset of labour to full cervical dilatation. Once cervix is 3cm dilated should then be at least 1cm/hr.
- *2nd stage:* time from fully dilated cervix to birth. Normal duration is 45–120min in a primiparous woman; 15–45min if multiparous. Active pushing during the second stage should not usually exceed 60–90min.
- *3rd stage:* time from birth to placental delivery.

Intrapartum foetal assessment
Intrapartum foetal heart monitoring detects signs of foetal compromise:
- In established low-risk labour intermittent auscultation (by Doppler USS, or Pinard stethoscope) should be undertaken for 1min after contractions, at least every 15min in the first stage and every 5min in the second stage.
- Continuous electronic foetal monitoring (cardiotocogram) should be undertaken in high risk pregnancies and when:
  - abnormal foetal HR detected;
  - meconium staining of liquor or bleeding in labour;
  - maternal pyrexia;
  - oxytocin use;
  - maternal request.
- Foetal blood sampling is indicated if foetal distress suspected.

Mode of delivery
Majority of term infants are delivered by normal vaginal delivery. Indications for caesarean section (CS) include:
- maternal ill health;
- acute foetal distress;
- antepartum haemorrhage (APH);
- placenta praevia;
- umbilical cord prolapsed;
- failure to progress;
- failed induction;
- previous CS;
- foetal malpresentation (including breech);
- multiple pregnancy;
- pregnancy-induced hypertension;
- maternal HIV or HSV;
- evidence of ongoing foetal compromise, e.g. severe IUGR.

Instrumental delivery (forceps or vacuum extraction) may be indicated when there is:
- prolonged 2nd stage;
- malpresentation, e.g. breech delivery or occipital-posterior;
- foetal distress.

Obstetric problems

It is desirable for a paediatrician to attend a birth if there is:
- foetal distress (including meconium-stained liquor);
- emergency CS;
- elective CS under general anaesthetic (GA);
- vaginal breech delivery;
- rotational forceps;
- preterm delivery <34wks gestation;
- severe IUGR;
- maternal IDDM;
- serious foetal abnormality; significant iso-immune haemolytic disease.

Small for gestational age

See 📖 p.111. Serial detailed US scans (including Doppler foetal umbilical and cerebral artery blood flow measurement) should be performed to determine:
- Whether growth reduction is symmetrical or asymmetrical. Symmetrical SGA is usually foetal in origin; asymmetrical suggests placental dysfunction.
- Foetal growth rate.
- Foetal health.

There is ↑ risk of foetal hypoxia or death, requiring close antenatal and intrapartum monitoring. Early delivery may be needed. Abnormal Doppler artery measurements (e.g. absent or reversed end diastolic flow) indicate an especially high foetal risk.

Large for gestational age

See 📖 p.112. A glucose tolerance test should be performed to detect maternal diabetes. Because of ↑ risk of obstetric complications, a senior obstetrician should supervise timing and mode of delivery and labour. Specialist input (diabetologist) should also be sought early.

Multiple pregnancy

There is an increased risk of:
- Perinatal mortality.
- Preterm delivery.
- Malformations.
- Malpresentation.
- Polyhydramnios.
- Pregnancy-induced hypertension.
- APH.
- Risk increases as foetus number increases. ◆ If ≥3, selective feticide may be indicated to improve outcome for survivors.

Oligohydramnios

Liquor volume <500mL. Causes:
- Placental insufficiency.
- Preterm prolonged rupture of membranes (PPROM).
- Foetal urinary tract obstruction or renal disease (e.g. Potter's syndrome: 📖 pp.370, 951).

Risks
- Pulmonary hypoplasia/dry lung syndrome.
- Contractures/developmental dysplasia of the hip.

Polyhydramnios

Liquor volume >2000mL. Causes:
- 50% 2° to foetal disease, e.g. upper GI tract obstruction.
- 30% idiopathic.
- 20% maternal diabetes mellitus.

Risks
- Preterm labour.
- Malpresentation.
- Umbilical cord prolapse.
- APH.

Amniotic fluid reduction and indomethacin may be beneficial.

Prolonged pregnancy

Longer than 42wks gestation.
- Significant ↑ perinatal mortality and morbidity (↑ risk of perinatal hypoxia due to placental insufficiency, obstructed labour due to larger foetus, meconium aspiration, reduced skull moulding).
- Induction of labour is usually advised after 41wks.

Antepartum haemorrhage

Uterine-placental bleeding after 24wks gestation.
- Associated with ↑ perinatal mortality and morbidity; preterm delivery.
- Major causes are placenta praevia, vasa praevia, placental abruption.
- Observation or immediate delivery performed depending on severity and gestation.

Umbilical cord prolapse

An obstetric emergency due to high risk of cord compression and perinatal asphyxia. Requires urgent delivery, usually by CS.

Preterm prelabour rupture of the membranes

- In 80% preterm labour rapidly follows.
- In remaining 20% there is significant risk of infection and, if PPROM occurs before 20wks, neonatal pulmonary hypoplasia.
- *Treatment*: Give mother corticosteroids. Consider antibiotics. Tocolysis is contraindicated.

Preterm labour See 📖 p.114 and p.116

Failure to progress

Neonatal and maternal morbidity increase with progressive delay.
- *Caused by:* passage obstruction (malpresentation, cephalopelvic disproportion, abnormal pelvic, or cervical anatomy) or uterine dysfunction.
- *Treatment:* artificial rupture of membranes (ARM), analgesia, and synthetic oxytocin to hasten delivery. CS may be necessary.

Disturbing/abnormal foetal heart rate patterns

May signify hypoxia. Foetal acidosis results if hypoxia prolonged or repeated.

Signs
- Loss of variability in baseline foetal heart rate (<5beats/min).
- Late decelerations (in heart rate) (lowest foetal heart rate is >30s after peak uterine contraction).
- Repetitive severe, variable decelerations.
- Prolonged foetal deceleration (2–9min below established baseline).
- Prolonged foetal bradycardia (<100/min).
- Persistent foetal tachycardia (>170/min).

Tests
- Foetal blood gas sampling (pH ≤ 7.24 = 'Borderline' - repeat ≤ 30min; ≤7.2 = 'Abnormal'—consultant obstetrician and delivery).
- Postnatal umbilical artery and venous blood gas are used to determine the actual level and nature of acidaemia.

Malpresentation

Most common form is breech (3% at term).
- *Types:* extended (hips flexed and knees extended); flexed (hips and knees flexed); footling (feet are presenting part).
- *External cephalic version:* may be successful in turning baby between 34 and 36wks.
- *Vaginal breech delivery:* associated with ↑ perinatal mortality and morbidity; CS is recommended.
- Other malpresentations are associated with ↑ risk of obstructed labour and CS rate (obligatory for brow and transverse presentation).

Shoulder dystocia

Inability to deliver shoulders after head has been delivered. Cord compression leads to rapid foetal asphyxia.
- *Treatment:* urgent delivery—experienced obstetrician, McRobert's manoeuvre (flexion + abduction maternal hips, thighs on abdomen), suprapubic pressure, posterior foetal arm extraction, +/– episiotomy
- *Risks:* perinatal asphyxia, humeral and clavicle fracture, Erb's palsy.

Maternal disorders causing neonatal disease

Any maternal disease can adversely affect foetal and neonatal health. Certain maternal illnesses, e.g. CHD, also raise the risk of inheritance in the newborn. Most common manifestations are:
- Spontaneous abortion.
- Foetal death.
- IUGR and/or preterm delivery.

Maternal drug ingestion
Maternal medications or substance abuse can affect the newborn:
- maternal anticonvulsants (□ p.951);
- alcohol abuse and foetal alcohol syndrome (□ p.951);
- tobacco;
- neonatal abstinence syndrome (□ p.186).

Hypertensive diseases
Pregnancy-induced hypertension (e.g. pre-eclampsia, eclampsia, haemolytic anaemia–elevated liver enzymes–low platelet count (HELLP) syndrome) is associated with increased foetal loss, the need for preterm delivery, IUGR, neonatal leucopenia, and thrombocytopenia. Maternal drug treatment may cause neonatal hypoglycaemia and hypotension.

Systemic lupus erythematosus
Associated with:
- ↑ Risk of spontaneous abortion.
- IUGR.
- Preterm delivery.
- Neonatal lupus syndrome (rare; associated with anti-Ro and –La antibodies): complete heart block, haemolytic anaemia, leucopenia, thrombocytopenia, and discoid erythematous skin rash.

Antiphospholipid syndrome Maternal antiphospholipid antibodies (e.g. lupus anticoagulant or anticardiolipin antibodies) are associated with spontaneous abortion, IUGR, foetal death, need for preterm delivery.

Thyroid disease See □ p.425.
In ~10% of women with Graves's disease, thyroid-stimulating hormone (TSH) receptor-stimulator antibodies cross the placenta causing neonatal thyrotoxicosis. Foetus most likely to be affected if high maternal IgG serum level develops, or mother requires treatment during pregnancy. Take cord blood for TSH, fT4, and TSH receptor antibody (TRAB). Repeat at D5 if results abnormal.

Myasthenia gravis
In ~10% transplacental passage of IgG antibodies to motor end-plate acetylcholine receptors causes transient neonatal myasthenia gravis.

Diabetes mellitus See □ p.112

Maternal infection See □ pp.184–185

Birth trauma

Risk factors
LGA, cephalic–pelvic disproportion, malpresentation, precipitate delivery, instrumental delivery, shoulder dystocia, prematurity.

Head
- *Caput succedaneum:* oedema of the presenting scalp. Can be particularly large following ventouse delivery (chignon). Rapidly resolves.
- *Cephalhaematoma:* common fluctuant swelling(s) due to subperiostial bleed(s). Most often occur over parietal bones. Swelling *limited* by suture lines. Resolves over weeks.
- *Subaponeurotic haematoma:* rare; bleeding not confined by skull periostium, so can be large and life-threatening. Presents as fluctuant scalp swelling, *not limited* by suture lines.

Skin
- *Traumatic cyanosis:* bruising and petechiae of presenting part.
- *Lacerations:* caused by forceps, ventouse cap, scalp electrodes, scalp pH sampling, or scalpel wounds during CS. Close with Steri-Strips® or suture if required.

Nerve palsies
- *Brachial plexus:* commonest is Erb's palsy (C5–C6 nerve routes). May result from difficult assisted delivery (e.g. shoulder dystocia); the arm is flaccid with pronated forearm and flexed wrist (waiter's tip position). Complete recovery occurs within 6wks in two-thirds of cases. X-ray clavicle to exclude fractures. Refer to physiotherapy for assessment and follow-up.
- *Facial nerve palsy:* follows pressure on face from either maternal ischial spine or forceps. Presents as facial asymmetry that is worse on crying (affected side shows lack of eye closure and lower facial movement; mouth is drawn to normal side). Majority recover in 1–2wks. May require eye care with methylcellulose and specialist referral.

Fractures
- *Clavicle* (commonest).
- *Long bone fractures:* usually lower avulsion fractures of the femoral or tibial epiphyses, or mid-shaft fractures of the femur or humerus. Infant presents as unsettled, with affected limb pseudo-paralysis, or obvious deformity or swelling. Confirm by X-ray.
- *Skull fracture:* associated with forceps delivery and usually require no treatment unless depressed in which case neurosurgical referral is required.
- *Treatment:* analgesia; limb immobilization (arm inside baby-grow), often do not require orthopaedic intervention, healed in a few weeks. Rapid healing and remodelling usually occur.

Soft tissue trauma

- *Sternocleidomastoid tumour:* overstretching of muscle leads to haematoma. Subsequent contraction of muscle results in non-tender 'tumour' and torticollis (head turns away from affected muscle). Physiotherapy almost always curative (see also 📖 p.883). Possible indication of malposition *in-utero*—consider increased risk of developmental dysplasia of the hip (DDH) (📖 p.748).
- *Fat necrosis* Tender, red, subcutaneous swelling caused by pressure over bony prominences, e.g. forceps. It usually resolves spontaneously. May be extensive with risk of ↑ Ca^{2+} and so there is a need to monitor serum level.

Non-specifically ill neonate

Early recognition of serious neonatal illness is an important skill. The nurse or parent may say that the infant is just 'not right'. Listen, examine the baby carefully, and act if in any doubt! Any serious disease can present non-specifically.

Major causes

- Infection (e.g. group B streptococcus or Guillain–Barré syndrome (GBS), septicaemia, meningitis; 📖 p.180).
- Hypothermia (may be sign of infection).
- Metabolic (e.g. hypoglycaemia, 📖 p.132; inborn errors of metabolism 📖 p.187).
- Cardiac (e.g. congenital heart disease, arrhythmias; 📖 pp.232, 250).
- GI (e.g. NEC; 📖 p.178).
- CNS (e.g. intracranial haemorrhage, seizures; 📖 pp.134, 176).

Presentation

- *Skin:* pallor, mottling, peripheral cyanosis, cool peripheries; capillary refill >2secs; rash; jaundice.
- *Temperature:* ↑ or ↓.
- *CNS:* lethargy, weak or unusual cry, generalized hypotonia, irritability, jittery, seizures.
- *Respiratory:* apnoea, expiratory grunting, flaring nostrils, tachypnoea (>60breaths/min), intercostal or subcostal recession, tracheal tug.
- *CVS:* tachycardia (>160/min), weak or absent pulses, (bradycardia <80 or hypotension should be considered late/pre-terminal signs).
- *GI:* vomiting, distended abdomen (ileus), diarrhoea, bloody stools; abdominal tenderness; bilious vomit or aspirate.
- *Metabolic:* ↑ or ↓ blood glucose.

Management of non-specifically ill neonate

- Quickly assess ABC. Secure airway, give O_2 if required, and provide ventilatory support if needed
- Transfer to neonatal unit as soon as safe to do so (get a nurse/midwife to accompany you on the move)
- Obtain vascular access (IV/UV/IO) and give bolus 0.9% saline 10–20mL/kg if circulatory compromise. Repeat if necessary
- Monitor breathing, SpO_2, heart rate, BP (consider arterial access), temperature
- Measure BP, blood glucose, urea and electrolytes (U&Es), FBC, blood gas. Consider clotting studies and C-reactive protein (CRP). Ventilate early if respiratory failure
- Full septic screen: blood culture; CXR/AXR; LP (only postpone if baby very unstable) for CSF, M, C&S, protein, glucose; stool culture and virology; urine (suprapubic, or midstream urine (MSU) if antibiotics can be delayed)
- Consider cranial ultrasound scan if preterm/at risk
- Start broad-spectrum antibiotics. IV benzylpenicillin and an aminoglycoside (e.g. gentamicin) unless possible listeria infection in which case substitute ampicillin for benzylpenicillin. If >48hr old, and particularly if indwelling lines were present before illness, consider flucloxacillin, or vancomycin, and gentamicin. If meningitis ensure broad spectrum cover and good CSF penetration—e.g. cefotaxime. If all cultures are negative and index of suspicion of sepsis is low, antibiotics can be stopped after 48hr. If not, treat for 5–7 days, changing antibiotics according to sensitivities of significant identified pathogens. Treat for 14–21 days if meningitis present. If any doubt consult microbiologist
- Specific treatment as appropriate, e.g. correct hypoglycaemia, inotropic support if persistently hypotensive, blood transfusion if significant haemorrhage, clotting factors to correct disseminated intravascular coagulation (DIC)

Neonatal jaundice

See also 📖 p.314. Jaundice is common (60% term, 80% preterm in first week), and is usually unconjugated. Significant jaundice may indicate underlying disease. High serum unconjugated free bilirubin is neurotoxic and can cause kernicterus (deafness, athetoid cerebral palsy (CP), seizures).

Physiological jaundice

Common and appears after 24hr, peaks around day 3–4, and usually resolves by 14 days. It is due to immaturity of hepatic bilirubin conjugation, but poor feeding (particularly in breast-fed infants) can also contribute. Jaundice progresses in a cephalic-caudal direction.

Measure bilirubin (transcutaneous or serum) in babies with jaundice. Action is required when serum bilirubin (SBR) is above gestation and age cut-offs (e.g. >300μmol/l in term infant at 72hr) or rapidly rising.

Causes of elevated SBR Exaggerated physiological jaundice (e.g. preterm, bruising); sepsis; haemolytic disorders; hepatic disease.

Treatment of elevated SBR

- Stop bilirubin rising to level that may cause kernicterus (📖 p.195).
- Treat any underlying cause, e.g. sepsis.
- Start 'blue light' phototherapy (converts bilirubin to water-soluble form that can then be excreted in urine).
- Use age/gestation specific charts to determine level to start phototherapy (see Fig. 6.2). Be aware of risk factors (family history, exclusive breast feeding, Rh or blood group incompatibility).
- Measure SBR frequently (4–24-hourly depending on circumstances) and stop when falls below treatment level.
- Ensure adequate hydration.
- Cover eyes (phototherapy side effects: ↓ or ↑ temperature; eye damage; diarrhoea; dehydration; rash; separation from mother).
- Exchange transfusion ± intravenous immunoglobulin (IVIG) if very high SBR (e.g. >450μmol/L in term infant at 48hr) or rapid rise (>8.5μmol/L/hr).
- In the UK the National Institute of Clinical Excellence (NICE) has produced guidance on investigation and management of newborn jaundice (see Fig 6.2)—the full guideline also includes gestation specific treatment thresholds and charts: ℘ http://guidance.nice.org.uk/CG98.

Jaundice in the first 24hrs

Assume it is pathological. Start phototherapy. Check SBR, FBC, direct coombs test (DCT), and blood group. Consider septic screen/ TORCH.

Causes Haemolysis (e.g. Rh disease), red cell enzyme defects (e.g. G6PD deficiency), red cell membrane defects (congenital spherocytosis, elliptocytosis), sepsis, severe bruising.

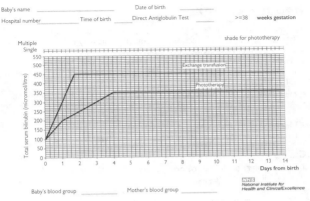

Baby's name _____ Date of birth _____
Hospital number _____ Time of birth _____ Direct Antiglobulin Test _____ >=38 **weeks gestation**

Baby's blood group _____ Mother's blood group _____

Fig. 6.2 Bilirubin thresholds for phototherapy and exchange transfusion in infants with hyperbilirubinaemia. Reproduced from: Neonatal Jaundice. National Collaborating Centre for Women's and Children's Health, May 2010, with the permission of the Royal College of Obstetricians and Gynaecologists.

Prolonged jaundice (>14 days in term infant; >21 days in preterm)

All infants require investigation and measurement of conjugated bilirubin. If conjugated hyperbilirubinaemia present, further specialized investigation will be required. Ask about pale stools/dark urine.

Causes Breastfeeding (benign, self-limiting, and usually resolves by 12wks), enclosed bleeding (e.g. cephalhaematoma), prematurity, haemolysis, sepsis, hypothyroidism, conjugated jaundice, hepatic enzyme disorders (e.g. Crigler–Najjar Syndrome, Lucy–Driscoll disease).

Initial investigations SBR (total and conjugated), U&E, FBC, DCT, blood group, thyroid function test (TFTs), LFTs, and glucose.

Treatment Depends on cause. Rarely phototherapy is beneficial, e.g. Crigler–Najjar Syndrome.

Conjugated jaundice (conjugated SBR >25µmol/L))

Stools may be clay-coloured in obstructive jaundice.

Causes Sepsis, TPN, biliary tract obstruction (e.g. biliary atresia, choledochal cyst), viral hepatitis; TORCH infections, α_1-antitrypsin deficiency, cystic fibrosis, inspissated bile syndrome after haemolytic disease, galactosaemia, other inherited metabolic disease, idiopathic giant cell hepatitis.

Initial investigations As for prolonged jaundice. Further investigations include radiology, enzyme testing, viral serology, liver biopsy, histology.

Treatment Depends on cause.

Hypoglycaemia

- Measurement of blood glucose using glucose reagent strips is unreliable. Use blood glucose analyser or laboratory measurement.
- In newborn period defined as <2.6mmol/L.
- Blood glucose drops naturally in first few hours after birth before normalising—newborns have increased ability to utilize ketones/lactate for energy.
- All infants should be encouraged to feed in first hour if well enough.
- At risk groups for hypoglycaemia include; infant of diabetic mother; <2500g or <3rd centile for weight; <37/40 gestation; maternal beta-blockers; birth asphyxia.
- Check blood glucose in all infants who are unwell/lethargic/jittery.

Causes

- *Reduced glucose stores:* preterm, IUGR, LBW, inborn errors of metabolism (IEM) (e.g. galactosaemia).
- *Increased glucose consumption:* sepsis, hypothermia, perinatal hypoxia, polycthaemia, haemolytic disease, seizures.
- *Hyperinsulinism:* maternal diabetes mellitus, BWS, pancreatic islet cell hyperplasia, transient.
- *Miscellaneous:* maternal ß blockers, tissued or malfunctioning IV infusion.
- *Other rare causes:* foetal alcohol syndrome, pituitary insufficiency, adrenal insufficiency.

Presentation

Commonly asymptomatic. Jitteriness, apnoea, poor feeding, drowsiness, seizures, cerebral irritability, hypotonia, macrosomia (if hyperinsulinism).

Investigation

Blood glucose should be measured in first hour in all high risk infants. Apart from regular blood glucose measurements, further investigation is not usually required if cause evident (e.g. IDM).

Suspicious patterns of hypoglycaemia meriting investigation include;
- Recurrent hypoglycaemia in term infant despite functioning intravenous infusion (IVI) of glucose 10%.
- Severe (<1mmol/L) and/or recurrent (>1) hypoglycaemia.
- Symptomatic hypoglycaemia.
- High glucose requirement (>8mg/kg/min).
- Hypoglycaemia and prolonged jaundice (panhypotpituitarism) or sodium abnormalities (adrenal problems).
- Hypoglycaemia with genital or midline abnormalities.

Calculating IV glucose infusion rate (mg/kg/min)

Infusion rate (mg/kg/min) equals:

$$\frac{\text{IV rate (mL/hr)} \times \% \text{ glucose in IV infusion} \times 0.167}{\text{weight in kg}}$$

First line tests (taken when hypoglycaemic):
- Blood for glucose, insulin, growth hormone, cortisol, β-hydroxybuyrate, free fatty acids, amino acids (consider C-peptide, lactate, and ammonia).
- Urine for urinalysis (ketones), amino and organic acids.
- Further investigations as guided by results/clinical biochemist.

Prevention of hypoglycaemia in at-risk infants (see list of causes on 📖 pp.98, 132).
- Adequate feed soon after birth (<1hr) and then at least 3-hourly.
- Monitor blood glucose levels (pre-feed), keep warm, support feeding.

Prognosis
Profound/prolonged hypoglycaemia can cause neurological damage—exact level/duration after which this may occur is unclear.

Treatment of hypoglycaemia

Symptomatic or severe hypoglycaemia (glucose<1.0mmol/L)
- IV bolus 3–5mL/kg of glucose 10%
- Follow with 10% glucose infusion IV (4–6mg/kg/min)

Asymptomatic (glucose <2.0mmol/L or 2.0–2.6mmol/L on 2 occasions)
- Enterally fed infants:
  - inspect feed chart (frequency/volume, etc.)
  - if reluctant to feed—consider NGT
  - if not tolerating milk—consider IV
  - give early milk feed (consider larger volume)
  - monitor with pre-feed blood glucose levels
- Infants on IV fluids:
  - check IV line is working
  - if glucose <1.0mmol/L—give bolus then increase infusion rate/concentration
  - if glucose >1.0mmol/L—increase infusion rate/concentration

Resistant hypoglycaemia (glucose requirement >8mg/kg/min)
- Seek specialist advice, as hyperinsulinism likely
- Increase background glucose infusion (central IV access needed)
- Glucagon 0.5mg IM can be given in emergency—rebound increased insulin secretion will occur
- Treatment options include:
  - diazoxide (given with chlorthiazide to counteract fluid retention)
  - somatostatin (octreotide)
  - nifedipine
  - surgery (subtotal pancreatectomy)
- Enteral feeding promotes normality. Aim to wean off IV as soon as able
- High concentrations of glucose (>12.5%) require central IV access
- Monitor plasma sodium if on IV fluids

Neonatal seizures

See also 📖 p.508. Incidence ~2–4/1000 live births. Usually occur 12–48hr after delivery. Can be generalized or focal, and tonic, clonic, or myoclonic. Subtle seizure patterns (lip-smacking, limb-cycling, eye deviation, apnoeas, etc.) can be difficult to identify or differentiate from other benign conditions that may mimic seizures:

- Startle or Moro reflexes;
- Normal 'jittery' movements (fine, fast limb movements that are abated by holding affected limb);
- Sleep myoclonus (REM movements).

A large proportion of clinically diagnosed seizures are not associated with electrical seizure activity and many electrical seizures do not manifest clinically.

Causes

- *Brain injury:*
  - hypoxic ischaemic encephalopathy (HIE);
  - intracranial haemorrhage;
  - cerebral infarction (ischaemic or haemorrhagic);
  - cerebral oedema;
  - birth trauma.
- *CNS infection:*
  - meningitis (e.g. GBS, coliforms);
  - encephalitis (e.g. HSV, CMV).
- *Cerebral malformation.*
- *Metabolic:*
  - hypoglycaemia;
  - hypo- or hypernatraemia;
  - hypocalcaemia, hypomagnesia;
  - pyridoxine dependent seizures;
  - non-ketotic hyperglycinaemia.
- *Neonatal withdrawal* from maternal medication or substance abuse.
- *Kernicterus* (📖 p.195).
- *Rare syndromes:*
  - benign familial neonatal seizures (autosomal dominant);
  - early myoclonic encephalopathy.

With improved access to neuroimaging, fewer infants are being categorized as 'benign' or 'idiopathic' seizures. Neonatal stroke is increasingly recognized.

Investigation and management

This should include family history, history of pregnancy and delivery, complete examination, evaluation for infection, serum electrolytes, calcium, magnesium, glucose, and blood gas. If available, cerebral function analysis monitoring (CFAM) should be commenced.

If appropriate, further investigation may include radiological evaluation, e.g. cranial MRI, toxicology screening, serum ammonia, urine organic acids, serum amino acids, karyotype, and TORCH screening.

Treatment of neonatal seizures

- *Immediate:* give O_2, maintain airway, insert IV, treat underlying cause. When to start anticonvulsants is controversial because risks and benefits of treatment have not been properly evaluated; usual indication is >3 seizures/hr or single seizure lasting >3–5min particularly if evidence of cardio-respiratory compromise.
- *First-line anticonvulsant:* IV phenobarbital (10–20mg/kg bolus; give further 10–15mg if seizures persist after 30min; maintenance dose 5mg/day).
- *Second-line* IV clonazepam, IV midazolam, or IV phenytoin.
- *For intractable seizures* consider therapeutic trial of parenteral pyridoxine (50mg). ☞ Depending on cause probably safe to stop treatment after a few days of no seizures, but many clinicians prefer to wait until several months before ceasing.

Prognosis

Prognosis varies with the cause of seizures, but is generally good for idiopathic seizures, sleep myoclonus, hypocalcemia, and benign familial neonatal seizures. There is a significant risk of adverse neurodevelopmental outcome after meningitis, HIE, hypoglycemia, cerebral infarction, hypo- or hypernatraemia, cerebral malformations, kernicterus, and some inborn errors of metabolism.

The floppy infant

See also 📖 pp.538–547 and p.944. It is often helpful to divide causes into those that are 'central' involving the CNS (so-called 'floppy strong') and 'peripheral' involving lower motor neurons, neuromuscular junction (NMJ), or primary muscle disease ('floppy weak').

Range of clinical features

- *Common to 'central' and 'peripheral' diseases*: generalized hypotonia; 'frog-leg' posture; respiratory failure; obstetric problems (e.g. polyhydramnios due to impaired swallowing, breech presentation); HIE.
- *Central conditions*: encephalopathy; dysmorphism; reasonable muscle strength; ↑ or normal tendon reflexes.
- *Peripheral causes*: normal conscious level; muscle signs (weakness, myotonia, fasciculations, or fatiguing); ↓ or normal tendon reflexes; little facial expression; micrognathia; high arched palate; ptosis; undescended testes; limb contracture/deformities (severe is arthrogryposis multiplex congenital); hip dislocation.

Management

- *Exclude severe systemic illness*: e.g. sepsis that requires prompt treatment.
- *Treat any respiratory failure* with O_2 or ventilatory support as required.
- *Examine* for above clinical features to help distinguish cause. Examine both parents for possible disease, e.g. maternal myasthenia gravis or myotonic dystrophy (possibly undiagnosed!).
- *Elicit family history* (e.g. maternal myotonic dystrophy); antenatal history (e.g. polyhydramnios).
- *'Central' cause*: consider—blood glucose; U&E; Ca^{2+}; Mg^{2+}; septic screen; ESR/CRP; TFT; karyotype; cranial ultrasound; CT/MRI; EEG; IEM screen; maternal drug screen; genetics opinion if dysmorphic.
- *'Peripheral' cause*: consider—serum creatinine phosphokinase; specific cytogenetics (e.g. myotonic dystrophy); electromyogram (EMG), nerve conduction studies; muscle or sural nerve biopsy; muscle ultrasound; edrophonium 20micrograms/kg test dose → followed 30s later (if no adverse reaction) with 80micrograms/kg IV (causes dramatic improvement in some forms of myasthenia gravis); echocardiogram (storage diseases).
- *Spinal cord damage (rare)*: consider in the infant who has a flaccid paralysis from birth. Associated with rotational forceps delivery. Immobilize neck. Seek specialist advice. MRI.
- Refer to paediatric neurologist.

Prognosis

Causation-dependent (see Box 6.1) and very variable. Some causes are fatal, e.g. type 1 SMA.

Box 6.1 Causes

'Floppy strong' or 'central' involving CNS
- Prematurity
- HIE
- Hypoglycaemia
- Sepsis
- Electrolyte disturbance
- Drug-related
- IEM
- Hypothyroidism
- Chromosomal disorders (e.g. trisomy 21)
- CNS malformations
- Benign congenital hypotonia
- Underlying syndrome (e.g. Prader–Willi syndrome)
- Cervical spinal cord trauma (birth injury)

'Floppy weak' or 'peripheral' involving lower neurology, NMJ, or primary muscle disease
- Spinal muscular atrophy (SMA), particularly type 1 (previously known as Werdnig–Hoffman disease)
- Myasthenia gravis (transient or congenital)
- Congenital myotonic dystrophy (autosomal dominant inheritance from mother)
- Congenital muscular dystrophies
- Congenital myopathies
- Metabolic myopathies
- Peripheral neuropathies
- Spinal cord injury

Hydrops foetalis

Abnormal accumulation of fluid in skin and body compartments. Results from rate of production of interstitial fluid exceeding absorption.

Characterized in the foetus by:
- Gross generalized oedema;
- Ascites;
- Pleural ± pericardial effusions.

If still present at birth, it results in severe illness. Incidence ~1/2500 to 1/4000 births.

Causes

Hydrops is due to underlying disease, singularly or in combination resulting in: ↑ capillary hydrostatic pressure; ↓ colloid osmotic pressure; lymphatic obstruction; capillary leaking (see Box 6.2 for summary).

> **Box 6.2 Some causes of hydrops foetalis**
>
> *Immune*
> Haemolytic disease of the newborn: alloimmune, Rh, Kell, other.
>
> *Non-immune*
> - Cardiac:
>   - *structure*—Ebsteins anomaly, *in-utero* closure of ductus arteriosus, hypoplastic left or right heart
>   - *arrythmia*—SVT, atrial flutter
>   - *cardiomyopathies*—TORCH or other viral infection
> - *Genetic:* Turners, Trisomy (21,13,18, etc.)
> - *Foetal anaemia:* twin-twin transfusion, α Thalassaemia, foeto-maternal haemorrhage
> - *Infection:* TORCH, Parvovirus B19
> - *Malformation:* congenital cystic adenomatoid malformation (CCAM), bowel atresia
> - AV malformation
> - Lymphatic (cystic hygroma)
> - Idiopathic

Associated complications
- Intrauterine/perinatal death.
- Obstetric complications, e.g. shoulder dystocia.
- Preterm labour.
- Pulmonary hypoplasia (pleural effusions).
- Perinatal asphyxia.

Management

Disorders treatable antenatally
- Intrauterine blood transfusion (IUT) for haemolytic disease/parvovirus infection
- Anti-arrhythmia drugs to treat foetal SVT
- Laser ablation of foetal vessels (twin-twin transfusion syndrome)

Birth planning
Before birth organize expert help
- If anaemia likely, have available fresh CMV −ve, O −ve blood, irradiated (if previous IUT), cross-matched blood against the mother
- Prepare for full resuscitation, ventilation, UVC insertion, paracentesis (ascites), or pleural effusion drainage

Neonatal management
- Resuscitation:
  - ventilation, intubation
  - paracentesis, thoracentesis
  - blood transfusion or partial exchange transfusion
- Supportive management:
  - cardiac support—pressors, ionotropes
  - respiratory support—mechanical ventilation
  - chest tube placement, drainage of ascites
  - fluid and electrolyte management
  - treatment of anemia: blood transfusion or partial exchange
  - transfusion
  - treatment of infections
  - octreotide to treat chylothorax and ascites

Prognosis
For foetuses or infants with non-immune hydrops, the survival rates are variable, in the range of 50%. Higher survival is reported in infants with SVT, chylothorax, and parvovirus infections, and lower rates in those with chromosomal abnormalities. Survival rates with immune hydrops is > 80%. Neurodevelopmental outcome depends on cause.

Routine care of the newborn

Routine measurements

Measure within 1hr of birth:
- Weight (term mean ~3.5kg);
- Head circumference (mean ~35cm);
- Body length (mean ~50cm).

Usually babies are not weighed again until day 3–5 and then alternate daily whilst they remain in hospital. It is normal to lose weight after birth due to water loss, but weight loss should not exceed 10% of birth weight. Birth weight should generally be regained by day 7. Subsequent mean growth is 20–30g/day until age 6mths.

Vitamin K (phytomenadione)

To prevent haemorrhagic disease of the newborn, vitamin K_1 is routinely given within 48hr of birth.

Dose 1mg IM (preferred) in term infants or alternatively 2mg orally on days 1 *and* 7, and, if breastfeeding, *also* on day 28.

Cord care

Immediately after birth clamp the cord with a purpose-made device. Keep the umbilicus clean and dry. Antibiotic powders or sprays are not routinely required. The cord usually detaches after 7–10 days. If umbilical granulomas develop, clean with alcohol wipes and consider chemical cautery (silver nitrate stick).

Thermal care

Babies should be delivered in a warm room, rapidly dried with a warm towel, and then immediately wrapped or placed skin to skin on the mother's front and then covered with a warm towel and a hat.

Routine observations

Record soon after birth and then daily whilst in hospital. Mean pulse is 120–160beats/min, respiratory rate 35–45breaths/min, and temperature 36.9 C. Infants should be nursed in an ambient temperature of 20–22 C.

Bathing

Not required until day 2 or 3. Use tepid water. Genitalia should be cleaned superficially only. Do not retract foreskin; it is attached to the glans.

Biochemical screening

In the UK, all infants should undergo a screening heel prick blood test placed on a specific card between day 3 and 10 ('Guthrie' test). Regional variation exists, but commonly screened diseases include:
- Phenylketonuria (↑ phenylalanine); congenital hypothyroidism(↑ TSH); cystic fibrosis (↑ immune-reactive trypsin).
- Medium chain acetyl-CoA deficiency.
- Sickle cell disease.

Positive tests require follow-up and more detailed testing.

Newborn hearing screening

All infants in the UK will have their hearing screened (otoacoustic emission—OAE) within the first 4wks of life. Automatic auditory brainstem response (AABR) testing is carried out if any uncertainty in OAE response.

Neonatal immunization

See also 📖 pp.728–729. In several countries hepatitis B immunization of all newborns is recommended. In the UK, immunization is only offered to infants of seropositive mothers. Similarly, in the UK, Bacille Calmette–Guérin (BCG) should be offered to babies born to parents of ethnic groups or communities with a high incidence of close contact with a sputum-positive case for tuberculosis (TB).

Milk feeding

Methods
- Bottle.
- Tube feeding (if too ill/immature to suck).
  - Naso/oro-gastic tube.
  - Silastic naso-jejunal tube (severe gastro-oesophageal reflux (GOR), aspiration, or recurrent apnoeas).
  - Gastrostomy (if required long term, older children).

Breastfeeding
Breast feeding is a learned skill for both mother and baby. Establishing feeding can take time, and it is vital that good support is available (breast feeding advisors or midwifes with appropriate training).

Advantages
- ↓ Maternal post partum haemorrhage.
- *Mild* maternal contraceptive effect.
- ↑ Bonding.
- ↓ Maternal breast cancer risk.
- Cheap.
- ↓ Infant mortality (less relevant in developed world).
- ↓ GI and respiratory infection rate.
- ↓ Later autoimmune disease incidence (e.g. type I diabetes mellitus, atopic diseases).
- ↑ later IQ.

Problems
- Cracked/sore nipples.
- Maternal anxiety (breast fed babies can gain weight slower than their bottle-fed couterparts—give reassurance and support).
- Small risk of hypernatraemic dehydration if low milk intake (suspect if weight loss >10%).

Contraindications
- +ve maternal HIV status (in developed countries).
- Certain maternal medications (e.g. amiodarone).
- Maternal herpes zoster over breast.
- Infantile galactosaemia or phenylketonuria (PKU).
- Primary lactose intolerance (very rare).

Expressed breast milk (EBM)
Usually mother's own breast milk, but some units have donor breast milk banks which can be of value, particularly in extreme preterm infants.

EBM is usually used to establish feeding in preterm infants, but is also useful when top-up feeds are required, if mother and baby are separated for any reason, or if there are other maternal problems e.g. cracked/sore nipples or breast engorgement.

Once expressed, can refrigerate and use within 24–48hr, or freeze and use for up to 3mths.

Formula milk

Normal volume required is 150mL/kg/day. See Box 6.3 for different types of formula milk available.

Advantages
• Paternal involvement.
• Milk intake determined.

Problems
• Constipation.
• Oral thrush.
• Milk bezoars.

> ### Box 6.3 Types of formula milk available
>
> • *Cow's milk formula:* standard milk used. Extensively modified, e.g. to ↓ solute load, ↑ iron and vitamins. Formula used from birth is predominantly whey protein, whilst 'follow on' milks (for 'hungrier' infants >6mths old) are predominantly casein-based
> • *Soya milk:* previously recommended for cow's milk protein allergy or lactose intolerance, but use **not** now recommended due to high levels of phyto-oestrogens and availability of other alternatives
> • *Hydrolysed cow's milk formula:* e.g. Nutramigen®. Contains short peptides. Indicated for prophylaxis or treatment of cow's or soya milk protein allergy.
> • *Elemental formulas:* e.g. Neocate®. Cow's milk protein is fully hydrolysed to amino acids. Indicated for severe milk protein allergy or malabsorption.
> • In addition, many specialized formula milks exist for conditions such as: preterm/LBW infants; gastro-oesophageal reflux (thickened with cornstarch); metabolic diseases; lactose intolerance (lactose-free milk); poor growth (high energy formulas); malabsorption, e.g. Pregestimil®.

Trophic feeding (gut-priming)

The term describes practice of feeding small milk volumes (0.5–1mL/kg/hr of EBM) to enhance gut structure and function in infants too ill or immature to tolerate substantive milk feeds. Evidence suggests that in the preterm infant it improves GI motility and function, as well as achieving clinical outcomes of ↑ weight gain, ↑ head growth, ↓ infection risk, and improved later milk tolerance.

Routine neonatal examination

Each baby must be examined at least once in the first week, usually on day 1 after birth. Such child health surveillance can be done by a hospital paediatrician, advanced neonatal nurse practitioner, general practitioner, or specially trained midwife/nurse.

Purpose
- Maternal reassurance.
- Health education; explaining common variations.
- Detecting asymptomatic problems, e.g. congenital heart disease, DDH.
- Screening for rare, but serious conditions.

Order of examination
- *Attending midwife:* ask if there are any concerns or problems.
- *Mother:* check patient notes for relevant details of the maternal medical history, family history, antenatal and obstetric history, and social history. Ask about feeding and whether baby has passed meconium/urine.
- *Baby:* when baby is <u>quiet</u> (if needed use calming techniques like pacifiers, sucking a clean finger, examination after a feed) note:
  - general posture and movements;
  - skin colour;
  - listen to the heart and lungs;
  - examine the eyes for size, strabismus (📖 pp.908–910);
  - using an ophthalmoscope examine the eyes for bilateral red reflexes to exclude cataract or retinoblastoma (see 📖 pp.614, 916).

The remaining examination should proceed as described in the box opposite.

Rest of routine neonatal examination

The baby should be completely undressed. Examination proceeds as follows in head to toe order:

- *Cranium:* measure maximum occipital-frontal circumference (normal 33–37cm at term), assess skull shape, fontanelle positions, tension, and size (anterior may be up to 4cm x 4cm, posterior 1cm)
- *Face:* assess any dysmorphism, nose, chin size. Inspect mouth. Visualize and palpate palate for possible clefts
- *Ears:* assess position, size, shape, and external meatus patency
- *Neck:* inspect and assess movements; palpate clavicles.
- *Chest:* assess shape, symmetry, nipple position, respiratory rate (normal 40–60/min), pattern, and effort. Palpate precordium and apex beat
- *Abdomen:* inspect shape and umbilical stump. Check for inguinal hernias. Palpate for masses, liver (normally palpable up to 2cm below costal margin), spleen (normally palpable up to 1cm), kidneys (normally palpable), bladder
- *Genitalia:*
  - girls—inspect (N.B. the clitoris and labia are normally large)
  - boys—assess size, shape, position of urinary meatus; palpate for descended testes (N.B. retractile testes are normal)
- Palpate the *femoral pulses* (absence or weakness may indicate aortic arch abnormalities)
- *Anus:* assess position and patency
- *Spine:* inspect for deformity and sacral naevi/dimple/pit/hair patch/ lipoma/pigmentation (may indicate underlying abnormality);
- *Limbs:* assess symmetry, shape, passive and active movements, digit number and shape. Assess palmar creases. Examine hips for DDH (see 📖 p.748)
- *CNS:* in addition to evaluation of above: assess tone during handling, pulling baby to sitting position by holding wrists, and ventral suspension (baby should be able to hold head almost horizontally), check moro reflex (symmetrical?) (see 📖 p.558)
- Finally, check that urine and meconium were passed within the first 24hr

Normal variations and minor abnormalities

Skin

- *Vernix:* normal 'cheesy' white substance on skin at birth.
- *Peripheral cyanosis:* normal in first few days after birth.
- *Post-mature skin:* dry peeling skin, prone to cracking, common in post-mature babies. Resolves, but topical emollients often beneficial.

Head

- *Skull moulding:* overriding skull bones with palpable ridges are part of moulding and are harmless. Resolves within 2–3 days.
- *Pre-auricular pits, skin tags, or accessory auricles:* usually isolated, but can be associated with hearing loss or other abnormalities. Test hearing and consider surgical referral for cosmetic reasons.
- *Caput succedaneum, chignon, and cephalhaematoma:* see 📖 p.126.

Eyes

- Blocked lacrimal duct leads to recurrent sticky eye; responds to regular eye toilet until ducts open. This may persist for months, but only consider surgery if >12mths. If purulent then secondary bacterial conjunctivitis is likely. Take swab for M, C&S (including swab for chlamydia). Treat with antibiotic eye drops (see also 📖 p.918).
- *Subconjunctival haemorrhage:* associated with precipitate deliveries or cord around the neck. Harmless and resolves within a few weeks.

Mouth

- *Epstein's pearls:* self-resolving white inclusion cysts on palate/gums.
- *Tongue-tie:* shortened tongue frenulum (see 📖 p.882).
- *Ranula:* self-resolving bluish mouth floor swelling (mucus retention cyst).
- *Oral candidiasis (thrush):* mucosal white flecks and erythema. Treat with oral antifungal, e.g. nystatin suspension 1mL 6-hourly.

Heart

See 📖 p.228. Murmurs are detected in 1–2% of all newborns, but only ~1 in12 will represent congenital heart disease.

If murmur heard, evaluate in context of other clinical findings (cyanosis, signs of heart failure, peripheral pulses). An innocent heart murmur is likely

- Murmur is grade 1–2/6, systolic, not harsh, loudest at the left sternal edge.
- Remaining cardiovascular examination is normal.

Good evidence exists to support the use of pre and post-ductal saturation readings (right arm = pre, foot = post) as part of assessment of a pathological murmur. ECG and 4-limb BP should also be performed. Echocardiography should be obtained in infants where there is clinical concern.

If murmur persists in an otherwise well infant, in whom no echocardiography has been performed, then arrange for repeat examination in a few days to weeks and consider referral for cardiac assessment.

Umbilicus

See also 📖 pp.874–875.

- *Umbilical hernia:* protuberant swelling involving the umbilicus. Rarely strangulates and almost all spontaneously resolve within 12mths.
- *Single umbilical artery:* usually isolated and of no significance, but can be associated with several syndromes and IUGR.

Genitalia

- *Undescended testes:* differentiate from retractile testes (can be 'persuaded' into the scrotum). If still undescended at 1yr refer to a surgeon (see 📖 p.878).
- *Hydrocele:* common and most resolve by a year. If persists refer to a surgeon (see 📖 p.868).
- *Vaginal mucoid or bloody discharge:* due to maternal oestrogen withdrawal. Almost always spontaneously resolves.
- *Vaginal/hymenal skin tags:* spontaneously shrink (📖 p.881).
- Inguinal hernias can rarely be present from birth. Refer to a surgeon. N.B. There is a relatively high likelihood of strangulation/incarceration.

Limbs

- *Single palmar crease:* found in ~2% of normal babies. May be associated with chromosomal abnormalities, e.g. trisomy 21.
- *Polydactyly:* can be isolated or associated with other abnormalities. Refer to a surgeon.
- *Syndactyly:* most common between the second and third toes. Often familial. If toes only are affected require no treatment.
- *Postural deformities:* common, especially after oligohydramnios or malpresentation, e.g. breech. Positional talipes is usually equinovarus or calcaneovalgus. If affected joint can easily be massaged back to normal neutral position, deformity will rapidly resolve. If fixed (structural) refer to orthopaedic surgeon/physiotherapist. These children are also at increased risk of DDH (see 📖 p.748).

Miscellaneous

- *Jaundice:* see 📖 pp.130–131.
- *Sacral coccygeal pits:* require no action if within natal cleft. Higher pits require spinal imaging.
- *Breast swelling:* almost always due to maternal hormones and may lactate. Spontaneously resolves over several weeks. If does not resolve then endocrinology investigation is warranted.

Newborn fluid and electrolyte balance

Normal

- The newborn baby is largely water (~75% term, ~85% at 26/40).
- There is a large extracellular compartment (65% of body weight at 26/40 compared to 40% by term, 20% in adult).
- There is a rapid loss of extracellular fluid after birth.
- Decreased pulmonary vascular resistance increases blood flow to left atrium, thereby inducing increased Atrial Natriuretic Peptide release (↑ GFR/↓ Na^+ reabsorbtion/ ↓ rennin-angiotensin aldosterone system).
- Physiological increased urine output at ~12–24hr after birth.
- Na/K ATPase activity is low at birth, but increases steadily (Na/K ATPase is responsible for reabsorbing Na+ from renal tubular lumen, in turn creating a gradient to allow reabsorption of Glucose, Na^+ and amino acids. Immature infants have lower enzyme activity.

Preterm babies have

- A variable ability to excrete a sodium load.
- An excellent ability to deal with water load.
- Modulated by ADH (osmo and baro-receptors).
- A tendency to lose sodium in urine over first weeks as the increased glomerular filtration rate (GFR) exceeds ability to resorb Na^+.
- A high transepidermal water loss (TEWL). Evaporation from immature skin, <28/40. To reduce nurse in incubator with 80% humidity
- Respiration related water losses (ventilated and spontaneously breathing infants) can be countered with warm-humidified gases.
- Sick infants (e.g. respiratory distress syndrome (RDS)) will have delayed dieresis;
    - giving additional Na^+ will further delay diuresis and may worsen outcome;
    - attempts to induce diuresis (e.g. with Furosemide) unlikely to be helpful.

Postnatal weight loss

- Weight loss after birth is normal;
    - up to 10 % in well term infants over the first week of life;
    - greater in preterm/VLBW.
- Rising sodium suggests dehydration (term and preterm infants).
- Failure to lose weight may suggest fluid retention/overload.
- Infants with >10% weight loss require further assessment of feeding;
    - risk of hypernatraemic dehydration;
    - usually breast-fed infants with unrecognized poor feeding;
    - weigh all babies day 3 (some suggest day 5);
    - check U&E if weight loss >12%;
    - support mother with breast expressing/top-up feeds;
    - may require admission/NG feeds/IV fluids

Specific disturbances

Hyponatraemia
- Na^+ < 130mmol/L.
- *Causes:*
  - water overload (most common in first-week);
  - maternal fluid overload;
  - iatrogenic;
  - sick infant (e.g. birth asphyxia, sepsis);
  - excess renal loss (common 'late' cause in preterm infants);
  - GI loss, e.g. diarrhoea, NG aspirates, high output stoma;
  - drainage of ascites/CSF;
  - other (e.g. hypoadrenalism of any cause, Bartter syndrome/Fanconi syndrome).
- *Symptoms:* irritability, apnoeas, seizures.
- *Treatment:* dependent on underlying cause (e.g. fluid restriction/ Na^+ supplementation)
- Take care as too rapid correction can cause neurological damage.

Hypernatraemia
- Risk of seizures if Na^+ >150mmol/L.
- *Causes:* water depletion (usual), excess Na^+ administration (unusual as normally retain water also).
- *Two major at-risk groups:*
  - extreme preterm infants in first days of life (excess water losses, e.g. TEWL);
  - breast-fed infants with poor intake (see 📖 p.142).
- *Treatment:* increase fluid intake (caution with rapid correction).

Hypokalaemia
- K^+ <2.5mmol/L—causes:
  - excess losses (diarrhoea, vomiting, NG aspirate, stoma, renal/ diuretics);
  - inadequate intake (failure to recognize daily requirement, e.g. TPN).
- *Correct with supplementation (IV or enteral):*
  - caution with enteral if GI disturbance;
  - extreme caution with IV infusion as risk of heart arrythmia.

Hyperkalaemia
- K^+ >7.5mmol/L OR >6.5mmol/L and ECG changes.
- *Causes:* Failure of K^+ excretion, e.g. renal failure.
- *Treatments:*
  - myocardial stabilization: calcium gluconate;
  - elimination: calcium resonium, dialysis;
  - re-distribution: salbutamol, insulin.

Respiratory distress syndrome

RDS refers to lung disease caused by surfactant deficiency. The disease is largely seen in preterm infants. RDS is rare >32wks gestation.

Causes

Surfactant deficiency causes alveolar collapse, increased work of breathing and hypoxia (due to intrapulmonary shunting of blood). Increased risk of RDS is associated with CS delivery; hypothermia; perinatal hypoxia; meconium aspiration; congenital pneumonia; maternal diabetes mellitus; past family history (see 📖 p.152).

Presentation

Cyanosis, tachypnoea, chest in drawing, grunting within 4hr of birth. If untreated, the disease worsens over 48–72hr and then (depending on severity) resolves over 5–7 days.

Investigations

- *CXR* (📖 p.156): bilateral, diffuse 'ground-glass' appearance (generalized atelectasis), airway bronchograms, reduced lung volume (see Fig. 6.3).
- SpO_2 monitoring and blood gases.

Management

- Good delivery room resuscitation. This may involve intubation and administration of surfactant (extremely preterm) or nasal CPAP.
- Respiratory support will depend on the severity. May need O_2, nasal CPAP (📖 p.160), or ventilation (📖 pp.162–165).
- Surfactant (Curosurf ® or Survanta®) requires intubation and ventilation, and should be considered in all extremely preterm (<27/40) infants and when oxygen requirement exceeds 30–40%.
  - given as bolus down ETT;
  - give 2nd dose if oxygen requirement remains high (FiO_2>0.3);
  - further doses are sometimes required.
- *Antibiotics*: e.g. penicillin and gentamicin, until congenital pneumonia has been excluded, as it can mimic or coexist with RDS.
- *Nutrition*: use IV fluids until the baby is stable. Then start gastric tube feeds with minimal volumes and slowly increase as tolerated. If unstable, start parenteral nutrition after 24–48hr.

Prognosis

The majority have a good recovery. Mortality is 5–10% and depends on severity and gestation. Bronchopulmonary dysplasia may develop (~15% of cases, inversely proportional to gestational age).

Prevention

- Corticosteroids (betamethasone/dexamethasone, 2 doses, 12-hourly) given to mother 1–7 days before birth decreases incidence and mortality by 40%. Maximum benefit 24hr after first dose and lasts 7 days.
- Treat co-existing morbidities that inhibit surfactant production developing, e.g. hypothermia, acidosis, infection.

Acute respiratory diseases

All of the diseases presented below have signs of respiratory distress (📖 p.150). Cerebral hypoxia, congenital heart disease, and metabolic acidosis can induce respiratory distress (suspect if CXR is normal).

Transient tachypnoea of the newborn (TTN)
- Caused by delayed clearance/absorption of lung fluid after birth.
- Presents within 4hr after birth. Common after elective CS. CXR: shows streaky perihilar changes and fluid in lung horizontal fissures.
- Treatment: supplemental O_2. Consider nasal CPAP and antibiotics.
- Spontaneously resolves within 24hr.

Congenital pneumonia
- Caused by aspiration of infected amniotic fluid.
- Associated with prolonged rupture of membranes (PROM), chorioamnionitis, foetal hypoxia.
- Usually group B streptococci, *Escherichia coli*, other Gram –ve bacteria, listeria, chlamydia.
- Presents in first 24hr. CXR: patchy shadowing and consolidation.
- *Respiratory support*: antibiotics (benzylpenicillin, or ampicillin if listeria, and gentamicin) after septic screen; chest physiotherapy.
- *Prognosis*: depends on severity and associated sepsis or persistent pulmonary hypertension of newborn (PPHN).

Meconium aspiration syndrome (MAS) (1–5/1000 live births)
- 5% of term infants with meconium-stained liquor develop MAS.
- Hypoxia results in gasping and meconium passage *in utero*, a combination that leads to aspiration. Meconium aspiration inhibits surfactant, obstructs the respiratory tract, and induces pneumonitis.
- Presents with respiratory distress soon after birth. Associated with pulmonary air leaks and PPHN. CXR: generalized lung over inflation with patchy collapse/consolidation +/– air leaks.
- *Prevention*: if liquor is meconium-stained, delivery should be expedited to prevent further hypoxia and gasping. If baby is apnoeic at birth, visualize the larynx and suck out any meconium from larynx/trachea. Tracheal suction is <u>not</u> recommended for vigorous infants.
- *Treatment*: supplemental O_2; intermittent positive pressure ventilation (IPPV) or high frequency oscillatory ventilation (HFOV) if ventilation required; surfactant; antibiotics (since listeria can cause antenatal meconium passage); treat any PPHN (📖 p.168); consider ECMO if severe.
- *Prognosis*: mortality <5%. Survivors do well, but there is ↑ risk of asthma and, if extracorporeal membrane oxygenation (ECMO) is needed, neurological sequelae.

Pulmonary air leaks
Commonly secondary to other respiratory disease (e.g. RDS, MAS) or to assisted ventilation.

Pneumothorax
Spontaneous pneumothorax occurs in ~2% term infants. Incidence is increased in prematurity and respiratory disease.
- *Features:* majority are small, asymptomatic, and resolve spontaneously. If large, present with respiratory distress. Tension pneumothorax (see 📖 p.214) is life-threatening (signs: respiratory distress, cyanosis, mediastinal shift away from affected side, ↓ chest movement and air entry on affected side, transillumination lights up affected side).
- *CXR:* shows ipsilateral translucency, lack of peripheral lung markings, collapsed lung (see Fig. 6.4).
- *Treatment:* none if asymptomatic. Give O_2 as required. If symptoms are severe or worsening, insert chest drain (📖 p.214). In emergency, perform needle aspiration before chest drain.
- *Prognosis:* excellent in term infants. Mortality is doubled in infants with RDS. Also ↑ risk of periventricular haemorrhage in preterms.

Pulmonary interstitial emphysema (PIE)
Air leak into lung parenchyma results in small airway and alveolar collapse. Follows high IPPV, particularly in preterm infants with severe RDS or MAS.
- *Signs:* respiratory distress; chest hyperexpansion; poor air entry; coarse inspiratory crackles.
- *CXR* (📖 p.157): hyperinflation; 'honeycomb' pattern of cystic lucencies/bullae, generalized or local (see Fig. 6.5).
- *Treatment:* high FiO_2, low PIP, low PEEP, fast rate IPPV; HFOV may be superior. Unilateral PIE: nurse infant with affected side down. In refractory cases consider selective intubation to ventilate the healthier lung.
- *Prognosis:* mortality 25–50%. There is an increased risk of bronchopulmonary dysplasia.

Pneumomediastinum
Often preceded by asymptomatic pneumothorax/PIE.
- *CXR:* translucency around the heart extending superiorly; thymus lifted and splayed from below ('sail' sign).
- *Treatment:* usually no treatment is required.

Pneumopericardium: usually occurs with other air leaks associated with IPPV and can lead to cardiac tamponade (with quiet heart sounds, hypotension, bradycardia, cyanosis).
- *CXR:* translucency around the borders of a small heart.
- *Treatment:* urgent needle drainage inserted under the xiphisternum.
- *Prognosis:* high mortality if symptomatic.

Pneumoperitoneum Air can occasionally track into the peritoneum from a pulmonary air leak. AXR confirms the diagnosis. Severe abdominal distention could impair ventilation. Drain if symptomatic.

Massive pulmonary haemorrhage (1/1000 live births)
Usually due to haemorrhagic pulmonary oedema in VLBW infants. Small bleeds are associated with tracheal trauma from ETT or suction. It is associated with: PDA, heart failure, PIE, hydrops foetalis, perinatal hypoxia, sepsis, coagulopathy, fluid overload, surfactant therapy.

Signs
- Rapid systemic collapse.
- Profuse bloodstained fluid welling up from upper airway.
- Respiratory crackles on auscultation.
- CXR. Virtual 'white out'. Consider echocardiography to detect PDA.

Treatment
- ↑ O_2 and ventilatory pressures.
- Frequent endotracheal suction.
- Correct hypovolaemia and coagulopathy.
- Consider blood transfusion.
- Consider surfactant.
- Treat known associations.

Milk aspiration

Term infants can accidentally aspirate a feed. The usual causes are:
- Swallowing incoordination, e.g. preterm, neurological disease.
- Upper airway or oesophageal disorders, e.g. tracheo-oesophageal fistula, gastro-oesophageal reflux.

Presentation
Sudden choking or respiratory distress during or after a feed, often with excessive milk in the mouth, or aspiration pneumonia.

CXR: normal or patchy collapse/consolidation in the upper lobes.

Treatment If well, observe only. If unwell, respiratory support and broad spectrum antibiotics are needed. Investigate cause and use gastric or naso-jejunal tube feeding. Period of IV fluids or feeding may be necessary.

Apnoea

Apnoea can result from any severe illness.

Management
- Support respiration.
- Investigate and correct primary cause.

Apnoea of prematurity
- Common below 34wks gestation (incidence ↑ as gestation ↓).
- Between episodes the infant is well.
- Consider and exclude other diagnoses (see 📖 pp.48, 128).

Treatment Tactile stimulation, blood transfusion, continuous tube gastric feeds, caffeine or theophylline, nasal CPAP, or IPPV.

Prognosis Short-lived apnoeas appear to cause no harm and should resolve by 34wks gestation.

Neonatal X-rays

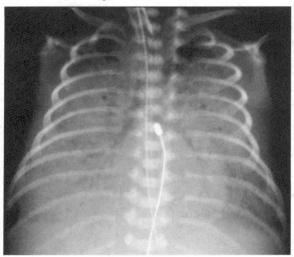

Fig. 6.3 Respiratory distress syndrome. Bilateral, diffuse 'ground-glass' appearance (due to generalized atelectasis), airway bronchograms, reduced lung volume.

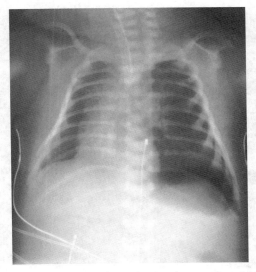

Fig. 6.4 Left tension pneumothorax. Left chest hyperlucency and hyperinflation, collapsed left lung (absence of peripheral lung markings), mediastinum shifted to the right.

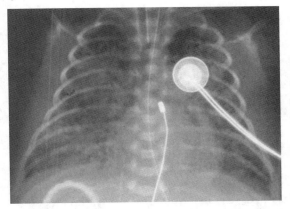

Fig. 6.5 Pulmonary interstitial emphysema. Bilateral lung hyperinflation (hyperlucency and downward displacement of diaphragm) with multiple radiolucent cystic areas. PIE may be unilateral. Isolated large bullae may appear. Cardiac compression may occur.

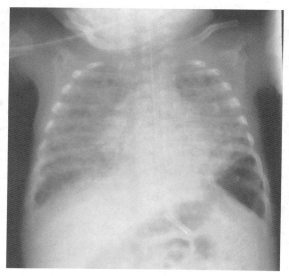

Fig. 6.6 Bronchopulmonary dysplasia. Hyperexpansion, diffuse patchy collapse and fibrosis interspersed by radiolucent cystic areas and area of emphysema in left lower lung.

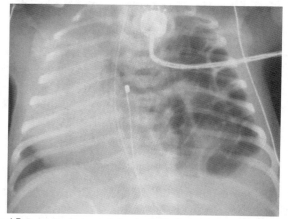

Fig. 6.7 Congenital diaphragmatic hernia. Air-filled bowels loops fill left hemithorax with absence of left lung markings and mediastinal shift to the right.

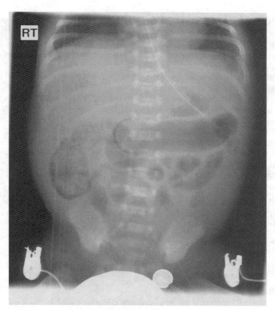

Fig. 6.8 Necrotizing enterocolitis. Dilated loops of thick walled bowel and pathognomonic appearance of gas in the gut wall (pneumatosis intestinalis) evident in the left lower abdomen (gut seen side on) and centre (gut seen end on – 'halo sign'). Gas evident in the portal venous system may also be seen and indicates severe disease (not present on this X-ray).

Neonatal respiratory support

Supplemental oxygen

Excess oxygen is toxic, particularly in preterm infants. All infants receiving supplemental oxygen should have SpO_2 monitoring as a minimum. If significant hypoxia, consider an arterial line to directly monitor PaO_2. Term infant's oxygen saturation levels should be >95% in air—usually ≥97%. ●
The 'correct' saturation range for preterm (≤32/40, ≤1500g) infants has not been determined. Maintaining SpO_2 around 90–95% and avoidance of 'swings' in either saturation or FiO_2 is reasonable whilst evidence from large RCTs is awaited. Supplemental oxygen can be given via:

- Head box (concentration easily monitored).
- Nasal cannula <2L/min (cannot monitor effective FiO_2—depends on gas flow rate, FiO_2 and tidal volume, can't humidify effectively).
- High flow nasal cannula >2L/min. Can be effectively humidified. Generates CPAP effect.

CPAP Prevents airway collapse and loss of lung volume. Maintenance of functional residual capacity above closing volume reduces work of breathing.

Uses

- RDS and respiratory support, particularly for preterm infants.
- Post-extubation.
- In upper airway obstruction.

Method

- Nasal mask or binasal prongs, rarely face mask or via ETT.
- Usual pressure is 5–6cmH$_2$O. Probable safe upper level is 8cmH$_2$O, but ↑ risk of pulmonary air leaks as pressure ↑.
- Some equipment can deliver bi-level CPAP with or without synchronization to spontaneous breaths.

Complications

- Pulmonary air leaks, e.g. pneumothorax. (particularly if treating RDS in an infant who has not received surfactant).
- Nasal trauma.
- Baby upset leading to hypoxia.
- ↑ Airway resistance and effort of breathing.
- Upper GI distension or perforation (insert gastric tube on free drainage to reduce risk, rarely seen with modern equipment).

Positive pressure ventilation

Intermittent positive pressure ventilation (IPPV) See 📖 p.162.

High frequency oscillatory ventilation (HFOV) See 📖 p.164.

Synchronized ventilation

Nomenclature confusing, but includes the following:

- *Synchronized intermittent positive pressure ventilation (SIPPV)/assist control/patient-triggered ventilation (PTV)*: every spontaneous patient breath can trigger time-limited positive pressure inflation.

- *Synchronized intermittent mandatory ventilation (SIMV)*: rate of triggered breaths are pre-set; any other spontaneous patient breaths are unassisted—in case of apnoea the set rate is given.
- *Pressure support:* all spontaneous breaths are supported by positive pressure for as long as inspiratory flow continues above a defined threshold. Can be combined with other modes.

Studies in newborn infants show no particular advantage for SIPPV or SIMV compared to conventional IPPV during acute stages of respiratory illnesses such as RDS. May be useful during weaning, or if infant is not synchronizing with ventilator. Smaller infants may not be able to trigger breaths (older ventilators). Autocycling can cause over ventilation in PTV.

Extracorporeal life support (ECLS)
Provided only in a very small number of specialist centres in the UK. Also known as extracorporeal membrane oxygenation (ECMO), ECLS reduces mortality in severe respiratory disease, e.g. meconium aspiration syndrome, persistent pulmonary hypertension of the newborn.[1] Early transfer to an ECLS centre is important as these infants are often critically unwell.

Criteria for eligibility: severe, but reversible cardiac or respiratory disease and oxygenation index persistently >30–40 where:

$$\text{Oxygenation index} = [(\text{mean airway pressure} \times \text{FiO}_2)/\text{PaO}_2\,(\text{kPa})] \times 100$$

FiO_2 is expressed as a decimal, e.g. 30% O_2 = 0.3

Contraindications
- Weight <1.8kg.
- Gestation <34wks.
- Severe congenital malformation.
- Intracranial haemorrhage or poor CNS prognosis (e.g. severe HIE).
- Coagulopathy.

Technique
Blood taken from a major cannula is passed through a membrane oxygenator and then returned to the body. Blood is heparinized (activated clotting time 2–3 × normal) and low level conventional ventilation is maintained. ECMO is maintained until adequate recovery. May be:
- *Venous–venous:* double lumen cannula in right jugular vein or right atrium;
- *Venous–arterial:* blood drawn from right jugular vein and returned to right carotid artery.

Outcome Survival rates are high for reversible lung pathologies. Up to 10% of ECMO survivors suffer major long-term problems. Complications include brain injury (secondary to neck vessel trauma, thromboembolism, CNS haemorrhage, complication of pre-ECMO disease/therapy) and peripheral thromboembolic phenomenon, e.g. may cause renal failure.

Reference
1 UK Collaborative Trial Group (1996). UK collaborative randomised trial of neonatal extracorporeal membrane oxygenation. *Lancet* **348**: 75–82.

Conventional positive pressure ventilation

IPPV via ETT with continuous flow of heated and humidified gas allows the non-paralysed baby to breathe spontaneously. The ventilator is time-cycled, pressure limited (TCPL) where the user sets the positive inspiratory pressure (PIP), inspiration time (Ti) and ventilator rate. In this mode the tidal volume is determined by the lung compliance. Some ventilators can adjust PIP within a set range to deliver a set tidal volume (volume guarantee). Some ventilators can terminate inspiration when a set volume is reached or when inspiratory flow is declining below a threshold level. Whichever method is chosen the user must be familiar with the operation and limitations of the ventilator.

Indications
- Worsening respiratory failure, e.g. RDS.
- Impending or actual respiratory arrest from any cause.
- Recurrent apnoeas.
- Massive pulmonary haemorrhage.
- Severe cardiac failure.
- Persistent pulmonary hypertension of the newborn.
- Severe congenital lung malformation, e.g. diaphragmatic hernia.
- Severe HIE.
- Anaesthesia.

Ventilation parameters
- Peak inspiratory pressure (PIP).
- PEEP.
- TI and expiratory (TE) time (often expressed as I:E ratio).
- Inspired O_2% or fraction inspired O_2 (FiO_2).
- Gas flow (L/min) through ventilator circuit (may not be adjustable).

Monitoring ventilation
- Review and adjust ventilation settings soon after commencement (see Box 6.4 for care principles).
- Monitor blood gases and adjust ventilation as appropriate. Acceptable limits will depend on the clinical situation, however, as a guide in preterm infants; pH 7.2–7.35, PCO_2 5–8kPa, PO_2 6–10kPa, saturation 90–95%, expired tidal volume around 5mL/kg.
  - *If PaO_2 is too low*—↑ FiO_2 or ↑ mean airway pressure (the latter by either ↑ PIP, ↑ PEEP, or ↓ TE which will ↑ rate as TI stays constant). Do the opposite if PaO_2 is too high.
  - *If $PaCO_2$ is too high*—↑ alveolar ventilation, i.e. minute volume, by ↑ PIP, or ↓ PEEP, or ↑ rate. Do the opposite if $PaCO_2$ is too low.

Box 6.4 Care principles in assisted ventilation in newborns

Endotracheal tube (ETT) Use correct size and secure appropriately.

Elective intubation Give prior sedation with opiate, e.g. morphine or fentanyl, and muscle relaxant, e.g. suxamethonium (ONLY if staff experienced in airway management are present).

Minimal handling Reduces episodes of deterioration.

Sedation/analgesia Evidence does not support routine use of morphine infusion for ventilated preterm infants.

● Prolonged neuromuscular relaxation (e.g. Vecuronium)
- Consider in specific circumstances, e.g. severe meconium aspiration
- Give sedation/analgesia to paralysed infants, e.g. morphine infusion

Feeding Once stable, ventilation is not a contraindication to careful gastric feeding. Very ill babies may not tolerate feeding as gastric distension can cause diaphragmatic splinting.

Humidify and warm inspired gas

Minimal routine suctioning

Continue monitoring
- Pulse, BP, respiratory rate
- SpO_2, $\pm TcO_2$, $TcCO_2$
- Tidal volume
- Intermittent blood gas analysis (capillary or arterial)

Acute deterioration during ventilation

May present as systemic collapse, $\Downarrow PaO_2$, or $\Uparrow PaCO_2$. Ventilate with manual system, e.g. T-Piece (preferably with PEEP), and O_2 as required. Rapid improvement suggests ventilator problem. Otherwise consider obstructed ETT, displaced ETT, pneumothorax, or non-respiratory disease, e.g. intraventricular haemorrhage (IVH), gut perforation.

Slow deterioration during ventilation

May present as slow deterioration in overall clinical condition, $\uparrow PaCO_2$, or $\downarrow PaO_2$. *Consider:* worsening respiratory disease; partial ETT obstruction; airway circuit leak; non-respiratory disease.

Ventilation weaning

As condition starts to improve aim to wean ventilation. Wean O_2 to lowest needed to maintain adequate PaO_2 ($\downarrow$ retinopathy risk). As lung compliance improves wean PIP to maintain appropriate expired tidal volume ($\downarrow$ risk of pulmonary air leak) in $2cmH_2O$ steps until $12\text{--}14cmH_2O$ (monitor blood gases). Then wean rate by 5 or 10 increments until 10–20breaths/min. Following extubation it is often helpful in preterm infants to start nasal CPAP $5cmH_2O$ (see 📖 p.160). Extubation without CPAP may be appropriate after short-term ventilation.

High frequency oscillatory ventilation

A continuous positive distending pressure (mean airway pressure) is applied and, around this pressure amplitude (or Δp) is oscillated by a diaphragm or an interrupter device in the ventilator circuit. High frequency oscillatory ventilation (HFOV) has an efficacy equivalent to IPPV in the primary treatment of RDS. It may be indicated for:

- Rescue treatment when IPPV has failed.
- Pulmonary air leaks.
- Meconium aspiration syndrome.
- PPHN.
- Pulmonary hypoplasia.
- Congenital diaphragmatic hernia (see Fig. 6.7).

Ventilation parameters

- Mean airway pressure (P_{aw}).
- FiO_2.
- Airway pressure difference generated around P_{aw} (amplitude or Δp).
- Oscillation frequency per second.
- Circuit gas flow.

Oxygenation (PaO_2) is dependent on both P_{aw} and FiO_2. As P_{aw} ↑, PaO_2 will improve as functional residual capacity (FRC) ↑. At some point, however, further P_{aw} ↑ will ↓ PaO_2 because of over distension.

CO_2 removal ($PaCO_2$) is dependent on alveolar ventilation and, so, on both the frequency and amplitude. Unlike IPPV, ventilator constraints make tidal volume inversely proportional to the frequency. It is normal for generated tidal volumes to be less than that physiologically required, yet adequate ventilation occurs—this apparent paradox is explained by complicated air flow physics of HFOV that augment CO_2 diffusion. Once the frequency is set, CO_2 removal is increased by ↑ amplitude and vice versa.

Commencing ventilation

If ventilating for the first time, appropriate initial settings at term are:
- P_{aw} 8cmH$_2$O.
- Amplitude 20cmH$_2$O.
- Frequency 10Hz.
- FiO_2 0.5, i.e. 50% inspired O_2 concentration.

If transferring from IPPV:
- Set initial HFOV P_{aw} 2cmH$_2$O higher then P_{aw} used in IPPV.
- Start on the same FiO_2, and set frequency at 10Hz.

Monitoring ventilation

- Once ventilated, observe the infant's chest expansion and oscillation, and alter settings as required.
- Perform a CXR after 1hr to assess chest expansion: 8 posterior ribs visible above the diaphragm is appropriate until the baby is stable.

Monitoring ventilation is otherwise as for IPPV (see 🕮 p.162). Be aware that rapid elimination of CO_2 can occur leading to over-ventilation. Anticipate and monitor blood gas/transcutaneous readings closely.

- If PaO_2 is too low: ↑ either the FiO_2 or mean airway pressure (MAP) by 1–2cmH$_2$O every 30–60min (avoid chest overexpansion), and vice versa.
- If CO_2 is too high: ↑ amplitude by 2cmH$_2$O increments and vice versa.
- Optimal CO_2 elimination occurs at 10Hz, and, hence, the frequency does not usually need to be changed.

Weaning ventilation

As clinical status improves: ↓ FiO_2 to 0.5 and then ↓ P_{aw} by 2cmH$_2$O steps until 6–7cmH$_2$O is tolerated. Also progressively ↓ amplitude to the minimum required to maintain normal CO_2.

Some babies will tolerate weaning to what is essentially CPAP, whilst others, below a certain P_{aw}, do better if changed to slow rate IPPV.

Bronchopulmonary dysplasia

See also p.276. Bronchopulmonary dysplasia (BPD) is a form of chronic lung disease that affects infants who have been born preterm. Over the last decade advances in neonatal care, including the increasing use of antenatal steroids, and early surfactant therapy, have modified a change in the underlying pathology in many cases. 'Old' BPD was described as a disease of scarring, and repair. This condition was associated with long periods of mechanical ventilation, often with high PIP, and high F_iO_2. 'New' BPD is a condition of impaired alveolar development, with less destruction and scarring. Mechanical, oxidative and inflammatory factors all contribute to lung injury. The radiographic appearances of more recent cases are less dramatic (see Fig. 6.6), however, the impairment in lung function continues through childhood, and is associated with a number of other impairments.

Definition

The definition of BPD has evolved with time. The most commonly used definition is 'Oxygen requirement at 36/40 corrected gestational age (CGA)'. This definition does not have any grading of severity, and encompasses a wide spectrum of disease.

NICHD/NHLBI Definitions (2001)

- *Mild:* need for supplemental O_2 at age 28 days, but not at 36/40 CGA
- *Moderate:* need for supplemental O_2 <30% at age 28 days and at 36/40 CGA
- *Severe:* mechanical ventilation or requiring >30% O_2 at ≥ 36/40 CGA

'Walsh' test (2003)

- Test at 36±1/40 CGA. Aim to maintain S_pO_2 > 88%
- BPD if need ≥ 30% O_2 to maintain SpO_2 >88% (or ventilated)
- If <30% O_2, then F_iO_2 is gradually decreased to air. BPD is defined as inability to maintain SpO_2 >88% for 1hr

Incidence and risk-factors

Incidence is dependent on definition used. Wide variations between centres with a range of 4–58% (mean 23%) of at-risk babies. BPD more likely with:
- Gestational immaturity.
- Low birth weight.
- Males.
- Caucasian heritage.
- IUGR.
- Family history of asthma.
- History of chorioamnionitis.

Prevention of BPD

No evidence of effect
- Surfactant and ANC steroids (effect may be off-set by increased survival?)
- Closure of PDA
- Diuretics
- Inhaled steroids
- Inhaled nitric oxide
- HFOV compared to conventional ventilation
- Treating *Ureaplasma urealyticum* (more research needed)

May be of benefit in certain infants
- Systemic corticosteroids ☛ (clinical trials needed as increased risk of CP)
- nCPAP vs. intubation ☛ (need for surfactant, risk of pneumothorax)

Evidence of effect
- Caffeine citrate for apnoea of prematurity in infants <1250g
- Vitamin A supplementation for infants <1000g

Treatment of established BPD

☛ No specific treatment has been demonstrated to show an improvement in outcome of BPD. Oxygen is the most commonly used therapeutic agent, although the 'correct' dose and what SpO_2 is acceptable has not been established. A number of large trials are ongoing and their results are awaited (Ref: NeOPrOM Collaboration).

Other treatments include; diuretics, corticosteroids, sildenafil, optimizing nutrition.

Immunization for at-risk infants with monoclonal respiratory syncytial virus (RSV) antibody has recently been recommended by the UK department of health. ☛ This involves monthly injections during the RSV season.

Outcome

Increased survival of preterm infants has led to an increase in the number surviving with BPD. Mortality has improved (previously 10–20% would die from cor-pulmonale or respiratory infection). Other problems include:
- Increased risk of CP.
- Poorer cognitive functioning and academic performance.
- High risk of re-hospitalization with respiratory illness.
- Poorer lung function.

Respiratory problems seem to lessen as children get older, perhaps reflecting the lung's continued growth and development.

Circulatory adaptation at birth

Foetal circulation

Oxygenated placental blood (PaO_2 ~5kPa) returns to the foetus via the umbilical vein. Blood bypasses the liver via the ductus venosus and flows into the inferior vena cava, and then the right atrium. This blood is then channeled to the left atrium and so to the left ventricle (via the foramen ovale). *Oxygenated* blood is then pumped to the cerebral and coronary vessels. The right ventricle mostly receives *deoxygenated* blood from the superior vena cava. About 15% is pumped to the lungs and the rest is diverted, via the ductus arteriosus, to the descending aorta so that it can go to the placenta via the umbilical arteries.

Postnatal circulation

At birth, oxygen inhalation leads to pulmonary arterial vasodilatation, leading to ↓ arterial resistance and ↑ pulmonary blood flow. At the same time systemic vascular resistance ↑ due to loss of the low resistance placental circulation. The ductus arteriosus constricts as PaO_2 ↑. The foramen ovale closes as pulmonary venous return to left atrium ↑ and right atrial pressure ↓. Although initially rapid, these changes consolidate over 2–3wks.

Persistent pulmonary hypertension of the newborn (PPHN)

Failure of pulmonary vascular resistance to fall after birth causes decreased pulmonary blood flow; incidence 1/1000–1500 live births.

Causes Rarely primary/idiopathic due to disease of pulmonary vasculature. More commonly, it is a secondary complication of severe illness.

Presentation

- Hypoxia disproportionate to any difficulty with CO_2 elimination.
- Discrepancy between pre- and post-ductal arterial oxygen saturations >10%.
- Mild breathlessness (as $PaCO_2$, not PaO_2, is the main physiological determinant of respiratory rate), acidosis, hypotension.
- Loud single second heart sound.

Echocardiography shows ↑ pulmonary arterial pressure, large right to left shunt at the level of the foramen ovale and ductus arteriosus.

Management

- Treat cause; minimal handling.
- Optimize BP, pH (aim high-normal), Hb, U&E, blood glucose.
- Ventilate (aim for high PaO_2 and normal $PaCO_2$). HFOV may be helpful.
- Inhaled nitric oxide (results in selective pulmonary vasodilatation): dose 20ppm for 6hr initially and monitor for toxic levels of NO_2 and methaemoglobin.
- ECMO, if severe.

Prognosis 10–30% mortality. Risk of neurodevelopmental impairment in survivors.

Patent ductus arteriosus

Defined as failure of ductus arteriosus to close normally after birth. The ductus is normally functionally closed within 1–3 days of birth in term infants. Common in preterms (>50% if VLBW).

Presentation
- *Small:* asymptomatic.
- *Large:*
  • poor growth, difficulty feeding, respiratory difficulty, systolic or continuous 'machinery' murmur at the upper left sternal edge radiating to back, heart failure;
  • CXR. Cardiomegaly, pulmonary plethora;
  • echocardiography confirms PDA and degree of shunt.

Complications Poor growth, heart failure, pulmonary haemorrhage, ↑ risk of BPD.

Management
♦ There is considerable uncertainty about whether preterm infants benefit from treatment for PDA and, if so, what is the optimal treatment. There is wide variation in practice with some units treating many cases and others almost none. An approach considered sensible by many is:

If asymptomatic Observe because most close spontaneously.

If symptomatic In a preterm infant consider the following:
- Restrict fluids, e.g. 100–120mL/kg/day.
- Optimize blood oxygenation, e.g. blood transfusion if anaemic.
- Treat heart failure, e.g. furosemide 1mg/kg 12-hourly PO or IV.
- Consider pharmacological closure (e.g. indomethacin or ibuprofen). If duct fails to close a repeat course may be given. Side effects: ↓ renal blood flow leading to oliguria, fluid retention, +/– hyponatraemia; ↓ cerebral blood flow; GI complications (bleeding, ulceration); bleeding (↓ platelet function); displaces protein bonding of bilirubin. Consequently, indomethacin is contraindicated if severe jaundice, necrotizing enterocolitis (NEC), thrombocytopenia, or renal failure. Pharmacological closure is also contraindicated when the PDA is necessary for pulmonary blood flow (e.g. some forms of congenital heart disease).
- Surgery may be necessary if medical management fails to control symptoms or if there is significant heart failure, ventilator dependence, or prolonged failure to close.

Prognosis
Generally good, but infants who require PDA treatment often have other morbidities that affect prognosis, including severe BPD. Surgery after failed medical treatment carries a significant risk of mortality. PDA is much less likely to close when present in term infants. Medical treatment in term infants is not likely to be effective.

CNS malformations

Overall incidence ~4–5/10 000 births. There has been a dramatic fall in last 50yrs.

Neural tube defects
- Failure of primary neural tube closure during 4th week of gestation.
- Prevalence decreasing due to:
  - prenatal diagnosis (↑AFP, USS) leading to termination;
  - maternal periconceptual folate therapy

Anencephaly Lethal condition comprising absence of skull bones, forebrain and upper brain-stem.

Encephalocele Midline skull defect with brain tissue herniation. The lesion is covered with skin and requires surgical excision and closure. Associated brain abnormality usually leads to poor neurodevelopment.

Spina bifida
Several types, all secondary to failure of midline fusion of dorsal vertebral bodies. All forms require specialist advice and treatment.
- *Spina bifida occulta:* no herniation of neural tissue. Often overlying dermal sinus, dimple, lipoma, or hairy naevus is present (perform spinal US or MRI). Associated with diastematomyelia or cord tethering.
- *Meningocele:* herniation of meninges and fluid only with skin covering. Requires surgical closure. Excellent prognosis.
- *Myelomeningocele:* herniation of spinal neural tissue, which may be covered by meninges/skin or be open. Adjacent spinal cord is always abnormal. Usually thoraco-lumbar, lumbar, or lumbo-sacral.
  - *problems include*—flaccid paralysis below the lesion; urinary and faecal incontinence; urinary tract dilatation; hydrocephalus; bulbar paresis secondary to Chiari malformation; and vertebral anomalies (e.g. kyphosis);
  - *treatment*—surgical closure and hydrocephalus drainage;
  - *prognosis* —related to severity of associated problems. Prognosis worst if lesion very large or high. Palliative care may be appropriate.

Congenital hydrocephalus
Excessive head growth caused by CSF accumulation (see also 📖 p.535).
- *Causes:* congenital (aqueduct stenosis, Dandy–Walker malformation, congenital infection, e.g. CMV, cerebral tumour); acquired (IVH, subarachnoid haemorrhage, CNS infection, e.g. meningitis).
- *Features:* OFC above the 97th centile with wide cranial sutures and bulging fontanelle, 'sun-setting' sign of eyes.
- Confirmed by cranial US or MRI.
- *Treatment:* surgical insertion of indwelling drainage device, e.g. ventriculo-peritoneal shunt.

Dandy–Walker malformation
- Cerebellar vermis hypoplasia associated with:
  - hydrocephalus;
  - posterior fossa CSF collection ('cyst') expanding into 4th ventricle.

- *Associated with variety of syndromes:* foetal alcohol, trisomy 13 + 18.
- *Prognosis:* depends on associated abnormalities/underlying condition.

Agenesis of the corpus callosum

- Non-specific feature of numerous conditions and is associated with a wide variety of conditions.
- May be total or partial.
- May be incidental finding.
- Prognosis depends on associated syndromes/features.

Hydrancephalus

- Absence of cerebral hemispheres with cavity filled with CSF. Brainstem and midbrain are usually spared.
- *Cause:* severe (vascular) cerebral insult leading to extensive cortical necrosis.
- *Prognosis:* usually lethal. Survivors have severe neurodevelopmental impairment.

Microcephaly

See also 📖 p.534. OFC progressively falls below 3rd centile.
- Primary defect is reduction in brain size.
- *Causes:* intrauterine infection, chromosomal defects, various syndromes, maternal drug/alcohol abuse, brain injury.
- *Prognosis:* generally poor neurodevelopmental outcome.

Holoprosencephaly

Severe developmental defect of the forebrain. There is a single central cerebral ventricular cavity with varying degrees of development and separation of the hemispheres. Midline facial defects are common. May be isolated or associated with chromosomal defects, particularly trisomy 13. Poor prognosis.

Neuronal migration defects

Includes lissencephaly (smooth brain), pachygyria (very few gyri), polymicrogyria (numerous underdeveloped gyri), schizencephaly (deep cerebral cleft), neuronal heterotopia (foci of neurones in abnormal locations within the brain). All are associated with poor neurodevelopmental outcome and seizures, but eventual outcome is dependent on severity of malformation.

Hypoxic–ischaemic encephalopathy

Clinical syndrome of brain injury secondary to a hypoxic-ischaemic insult. In developed countries the incidence is ~2–5/1000 live births (moderate to severe incidence is 1–2/1000 live births).

Causes
- ↓ Umbilical blood flow, e.g. cord prolapse.
- ↓ Placental gas exchange, e.g. placental abruption.
- ↓ Maternal placental perfusion.
- Maternal hypoxia from whatever cause.
- Inadequate postnatal cardiopulmonary circulation.

Presentation
Varies depending on severity of cerebral hypoxia. An infant may have a range of symptoms and signs affecting: level of consciousness, muscle tone, posture, tendon reflexes, suck, heart rate and central nervous system homeostasis.[1]

Before concluding that an infant may have HIE secondary to an *intrapartum* hypoxic-ischaemic event, assess for evidence of an *intrapartum* problem (e.g. CTG abnormality, sentinel event such as abruption or cord prolapse). There should be respiratory depression at birth and a need for resuscitation, including IPPV (Apgar score at 5min < 5). There should be moderate to severe acidosis soon after birth (pH<7.0, base excess worse than −12). The baby should develop encephalopathy within 24hr of birth. Other causes of encephalopathy should be excluded.

Management
- Resuscitate at birth; insert IV ± arterial lines. Avoid hyperthermia.
- Assess eligibility for therapeutic hypothermia (TH) (see Box 6.5).
- Start cerebral function analysis monitoring (CFAM).
- Assess for features of dysmorphism and birth trauma.
- Assess neurological features.
- Exclude other causes of encephalopathy, e.g. meningitis, metabolic disturbances, maternal drugs, CNS malformation, and haemorrhage.
- Expect and manage associated multi-organ failure, e.g. cardiac or renal.
- Monitor and maintain homeostasis, e.g. U&E, Ca^{2+}, Mg^{2+} blood glucose, Hb, blood gases, coagulation. Support BP.
- Mild fluid restriction initially (e.g. 40mL/kg/day 10% dextrose) as there may be oliguria. Omit milk feeds for 1–2 days if HIE severe and then feed slowly.
- Treat seizures ✒.

Therapeutic hypothermia
This is now the standard of care for term infants with moderate/severe hypoxic ischaemic encephalopathy.[2] Cooling is achieved using a temperature controlled mattress or wrap, and eligible infants have their temperature lowered to 33–34°C within 6hr of insult. Hypothermia is maintained for 72hr before gradual re-warming.

Box 6.5 Criteria for therapeutic hypothermia:

(A) Infants >36/40 and >1800g and <6hr old with one of
- Apgar ≤ 5 or continued need for resuscitation at 10min
- *Acidosis:* cord pH (or any blood gas in first hour) <7/BE≤–16

(B) Moderate or severe encephalopathy
Altered level of consciousness (lethargy/stupor/coma) and one of:
- Hypotonia
- Abnormal reflexes, e.g. moro, suck, gag, papillary, oculovestibular
- Clinical seizures

If criteria A and B both met then assess for criterion C (CFAM)

(C) At least 30min of CFAM recording which shows either abnormal background activity or seizures (clinical or electrical).
If CFAM not available and criteria A&B are met, cooling can be started after senior doctor discussion (e.g. before or during transport).

Cerebral function analysis monitoring (CFAM)

Single or 2 channel machines available (2 channel = left and right hemispheres). Displays 'raw' EEG and a compressed 'amplitude integrated' recording. Pattern of a EEG is used for classification of background activity (see Figs 6.9–6.12). Normal CFAM (aEEG) recording (term infants):
- Lower margin ≤5µV (when awake), upper margin ≥10µV.
- Evidence of sleep-wake cycling, no seizures.

Prognosis

Without cooling, risk of later disability or death is: grade I <2%; grade II 24%; grade III 78%. Disabilities are likely to be one or more of the following: spastic quadriplegia, dyskinetic cerebral palsy, severely reduced IQ, cortical blindness, hearing loss, and epilepsy.

References

1 Sarnat HB, Sarnat MS (1976) Neonatal encephalopathy following foetal distress. A clinical and electroencephalographic study. *Arch Neurol* **33**: 696–705.
2 Edwards AD, Brocklehurst P, Gunn AJ, et al. (2010) Neurological outcomes at 18 months of age after moderate hypothermia for perinatal hypoxic ischaemic encephalopathy: synthesis and meta-analysis of trial data. *Br Med J* **340**: c363.

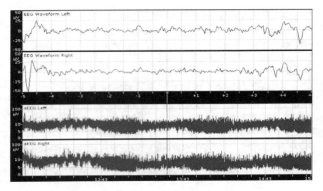

Fig. 6.9 Normal CFAM trace. Note sleep-wake cycling (narrowing and widening of trace).

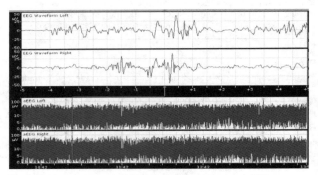

Fig. 6.10 Moderately abnormal CFAM trace. Note the widened aEEG trace (baseline <5) and suppressed raw EEG with periodic high-voltage complexes.

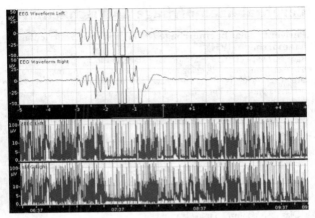

Fig. 6.11 Severely abnormal CFAM trace—burst suppression. Note the very low baseline voltage (<5) with high voltage discharges (as seen on raw trace below) giving a spiked pattern to the aEEG.

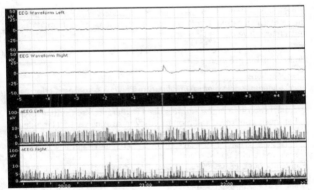

Fig. 6.12 Severely abnormal CFAM trace – continuous low voltage. Note that there is almost no electrical activity.

Cerebral haemorrhage and ischaemia

Periventricular haemorrhage (PVH) and intraventricular haemorrhage (IVH)

Rare >32wks gestation. Haemorrhage starts in the vascular germinal matrix (subependymal). Bleeding may then extend into, and may dilate, the lateral ventricles (IVH). Haemorrhagic periventricular infarction may then occur secondary to impairment of cerebral venous drainage by intraventricular haemorrhage.

Incidence: ~10–15% of infants born <32wks. Risk ↑ with ↑ prematurity.

Causes: related to rapid alteration in cerebral blood flow, e.g. severe RDS, pneumothorax, hypotension, hypoxia, ↑/↓ $PaCO_2$.

Presentation: most occur within 72hr of birth. Seldom occur before birth unless there is alloimmune thrombocytopenia. Up to 50% are asymptomatic. Larger bleeds may present as sudden catastrophic systemic collapse, bulging fontanelle, neurological dysfunction (e.g. seizures or paucity/abnormal movements), anaemia, and jaundice.
- Diagnosis confirmed using cranial US.
- At risk groups or preterm infants <32wks should be screened by cranial US (at 1wk, and at 1mth, or after sudden deterioration). Several grading systems exist, but it is better to describe the location and extent of haemorrhage as one of:
  - subependymal only; or
  - IVH ± ventricular dilatation; or
  - IVH ± parenchymal involvement.

Prevention Antenatal steroids reduce incidence. Prophylactic neonatal indometacin treatment reduces incidence, but does not improve long term neurodevelopmental outcome.

Treatment Supportive. Irrigation of lateral ventricles following surgical drain insertion is experimental.

Complications
- *Post-haemorrhagic ventricular dilatation (PHVD):* 2° to obstruction of CSF flow or absorption. Clinical features include: increasing OFC; wide cranial sutures; apnoea; seizures; feed intolerance; 'sun setting' eyes. Diagnosis confirmed and monitored by measuring ventricular index on cranial US. 50% resolve spontaneously. Progressive symptomatic PHVD requires CSF drainage either by serial LP or intracranial reservoir and then by insertion of ventriculo-peritoneal shunt.
- *Haemorrhagic periventricular infarction:* occurs in 15%. Blood in the lateral ventricles impairs adjacent venous drainage, which results in adjacent cerebral infarction. *Cranial US:* cystic parenchymal area(s) adjacent and communicating with lateral ventricle (porencephalic cyst).

Prognosis Sub-ependymal or uncomplicated IVH does not affect neurodevelopment. Cerebral palsy is common if either PHVD present and treatment is required (50%), or there is parenchymal extension (80%).

Term intracranial haemorrhage

- *Subdural:* increased risk with difficult extraction.
- *Subgaleal:* potential massive blood loss with systemic collapse. Boggy swelling all over scalp, not limited by sutures.
- *Subarachnoid:* asymptomatic, or may present with seizures/irritability.
- *Parenchymal or intraventricular:* is usually haemorrhagic infarction—seizures possible.
- *Cephalohaematoma:* subperiosteal bleed, limited by suture lines, may take weeks to resolve, and may partially calcify.

Periventricular leucomalacia (PVL)

Severe HIE can lead to cortical neuronal necrosis, basal ganglia injuries, focal cerebral infarctions or subcortical leukomalacia. PVL is characterized by periventricular white matter lesions: ↑ echogenicity; cysts.
- *Cause:* poor cerebral perfusion or ischemia, inflammation.
- *Risk factors:* extreme prematurity; hypotension; severe illness; hypocarbia.
- May not be apparent for several weeks after birth.
- *Diagnosis:* periventricular echodensities or cysts seen on cranial US.
- *Prognosis:* higher risk of cerebral palsy (especially spastic diplegia), particularly if there is cyst formation.

Cerebral infarction (perinatal stroke)

- *Incidence:* 1:1600 to 1:5000 births.
- Neurological signs and symptoms caused by a vascular event around the time of delivery.
- Presentation depends on timing and nature of event; focal seizures, encephalopathy, apnoea, poor feeding, asymmetrical reflexes/movement/tone.
- May be associated with maternal/neonatal coagulation disorders (e.g. Factor V Leiden, Protein C or S deficiency).
- *Management:* supportive, cover infection, correct any metabolic (e.g. hypoglycaemia) or haematological (e.g. polycythemia) abnormalities. Start CFAM and treat any seizures.
- *Investigation:* FBC/Coag/U&E(Ca^{2+}, Mg^{2+})/LFTs/Glucose/CFAM/ MRI/ EEG.
- *Prognosis:* depends on site and nature of lesion. ~50% of affected children will carry some neurological impairment into childhood.

Necrotizing enterocolitis

Incidence

The most common neonatal surgical emergency. Incidence 1–3/1000 live births (5–10% in VLBW infants). Incidence is reduced 6-fold in preterm infants fed breast milk. Typically a sporadic condition affecting preterm infants (~90% of cases), but can be epidemic or occur in term infants. The disease may just involve an isolated area of gut, or be extensive. Distal terminal ileum and proximal colon are most frequently affected. Multi-organ failure is associated with diffuse disease.

Cause

Multifactorial. Severe intestinal necrosis is end result of an exaggerated immune response within the immature bowel leading to inflammation and tissue injury. NEC rarely occurs before milk feeding commences, but timing of first feed appears not to be relevant. Predisposing factors:
- Prematurity.
- IUGR (causes chronic bowel ischaemia).
- Hypoxia.
- Polycythaemia.
- Exchange transfusion.
- Hyperosmolar milk feeds.

Presentation

Most common in the second week after birth.

Early
- Non-specific illness.
- Vomiting/bilious aspirate from gastric tube.
- Poor feed toleration (increasing gastric aspirates).
- Abdominal distension.

Late
- Additional abdominal tenderness.
- Blood, mucus, or tissue in stools.
- Bowel perforation.
- Shock.
- DIC; multi-organ failure. AXR shows intestinal distension (see Fig. 6.8).
- Pneumatosis intestinalis.
- Hepatic portal venous gas.
- Signs of intestinal perforation, e.g. free peritoneal gas or gas outlining of falciform ligament ('football' sign).

Management
- *Prophylaxis:* antenatal steroids and breast milk are protective. Emerging evidence for prevention by administration of probiotic bacteria.
- *Investigations:* FBC; U&E; creatinine; coagulation screen; albumin; blood gas; blood culture; AXR; Group and cross match.
- Stop milk feeds for 10–14 days ☞. Insert gastric tube on free drainage.
- 'Bell staging' (see Table 6.2) may be useful in grading severity.

- IV antibiotics for 10–14 days, e.g. benzylpenicillin, gentamicin, and metronidazole.
- *Systemic support:* e.g. assisted ventilation, correct BP and DIC, parenteral nutrition (PN).
- *Surgical opinion:* indications for surgery are GI perforation, deterioration despite above medical treatment (necrotic bowel likely), GI obstruction secondary to stricture formation (late). If localized disease, surgical resection of involved bowel with primary repair. If more extensive, two stage repair with bowel resection(s) and enterostomy, followed later by intestinal re-anastomosis.

Prognosis

Overall mortality is ~22%. Increased mortality is associated with:
- VLBW.
- Extensive intestine involvement.
- Multi-organ failure.
- Intrahepatic portal gas.

Extensive bowel resection may result in short bowel syndrome. Excellent prognosis is seen in those who respond to medical treatment, but subsequent stricture may develop.

Table 6.2 Bell staging of NEC

Stage I (suspected NEC)	Predisposed infant Systematic manifestations: temperature instability, lethargy, apnoeas, bradycardias *GI manifestations:* feed intolerance, vomiting (may be bilious), occult blood in vomit or stool, mild abdominal distension *Abdominal radiographs:* bowel distension only
Stage II (definite NEC)	As above plus mild/moderate acidosis and/or thrombocytopaenia Persistent occult or gross GI bleeding, marked abdominal distension Abdominal radiographs show distension and bowel wall thickening, intramural gas (portal vein or a fixed bowel loop)
Stage III (advanced NEC)	As above plus shock, severe acidosis, electrolyte abnormalities, thrombocytopaenia, DIC Marked GI bleeding Abdominal radiographs may show pneumoperitoneum

Neonatal infection

Neonatal infection can be acquired transplacentally (congenital, see 📖 p.182), by ascent from the vagina, during birth (intrapartum infection), or postnatally from the environment or contact with others. Infections are categorized as early-onset (first 48hr of age) vs. late-onset sepsis (>48hr). Preterm infants are at greater risk for both types of infections.

Risk factors for early-onset neonatal sepsis

- Prolonged rupture of membranes >18hr, especially if preterm.
- Signs of maternal infection, e.g. maternal fever, chorioamnionitis, UTI.
- Vaginal carriage or previous infant with GBS.
- Preterm labour; foetal distress.
- Skin and mucosal breaks.

Risk factors for late-onset sepsis

- Central lines and catheters.
- Congenital malformations, e.g. spina bifida.
- Severe illness, malnutrition, or immunodeficiency.

Early-onset neonatal infection (2–5/1000 live births)

Infection is caused by organisms acquired from the mother, usually GBS, *E. coli*, or *Listeria*. Other possibilities include herpes virus, *H. influenza*, anaerobes, *Candida*, and *Chlamydia trachomatis*.

Presentation (symptomatic)

Includes temperature instability, lethargy, poor feeding, respiratory distress, collapse, DIC, and osteomyelitis or septic arthritis.

Initial investigations

- These include blood culture, cerebrospinal fluid (glucose, protein, cell count and culture), FBC, CXR.
- The diagnostic value of CRP in early neonatal sepsis is unclear 💣.
- Failure to respond within 24hr should prompt further investigation.

Treatment

- Supportive (may require ventilation, volume expansion, inotropes).
- Broad-spectrum antibiotics, e.g. penicillin and gentamicin (consider ampicillin/amoxicillin if *listeria* a possibility).
- If meningitis confirmed or strongly suspected then treatment with cefotaxime (+/– amp/amoxicillin) should be commenced.
- Length of antibiotic course and choice of antibiotics will depend on local sensitivities/policy as well as the age/gestation of baby.
- If infant has remained well, and initial index of suspicion was low, then consider stopping antibiotics if culture results are negative (~48hr), and observe.

Length of treatment in CSF positive meningitis ranges from 14 to 21 days (or greater). A repeat LP demonstrating resolution at the proposed end of treatment may be of value in deciding length of course.

Prognosis

Up to 15% mortality (up to 30% if VLBW).

Late-onset neonatal infection (4–5/1000 live births)

Infection is caused by environmental organisms such as coagulase –ve staphylococci, *Staph. aureus*, *E. coli*, and other Gram –ve bacilli, *Candida* spp., and GBS.

Investigation

FBC, blood culture, urinalysis (clean catch) and urine culture, CSF glucose, protein, cell count and culture.

Treatment

- Give broad spectrum antibiotics, e.g. flucloxacillin and gentamicin IV.
- Consider cefotaxime if meningitis is likely.
- Vancomycin if coagulase –ve *Staph.* sepsis likely, e.g. preterm infant with indwelling central venous catheter. Decisions on removing/ continuing to use any central catheter should be made by a senior doctor.
- Fungal sepsis is relatively uncommon in the UK (1% of VLBW infants), however, should be considered in any infant who fails to respond to standard therapy or has additional risk factors.

Transplacental (congenital infection)

Causes
- 'TORCH' infections.
- Herpes zoster.
- Parvovirus B19.
- Syphilis.
- Enterovirus.
- HIV; hepatitis B.
- Rarely bacterial, e.g. GBS, *Listeria monocytogenes*, *N. gonorrhoeae*.

Presentation
- *TORCH infection:* SGA, jaundice, hepatitis, hepatosplenomegaly, purpura, chorioretinitis, micro-ophthalmos, cerebral calcification, micro/macrocephaly, hydrocephalus.
- *Rubella and CMV:* also cause deafness, cataracts, congenital heart disease, osteitis (rubella only).
- *Parvovirus B19:* rubella-like rash, aplastic anaemia +/– hydrops.
- *Herpes zoster:* cutaneous scarring, limb defects, multiple structural defects.
- *Congenital syphilis:* SGA, jaundice, hepatomegaly, rash, rhinitis, bleeding mucous membranes, osteochondritis, meningitis.
- Bacterial infections present with features that may be non-specific or even result in multi-organ failure. Gonorrhoea causes purulent conjunctivitis (ophthalmia). Listeriosis causes preterm labour and meconium-stained liquor.

Investigation
Consider:
- Blood culture.
- Pathogen-specific IgM and IgG (paired for Herpes zoster, *Toxoplasma*).
- Venereal Disease Research Laboratory (test)(VDRL).
- Maternal-specific serology.
- Urine CMV culture.
- Throat swab viral culture.
- CSF culture and latex particle agglutination (GBS).
- Stool viral culture.
- Skin vesicle viral culture and electron microscopy.

Treatment
- Most congenital infections have no specific treatment.
- General treatment is supportive and involves careful follow-up to identify sequelae, e.g. deafness and CMV.
- *Toxoplasma:* spiramycin (4–6wks 100mg/kg/day) alternating with pyrimethamine (3wks 1mg/kg/day) plus sulfadiazine (1yr 50–100mg/kg/day).
- *Syphilis:* benzylpenicillin 14 days 30mg/kg 12-hourly IV.
- *Symptomatic CMV:* consider IV ganciclovir then oral valganciclovir ♠.

Prognosis Variable and depends on disease severity.

Prevention of neonatal infection

General measures
- Good hand washing with antiseptic solutions and use of gloves.
- Avoidance of overcrowding.
- Low nurse to patient ratio.
- Nurse cohorting.
- Patient isolation and barrier nursing.
- Minimal handling.
- Rational antibiotic use.
- Minimize indwelling vascular access.

Group B streptococcal disease
The best approach to minimize early onset sepsis due to Group B strepto-coccal infection is uncertain because there have not been trials that permit the overall risks and benefits of intrapartum antibiotic prophylaxis (IAP) to be judged. IAP reduces the number of newborns with positive blood cultures, but with a very low disease incidence and a very high rate of maternal GBS colonization (around 25%) a very large number of women must be treated to prevent a case if bacteriological screening programs are implemented. Routine bacteriological screening of pregnant women is not presently recommended in the UK. Current practice follows a risk factor based approach. The incidence of early-onset GBS disease in term infants without antenatal risk factors in the UK is 0.2cases/1000 births.

The Royal College of Obstetrics and Gynaecology[1] recommend that intrapartum IV penicillin (or clindamycin) should be offered to women with a previous baby with neonatal GBS disease. Other risk factors that should prompt consideration of IAP are:
- intrapartum fever >38 C;
- preterm (<37/40);
- PROM >18hr;
- GBS maternal carriage detected on low vaginal swab culture or GBS bacteriuria.

Management of the newborn is not well evidenced. Any ill newborn infants should have cultures taken and be treated with broad spectrum antibiotics that are effective against Group B streptococcus and other common neonatal pathogens.

Well infants exposed to the above risk factors should be evaluated clinically and observed. Because more than 90% of cases of early onset GBS disease present in the first 12–24hr after birth. Infants who remain well after this time are not at increased risk of disease in comparison with infants without risk factors. There is no need to send investigations on infants who are not ill. If there are multiple risk factors, or a previous child has been affected by Group B streptococcal sepsis many would consider blood culture and starting antibiotics appropriate.

Hepatitis B

Usually contracted at birth. Routine antenatal screening detects maternal carrier state (hepatitis B (HBsAg) +ve). Transmission risk ~10% if mother is a low-risk carrier, (i.e. anti-HBe +ve). To reduce vertical transmission give hepatitis B vaccine to infant within 24hr of birth. *Also give* specific hepatitis B immunoglobulin 200IU IM *if mother is a high-risk carrier*, (i.e. mother HBeAg +ve, or, anti-HBe −ve, or, antibody/antigen status unknown), since the untreated transmission risk is 90%. In both groups, subsequent hepatitis B vaccine is required at 1, 2, and 12mths (UK schedule).

Human immunodeficiency virus (HIV)

See 🕮 p.726. Vertical transmission rate ~15–25%. Risk markedly reduced by:
- Maternal antiretroviral drug therapy to minimize viral load during third trimester and labour and then postnatal treatment of baby for 6wks.
- Elective lower segment Cesarean section (LSCS).
- Avoidance of breastfeeding (in developed world).

Infants are usually asymptomatic at birth. Test at birth and 3 and 6mths for:
- HIV viral PCR;
- P24 antigen;
- specific IgA.

Infection is very unlikely if all negative at 6mths and baby well.

Herpes simplex

85% of neonatal HSV is contracted at birth from active maternal genital lesions. Elective LSCS reduces transmission if mother has *active genital* herpes. Treat infant with prophylactic IV aciclovir if born by vaginal delivery and there is *primary* maternal herpes (transmission risk of 50% compared with 3% in secondary herpes). To prevent infection from carers with cold sores, the lesions should be covered with a mask and the sores treated with topical aciclovir.

Herpes zoster

Perinatal infection can cause severe disseminated disease with high mortality (30%) if:
- Maternal rash occurs in the period between 7 days antenatally and 7 days postnatally;
- A LBW infant (<1mth old) has contact with varicella and whose mother is non-immune (i.e. check maternal antibody status if unsure).

Prevention Oral aciclovir and specific zoster immunoglobulin (ZIG) 100mg IM given soon after delivery.

Reference

1 Royal College of Obstetrics and Gynaecology (2003). *Prevention of early onset neonatal group B streptococcal disease*, RCOG Guideline No. 36, November 2003. London: RCOG Press.

Neonatal abstinence syndrome

A cluster of symptoms caused by withdrawal from a dependency-inducing substance. In the UK this is commonly related to methadone (+/– heroin), or benzodiazepines, however, withdrawal is well documented with a number of other substances, for example; cocaine, amphetamine, SSRIs (e.g. fluoxetine), alcohol, caffeine, and nicotine.

Presentation
- *Timing depends on substance:* heroin and SSRIs often present soon after birth, methadone within 24hr, and benzodiazepines later.
- *CNS symptoms:* include irritability, sleepiness, hyperactivity, tremors, seizures.
- *Non-CNS:* poor/disorganized feeding, vomiting, diarrhoea (can cause severe nappy rash), sneezing, tachycardia, sweating, respiratory depression, fever (be cautious—sepsis may co-exist or present with similar symptoms).

Management
- Observe 'at risk' infants for signs of withdrawal for several days after birth. Several scoring systems exist for quantifying withdrawal.
- *General and supportive measures:* swaddling, minimal handling, dark and quiet environment, frequent low volume feeding.
- A pragmatic approach to starting drug treatment (low dose oral morphine) would be to start if *significantly symptomatic,* e.g. sleeping <1hr after feeds, continuous high-pitched cry, unable to feed. Once stable, wean morphine slowly over several days.
- Start apnoea monitor if preterm or require large doses of morphine.
- Seizures should be controlled by phenobarbital (also drug of choice to treat barbiturate withdrawal).

Other points to consider are:
- Does baby need a urine screen (remember this will effectively drug-test the mother)?
- Ensure Social Services are aware as child protection and family support issues must be considered.
- Consider associated pathologies, e.g. HIV or hepatitis B or C infection.
- Breastfeeding is not contraindicated unless mother is taking high doses of methadone (>20mg/day), amphetamines, cocaine, or is HIV +ve.

Prognosis
It is difficult to establish whether any adverse outcomes are directly related to drug exposure as literature is confounded by social and environmental factors. There is an increased risk of:
- prematurity;
- IUGR;
- sudden infant death syndrome (SIDS);
- congenital HIV/hepatitis B/C infection;
- social problems;
- neurodevelopmental impairment.

Inborn errors of metabolism

See also 📖 pp.102–105, Chapter 26. The common presentations of IEM are as follows:

- *Encephalopathy without metabolic acidosis:* e.g. pyridoxine-dependent seizures, urea cycle enzyme defects (hyperammonaemia; see 📖 pp.960, 964);
- *Encephalopathy with metabolic acidosis:* e.g. organic acidurias (see 📖 p.958);
- *Hepatic failure:* e.g. galactosaemia (see 📖 pp.342, 960);
- *Non-immune hydrops:* can be haematological, e.g. β-thalassaemia, or due to lysosomal storage disorder, e.g. Gaucher disease (see 📖 p.968);
- *Significant dysmorphism:* these can be divided into: lysosomal disorders, e.g. mucopolysaccharidosis; peroxisomal disorders, e.g. Zellweger syndrome; mitochondrial disorders; biosynthetic defects, e.g. albinism; receptor defects, e.g. pseudo-hypoparathyroidism;
- *Other:* non-specific illness (see 📖 p.128); severe hypotonia; resistant hypoglycaemia; cataracts; odours; cardiomyopathy; severe diarrhoea.

Investigations

- *Initial:* blood for U&E, SBR, gas analysis, glucose, Ca²⁺, Hb, ammonia, and anion gap (normal range 12–16mmol/L). Urine for ketones and reducing substances.
- *'Metabolic screen' (for amino acid and organic acid analysis):* take and save blood in heparinized (1–2mL) and EDTA (3–5mL) tubes and save urine (5–10mL) in sterile container with no preservatives.
- *Subsequent investigation after discussion with expert:* if child dies prior to diagnosis, seek permission to take:
  - further blood for storage (clotted and heparinized);
  - skin biopsy placed in sterile saline;
  - liver and muscle biopsy;
  - send immediately to pathology laboratory for preservation.

Acute management

- Supportive.
- Stop all protein intake, including milk, and start 10% glucose IV infusion.
- Correct electrolyte/acid-base imbalance.
- Broad spectrum antibiotics in case crisis was precipitated by infection.
- Specific treatments after expert advice.

Prognosis

Depends on disease.

Retinopathy of prematurity

See also 📖 p.920. Retinopathy of prematurity (ROP) is a leading cause of preventable blindness. Infants born <32/40 and those weighing <1500g at birth are at greatest risk. The incidence is decreasing and recent data suggest that around 90% of infants born weighing >1000g will have no ROP, however, this number drops to only 38% for those <750g at birth. The cause is multifactorial. In utero, the retinal vasculature develops in a relatively hypoxic environment, with vessels stimulated to grow towards the most hypoxic regions. This development is disrupted with preterm delivery. ROP is associated with retinal arterial hyperoxic vasoconstriction and retinal ischaemia during retinal development before 32wks gestation. It is therefore, essential to monitor and prevent hyperoxia in infants requiring supplemental O_2. Minimizing variability in oxygenation may also be important.

Classification

ROP is a proliferative retinopathy that is classified according to internationally accepted guidelines (see Box 6.6).[1]

Screening criteria

- ≤27/40: first screen at 30–31/40 CGA.
- 27–32/40: first screen at day 28–35 of life.
- Screen 2wkly thereafter unless:
  - any stage 3 disease;
  - any plus/pre-plus disease;
  - vessels end in zone 1, or posterior zone 2;
  - weekly screening if present.
- Screening is performed by indirect ophthalmoscopy after pharmacological pupil dilatation or increasingly by wide field digital retinal imaging.
- Screening continues until vascularization has progressed into zone 3 (usually >36/40).

Treatment

Diode laser treatment within 72hr (48hr if aggressive disease) of meeting any of the treatment criteria (see Box 6.6).

Babies should be ventilated, adequately sedated, and given a muscle relaxant. Atropine should be available.

Side effects of treatment include:
- Need for re-ventilation.
- Bradycardia.
- Apnoea.
- Ocular haemorrhage.
- Eyelid trauma.
- Laser burns.

Infants should be re-examined 5–7 days following treatment, and if no regression, re-treatment should be performed at 10–14 days after initial therapy. Steroid eye drops may be useful in decreasing post-operative swelling. Direct injections of monoclonal antibodies against vascular endothelial growth factor (VEGF) are showing promise as an alternative.

Prognosis

Almost all cases can be treated effectively so blindness is a rare outcome. There may be reduced visual fields in severe cases. Refractive errors are common.

Box 6.6 Classification of ROP[1]

Severity
- *Stage 1:* demarcation line visible
- *Stage 2:* ridge evident
- *Stage 3:* ridge with extraretinal fibrovascular proliferation
- *Stage 4:* subtotal retinal detachment (4A, extrafoveal; 4B involves the fovea)
- *Stage 5:* total retinal detachment

Location
- Zone 1 extends a radius of 30   from the optic disc
- Zone 2 extends from the nasal retina periphery in a circle around the anatomical equator
- Zone 3 involves the anterior residual crescent of temporal retina

Extent Recorded as clock hours in each eye in the appropriate zone.

'Plus' (+) disease Indicates aggressive disease and is used when there is: engorgement and tortuosity of posterior pole retinal vessels; iris rigidity or vessel engorgement; vitreous haze.

Treatment criteria
- Zone 1, any stage if 'Plus' disease present
- Zone 1, stage 3 (no plus)
- Zone 2, stage 3 with 'Plus' disease
- Seriously consider if Zone 2, stage 2 with 'Plus'

Reference

1 Royal College of Ophthalmologists/RCPCH Medicine Joint Working Party (2008) *Retinopathy of prematurity: guidelines for screening and treatment.* London: Royal College of Ophthalmologists and British Association of Perinatal Medicine.

Metabolic bone disease

Also known as osteopenia of prematurity, the incidence is 32–90% in pre-term infants (mostly ELBW).

Cause

Chronic substrate deficiency—usually phosphate, rarely calcium or vitamin D. Risk is increased if:
- prolonged PN;
- breastfed (low in phosphate);
- chronic diuretic treatment.

Presentation

- Bone mineral biochemical derangement (see 📖 Investigations); measure serum Ca^{2+}, PO_4^{3-} and alkaline phosphatase weekly in all infants under 33wks gestation.
- ↓ Linear growth.
- Rib or distal long bone fractures.

Investigations

- *Biochemistry:* PO_4^{3-} <1.2mmol/L; Ca^{2+} >2.7mmol/L; alkaline phosphatase >1000IU/L.
- *Bone X-ray:* osteoporosis, features of rickets, fractures.
- Urine Ca^{2+}/PO_4^{3-} ratio >1 after 3wks of age (high renal PO_4^{3-} reabsorption).

Treatment

- Oral PO_4^{3-} 1mmol/kg/day supplement if milk fed.
- Increase TPN Ca^{2+} and PO_4^{3-} (consult pharmacist).

Prevention

In infants <2kg or <33wks gestation:
- Supplement breast milk with oral PO_4^{3-} 1mmol/kg/day (not required if fed preterm formula as already contains added PO_4^{3-});
- Oral vitamin D 400IU/day;
- Ensure TPN contains Ca^{2+} 2mmol/kg/day and PO_4^{3-} 2.5mmol/kg/day (organic phosphate solution avoids mineral precipitation);
- 10min/day of passive exercise appears beneficial.

Prognosis

Stature is reduced at age 18mths. Bone mineralization and fracture risk appear to be normal by 2yrs.

Orofacial clefts

See also 📖 p.846. Orofacial clefts are due to failure of fusion of maxillary and pre-maxillary processes. They may be unilateral or bilateral and result in cleft lip and/or cleft palate. The incidence is ~1/1000 live births.

Causes

Multifactorial and includes genetic and environmental factors. 66% of clefts are isolated. Majority have no obvious cause.

- *Enviromental factors:* maternal folic acid deficiency; maternal exposure to alcohol, tobacco, steroids, anticonvulsants, and retinoic acid.
- ~30% are syndromic, e.g. Pierre–Robin syndrome (large midline posterior cleft palate, mandible hypoplasia, prone to upper airway obstruction due to a posteriorly displaced tongue).

Treatment

- Refer to specialized 'cleft lip and palate' multidisciplinary team.
- Possible upper airway obstruction is a recognized complication of a large cleft palate, e.g. Pierre–Robin syndrome. If it occurs or is likely:
  - nurse prone;
  - nasopharyngeal airway may be helpful;
  - monitor SpO_2—a low or worsening SpO_2 is an ominous sign and should be taken very seriously;
  - intubation may be difficult and require specialist (ENT) support.
- Feeding problems are common. Specialist nursing input, special feed devices and prosthetic plate (obdurator) may all be required if cleft palate is too large to allow adequate suck.
- Be aware of increased risk of infections (aspiration pneumonia and, later, secretory otitis media with conductive hearing loss). Treat as appropriate.
- Surgical repair of lip is usually at 3mths; palate at 6–12mths.
- Later speech defects and dental problems can occur requiring speech therapy and dental input respectively.

Prognosis

Repair of unilateral complete or incomplete lesions usually produces a good result. As well as those complications described above later problems may include:

- Hindered parental bonding.
- Psychological morbidity.

Neonatal haematology

Anaemia See also 📖 pp.610–629.

Causes

Antenatal
- Alloimmune haemolytic disease, e.g. Rhesus disease.
- Twin to twin transfusion syndrome.
- Parvovirus B19 infection.
- Antepartum haemorrhage.
- Red cell defects or aplasia.

Postnatal
- Nutritional deficiency.
- Chronic illness.
- Anaemia of prematurity occurs 6–12wks after preterm delivery and is caused by:
  - repeated and frequent blood sampling;
  - shorter hbf red cell half-life;
  - ↓ erythropoietin;
  - fast growth rate.

Presentation
- Pallor and tachycardia.
- ↑ O$_2$ requirement or apnoea.
- Poor feeding 💣.
- Growth failure 💣.

Treatment
- Start iron supplement at 4wks old for 12mths if <35wks gestation.
- Further research is required to establish appropriate blood transfusion thresholds for preterm infants. Transfuse if clinically indicated. Volume to transfuse (mL) = desired rise in Hb (g/dL) × weight (kg) × [4 (packed cells) or 6 (whole blood)]. Alternatively, give 20mL/kg over 4hrs. Blood should be CMV –ve and irradiated.
- Erythropoietin is useful, but not cost-effective for routine use and may increase the risk of retinopathy of prematurity. Use is limited to infants from Jehovah's witness families.

Polycythaemia

See also 📖 p.630. Defined as arterial or venous packed cell volume (PCV) >65%. More common if placental insufficiency, maternal diabetes mellitus, Down's syndrome, or after twin to twin transfusion. Risk of complications due to thrombosis and or microvascular sludging.

Treatment
- *If symptomatic:* (lethargy, seizures, respiratory distress, poor feeding, thrombocytopenia, stroke, renal failure, NEC) perform dilutional exchange transfusion with 20–30mL/kg of normal saline over 30–60min.
- *If asymptomatic:* it is probably wise to perform dilutional exchange transfusion if PCV >70% to prevent complications.

Thrombocytopenia

See also p.642. Common neonatal causes include:
- Sepsis, including congenital infection.
- NEC.
- IUGR.
- Maternal idiopathic thrombocytopenic purpura (ITP) (due to passive transfer of autoimmune IgG antiplatelet antibodies).
- Neonatal alloimmune thrombocytopenia (NAIT) resulting from transplacental passage of maternal specific IgG antiplatelet antibodies sensitized to differing foetal human platelet antigen (HPA). In 85% antibody is to HPA1 antigen.
- Placental dysfunction.
- Pre-eclampsia.
- DIC.

Presentation
- Petechiae.
- Thrombocytopenia.
- Intracranial haemorrhage (10–20%) particularly with NAIT.

Treatment
Platelet transfusion 10–15mL/kg if platelet count is <50 and active bleeding or <30 plus additional haemorrhagic risk factor or <20 in a well baby.

NAIT-specific treatment
- *Antenatal:* foetal platelet transfusion. Maternal IV immunoglobulin.
- *Postnatal:* observe if platelets >40 × 10^9/L. If platelets less or infant symptomatic, give platelet transfusion (HPA1-negative if relevant) and consider corticosteroids, IV immunoglobulin, or even exchange transfusion (liaise with blood transfusion/haematology).

Coagulation disorders

See also pp.632–640. The most common neonatal cause is DIC. Rarely, there is a specific coagulation defect, e.g. haemophilia, or haemorrhagic disease of newborn.

Haemorrhagic disease of newborn
Bleeding is due to deficiency of vitamin K dependent factors resulting from:
- Poor transplacental supply.
- Lack of enteric bacteria.
- Maternal anticonvulsants.
- Low vitamin K levels in breast milk.

Typical presentation: is at age 2–7 days with bruising and spontaneous bleeding, e.g. from umbilicus, GI tract, or intracranial.

Investigation: shows ↑ prothrombin time (PT) and partial thromboplastin time (PTT), whilst platelet count is normal.

Prevention: vitamin K$_1$ at birth (see p.140).

Treatment: immediate IV vitamin K$_1$ 1mg and fresh frozen plasma 10mL/kg.

Rh disease (rhesus haemolytic disease)

Haemorrhage of foetal blood of differing rhesus group into the maternal circulation leads to maternal anti-D IgG production (usually foetus RhD +ve, mother RhD −ve). Transplacental passage of this antibody leads to foetal RBC haemolysis. The condition is usually asymptomatic or only mild in the first affected pregnancy. Severity usually increases with subsequent pregnancies. Maternal blood group and rhesus antibody status are routinely checked in early pregnancy. Elevated or rising titres indicate that further foetal investigation is warranted, e.g. serial anti-Rh titres, foetal US, foetal blood sampling. The risk of disease is predicted by maternal anti-Rh titre:

- Unlikely when maternal anti-Rh titre <4u/mL.
- 10% when titre is 10–100u/mL.
- 70% when foetal Hb <7g/dL or titre >100u/mL.

Iso-immunization may also occur with other blood group incompatibilities, (e.g. ABO—usually baby A or B and mother O), other rhesus groups (e.g. c, C, e, E), Kell, Kidd, Duffy. Clinical presentation is usually milder than with RhD (particularly ABO).

Presentation

- *Antenatal:* foetal anaemia, hydrops foetalis.
- *Postnatal:* hydrops foetalis, early jaundice, kernicterus
  (□ p.195), cutaneous haemopoietic lesions ('blueberry muffin'), hepatosplenomegaly, coagulopathy, thrombocytopenia, leucopenia.
  Late: anaemia, inspissated bile syndrome.

Investigations

- *Maternal blood for:* group (usually RhD −ve), ↑ anti-Rh titre.
- *Initially, cord or neonatal blood for:* ↓ Hb, ↑ reticulocytes, ↓ platelets, DCT +ve, group (usually RhD +ve), ↑ SBR.
- After diagnosis monitor SBR 4-hourly (until rate of rise known), blood glucose, rate of Hb fall. Check coagulation screen.

Treatment

See also hydrops foetalis, □ p.138.

- Close antenatal supervision +/− intrauterine blood transfusion.
- After birth check cord SBR and Hb, start high risk infants on intensive phototherapy whilst awaiting results. If SBR>100µmol/L then prepare infant for exchange transfusion, consider IVIG (see □ pp.130, 646).
- Supportive treatment as required, e.g. correct any coagulopathy.
- If treatment required, oral folic acid 250mcg/kg/day for 6mths.
- Check Hb every 1–2wks to detect anaemia for up to 12wks. Transfuse if symptomatic or Hb <7g/dL.
- Perform audiology screening if exchange transfusion required.
- *Prophylaxis:* Rh anti-D IgG given to RhD −ve mothers after birth of Rh +ve foetus or possible foeto-maternal haemorrhage.

Prognosis

Mortality <20% even if hydropic. Risk of late onset anaemia.

Bilirubin encephalopathy (kernicterus)

A clinical syndrome resulting from the development of excessive neurotoxic unconjugated bilirubin levels. Toxic levels lead to selective damage of the cerebellum, basal ganglia, and brainstem auditory pathways. It may occur in the healthy neonate if serum bilirubin is >360µmol/L , but usually only occurs at significantly higher serum levels (>430µmol/L after 48hr of life) unless:

- Infant is <24hr old.
- Infant is preterm.
- Infant is severely ill (any cause).
- Infant is acidotic.
- Caused by iso-immunization haemolytic disease.
- Reduced albumin binding caused by drugs or hypoalbuminanaemia.

Presentation

- Lethargy progressing to hypertonia then hypotonia.
- Poor feeding.
- Fever.
- High-pitched cry.
- Opisthotonos.
- Seizures and coma.

Main differential diagnosis is meningoencephalitis/sepsis. Neonatal tetany may also present with opisthotonos.

Treatment

- Supportive (likely to require full intensive care).
- Urgent reduction of serum bilirubin by intensive phototherapy and exchange transfusion.
- Give IV immunoglobulin.
- Treat underlying cause.

Prognosis

Majority survives, but there is a high risk of athetoid cerebral palsy, deafness, and low IQ.

Neonatal dermatology

Neonatal skin is covered with vernix at birth and is poorly keratinized. There is reduced resistance to bacterial infection, increased water loss, increased absorption of drugs (all more pronounced with prematurity.)

The following conditions are all benign and resolve without treatment, often within a few weeks of birth.

- *Milia:* <2mm yellowish-white spots, usually on the face, secondary to blocked sebaceous/sweat glands.
- *Erythema toxicum (erythema neonatorum):* erythematous macular–papular discrete lesions, often with a white centre, mostly present over the knees, elbows, trunk, and face. Very common particularly in post-mature infants.
- *Harlequin colour change:* marked erythema or pallor in different halves, or quadrants, of body. 2° to vasomotor immaturity.
- *Cutis marmorata (livedo reticularis):* marble-like colour change in well baby, secondary to vasomotor immaturity.
- *Sucking blisters:* common on hand, wrist, or upper lip.
- *Superficial capillary haemangioma (salmon-patches, stork marks):* erythematous vascular marks common on eyelids, face midline, and posterior scalp, particularly over the nape of neck (tends to persist at latter site).
- *Mongolian blue spots:* bluish-black macules, most often in lumbar–sacral region, common in non-Caucasians. May last several years.

Nappy rash

Usually a contact dermatitis from ammonia released by bacterial breakdown of urine.

Treatment

Includes:
- Frequent nappy changes.
- Barrier cream, e.g. zinc and castor oil cream; expose to air.
- Suspect secondary *Candida* infection if worse in flexures or satellite lesions present. Treat with topical antifungal, e.g. nystatin ointment 6-hourly (if severe may benefit from oral antifungal simultaneously).

Infantile seborrhoeic eczema

Very common. Usually appears after a few weeks. Erythema and scaling rash affects face, neck, behind ears, axillae, scalp (cradle cap), upper trunk, napkin area, and flexures. Majority spontaneously resolve within weeks. Minority will go on to develop atopic eczema, particularly if there is a family history.

Treatment

- Avoid detergents (i.e. soap).
- Use topical emollients.
- Mild topical steroid/antifungal preparation (e.g. 1% hydrocortisone cream).

Perinatal death

Causes
- Extreme prematurity (40%).
- Congenital abnormalities (30%).
- RDS.
- Sepsis.
- Perinatal asphyxia.
- Pulmonary hypoplasia.
- Miscellaneous.

After death
- Take photographs and mementos, e.g. footprints, according to parents' wishes.
- Inform all relevant professionals, (e.g. GP, obstetrician).
- Refer to coroner (Procurator Fiscal in Scotland) if required. UK criteria are:
  - cause of death unknown;
  - no medical practitioner attended illness leading to death;
  - intraoperative death or prior to recovering from anaesthetic;
  - suspicious circumstances.
- Explain and offer post-mortem to parents. Possible benefits include:
  - determines cause of death;
  - identifies unknown comorbidities;
  - determines degree of normality;
  - audits clinical care;
  - research;
  - medical education.
- Unexpected/unexplained death. As soon as possible consider (with consent!):
  - blood for culture—save serum for possible later testing (iem);
  - throat, eye, ear surface swabs for bacterial and viral culture;
  - suprapubic aspiration (spa) of urine to be saved (iem);
  - axilla skin biopsy for fibroblast culture (send in sterile saline).
- Currently, no neonatal organ or tissue is harvested for transplantation in UK.
- If able, issue completed death certificate to parent/guardian who is then responsible for registering the death. In the UK there is a specific certificate required for a neonatal death (i.e. <28 days old).
- Offer follow-up appointment with senior doctor at 4–6wks to discuss issues surrounding death, post-mortem findings, bereavement.

Withholding or withdrawal of life support
Up to 70% of deaths on UK neonatal units follow withholding or elective withdrawal of life-sustaining treatment. In UK the Royal College of Paediatrics and Child Health states that there are 5 situations when withholding or withdrawal of life sustaining treatment may be appropriate. Three are relevant to newborns and are summarized here:

- *'No chance'*: life-sustaining treatment simply delays death without significant alleviation of suffering, e.g. spinal muscular atrophy type 1.
- *'No purpose'*: although the baby may be able to survive with treatment, the degree of physical or mental impairment will be so great that there is no quality of life, e.g. severe permanent brain injury after perinatal hypoxia.
- *'An unbearable situation'*: treatment is more than can be borne by the baby and/or family when the illness is progressive and irreversible, e.g. recurrent cardiopulmonary resuscitation in an infant with irreversible and progressive cor pulmonale.
- The other two situations relating to 'brain death' and 'permanent vegetative state' cannot currently be diagnosed in the newborn.

Withholding or withdrawing life-sustaining treatment must be first discussed with the parents. Almost always a joint decision can be made in the child's best interests. Time, rather than court proceedings, is usually the best approach, the latter being best reserved for extreme situations.

Procedure for withdrawal of life-supporting treatment

Remember, withdrawal of life-sustaining treatment does not equal withdrawing care:

- If possible, allow parents and family to say their good-byes, spend time alone with baby, have appropriate religious services conducted.
- Parents may wish to be present at the time of withdrawal. Offer options of being present or holding the child in a private quiet room during withdrawal or afterwards.
- Stop all non-palliative infusions and remove all peripheral vascular lines and gastric tubes. Clamp central lines and chest drains.
- Switch off all alarms/monitors.
- If ventilated, disconnect and remove ETT.
- Dress or swaddle infant and then allow parents to cuddle infant.
- Give parents/family space and privacy.
- After death undertake relevant tasks as outlined in 📖 'After death', above.

Practical procedures

Note: All practical procedures should be performed whilst observing appropriate practices to minimize the risk of infection for both the patient and the operator, including aseptic technique, wearing protective clothing, such as gloves, and safe disposable of all contaminated sharp equipment, e.g. needles.

Capillary blood sampling

Capillary blood sampling is used when small volumes of blood are necessary for analysis, e.g. FBC, blood gas, blood glucose. An automated device to pierce the skin is preferred over a lancet, as it causes less pain and punctures to a predetermined depth, thereby reducing the risk of underlying bone damage or infection.

Equipment
- Alcohol impregnated swab.
- Automated device or sterile lancet.
- Appropriate sample bottles or capillary tubes.
- Cotton wool or gauze swab.

Site
- Plantar heel surface outside the medial and lateral limits of calcaneous bone in the young infant (Fig. 7.1).
- Finger site in the older child.

Procedure
- Warm the heel or finger.
- In the case of foot, hold dorsiflexed.
- Clean with an alcohol impregnated swab.
- Gently massage area to improve blood flow and use your hand as a tourniquet.
- Puncture skin with an automated device or sterile lancet.
- 'Scoop' droplets of blood into an appropriate sample container or on to blood glucose-measuring strip. Note that excessive squeezing leads to falsely high serum potassium and haematocrit levels, and bruising.
- Once sample has been collected stop any residual bleeding by local pressure with a cotton wool ball or gauze swab.

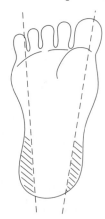

Fig. 7.1 Site for capillary blood sampling on plantar surface of foot. Sampling area is indicated by shaded area.

Venepuncture

Venepuncture is preferable to capillary blood sampling when a significant volume of blood is needed for testing, e.g. coagulation studies, or when sterility of sample is important, e.g. blood culture.

Equipment

- In older child, as in adults, a 21–23G needle and syringe or vacuum tube should be used.
- In infants and small children use either a 23G butterfly needle and syringe or 21–23G butterfly needle without the normal tubing.
- An alcohol impregnated swab.
- Appropriate sample bottles or capillary tubes.
- Cotton wool or an occlusive plaster.

Procedure

- Suitable sites include the antecubital fossa, dorsum of the hand, and dorsum of the foot. Sometimes, necessity demands that other sites such as the scalp are used, particularly in infants.
- Identify suitable vein and warm limb if necessary.
- Topical local anaesthetic cream can be applied under an occlusive dressing for 30–60min reduces pain and may be appropriate in young children.
- Apply a tourniquet proximal to the intended venepuncture site. In infants this is often best done using your own gloved fingers or asking an assistant to squeeze the limb. Also use your fingers to stretch the overlying skin to stabilize the vein. In young children an assistant may be required to keep the child's limb steady.
- Clean overlying skin with an alcohol impregnated swab.
- Along the line of the vein and in a proximal direction, insert needle through overlying skin at 20–30° into the vein until blood flashes back into the needle.
- Stabilize needle/butterfly with your fingers and then aspirate into syringe or, if using a butterfly with no tubing, allow blood to drip into sample bottles. Repeated gentle release and retightening of tourniquet often increases blood flow.
- Once blood has been collected, release the tourniquet, remove needle and then apply gentle pressure to puncture site for a few minutes with cotton wool.
- Once bleeding has stopped, an occlusive plaster is optional, but is often appreciated!

Intravenous cannulation

IV cannulation is required for the infusion of fluids or drugs. Any blood sampling necessary may also be done at the time of insertion. This 'combined' technique will save puncturing the child twice.

Equipment
- An alcohol impregnated swab.
- *IV cannula:* 24G in newborns, 21G in older children.
- IV extension set and 3-way tap with Luer lock flushed with 0.9% saline.
- Tourniquet (older children).
- Fixing tape or transparent occlusive dressing to fix cannula in site.

Procedure
- Carefully identify a suitable vein. The dorsum of the hand or foot or antecubital fossa is ideal. Other suitable sites include the anatomical snuff box, volar aspect of forearm, great saphenous vein at the medial malleolus or knee. Whilst not ideal, scalp veins can be used, but the hair usually needs to be shaved. If possible, avoid larger veins if a percutaneous central line insertion is likely to be needed later.
- *Tip:* transillumination of hand or foot with a 'cold' light source can be very useful for locating 'hidden' veins, particularly in the newborn. In an emergency, or if one or more normal sites have been used, scour the whole body and use whatever vein you can find!
- Consider at least 45min of local anaesthetic cream applied under an occlusive dressing over the intended vein before starting. Remove the cream before starting.
- Ensure good vein perfusion, e.g. warm extremity before cannulation.
- If needed, ask an assistant to help with keeping the child's limb steady. This may require wrapping a young child in a towel or sheet.
- In older children, apply a tourniquet proximal to the vein. In infants, if attempting the hand dorsum, apply compression and immobilization by flexing the wrist, then grasping with the index and middle fingers over the dorsum, whilst the thumb is placed over the child's fingers.
- Clean site with an alcohol impregnated swab.
- Insert cannula at an angle of 10–15° to the skin with the bevel upright, just distal and along the line of the vein.
- When the stylet tip penetrates into the vein lumen blood will flash back (not always if the vein is small!).
- Once vein lumen is entered advance 1–2mm, to ensure the cannula is also in vein, and then advance the cannula over stylet up into the vein.
- Remove stylet, and collect any blood required from the cannula hub.
- Flush cannula with 0.9% saline to confirm IV placement (fluid should infuse without resistance) and to prevent clotting, then connect IV line.
- Secure cannula with appropriate adhesive tape or dressing leaving the skin over the cannula tip visible so that extravasation can be observed.
- Splint extremity to prevent the cannula kinking.
- This is a difficult procedure to master, particularly in the newborn. *Do not be afraid to ask for senior help if unsuccessful after 2 or 3 attempts.*

Peripheral arterial blood sampling

Used for determination of blood gases, acid–base status, or when large volumes of blood are required and venous access is difficult.

Equipment
- As for venepuncture.
- Heparinized arterial blood syringe, if blood gas analysis intended.

Procedure
- In descending order of appropriateness, the suitable sites are: radial artery, posterior tibial artery (in newborns), dorsalis pedis artery (newborns) and ulna artery (only if Allen's test confirms patent adjacent radial artery). If the femoral artery is to be used in the older child, cannulation is preferable before sampling. Brachial artery should rarely, if ever, be used because of its 'end arterial' distribution.
- Identify artery by pulse or 'cold' light.
- Partially extend limb, (e.g. extend wrist for radial artery sampling), and with a finger slightly stretch skin over artery to stabilize its position.
- Clean overlying skin using an alcohol impregnated swab.
- Insert needle through overlying skin at 15–30° angle into artery until blood flashes back; if after inserting needle there is still no flash back withdraw slowly as often blood will then appear.
- Collect blood by aspirating into the syringe.
- Remove needle and apply pressure with cotton wool or gauze swab to puncture wound for at least 5min and bleeding has stopped.

Peripheral arterial cannulation

This procedure is indicated when repeated arterial blood sampling or arterial pressure monitoring is required. The most common arteries used are those described for peripheral arterial blood sampling.

Equipment As for IV cannula (see 📖 p.204).

Procedure
- Identify selected artery by method described above and follow the procedure described, but use a cannula instead of a needle.
- When blood flashes back into the hub, advance the cannula smoothly over the stylet and into the artery.
- Remove the stylet and immediately stop the bleeding by applying pressure over the artery and the tip of the catheter with your finger.
- Connect a 3-way tap that has been previously flushed with heparinized saline. Samples can be obtained from the unused ports.
- Flush the arterial line with heparinized saline (1U/mL) and connect the saline infusion line at 1–2mL/h (1U heparin/mL).
- A pressure transducer may be attached to continuously monitor arterial BP.

Umbilical arterial catheter

An umbilical arterial catheter (UAC) can be used in newborns up to 48hr old for invasive BP monitoring, continuous blood gas monitoring, blood sampling, fluid infusion, and/or exchange transfusion.

Site

To avoid the origins of the coeliac, mesenteric, and renal arteries, the tip of the catheter should be positioned in the aorta above the diaphragm at the T8–T10 vertebral level or in the distal aorta at the L3–L4 level.

Equipment

- Antiseptic solution, e.g. 0.5% chlorhexidine.
- Sterile surgical instruments including fine forceps, blunt-ended dilator probe, scalpel, artery forceps, scissors, suture forceps, sutures.
- Sterile drapes, gown, gauze swabs, and gloves.
- *Umbilical catheters:* 3.5Fr if birth weight <1500g; 5.0Fr for newborns ≥1500g. Catheters with a terminal electrode can be used for continuous measurement of arterial O_2 and CO_2 concentrations.
- 3-way taps, IV extension sets, syringes, cord ligature.
- 5–10mL syringes, one containing heparinized saline (1Ut/mL).
- BP transducer if monitoring is intended.

Procedure

- Monitor baby closely during procedure, e.g. O_2 saturation monitoring.
- An assistant should hold the baby's legs down with the infant supine.
- Calculate the distance (cm) to insert the catheter from the *umbilicus* to the aorta at T8–10 level using the formula:

  Insertion distance = 3 × weight (kg) + 9 + umbilicus stump length.

- To control bleeding, tie a cord ligature around the umbilicus stump.
- Catheter insertion should be performed using strict aseptic technique.
- Wash hands and put on sterile gloves, gown, +/– surgical mask.
- Connect a 3-way tap to catheter and prime with heparinized 0.9% saline (do not use heparinized saline if coagulation testing is required).
- Clean cord and periumbilical area with antiseptic solution.
- Surround periumbilical area with sterile towels to create sterile field.
- Clamp the umbilical cord horizontally with artery forceps 0.5–1cm above umbilical skin. Using the artery forceps as a guide, cut the umbilical cord horizontally and immediately below with the scalpel.
- Identify the two umbilical arteries and umbilical vein (see Fig. 7.2).
- Dilate the end of one of the arteries with fine forceps or a probe until wide enough for the catheter tip to be easily introduced.
- Gently advance catheter the calculated distance (see formula). If resistance is met put gentle traction on the umbilicus using artery forceps as this often eases insertion down the spiral umbilical artery.
- Aspirate blood to confirm position and take required samples. *Note:* arterial blood should pulsate and still bleed if catheter hub is held above infant (unlike blood from the umbilical vein).

- Secure catheter by fixing a zinc oxide flag around the catheter and then suture it to the stump (see Fig. 7.2). Ligate remaining vessels with a separate purse string suture. Remove cord ligature and check for bleeding.
- Connect catheter to 3-way tap and IV infusion set. BP monitoring can be performed by connecting appropriate pressure transducer.
- Confirm correct placement with a combined CXR/AXR. Catheter should loop initially downwards to the pelvis as it traverses the iliac arteries before ascending up the aorta.
- Check perfusion of the perineum and lower limbs. If ischaemia occurs, this usually may be corrected by an IV bolus of 0.9% saline or albumin. If ischaemia remains, remove the catheter immediately.
- Following insertion, the abdomen should remain exposed to allow immediate observation of any haemorrhage, e.g. from accidental removal of catheter.
- As soon as the catheter is no longer required, it should be removed. Cut the surrounding suture, then slowly withdraw it, taking several minutes to remove the final few centimetres from the artery. Then apply pressure or suture to limit any bleeding.

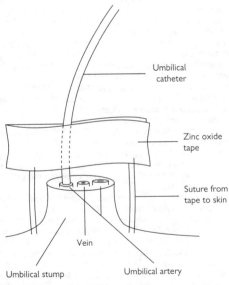

Fig. 7.2 One method of umbilical catheter fixation.

Umbilical venous catheter

A UVC is indicated in newborns up to 5 days of age for: emergency vascular access during resuscitation; vascular access when it is difficult to obtain otherwise; prolonged fluid or drug infusion; exchange transfusion; central venous pressure (CVP) measurement.

Equipment

- 5 or 6 Fr umbilical venous catheter.
- Remaining equipment as for umbilical arterial catheter (📖 p.206).

Procedure

- Measure distance from umbilicus to mid-sternum (= insertion distance).
- Catheter insertion should be performed using strict aseptic technique.
- Wash hands and put on sterile gloves, gown, +/– surgical mask.
- Clean and prepare umbilical stump and create sterile field as detailed on 📖 p.206.
- Identify umbilical vein (see Fig. 7.2) and then dilate opening with fine forceps or a dilating probe.
- Insert catheter the measured distance (see Procedure, first bullet point).
- Aspirate blood to confirm insertion. Blood from the umbilical vein should not pulsate and, when the catheter hub is held open to the air above the infant, blood will slowly fall back to the infant. Do not do this for long or an air embolus will result!
- If blood will not aspirate or resistance is felt before the catheter is inserted the measured distance, it is likely that the catheter tip has lodged in the hepatic portal veins or sinus. Withdraw the catheter and then reinsert as far as it will go while still allowing blood aspiration.
- Flush umbilical catheter with heparinized saline (1Ut/Ml).
- Secure catheter and ligate unused other umbilical vessels using method described for umbilical arterial catheter (📖 p.206).
- Remove cord ligature and check for bleeding.
- Confirm correct position by a combined CXR/AXR. UVC should only follow a direct course proximally through the liver (unlike a UAC) Ideally, tip should lie in the inferior vena cava (IVC) just above diaphragm.
- The catheter can then be used for blood sampling, fluid or drug administration, or CVP monitoring (the later only if the catheter tip is above the diaphragm).
- As soon as the catheter is not needed, remove it slowly and then gently compress umbilical stump until bleeding stops.
- In an emergency (e.g. resuscitation at birth) the procedure is simplified. Simply, cut the umbilical cord with a scalpel blade 1–2cm distal to the umbilical skin and rapidly insert the umbilical catheter until blood can be aspirated. Resuscitation drugs and fluids can then be given safely. Don't worry about haemorrhage as cardiac output will be minimal or absent in such an emergency! Besides, any bleeding can be easily controlled by squeezing the base of the umbilicus between the thumb and index finger. *Note:* Caution is needed as air embolism will occur if an umbilical catheter is left open to the air for any significant time.

Central venous catheterization via a peripheral vein

For administration of prolonged or concentrated IV fluids or drugs.

Sites

Suitable sites include the veins of the antecubital fossa, or long saphenous vein anterior to the medial malleolus or inferior–medial to the knee. Less preferred sites include the axillary or scalp veins.

Equipment

- Sterile surgical instruments including fine forceps and scissors.
- Sterile gloves, gauze swabs, gown, and drapes.
- Antiseptic solution, e.g. 0.5% chlorhexidine.
- 23 or 27G silastic long line catheter. 27G should only be used when a 23G line cannot be inserted.
- 2–5mL syringe and heparinized (1U/mL) saline solution.
- Introducer, e.g. 19G butterfly needle, 20G IV cannula.
- Sterile adhesive tape and transparent occlusive dressing.

Procedure

- Measure distance from insertion site to just above the right atrium. Placing the catheter tip in the right atrium risks pericardial tamponade.
- Catheter insertion should be performed using strict aseptic technique.
- Wash hands and put on sterile gloves, gown, +/– surgical mask.
- Set out equipment and prime catheter with sterile heparinized saline.
- Apply tourniquet proximal to selected insertion point.
- Immobilize relevant limb, then clean insertion site with antiseptic.
- Place sterile drapes around insertion point to create sterile field.
- Insert introducer needle into the vein until blood flashes back. If using a cannula, remove stylet.
- With fine forceps advance catheter through introducer needle/cannula.
- Continue to advance catheter into vein until the desired distance is reached. *Tip:* often the catheter will meet resistance as it becomes wedged against a kinked vein or valve. Milking in a proximal direction with a finger over the catheter tip may facilitate further advancement.
- Remove tourniquet and then flush catheter with heparinized saline.
- Once fully inserted, withdraw introducer needle/cannula. Remove from line after unscrewing catheter hub. Reconnect hub to catheter.
- Ensure haemostasis at puncture site by applying gentle pressure with sterile gauze swab. This may take some considerable time!
- Secure line in place by using thin strips of sterile adhesive tape and sterile transparent occlusive dressing.
- Start infusion of heparinized saline (1U/mL) to keep line patent.
- Confirm catheter tip placement with CXR. This may be aided by the injection into the line of 0.5mL of contrast solution immediately before X-ray. Ideally, the catheter tip should lie just proximal to the right atrium. Withdraw the catheter before use if it is in the right atrium.

Airway management

Before effective ventilation can take place, the airway must be patent. This can be ensured in various ways, alone or in combination.

- *Head tilt:* tilt the head back gently to a neutral position in newborns, slightly extended in older children.
- *Chin lift:* using 1 or 2 fingers apply forward pressure to just under the chin to pull the tongue forward.
- *Jaw thrust:* apply forward pressure behind one or both angles of the jaw to pull the tongue forward.
- *Guedel oro-pharyngeal airway:* slip the airway over the tongue until the flange reaches the lips. Be careful not to push the tongue back. To determine the correct size, hold the airway along the line of the jaw with the flange in the middle of the lips. The end of the correctly sized airway should be level with the angle of the jaw.
- *Endotracheal intubation:* see 📖 p.212.
- *Suction:* not routinely required, especially in newborn resuscitation. However, if the methods described above are not successful in obtaining an adequate airway, check that the airway is not obstructed by secretions, vomitus, blood, meconium, etc. If there is obstruction on inspection, or it is obvious from the start, suction should be performed using an appropriate suction catheter connected to a suction source.
- *Tracheotomy:* bypasses upper airway obstruction and when oral oro-nasal endotracheal intubation fails or is contraindicated. Perform *only* if already trained by a senior doctor. The description of this technique is beyond the scope of this book.

Mask ventilation

This procedure is useful during resuscitation or for short periods of assisted ventilation. It can be performed using a self-inflating bag and face mask with an appropriately-sized reservoir bag; alternatively, use a mask connected to a 'T' piece and a continuous supply of gas, as well as a pressure-limiting device. In the latter, a breath is given by occluding the open aperture of the 'T' piece.

Procedure

- Ensure patent airway (see 📖 p.210).
- Select appropriate size mask. It should be big enough to be able to cover the face from the bridge of the nose to below the mouth, but not extend over the edge of the chin or over the orbits. In infants a round mask, e.g. *Laerdal*® or Bennett's mask, is most appropriate. In older children the *Laerdal*® moulded mask is more suitable.
- Connect face mask to an appropriate self-inflating bag or tubing with a 'T' piece and then to an oxygen or air supply at an adequate flow rate, e.g. 5–8L/min in the newborn.
- In newborns, a pressure-limiting valve should used and initially be set at ~25–30cmH$_2$O.
- Apply mask to face over mouth and nose, and apply enough downward pressure to make an effective seal.
- Give inflation breaths by either compressing self-inflating bag or occluding open aperture of 'T' piece.
- Observe and ausculate chest wall for adequate inflation. Note whether condition of child is improving or deteriorating.
- If inflation is poor or child deteriorating, check airway is not obstructed and use one or more techniques described on 📖 p.210 to ensure patent airway.

Prolonged mask ventilation is likely to lead to a distended stomach. Insert an oro-gastric tube on free drainage to decompress the stomach and prevent diaphragmatic splinting.

Endotracheal intubation

Indications This procedure is used as part of advanced resuscitation and care.

Equipment

- *Appropriately-sized laryngoscope:* neonatal laryngoscopes are straight; blade size starts at 0 (7.5cm long) for use in preterm infants. Use size 1 (10cm) in term infants. In older children use curved blade laryngoscopes (Macintosh).
- *ETT size:* 2–2.5mm (internal diameter) in infant <1000g; 3mm when 1000–3000g; 3.5mm when >3000g. The appropriate size then increases as child size increases up to male adult size of 8–9mm. Cole (shouldered) ETTs are suitable for oral intubation in newborns. Straight (non-shouldered) tubes can be used for oral or nasal intubation.
- Appropriately-sized introducer if required.
- Lubricating jelly if attempting nasal intubation.
- Magill forceps if attempting nasal intubation.
- Suction catheter and tubing connected to suction source.
- Appropriate ETT connection adaptors, tubing, and O_2 source.
- Fixation device and tape.

Procedure

- Oral intubation is preferred during short-term intubation or during resuscitation. Nasal intubation has advantages if ventilation is prolonged.
- Check laryngoscope light, O_2 supply, and suction.
- Connect child to pulse oximeter and cardiac monitor.
- Sedation or anaesthesia should be given prior to elective intubation.
- Pre-oxygenate the child by hyperventilation with 85% O_2 for 15–30s prior to elective intubation.
- Place the child in the supine position with the head in the neutral position and the neck slightly extended.
- Stand immediately behind the child's head.
- If nasal intubation is being performed, a prelubricated ETT should be passed into one nostril as far as the nasopharynx prior to insertion of laryngoscope. If the ETT will not pass easily, do not try force, as this may lead to penetration of the cribriform plate.
- Open the mouth and use suction to clear airway secretions.
- Holding the laryngoscope in the left hand, initially insert the blade to the right side of the mouth and advance to the base of the tongue.
- Once inserted move the laryngoscope blade into the centre of the mouth, thereby pushing the tongue to the left.
- Advance the blade further until epiglottis is seen and then insert blade tip into the valleculla (space between base of tongue and epiglottis).
- Vertically lift up the whole blade, thereby exposing the vocal cords (see Fig. 7.3). Apply cricoid pressure with the little finger of the left hand to see the vocal cords. Perform suction if needed.

- If the vocal cords cannot be seen after 30s do not try to attempt blind intubation. Abandon the attempt, maintain patent airway (📖 p.210), and perform mask ventilation (📖 p.211), before trying again.
- Once the vocal cords are seen, insert the ETT between the vocal cords. If difficult, or performing nasal intubation, use the Magill forceps with the right hand to advance the ETT tip.
- If using a straight tube, the ETT should be advanced until the thick black line at the tip is level with the vocal cords. If using a Cole ETT, advance it until the shoulder just reaches the vocal cords.
- If using a cuffed tube advance until the cuff is just below the vocal cords and no further. Then inflate the cuff with air using a syringe.
- Once intubation is successful, connect tubing and ventilate.
- Visually check chest movement and auscultate over each lung to ensure appropriate and equal bilateral air entry.
- If this procedure is successful, SpO_2 and heart rate should improve.
- Fix ETT in place appropriately following local institutional guidelines.
- Perform a CXR to confirm position of ETT, which should ideally be 1–2cm above the carina, depending on the childs' size.
- Causes of failure to intubate include: poor visualization of vocal cords due to over extension of neck or advancement of laryngoscope too far into the oesophagus; spasm of vocal cords (wait, as almost certainly vocal cords will open eventually—do not attempt to force ETT through as this may cause damage); anatomical abnormalities, e.g. laryngeal atresia; vocal cord oedema.
- Conditions that may give an impression of failed intubation (little or no chest movement on ventilation after intubation) include: thoracic pathology (e.g. tension pneumothorax, diaphragmatic hernia); intubation of the right main bronchus (detected by unequal air entry); and particulate obstruction of airway or ETT.

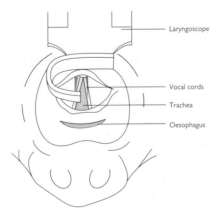

Fig. 7.3 Anatomy of laryngeal intubation.

Insertion of a chest drain

Indications

This procedure is used to drain a pneumothorax, pleural effusion or chylothorax. In an emergency (most commonly due to a tension pneumothorax), drainage should first be performed by inserting 21–23G butterfly into the affected side at the second intercostal space in the mid-clavicular line. The butterfly tubing can be placed under water following insertion; alternatively, a 3-way tap can be attached allowing aspiration with a syringe. Once the child is stable, a formal chest drain should be inserted.

Equipment

- *Antiseptic solution:* e.g. 0.5% chlorhexidine.
- *Local anaesthetic:* e.g. 1% lidocaine, needle, and 10mL syringe.
- *Intercostal drain:* size ranges from 8–12Fr for newborns up to 18Fr for young adults.
- Straight surgical scalpel blade, artery forceps, and suture.
- Sterile dressing pack (including gauze, gloves, drapes).
- Underwater drainage system and suction pump.
- *Steri-Strips®* and plastic transparent dressing, e.g. *Tegaderm®*.

Procedure

- Lie the child supine with the affected side raised by 30–45° using a towel.
- Raise the arm towards the head.
- Suitable sites are the fourth intercostal space in the mid-axillary line (be careful to avoid the nipple), and second intercostal space in mid-clavicle line.
- Chest drain insertion should be performed using strict aseptic technique.
- Wash hands and put on sterile gloves, gown, +/– surgical mask.
- Clean skin over the insertion site with antiseptic solution.
- Prepare sterile field, then infiltrate small amount of local anaesthetic into the tissues down to the pleura.
- Wait 1–2min, then make a small skin incision with the scalpel just *above and parallel to* rib. *Note:* Blood vessels lie just *below* each rib.
- Using artery forceps make a blunt dissection down to and through the parietal pleura.
- Using forceps clamp chest drain and then insert into pleural space. Most clinicians remove the trocar before insertion.
- Aim to push the chest drain tip towards the lung apex. In the event of a small pneumothorax aim the tip in the direction of the pneumothorax remembering to aim anteriorly (air rises in the ill child lying supine).
- Connect the drain tightly to the underwater drainage system, unclamp drain, and apply negative pressure of 5–10cmH$_2$O. Bubbling should start to occur.

- Using single sutures close skin wound closely around chest drain. Do not use a purse string suture as this will increase scarring.
- Apply zinc oxide tape to chest drain and fix to skin using sutures.
- Perform a CXR to check drain position and pneumothorax or effusion drainage.
- Remove drain when confident it is no longer required, e.g. pneumothorax has resolved and there has been no bubbling for >24hr. This is done by releasing holding sutures, then rapidly removing drain followed by immediate pressure and gentle rubbing with a gauze swab to close the underlying tissues. Apply *Steri-Strip*® across skin incision to provide air-tight seal. Perform a CXR to confirm that a significant pneumothorax has not re-accumulated.
- *Note:* If pleural fluid is required for diagnostic purposes only, then simple needle aspiration at the above sites is the technique of choice.

Intraosseous infusion

Indication
This procedure is used for emergency vascular access to give resuscitation drugs or fluids, or for blood sampling when vein cannulation difficult.

Equipment
- 22G IO needle or 1.5G spinal needle in neonates.
- Alcohol impregnated swab.
- 5mL syringe.
- Local anaesthetic, e.g. 1% lidocaine, 2mL syringe and a small gauge needle if patient conscious and local anaesthetic appropriate.

Sites
- *≤3 years old:* anteromedial proximal aspect of tibia, 1–2cm below tibial tuberosity, or anterolateral surface of femur, 2–3cm above lateral condyle.
- *Any age:* medial malleolus of the tibia above the ankle.

Procedure
- Identify site and inject local anaesthetic if the patient is conscious.
- Clean skin with an alcohol impregnated swab.
- Insert at 90° to the skin. Advance into bone using a rotary action.
- Advance trocar until bone cortex is reached, when a give will be felt.
- Remove stylet, attach syringe, and aspirate to confirm position. Obtain any required blood samples.
- Flush needle with 0.9% saline to again confirm position. Swelling outside the bone indicates needle displacement.
- Infuse any required fluids (any fluid that can be given IV can be used).
- Obtain conventional vascular access as soon as possible and then remove IO needle.

Intracardiac injection

Indicated only during resuscitation when all other attempts at securing vascular access have failed.

Equipment
- Alcohol impregnated swab.
- 21G needle and syringe containing resuscitation drug.

Procedure
- Attach needle and syringe. Flush needle with drug to expel air.
- *Locate site:* 4th intercostal space immediately lateral to the left sternal edge (immediately below the line joining the nipples).
- Clean site with an alcohol impregnated swab.
- Insert needle and aspirate syringe as needle is inserted.
- Once blood flashes back, stop advancing.
- Inject resuscitation drug(s).

Pericardiocentesis

Indications
Therapeutic drainage of a pericardial effusion or for diagnostic purposes.

Equipment
- Alcohol impregnated swab/antiseptic solution, e.g. 0.5% chlorhexidine.
- 21G needle or IV cannula and 10–20mL syringe.
- Sterile gloves, drapes, gown, and adhesive plaster.
- Sterile sample containers if pericardial fluid analysis intended.

Procedure
- Lay child on a 30° slope to cause effusion to pool inferiorly.
- Locate insertion site; this lies just below the angle between the sternum and the left costal margin.
- Use sterile gloves and gown. Clean the site with antiseptic and place sterile drapes around insertion site.
- Local anaesthetic infiltration may be appropriate.
- Insert needle connected to syringe at an angle of 30° to the skin and advance slowly, aiming towards the left shoulder. Gently aspirate the syringe as needle is inserted.
- Stop when pericardial fluid (usually straw-coloured) is aspirated and remove desired amount as indicated.
- Once drainage is complete, remove needle and apply adhesive plaster.

Abdominal paracentesis

This is indicated for drainage of ascites when it compromises breathing, e.g. hydrops fetalis, or for diagnostic purposes, e.g. following trauma.

Equipment As for 📖 p.217, Pericardiocentesis.

Procedure
- In infants, the left iliac fossa is the preferred site (which avoids liver and spleen). In older children, a midline site between the symphysis pubis and the umbilicus is preferred because of less vascularity.
- Lay the child supine. If ascites is minimal also tilt towards the left side.
- Except in emergencies, clean and prepare the site as described in 📖 p.217, Pericardiocentesis.
- Attach needle to the syringe and carefully insert it at 90° to the skin.
- Aspirate fluid and place it in sample containers. If large amounts of fluid are to be drained use an IV cannula. Once inserted, remove the stylet, and leave the cannula in place to reduce the risk of bowel perforation. If prolonged drainage is needed, attach the cannula to the skin using adhesive tape or stitches.
- Once complete, remove needle and apply sterile plaster to site.
- If a large amount of fluid is withdrawn, drainage should be followed by IV infusion of albumin.

Urethral bladder catheterization

Indications
This procedure is used for bladder decompression, e.g. potential obstruction, accurate measurement of urine output, and collection of urine for bacteriological investigation in suspected urinary tract infection.

Equipment
- 3–8Fr urinary catheter (depending on child's size).
- Anaesthetic lubricating gel, e.g. 0.1% lidocaine gel.
- Water-based antiseptic solution, e.g. 0.5% chlorhexidine.
- Sterile urine sample container.
- Sterile gloves and adhesive tape.

Procedure
- Lay child in supine position with hips abducted, with an assistant holding the child.
- Clean penile tip or vulval area with antiseptic solution.
- Apply anaesthetic lubricating gel to catheter tip and urethral opening.
- Partially withdraw foreskin in males. Part the labia in females.
- Insert and advance catheter into urethra in a posterior manner until urine is obtained, indicating that the bladder has been entered.
- Once in the bladder, inflate the catheter balloon with saline if the catheter is intended to be indwelling.
- Use adhesive tape to secure the catheter to the thigh.
- Connect catheter to the urine collection bag or aspirate urine for analysis.

Suprapubic aspiration of urine

Optimal method for obtaining urine for bacteriology in a child <2yr old.

Equipment

- 21–23G needle.
- 2–5mL syringe.
- An alcohol impregnated swab.
- Sterile urine sample container.
- Cotton wool or gauze swab and adhesive plaster.

Procedure

- Wait at least 30min from last urination.
- If in doubt as to whether the bladder contains adequate urine, perform bladder US to confirm.
- Place child supine (with an assistant holding hips abducted) and then identify site—midline anterior lower abdominal wall 1cm above the pubic bone.
- Clean site with an alcohol impregnated swab.
- Insert needle connected to the syringe at 90° to the skin, aspirating continuously until urine is obtained.
- Insert to almost the depth of the needle. If no urine is obtained, partially withdraw it before inserting again at different angle.
- Once required urine is aspirated, remove the needle, press on puncture site with cotton wool or gauze swab, and then apply an adhesive plaster.
- Place urine in sterile container.
- If unsuccessful, repeat the procedure 30–60min later.

Lumbar puncture

Indications To obtain sample of CSF for microbiological, biochemical, or metabolic analysis; therapeutically drain CSF in communicating hydrocephalus.

Contraindications Include thrombocytopenia or coagulation defect, raised intracranial pressure, and significant cardiorespiratory compromise, as positioning may risk cardiorespiratory arrest (see also 📖 p.109).

Site L3–L4 intervertebral space (spinal cord may be as low as L2 in neonates).

Equipment
- 24–22G 1.5 inch spinal needle.
- Antiseptic solution, e.g. 0.5% chlorhexidine.
- Sterile dressing pack (including gauze, gloves, drapes).
- Sterile sample containers; usually 3 are needed for M,C&S, protein, and glucose, but sometimes also for virology, cytology, or immunology.
- Adhesive plaster or aerosol plastic dressing spray.
- Pressure manometer and 3-way tap if measuring CSF opening pressure.

Procedure
- Apply topical local anaesthetic cream to site under an occlusive dressing for 45min before the procedure.
- Place child on their side with back along an edge of a firm surface.
- Ask an experienced assistant to firmly, but gently, hold child with the spine maximally flexed. Beware compromising respiration!
- Locate site. L4 spinous process lies on a line joining the iliac crests.
- Using strict aseptic technique, clean the site with antiseptic solution and then create a sterile field by surrounding it with sterile drapes.
- Inject local anaesthetic into site if child is ≥6mths old.
- Insert spinal needle into intervertebral space slowly at 90° to the skin and aim in the direction of the umbilicus, i.e. slightly cephalad.
- Advance needle slowly until there is a sudden give, which occurs as the dura is penetrated.
- Remove stylet; wait for CSF to drain. If no CSF drains, advance needle very slowly and withdraw stylet every 1–2mm to check for drainage. If bone is struck or needle is fully inserted and no CSF obtained, remove the stylet and then withdraw cannula very slowly in case CSF appears.
- Allow 10 drops of CSF to drain into each sample bottle.
- If measuring CSF pressure, connect 3-way tap before collecting samples and direct fluid up attached manometer. Once opening pressure is measured, turn 3-way tap to allow CSF to drain.
- If therapeutic CSF drainage is required, drain required amount.
- Once drainage is complete, remove the needle and rub the puncture site with a sterile gauze swab while applying pressure.
- Cover site with an adhesive plaster or aerosol plastic dressing.
- The child should lie flat for the next 6hr and have hourly neurological observations and BP measurement.

Cerebral ventricular tap

Indications

This procedure is done for drainage of CSF in non-communicating hydrocephalus, to obtain CSF for microbiological testing, e.g. to diagnose ventriculitis, and to administer intraventricular antibiotics.

Equipment As for lumbar puncture (📖 p.220).

Procedure

- Before the procedure is undertaken, cerebral lateral ventriculomegaly must be confirmed by cranial US.
- Place the baby supine, with an assistant firmly holding the baby's head.
- Measure the necessary depth required for needle insertion.
- Palpate and locate the lateral corner of the anterior fontanelle on the intended side to drain.
- Shave a small area of the scalp at the needle insertion point if required.
- Set out sample containers +/– CSF pressure manometer if needed.
- Full aseptic technique should be used.
- Wash hands and put on sterile gloves, gown, +/– surgical mask.
- Clean area with antiseptic solution and create a sterile field with sterile drapes.
- Insert needle into the lateral corner of the fontanelle in a direction slightly forward and inward, aiming toward the inner canthus of the ipsilateral eye.
- After the needle is inserted to the predetermined distance, remove stylet and CSF should drip out.
- If CSF pressure measurement is required, attach manometer and allow it to fill until measurement is complete.
- If CSF drainage or sample is required, then allow fluid to drip out spontaneously into containers until required amount is drained.
- Once required CSF has been drained, remove the needle and then cover with adhesive plaster or spray with plastic dressing to seal.
- The child should lie flat for the next 6hr and have hourly neurological observations and BP measurement.

Exchange transfusion

Indications

- Severe or rapidly rising hyperbilirubinaemia, e.g. due to severe rhesus or other haemolytic disease (see 📖 p.194).
- Cardiac failure secondary to severe anaemia (with normal or increased plasma volume), e.g. hydrops fetalis due to rhesus haemolytic disease.
- Disseminated intravascular coagulation.
- Polycythaemia with a venous haematocrit >70% and/or symptomatic.
- Acute poisoning, including that due to metabolic disease.

Exchange is achieved by sequentially removing 10–15mL of blood from the child and then infusing warmed (37°), cross-matched, fresh (<72hr old), rhesus –ve, cytomegalovirus (CMV) –ve, irradiated or leucocyte filtered (to prevent graft vs. host disease), partially packed or whole blood. Exchange transfusion can be performed by either both withdrawing and then infusing blood via a single central venous catheter (e.g. umbilicus venous catheter), or withdrawing blood via a central catheter (arterial or venous) or peripheral arterial catheter and replacing it via a second central or peripheral venous catheter.

Blood volume (mL) to remove and then replace (i.e. exchange) is:
- Severe anaemia with hydrops requires a *single volume* exchange, i.e. 80mL/kg body weight. Should be performed over a minimum of 1hr.
- Removal of toxins, e.g. bilirubin or ammonia, requires a *double volume* exchange, i.e. 160mL/kg in newborns. This replaces ~90% of total blood volume and should be performed over a minimum of 2hr.
- To treat polycythaemia, a dilutional exchange transfusion is performed. The required exchange volume depends on the haematocrit (Hct) and can be calculated using the formula:

  Volume = [measured Hct – desired Hct] × blood volume measured Hct

- In a dilutional exchange replace blood with 0.9% saline 0.45% albumin.

Equipment

- Venous and arterial catheters, either central or peripheral.
- Two 20mL syringes and 3-way taps.
- Blood administration set and warming coils.
- Calibrated waste blood container.
- +/– High flow rate infusion pump.
- Appropriately cross-matched blood (see Indications).
- ECG and BP monitor.
- Sterile dressing pack (including gown, gauze swabs, drapes, and gloves).

Procedure

- If not already present, insert central or peripheral venous/arterial catheters.
- Start continuous ECG and frequent BP monitoring.
- As a baseline, measure serum FBC, U&E, Ca^{2+}, glucose, and blood gases.
- Prime blood administration set and warm blood to 37°C.
- Arrange for an assistant to keep a constant accurate log of volumes removed and replaced throughout the procedure.
- Use a full aseptic technique throughout the procedure.
- Wash hands and put on sterile gloves, gown, +/− surgical mask.
- Connect 3-way taps into the system (exact arrangement depends on choice of method; see the following bullet points).
- If using a single central venous catheter, e.g. UVC, use two sequential 3-way taps to perform the following in order:
  - Withdraw 5–20mL blood from the baby using a syringe *over a few minutes*.
  - Turn first 3-way tap to allow blood to be syringed into a waste bag.
  - Turn second 3-way tap to allow 5–20mL, fresh, warmed blood to be drawn from pack.
  - Turn tap and syringe fresh blood *slowly* into baby (2–3min).
- If using two catheters together, remove 5–20mL aliquots of blood from the central or arterial catheter over 5–10min and then turn a single 3-way tap to allow blood to be pushed into the waste bag. Simultaneously, the same volume of fresh warmed blood is infused into the patient via the other venous catheter using a high rate flow infusion pump.
- A safe volume to remove each turn varies depending on size of infant. Remove 5mL aliquots for ELBW infants, increasing up to 20mL for full term infants.
- Apart from continuously monitoring pulse, ECG, BP, and temperature, every 30–60min during the procedure measure blood gases, FBC, U&E, serum Ca^{2+}, and glucose. Measure again at the end of the procedure, as well as a coagulation profile. Correct any abnormality found.
- Once procedure is completed, leave catheters in place in case repeat exchange transfusion is required.

Complications of exchange transfusion

- Catheter-induced thrombotic or embolic phenomenon, e.g. portal vein thrombosis or NEC.
- Haemodynamic compromise, e.g. cardiac arrhythmia or hypotension.
- Metabolic, e.g. hypoglycaemia (transfused plasma often has a low blood glucose concentration due to red cell consumption), hypokalaemia, hypocalcaemia, hypomagnesaemia, acidaemia.
- Coagulopathy or thrombocytopenia.
- Hypothermia.
- *Infection:* bacteraemia, HIV, CMV, hepatitis B or C. Blood must be screened prior to transfusion.
- *Graft vs. host disease:* risk reduced by irradiation or leucocyte filtration.

Cardiovascular

Common presentations

The cardiovascular examination in children is described on 📖 p.32. The majority of children with cardiovascular disease will present with one or more of the following three clinical problems:
* cyanosis;
* heart failure (📖 p.226);
* heart murmur (📖 p.228).

Cyanosis

Distinguishing between respiratory and cardiac causes of cyanosis is important (see 📖 pp.55, 60–62).

Heart failure

Heart failure may be manifested by symptoms of poor tissue perfusion alone (e.g. fatigue, poor exercise tolerance, confusion) and/or by symptoms of congestion of circulation (e.g. dyspnoea, pleural effusion, pulmonary oedema, hepatomegaly, peripheral oedema), without evoking compensatory mechanisms.

The underlying pathophysiology mechanisms that lead to compromise of cardiac stroke volume, cardiac decompensation, and heart failure include:
* increased afterload (pressure work);
* increased preload (volume work);
* myocardial abnormalities;
* tachyarrhythmias.

Causes of heart failure

In children the most common cause of heart failure is congenital structural defects of the heart.
* *Large left to right shunt:* e.g. large VSD (not in first few days of life).
* *Left-sided obstructive lesions:* coarctation of aorta; hypoplastic left side of heart (within first few days of life).
* *Cardiomyopathy:* hypertrophic; dilated; restrictive.
* *Myocarditis:* viral; rheumatic fever.
* Endocarditis.
* *Myocardial ischaemia:* anomalous left coronary artery; Kawasaki disease.
* *Tachyarrhythmias:* supraventricular tachycardia.
* Acute hypertension.
* *High-output:* severe anaemia; thyrotoxicosis; AV malformations.

Clinical features
The clinical features of heart failure depend on the degree of cardiac reserve. The most common symptoms and signs are those in keeping with increased compensatory sympathetic drive:
- sweating;
- breathlessness, tachypnoea, coughing, lung crepitations;
- poor feeding (infant), poor weight gain, and failure to thrive;
- hepatomegaly;
- cardiomegaly;
- tachycardia/'gallop' heart rhythm.

There are usually few signs of systemic congestion as observed in adults. Only children with chronic heart failure, or adolescents, may have 'adult' signs such as oedema, orthopnoea, paroxysmal nocturnal dyspnoea, ankle oedema and elevated JVP.

Investigations
These are directed at finding a cause and quantifying function.
- *Chest radiograph:*
  - cardiac enlargement;
  - lungs—oligaemic/oedema.
- *Echocardiography:* congenital heart defects.
- *Arterial blood gas:* reduced PO_2/metabolic acidosis.
- *ECG:* not diagnostic, but may assist in establishing aetiology.
- *Serum electrolytes:* hyponatraemia due to water retention.

Management
The underlying cause of heart failure must be treated.

General measures
- Bed rest and nurse in semi-upright position: infants in chair/seat.
- Supplemental oxygen (not in left to right shunt).
- *Diet:* sufficient calorie intake.
- Diuretics.
- Angiotensin converting enzyme inhibitors.

Heart murmurs

Heart murmurs should be characterized in terms of type, location, radiation, and quality of sound.

Murmurs are classified as follows:

- *Systolic:* pansystolic; ejection systolic.
- *Diastolic:* early diastolic; mid-diastolic.

The location where a murmur is best heard may give a clue to the underlying aetiology.

- *Lower sternal edge:* VSD—often loud; innocent heart murmur—soft.
- *Upper sternal edge:* aortic stenosis; pulmonary stenosis.
- *Base of neck:* aortic valve lesion.

Pathological heart murmur

Characteristic features of pathological heart murmurs:

- All diastolic murmurs.
- All pansystolic murmurs.
- Late systolic murmurs.
- Loud murmurs >3/6.
- Continuous murmurs.
- If there are associated cardiac abnormalities.
- Abnormal symptoms or signs:
  - shortness of breath (SOB);
  - tiredness/easy fatigue;
  - failure to thrive (FTT);
  - cyanosis;
  - finger clubbing;
  - hepatomegaly.

Innocent heart murmurs

This is the commonest cause of a heart murmur in children. It arises due to the rapid flow and turbulence of blood through the great vessels and across normal heart valves. It does not signify the presence of any underlying cardiac abnormality or any other pathology.

Characteristics of innocent heart murmur

- Systolic in timing—always. *Never* diastolic.
- Short duration/low intensity sound.
- Intensifies with increased cardiac output (e.g. exercise/fever).
- May change in intensity with change in posture and head position.
- No associated cardiac thrill or heave.
- No radiation.
- Asymptomatic patient.

Types of innocent heart murmur

Venous hum (uncommon)

- 'Machinery' quality sound. Upper left sternal edge.
- Due to blood flow in great veins.

Flow murmur

- Short systolic murmur. Mid-left sternal edge.

- Often heard during acute illness with fever, disappears when fever resolves.

Musical murmur
Systolic murmur. Lower left sternal edge.

Murmurs: clinical features

A likely diagnosis can be assessed using the clinical examination and features from CXR and ECG. Tables 8.1 and 8.2 summarize likely diagnoses given the characteristics of the murmur and the findings from your initial investigations.

Table 8.1 Likely diagnoses based on clinical features of murmur

Location of murmur	Diagnoses	Features
Continuous murmur		
Left clavicular (machinery) in child; LSE in preterm infant	PDA (📖 p.234)	Acyanotic; bounding pulse;
Long systolic murmur		
Lower LSE (pansystolic) parasternal thrill	VSD (📖 p.234)	Acyanotic
Apex	Mitral regurgitation	Acyanotic Rheumatic fever
Mid-LSE	Tetralogy of Fallot (📖 p.235)	Cyanotic; single S2
Ejection systolic murmur		
Upper LSE	ASD secundum (📖 p.233)	Acyanotic; fixed split S2;
	AVSD partial (📖 p.233)	Acyanotic; fixed split S2; + Apical pansystolic murmur
Upper LSE +/- thrill	PS (📖 p.238)	Acyanotic
Upper LSE	CoA (📖 p.238)	Acyanotic; weak or absent femoral pulses (if neonate); *hypertensive* in right arm (if older)
Upper RSE	AS (📖 p.237)	Acyanotic; carotid thrill; delayed soft S2; small volume & slow rising pulse

Key: AS, aortic stenosis; ASD, atrial septal defect; AVSD, atrioventricular septal defect; CoA, coarctation of the aorta;; LSE left sternal edge; RSE right sternal edge; LV, left ventricle; PDA, persistent ductus arteriosus; PS, pulmonary stenosis; PV, pulmonary valve; S1, first heart sound; S2, second heart sound; VSD, ventricular septal defect.

Investigation of suspected heart problem using CXR and ECG

Table 8.2 Likely diagnoses based on CXR and ECG findings

CXR findings	ECG findings	Diagnosis
Normal	Normal	Normal or small VSD (📖 p.234)
Mild cardiomegaly + increased pulmonary markings	RVH + LVH + RAD RBBB + LAD + RBBB prolonged PR	VSD (📖 p.234) ASD secundum (📖 p.233) AVSD partial (📖 p.233) PDA (📖 p.234)
	Normal or LVH	
Cardiomegaly	Normal LVH	HLHS (📖 p.239) HOCM (📖 p.240)
Enlarged LV	LVH	AS (📖 p.237)
Small boot-shaped heart + oligaemic lung fields	RAD, RVH	ToF (📖 p.235)
Narrow mediastinum, heart 'egg on side', + increased pulmonary vascular markings	Normal	TGA (📖 p.238)
Rib-notching	RVH (neonate); LVH	CoA (📖 p.238)
PA post-stenotic dilatation	Normal or RVH	PS (📖 p.238)

Key: HLHS; hypoplastic left heart syndrome, LAD; left axis deviation; LV left ventricle; LVH, left ventricular hypertrophy; PA, pulmonary artery; RAD, right axis deviation; RBBB right bundle branch block; RVH, right ventricular hypertrophy; ToF, tetralogy of Fallot. For key to diagnoses see footnote to Table 8.1.

Acyanotic: congenital heart disease

Definition Failure of normal cardiac development or persistence of the foetal circulation after birth.

Incidence
- 8/1000 live births.
- 10–15% complex lesions with >1 abnormality.
- 10–15% of CHD also have a non-cardiac abnormality.

Causes
This is unknown in the majority of cases, but commonly associated with following conditions:
- *Chromosomal defects:* e.g. Down, Turner syndromes.
- *Gene defects:* e.g. 22q deletion, Noonan syndrome
- *Congenital infections:* e.g. rubella.
- *Teratogenic drugs:* e.g. phenytoin, warfarin, alcohol.

Classification
CHD can be classified into acyanotic or cyanotic types depending on whether predominant presentation is with or without central cyanosis. The latter is caused by deoxygenated blood gaining abnormal access to systemic side of the circulation via the left side of the heart or the aorta.

Acyanotic CHD
- VSD.
- ASD.
- PDA.
- Pulmonary valve stenosis.
- Coarctation of the aorta.
- Aortic stenosis.
- Hypoplastic left heart syndrome.
- Hypertrohpic obstructive cardiomyopathy.
- Dextrocardia.

Cyanotic CHD
- Tetralogy of Fallot.
- Transposition of the great arteries.
- Tricuspid atresia.
- Total anomalous pulmonary drainage.

The diagnosis of a specific lesion is made after clinical examination; CXR, ECG, and echocardiography (see 📖 pp.226–231).

Left to right shunt: atrial septal defect

ASD may be subtyped as ostium secundum or partial atrioventricular septal defect (ostium primum).

Ostium secundum defect

This defect is in the region of the foramen ovale. The atrioventricular (AV) valves are normal. The defect is usually isolated, found incidentally, and 3 times more common in girls.

- *Clinical features:* most children are asymptomatic. ASDs may rarely result in heart failure.
- *Prognosis:* ostium secundum defects are well tolerated and symptoms and complications usually only present in 3rd decade or later.
- *Treatment:* ASD closure is required and advised for all patients, even if asymptomatic. This is achieved usually by insertion of an occlusion device at cardiac catheterization or by open heart surgery. Intervention should be performed in early childhood, before school entry.

Partial atrioventricular septal defect

This is the more serious ASD, affecting the endocardial cushion tissue that gives rise to the mitral and tricuspid valves. It is located in the lower atrial septum and is associated with a three leaflet mitral valve. These abnormalities result in a left to right shunt with valve incompetence. AVSD are often seen in Down syndrome.

- *Clinical features:* most children with small defects are asymptomatic. Those with larger defects are predisposed to recurrent chest infections and to heart failure.
- *Prognosis:* depends on the degree of left to right shunt, pulmonary hypertension, and severity of mitral regurgitation. Without surgical repair congestive cardiac failure may develop in infancy/early childhood.
- *Management:* definitive treatment with surgical closure of the defect is indicated pre-school.

Ventricular septal defect

VSDs account for 25% of all CHD (2/1000 live births). They may occur in isolation or as part of complex malformations. The clinical features depend on the size and location of the defect.

Subtypes
- Large/small VSD.
- Perimembranous.
- Muscular.
- Multiple/small defects (maladie de Roger).

Clinical features
- Asymptomatic (typical/early).
- Heart failure (breathlessness—after the first few days of life).
- Recurrent chest infections.
- Cyanosis (rare after 1st decade of life)—2° to Eisenmenger syndrome.
- Endocarditis (late).

Examination Pansystolic murmur—lower left sternal edge parasternal thrill.

Prognosis The majority of defects will close spontaneously.

Management
- *Medical:* treat heart failure if present.
- *Surgery:* indicated if severe heart failure; pulmonary hypertension. This is performed at 3mths of age, before the pulmonary hypertension causes pulmonary vascular disease (Eisenmenger syndrome).

Persistent ductus arteriosus

PDA is common and seen in 1–2/1000 live births. Sometimes it follows on from a preterm delivery. It is defined as a duct still being present 1mth after the date that the child should have been born.

Clinical features
PDA results in a low diastolic pressure, due to blood flowing back into the pulmonary artery. There may be heart failure (breathlessness).

Examination
- A wide pulse pressure or bounding peripheral pulses.
- A continuous or machinery murmur in the left infraclavicular area.

Prognosis The majority of defects will close spontaneously.

Management
- *Medical:* diuretics.
- *Cardiac catheter:* device closure usually at 1yr.
- *Surgical:* ligation (rarely).

Right to left shunt: tetralogy of Fallot

This, the most common cyanotic CHD, is characterized by 4 cardinal anatomical cardiac anomalies:
- Large VSD.
- Overriding aorta.
- Right ventricular outflow obstruction (infundibular and valvular pulmonary stenosis).
- Right ventricular hypertrophy.

Systemic venous return to the right side of the heart is normal. In the presence of pulmonary stenosis, however, blood is shunted across the VSD into the aorta and arterial desaturation and cyanosis result. The severity of cyanosis is dependent on the degree of right ventricular outflow obstruction and, when this is moderate, a balanced shunt across the VSD occurs and cyanosis may be mild or absent.

Clinical features

Tetralogy of Fallot presents in early infancy with the following.
- *Cyanosis:* usually not present at birth and leading to clubbing.
- *Paroxysmal hypercyanotic spells (infancy):* spontaneous/unpredictable onset; tachypnoea; restlessness; and increasing cyanosis, then becoming white and floppy. Potentially dangerous. Duration ranges from a few minutes to hours; severe episodes result in syncope and occasionally convulsions/hemiparesis.

Treatment

Severe tetralogy of Fallot with worsening cyanosis in early neonatal period requires prostagladin E infusion; (see 📖 p.58) and surgery (e.g. modified Blalock–Taussig shunt) in order to maintain pulmonary blood flow and oxygenation. Definitive surgery to repair the underlying heart defects is carried out from 4mths of age onwards.

Management of hypercyanotic spells See 📖 p.63.

Prognosis

Untreated, the combination of right to left shunt, chronic cyanosis, and polycythaemia predispose to:
- Cerebral thrombosis and ischaemia.
- Brain abscess.
- Bacterial endocarditis.
- Congestive cardiac failure.

Patients are often asymptomatic after surgical corrections. Long-term follow-up (up to 30yrs) suggest that improved quality of life is maintained and most are able to lead unrestricted lives. Some will require pulmonary valve replacement in teenage years. Cardiac conduction defects, including complete heart block, are seen post-operatively and require treatment.

Transposition of the great arteries

The normal 'figure of eight' systemic/pulmonary blood flow circuit is replaced by two separate parallel circuits, i.e. systemic venous blood passing through the right side of heart returns directly to the systemic circulation via a connecting aorta. Pulmonary venous blood returning to the left side of the heart is retuned directly to the pulmonary circulation via a connecting pulmonary artery. This condition is not compatible with life unless there is adequate mixing of the blood from both circulations via an ASD or PDA.

Clinical features

Infants usually present in the first few hours or days with worsening duct-dependent cyanosis. Hypoxia is usually severe, but heart failure is not a feature. This is a medical emergency and early diagnosis and intervention are required to avoid severe hypoxia.

Treatment

Once diagnosed care is needed to maintain body temperature as hypothermia will worsen the metabolic acidosis of hypoxaemia. Prompt correction of acidosis and hypoglycaemia is essential. Before cardiac surgery, systemic arterial oxygenation can be improved with prostaglandin E infusion (see 📖 p.58) and balloon atrial septostomy. Definitive arterial switch procedure is performed in the first 2wks of life.

Common mixing: complete atrioventricular septal defect

Complete AVSD is often found in conjunction with Down syndrome. There is a large defect often from the middle of the atrial septum down to the middle of the ventricular septum. In addition there is not a separate mitral and tricuspid valve, but there is a common atrioventricular valve of 5 leaflets guarding the atrioventricular junction.

Clinical features

Most patients with Down syndrome are screened for congenital heart disease with an echocardiogram. An ECG will show a superior axis.

Treatment

• *Medical*: treat heart failure if present.
• *Surgery*: is performed at 3mths of age, before pulmonary hypertension causes pulmonary vascular disease (Eisenmenger syndrome).

Tricuspid atresia

In tricuspid atresia (TA) there is no connection between the right atrium and the right ventricle. Venous blood is diverted to left side via a patent foramen ovale. Pulmonary blood flow is dependent on associated VSD or PDA.

Clinical features

Most patients with TA present in the first few days to early months of life with increasing cyanosis. The clinical features will vary depending on other associated cardiac abnormalities. The ECG shows a superior axis.

Treatment

In an emergency, duct patency is achieved with prostaglandin E infusion (see 📖 p.58). Surgical palliation and procedures include:
- Blalock–Taussig shunt (neonatal period).
- Pulmonary artery banding (neonatal period).
- Glenn shunt (6mths of age).
- Fontan procedure (pre-school).

Aortic stenosis

Congenital aortic stenosis accounts for about 5% of all causes of CHD and is the commonest cause of left ventricular outflow obstruction. It is due to thickening of the aortic valves, although subvalvular (subaortic) stenosis is also an important form of obstruction. Congenital aortic stenosis is more common in boys (3:1). A supravalvular form of aortic stenosis is also recognized, which may be sporadic or familial. Supravalvular aortic stenosis is also associated with Williams syndrome (📖 pp.373, 941).

Clinical features

Are dependent on the severity of obstruction and age at presentation. Mild stenosis is usually asymptomatic and found on routine examination. Severe defects in the neonate may present with heart failure and collapse. In the older child sudden unexpected syncope and chest pain on exertion may occur.

Management

Surgical or balloon dilatation is indicated if symptomatic, or if a high resting pressure gradient of >64mmHg is present; avoidance of competitive sports recommended if severe.

Prognosis

Good in the majority with mild or moderate stenosis. In severe stenosis sudden death may occur. Eventually, aortic valve replacement will be required.

Pulmonary stenosis

This is a common form of CHD due to the following:
- Isolated thickened deformed pulmonary valves (usually).
- Isolated infundibular stenosis; supravalvular pulmonary stenosis.
- Branch pulmonary artery stenosis.

Pulmonary valve stenosis is seen in Noonan syndrome (📖 p.941).

Clinical features

- Asymptomatic (mild to moderate stenosis).
- Poor exercise tolerance (severe stenosis).
- Right ventricular failure/cyanosis (critical stenosis).

Prognosis

Mild to moderate stenosis is compatible with normal activities, but patients require monitoring because worsening obstruction and significant pressure gradients may develop, which will predispose to heart failure when very severe.

Treatment Severe pulmonary valve stenosis requires treating by transvenous catheter balloon dilatation.

Coarctation of the aorta

Constrictions of the aorta (CoA) may occur at any point. In the majority (98%) of cases, it is usually distal to the origin of the left subclavian artery at the level of the ductus arteriosus.

Most often, this occurs in the neonatal period and the infants present at 48hr old when the duct closes. In older children, the BP is elevated in blood vessels proximal to the obstruction and an extensive collateral circulation develops. CoA is seen more often in boys than girls (2:1), although it is common in Turner syndrome (📖 p.948). In ♀, 0% an abnormal bicuspid aortic valve is present.

Clinical features

In severe defects a PDA is required to maintain the systemic circulation; heart failure and collapse may occur in the neonatal period. CoA results in a disparity in pulse volume with weak or absent femoral pulses. Mild defects may present later with hypertension (right arm).

Prognosis

Outside the neonatal period, mortality from untreated hypertension is high and usually occurs when aged 20–40yrs. Complications include premature coronary artery disease, congestive cardiac failure, hypertensive encephalopathy, and intracranial haemorrhage.

Treatment Neonates require resuscitation and early surgery. Older children or adolescents require stent insertion at cardiac catheter or surgical resection.

Hypoplastic left heart syndrome

This term is used to describe a group of disorders associated with under-development of the left side heart structures. The left ventricle is small and non-functional and the right ventricle maintains both pulmonary and systemic circulations. The latter is achieved by pulmonary venous blood passing through an ASD or patent foramen ovale, or via retrograde flow through a PDA.

Clinical features

Hypoplastic left heart syndrome (HLHS) presents with early onset (days) of cyanosis and heart failure leading to collapse and death within the first few days of life. Most infants will appear sick (greyish-blue colour) with poor peripheral perfusion and weak peripheral pulses. Central cyanosis and evidence of heart failure will be present.

Treatment

Medical management aimed at maintaining patency of the ductus is necessary to support systemic blood flow. Surgery is either palliative (2–3 stages, Norwood operation or Hybrid procedure) or definitive (heart transplantation).

Total anomalous pulmonary venous connection

All blood returning to the heart (systemic and pulmonary) returns to the right atrium, and an obligatory patent foramen ovale or ASD is necessary for survival. The pulmonary veins form a single channel and join the systemic venous circulation through either a supracardiac superior vena cava (SVC), intra- or infracardiac IVC connection.

Clinical features

Infants usually present in the first few days of life with varying degrees of obstruction, cyanosis, and congestive cardiac failure. Presentation will depend on the degree of obstruction to the pulmonary venous return.

Treatment

This is often a surgical emergency and anastomosis of the common pulmonary channel to the left atrium, with closure of ASD, and interruption of connections to the systemic venous circuit are required.

Hypertrophic obstructive cardiomyopathy

This condition is characterized by massive ventricular hypertrophy principally involving the septum. All portions of the left ventricle are affected, although the right ventricle may also be involved. There is myocardial fibrosis resulting in a stiff muscle with decreased distensibility. Ventricular filling is decreased, but systolic pumping is maintained until late in the course of disease. Hypertrophic obstructive cardiomyopathy (HOCM) has been recognized in all age groups and may occur in members of the same family. A dominant pattern of inheritance sometimes is observed.

Clinical features

Most children with HOCM are asymptomatic and are only detected following routine clinical examination and the discovery of an incidental heart murmur. Symptoms when present include fatigue and dyspnoea and chest pain and syncope on exertion. HOCM is an important cause of sudden unexpected death.

Prognosis Unpredictable, especially in those without symptoms.

Treatment

Avoidance of competitive sports and strenuous activity is encouraged. Therapy is aimed at reducing the outflow obstruction:
- *Medical therapy:* beta blocking agents; calcium antagonists, pacemaker.
- *Surgical therapy:* ventricular septal myotomy, transplantation.

Dextrocardia

Abnormal position of the heart, with location of left atrium on right side and vice versa (i.e. situs inversus), is classified according to the position of the left atrium, the main bronchi, and the abdominal organs. Inversion of viscera (abdominal situs inversus) is always associated with atrial inversion. Major malformations of heart structures are usually found in either of the following:
- Dextrocardia + normal position of abdominal organs.
- Normal position of heart (laevocardia) + abdominal situs inversus.

Characteristic heart malformations include—pulmonary stenosis; tricuspid atresia; transposition of the great arteries; anomalous pulmonary venous drainage; atrioventricular septal defects; single ventricle.

No malformations of the heart structures are found when dextrocardia and abdominal situs inversus (i.e. mirror-image dextrocardia) are present in combination.

Infection: infective bacterial endocarditis

There are both acute and subacute forms of infection of the endocardium. Children at risk are those with turbulent blood flow through the heart or where prosthetic material has been inserted following surgery: e.g.
• PDA or VSD;
• coarctation of aorta;
• previous rheumatic fever.

The most common pathogens associated with infective bacterial endocarditis are:
• *Streptococcus viridans (50% cases):* often after dental procedures.
• *Staphylococcus aureus:* often related to central venous catheters.
• *Group D streptococcus (enterococcus):* often after lower GI surgery.

An organism is not found in up to 10% of cases.

Clinical features
• In the early stage symptoms are mild.
• Prolonged fever persisting over several months may be the only feature.
• Alternatively, rapid onset of high intermittent fever can occur.
• Non-specific symptoms include:
  • myalgia and arthalgia;
  • headache, weight loss, night sweats.

Examination
This may be variable, but classic signs include:
• pallor/anaemia;
• nail bed—splinter haemorrhages;
• tender nodules—fingers/toes (Osler's nodes);
• erythematous palms/soles of feet (Janeway lesions);
• finger clubbing (late);
• necrotic skin lesions;
• splenomegaly;
• haematuria (microscopic)
• retinal infarcts (Roth's spots);
• heart murmurs (change in character with time).

Diagnosis
A high index of suspicion is required. Blood tests include FBC (raised WCC), ESR (raised), CRP (raised) and repeated blood cultures. Echocardiography is needed to look for valve 'vegetations'.

Prophylaxis This is no longer routinely advised.

Treatment
- *Antibiotic therapy:* should be started as soon as possible. Delays may result in progressive endocardial damage and deterioration in cardiac function. High dose IV antibiotics (e.g. penicillin/vancomycin) are required for a minimum of 6wks.
- Bed rest is recommended and heart failure should be treated.
- Surgery will be necessary for removal of infected prosthetic material.

Prognosis
Even with antibiotic treatment mortality may be as high as 20% and complications (50–60%) include heart failure. Systemic emboli from left-sided vegetations may result in brain abscess and stroke.

Rheumatic fever

This is an important cause of heart disease worldwide, but rarely seen in developed countries. Acute rheumatic fever (ARF) develops in response to infection with group A β-haemolytic streptococcus. It is seen in children aged 5–15yrs and incidence is highest in those from socially and economically disadvantaged areas.

Clinical features

- There is a latent period of 2–6wks between onset of symptoms and previous streptococcal infection (e.g. pharyngitis).
- Symptoms are non-specific.
- The grouping together of clinical features makes the diagnosis more likely (Jones criteria).
- These are categorized into major or minor (see Box 8.1).

Box 8.1 Jones criteria

Major features
- *Pancarditis (50%):* endocarditis/myocarditis/pericarditis
- *Polyarthritis (80%):*
  - *flitting*—<1wk
  - *migratory*—to other joints over 1–2mths
  - *joints*—knees/ankles/wrists
- *Erythema marginatum (<5%):*
  - early/trunk and limbs
  - pink border/fading centre
- *Subcutaneous nodules (rare):* pea size/hard/extensor surfaces
- *Sydenham's chorea (10%) (see* 📖 *p.524):*
  - *late feature*—2–6mths post-infection
  - *involuntary movements*—choreoathetoid
- Emotional lability

Minor features
- Fever
- Arthralgia
- *Abnormal ECG:* prolonged P–R interval
- Elevated ESR/CRP
- *Evidence of streptococcal infection:* e.g. raised ASO titres
- History of previous rheumatic fever

Diagnosis of ARF

- Two major features; *or*
- One major + two minor features; *and*
- Evidence of previous group A streptococcal infection.

Management

- In the acute phase treatment will include:
  - bed rest;
  - anti-inflammatory drugs (e.g. aspirin);
  - corticosteroids (2–3wks);
  - diuretics/ACE inhibitors if in heart failure;
  - antibiotics (e.g. penicillin V for 10 days).
- Long-term therapy is aimed at 2° prevention of further attacks of acute rheumatic fever and the development of chronic rheumatic heart disease. Antibiotic prophylaxis (daily oral penicillin, or monthly IM penicillin G) is recommended.

Chronic rheumatic heart disease

Recurrent bouts of ARF with associated carditis result in scarring and fibrosis of the heart valves (most commonly mitral valve) and may result in incompetent valves requiring replacement.

Pericarditis

Inflammation of the pericardium may be 1° or a manifestation of more generalized illness. The principal causes of pericardial inflammation are:
- *Infections:*
  - viral, e.g. coxsackie B, Epstein–Barr virus (EBV);
  - bacterial, e.g. streptococococcus, mycoplasma;
  - tuberculosis;
  - fungal, e.g. histoplasmosis;
  - parasitic, e.g. toxoplasmosis.
- *Connective tissue:*
  - rheumatoid arthritis;
  - rheumatic fever;
  - systemic lupus erythematosus (SLE);
  - sarcoidoisis.
- *Metabolic:*
  - hyperuricaemia;
  - hypothyroidism.
- *Malignancy.*
- *Radiotherapy.*

Clinical features

The features depend on the extent of involvement of the pericardium. The predominant symptom is precordial pain that is typically sharp, exacerbated and exaggerated by lying down, and relieved by sitting or leaning forward. The pain is often referred to the left shoulder. Other symptoms include cough, dyspnoea, and fever.

The accumulation of sufficient fluid to cause cardiac tamponade and heart failure is rare.

Examination

Specific diagnostic findings will relate to the amount of fluid within the pericardial sac, including pulsus paradoxus, pericardial rub, quiet/distant heart sounds.

Investigations

Investigations directed at confirming the diagnosis include:
- echocardiogram;
- ECG (typical low voltage QRS complexes).

Other investigations should be directed at identifying the underlying cause of the pericarditis and will include: pericardiocentesis, bacterial/viral culture and biochemical analysis; blood serology for viral studies, ASOT, and connective tissue disease.

Management

Treatment is directed both at the underlying cause, e.g. antibiotics, and symptoms, e.g. the following:

- Analgesia for pain relief.
- Anti-inflammatory drugs to reduce pericardial inflammation.
- Pericardiocentesis for pericardial effusion causing cardiac tamponade and heart failure.

Constrictive pericarditis

Previous pericardial inflammation may predispose to this condition. However, most cases of constrictive pericarditis occur in the absence of any preceding illness or generalized systemic disease. The fibrosed restrictive pericardium impairs cardiac contractility.

Clinical features

Include evidence of heart failure, hepatomegaly, and neck vein distention. On auscultation, heart sounds are distant and a characteristic pericardial 'knock' is often heard. CXR may reveal calcification of the pericardium.

Treatment Requires pericardiectomy.

Myocarditis

Myocarditis may be due to:
- *Infections:* viral, e.g. coxsackie B, EBV.
- Kawasaki disease (see 📖 p.716).
- *Drugs:* adriamycin.
- *Connective tissue disease:* SLE (see 📖 p.780); rheumatoid arthritis (see 📖 p.774); rheumatic fever (see 📖 p.244); sarcoidosis.

Clinical features

Variable and will depend on the age of the patient and on the time course of underlying disease. Specific cardiovascular symptoms include progressive worsening of dyspnoea and congestive cardiac failure. Sudden onset of ventricular arrhythmia may occur.

Examination

Typical cardiovascular examination includes:
- weak pulses;
- tachycardia;
- gallop heart rhythm;
- distant heart sounds.

Diagnosis

Echocardiography shows poor ventricular function. Definitive histological diagnosis is made after percutaneous endomyocardial biopsy. CXR shows cardiomegaly; ECG shows reduced QRS complex size.

Treatment

This is directed at the underlying cause and at controlling symptoms of congestive heart failure. Arrhythmias should be treated. Cardiac transplantation is needed in patients with refractory heart failure.

Cardiomyopathy

Cardiomyopathy may be primary, or secondary to systemic or metabolic disease (see 📖 p.962). Primary cardiomyopathy may be classified as:
- hypertrophic (obstructive; see 📖 p.240);
- dilated (congestive);
- restrictive (see 📖 p.249).

Dilated (congestive) cardiomyopathy

This condition is rare and characterized by massive dilatation of the ventricles and cardiomegaly. The cause is unknown in most cases, although it is seen in association with other conditions:
- post-viral infection phenomenon;
- metabolic (e.g. mitochondrial disease, 📖 p.971).

Clinical features
- Insidious onset of progressive congestive cardiac failure is common.
- The course is usually progressive and the prognosis poor.

Management
Mainly directed at treating heart failure and, where possible, any underlying cause. Heart transplantation if severe heart failure.

Restrictive cardiomyopathy

This condition is rare and characterized by poor ventricular compliance and inadequate ventricular filling. The clinical features are similar to constrictive pericarditis (📖 p.247). It is sometimes seen in the Löffler hypereosinophilic syndrome (multisystem disorder of skin, lungs, nervous system, and liver) and results in endocardial fibrosis of the AV valves and the ventricles. Prognosis is poor and cardiac transplantation often required.

Cardiac arrhythmias

See pp.42–43, 55–57. Sinus arrhythmia is normal in children and adolescents. Other arrhythmias are rare in childhood and may be transient or permanent. Congenital arrhythmias may occur in structurally normal or abnormal hearts. They may be secondary to myocardial disease (e.g. rheumatic fever, myocarditis) or follow exposure to toxins, drugs or surgery to the heart. Children with suspected arrhythmia require a detailed history and examination. The arrhythmia should be identified and characterized by ECG. Intermittent arrhythmias may be detected by 24hr ECG. Underlying congenital heart disease should be excluded by echocardiography.

Supraventricular tachycardia

The most common abnormal arrhythmia in childhood. Re-entry within the A–V node is the most common mechanism of SVT.

Clinical features

Sudden onset (and cessation) lasting from seconds to hours; heart rate 250–300beats/min. SVT is well-tolerated in older children, but heart failure may occur in the young infant. Often precipitated by febrile illness.

Wolff–Parkinson–White syndrome

Pre-excitation syndrome predisposing to SVT. This is due to an abnormal re-entry circuit of the AV node and an accessory conduction pathway connecting atrium to ventricle on the right or left lateral cardiac border, or within the ventricular septum. It may be associated with Ebstein anomaly, post-surgical repair, and cardiomyopathy. ECG shows short PR interval and delta wave (slow upstroke of QRS complex).

Treatment

- *Medical:* adenosine (emergency) β-blocking medication, flecainide, amiodarone.
- *Interventional:* electrophysiological studies and intracardiac ablation when a teenager.

Ventricular tachycardia

Long QT syndrome may be associated with sudden loss of consciousness during exercise, stress or emotion, usually in late childhood. If unrecognized, sudden death from VT may occur. Inheritance is autosomal dominant; there are several phenotypes. Prolongation of the QT interval on ECG is associated with many drugs, electrolyte disorders, and head injury.

Long QT syndrome is a channelopathy caused by specific gene mutations with gain or loss of function. There is a range of effect from Long QT, Short QT, Brugada syndrome and cardiomyopathy. Anyone with a family history of sudden unexplained death, or syncope on exertion must be assessed for these.

Congenital complete heart block

Rare. Mothers of affected children are usually positive for serum anti-Ro or anti-La antibodies and have underlying connective tissue disorder.

Clinical features
- Foetal hydrops and intrauterine death.
- *Neonate:* heart failure.
- *Childhood:* asymptomatic; syncope.

Management Endocardial/epicardial pacemaker.

Respiratory medicine

Introduction

Disorders of the respiratory tract account for a major part of paediatric medicine both in hospital and in general practice. There are 5 key common presentations that the practitioner should be familiar with and we will focus on these first. Next, we will discuss the investigations we use in the care of children. Last, we provide a mini-catalogue of diseases and conditions that you will need to know about, and be able to treat.

We have discussed in Chapters 3 (📖 p.31) and 5 (📖 pp.48–50) the general approach to history and examination for patients with respiratory illness. Here are some additional points that you will need to take note of during your consultation.

History
- *General information:* neonatal period and any prior endotracheal intubations; growth and general body proportions; weight loss; immunizations.
- Age of onset of symptoms or problem.
- Have there been any triggers to this illness?
- What makes the problem worse? Exercise (e.g. asthma), sleep (e.g. adenotonsillar hypertrophy and snoring)?
- What makes the problem better? (Bronchodilators in asthma.)
- *Other symptoms:* haemoptysis; cough; sputum production; choking; gastro-oesophageal reflux; apnoea; coryza; chest/abdominal pain.

Examination
See also 📖 p.31.
- *General information:* growth parameters; clubbing; lymphadenopathy; temperature; level of consciousness; colour; and arterial pulse oximetry saturation; pulse rate.
- Rate, pattern of breathing (episodic, periodic, apnoea), duration of expiration, and use of accessory muscles (+/– recession).
- *Nose and speech:* crease across the bridge of the nose and nasal discharge (e.g. allergic rhinitis); hyponasal speech (e.g. palate and nasal problems); nasal or mouth breather; nasal flaring.
- *Facial appearance:* size of midface, lower jaw, tongue (e.g. craniofacial syndrome).
- Tonsillar hypertrophy.
- Cough (paroxysms, barking, high-pitched).
- Neck retraction and external compressive mass.
- *Breathing cycle:* inspiratory stridor indicates extrathoracic airway obstruction; expiratory prolongation or wheeze indicates intrathoracic airway obstruction.
- Breath sounds.
- Chest appearance (Harrison's sulcus), and percussion.
- Sputum pot.

Common presentation: wheeze

Wheeze is a breath sound that is heard during expiration. It is often associated with prolongation of the expiratory phase of the breathing cycle. Wheeze indicates obstruction to airflow within the thorax. It can be high- or low-pitched; this differentiation indicates that the obstruction is likely to be in the smaller and larger airways, respectively. Also, wheezes can be monophonic or polyphonic; identifying these sounds will tell you whether the obstruction is likely to be in one or multiple airways.

Differential diagnosis

Extrinsic lower airway compression

- *Lung parenchyma:* e.g. pneumonia, pulmonary oedema, bronchogenic cyst.
- *Vascular:* e.g. enlarged left atrium compressing left mainstem bronchus, pulmonary artery vascular ring.
- *Lymphatic:* e.g. enlarged hilar lymph nodes (🕮 pp.290–291, 654).
- *Chest deformity:* e.g. scoliosis (🕮 p.746).

Intrinsic change in lower airway dimension

- Asthma (🕮 p.262).
- Bronchiolitis (🕮 p.288).
- Bronchitis and bronchiectasis (🕮 pp.257, 291).
- Cystic fibrosis (🕮 pp.270–273).
- Ciliary disease.
- Haemangioma.
- Polyps.
- Tracheobronchomalacia.

Intraluminal lower airway obstruction

- Aspiration of food or milk from gastro-oesophageal reflux (🕮 pp.276, 295, 326).
- Foreign body inhalation (🕮 p.51).
- Mucus, pus, and blood.

Each of the conditions in the list above will require specific investigation and treatment. Wheeze due to asthma will require both acute and chronic treatment (see 🕮 pp.264–269).

Common presentation: stridor

Stridor is a noise heard during the inspiratory phase of breathing. It indicates either dynamic or fixed extrathoracic airway obstruction (anywhere from the nose to the thoracic inlet). When it arises acutely and is associated with respiratory distress, immediate attention is required (📖 pp.48–50, 284–285). The differential diagnosis of stridor is as follows.

Nose and nasopharynx
- Congenital obstruction, e.g. choanal atresia (📖 p.846).
- Inflammation, e.g. rhinitis and sinusitis (📖 p.280).

Mouth, oropharynx, and hypopharynx
- *Congenital obstruction:* e.g. macroglossia and glossoptosis.
- *Inflammation:* e.g. tonsillar hypertrophy (📖 p.279).
- *Masses:* e.g. cystic hygroma or other malformation.
- *Foreign body* (📖 p.51).

Larynx
- *Congenital obstruction:* e.g. laryngomalacia, laryngeal web or cleft, vocal cord paralysis.
- *Inflammation:* e.g. gastro-oesophageal reflux.
- *Infection:* e.g. epiglottitis, laryngotracheobronchitis (📖 p.284).
- *Masses:* e.g. haemangiomas, abscess.
- *Trauma:* e.g. subglottic stenosis, foreign body inhalation (📖 p.51).

Trachea
- *Congenital obstruction:* e.g. tracheomalacia, tracheo-oesophageal fistula.
- *Infection:* e.g. bacterial tracheitis.

There are specific treatments for many of these conditions. In persistent, non-medical causes of stridor, airway surgery may be required after endoscopy.

Common presentation: cough

Cough is a protective response for removing secretions and particulate matter from the airway. Main feature sudden expulsion of air from lungs.

Differential diagnosis of acute cough

Upper airway disease
- *Common cold*: e.g., rhinovirus.
- *Other infections*: e.g. viral influenza and parainfluenza, sinusitis, tonsillitis, laryngitis, croup.
- *Allergy.*
- *Vocal cord dysfunction.*

Lower airway disease
- Asthma (📖 p.262).
- *Infection*: e.g. respiratory syncytial virus bronchiolitis, bronchitis due to adenovirus, influenza, and parainfluenza.

Lung parenchymal disease
- *Infection*: e.g. viral and bacterial pneumonia, empyema (📖 p.293).
- *Atypical pneumonia*: e.g. *Mycoplasma pneumoniae* infection.

Treatment In general, we do not treat cough, but focus on underlying cause.

Differential diagnosis of chronic cough

A chronic cough is one that has persisted for more than 8wks (British Thoracic Society 2008 guideline[1] for the assessment and management of children with chronic cough). Its causes are as follows:
- *Upper airway disease:*
  - infection—e.g. chronic sinusitis, tonsillitis, *Bordetella pertussis* (📖 p.286);
  - inflammation—e.g. gastro-oesophageal reflux (📖 p.276).
- *Lower airway disease:*
  - congenital abnormalities—e.g. tracheo-oesophageal fistula, cleft larynx, pulmonary artery sling;
  - asthma;
  - infection: e.g. post-bronchiolitis symptoms, atypical infections;
  - foreign body
  - bronchiectasis: e.g. damage to the airway from chronic infection and tuberculosis, or immunodeficiency;
  - cystic fibrosis (📖 p.270).
- *Lung parenchymal disease:* infection, e.g. pneumonia and empyema.
- *Central causes:*
  - Psychogenic cough.
  - Tourette disease: with a tic involving throat clearing or cough.
- *Treatment:* in common with acute cough, when treating chronic cough, try and identify the underlying cause and focus on its treatment.

Reference
1 Shields Bush A, Everard ML, *et al.* (2008). BTS guidelines: recommendation for the asssessment and management of cough in children. *Thorax* **63**(Suppl. 3): 1–15.

Common presentation: breathlessness

Being short of breath can be due to heart or lung disease. In lung disease, this sensation arises because of lack of oxygen, difficulty breathing due to airway obstruction, or abnormal lung mechanics. Infants may not be able to express their discomfort—in this instance you will need to be able to identify signs of respiratory distress. The causes include the following.

Differential diagnosis

Airway obstruction
- *Upper airway* (see 📖 pp.48, 282).
- *Lower airway* (see 📖 p.48).

Abnormal lung mechanics

- *Restrictive lung disease:* e.g. chest wall (obesity), chest deformity, kyphoscoliosis (📖 pp.744–747).
- *Parenchymal lung disease:* e.g. pneumonia, pulmonary hypertension.
- *Muscle weakness:* e.g. Duchenne muscular dystrophy, diaphragmatic paralysis (📖 pp.546–548).

Hypoxia

- *Ventilation perfusion mismatch:* e.g. lung disease, pneumonia, pneumothorax, pulmonary embolism.
- *Heart disease:* e.g. cyanotic congenital heart disease, pericarditis and myocarditis (📖 pp.231, 246–248).

Emergency treatment and care Discussed in Chapter 5 (📖 p.50).

Common presentation: snoring

We are concerned about snoring in children when it indicates that the child has obstructive sleep apnoea (OSA), i.e. snoring in association with periods of ineffective breathing lasting longer than 2 breaths (e.g. breathing at a rate of 20/min, this would be 6s). This is as opposed to central apneas, which are a pause >20s in an otherwise well child. The most common cause of OSA is adenotonsillar hypertrophy. The other causes are as follows.

Differential diagnosis

Congenital anatomical
- *Midface:* e.g. hypoplasia in achondroplasia.
- *Choanal atresia* (📖 p.846).
- *Tongue:* e.g. macroglossia in Beckwith syndrome (📖 p.949), trisomy 21 (📖 p.936).
- *Lower jaw:* e.g. retro- and micrognathia.
- *Syndromes:* e.g. Pierre–Robin sequence (📖 p.847), Treacher–Collins, Goldenhar, Apert.

Inflammation
- Adenotonsillar hypertrophy.
- Allergic rhinosinusitis.
- Nasal polyposis.
- Gastro-oesophageal reflux.

Masses
- Encephalocele.
- Nasal gliomas.

Central causes of pharyngeal hypotonia during sleep
- Cerebral palsy (📖 p.550).
- Seizures (📖 p.505).
- Hydrocephalus (📖 p.535).
- *Obesity* (📖 p.400)

Treatment

When snoring is associated with OSA, the underlying cause needs to be treated.

Investigations

Chest X-ray

CXR is a key investigation in respiratory disease. It will give you information about lung volume (e.g. hyperinflation in asthma), signs of chronic inflammation (e.g. peribronchial cuffing), and evidence of congenitial lesions (e.g. lung cysts). However, it is an investigation that can be overused. It should not replace a thorough clinical examination, and think hard before requesting repeat studies.

A CXR is used to glean more clinical evidence about what the child's underlying problem is. So, in each presentation consider why you have requested the test. Here are some examples.

Wheeze

A CXR is not needed every time a patient presents with 'asthma'. However, if that child has never had an X-ray, or there is something atypical about the history, consider other possibilities:

- *Suspected foreign body inhalation:* i.e. inspiratory and expiratory film (object often radiolucent).
- *Suspected gastro-oesophageal reflux with aspiration, or aspiration from abnormal swallowing:* i.e. looking for different lobes affected at different times.
- *Monophonic wheeze:* i.e. looking for hilar lymph nodes compressing on the right main-stem bronchus, or a large left atrium compressing the left main-stem bronchus, or mediastinal mass.

Stridor Suspected tracheal lesion around the thoracic inlet.

Cough

- Suspected typical and atypical pneumonia, or empyema.
- Suspected bronchiectasis.

Breathlessness

- Suspected pulmonary parenchymal disease.
- Pneumothorax.
- Suspected heart disease, e.g. heart failure.

Snoring with sleep apnoea Suspected cardiopulmonary disease or cor pulmonale from chronic upper airway obstruction.

Bedside tests in respiratory medicine

Four tests are frequently performed at the bedside or in the laboratory are lung function testing, sweat test, and arterial blood sampling.

Lung function testing

Spirometry can be achieved in ≥5-yr-olds, but measurements are easier in ≥7 year olds. Peak expiratory flow rate (PEFR) monitoring is useful in asthma. Other measurements include:

- FEV_1/FVC: the forced expired volume in 1s as a fraction of forced vital capacity.
- Exercise testing.
- Bronchodilator responsiveness (i.e. reversibility).

Sweat test

This test is used in the diagnosis of cystic fibrosis. Sweating is induced in an area of the forearm using pilocarpine, and a capillary tube is used to collect the sweat. A minimum of 15µL (and preferably >30µL) of sweat should be collected. In cystic fibrosis abnormal function of the sweat glands results in higher concentrations of chloride in the sweat:

- *Suspicious:* >40mmol/L (>30mmol/L in newborn screened babies).
- *Diagnostic:* >60mmol/L.

Pulse oximetry Assessment of oxygen saturation (SpO_2) using a pulse oximeter is a non-invasive way of assessing a child's oxygenation using a probe attached to a finger or toe.

Arterial blood gas Assessment of blood O_2, CO_2, and acid–base are important in critically ill children, or in those where you suspect significant lung disease.

Further investigations

Sometimes more detailed investigations are needed before you can select the best treatment for your patient. These include the following:

Imaging

- *Chest computed tomography:* useful for assessing abnormalities in airways as well as abnormalities in parenchymal tissue density.
- *Thoracic MRI:* useful for looking at airway–blood interface, and vascular and mediastinal anatomy.
- *Nuclear imaging:* useful for assessing regional ventilation (V) and perfusion (Q), as well as V/Q matching.

Direct visualization of structure

- *Flexible bronchoscopy:* used to assess directly the airway from nose to distal bronchus; used to lavage the lung for microscopy and culture

Asthma

Asthma is a disease of chronic airway inflammation, bronchial hyper-reactivity, and reversible airway obstruction. It affects 10% of the population and can develop at any age, but typically half of the paediatric cases present before the age of 10yrs. There is often a family history of asthma or atopic disease.

Diagnosis

History
- Cough after exercise or sometimes in the early morning, disturbing sleep.
- Shortness of breath.
- Limitation in exercise performance.

Examination
In the child with chronic problems consistent findings include:
- Barrel-shaped chest.
- Hyperinflation.
- Wheeze and prolonged expiration.

Chest X-ray
Not needed if there has been recent imaging. It may show:
- Hyperinflation.
- Flattened hemi-diaphragms.
- Peribronchial cuffing.
- Atelectasis.

Spirometry
- Peak expiratory flow rate (PEFR) <80% predicted for height.
- FEV_1/FVC <80% predicted.
- Concave scooped shape in flow volume curve.
- Bronchodilator response to β-agonist therapy (i.e. 15% increase in FEV_1 or PEFR).

Medication

The main medications used for maintenance are bronchodilators, which give short-term relief of symptoms, and prophylactic therapy, which reduces chronic inflammation and bronchial hyperreactivity. In the outpatient clinic our aim is to titrate these treatments so that the child can function normally, yet still avoid any detrimental effect on growth and development. See p.267 for stepwise manner in which these drugs may be used.

Bronchodilators
- *Short-acting β2-agonists:* salbutamol, terbutaline.
- *Long-acting β2-agonists:* salmeterol, formoterol.
- *Short-acting anticholinergic:* ipratropium bromide.

Chronic treatment of inflammation and hyperreactivity
- *Inhaled steroids:* budesonide, beclometasone, fluticasone.
- *Oral steroids:* prednisolone.
- *Sodium cromoglicate:* rarely used.
- *Methylxanthines:* theophylline.
- *Leukotriene inhibitors:* montelukast and zafirlukast may reduce the amount of steroid therapy that is needed to control symptoms.
- Combination inhalers containing inhaled steroids and long-acting β_2-agonists.

Side-effects of chronic treatment

Steroids
When long-term oral steroids or high-dose inhaled steroids are used, special attention will need to be given to unwanted effects including:
- *Impaired growth:* can affect growth in height, but also ask about frequency of hair-cuts, or changing shoe size, as these are early indicators of poor growth.
- *Adrenal suppression.*
- *Oral candidiasis.*
- *Altered bone metabolism.*

Theophylline
Now rarely used in children, but you should be aware that there are a number of problems related to toxic blood levels, including:
- Vomiting
- Sleep disturbance or increased sleeping.
- Headaches.
- Poor concentration and deterioration of performance at school.
- Arrhythmias.

Asthma: drug delivery devices

There are a number of drug delivery devices that are available for use in children:

- *Nebulizer:* use in emergency treatment at all ages for delivery of bronchodilator (although a spacer device is often used instead).
- *Large or small volume spacer with metered dose inhaler (MDI):* use in infancy to any age (facemask for under 3yrs and mouthpiece for older children). This device uses a plastic 'bubble' with a valve at one end and a place where an MDI can be inserted at the other end. The spacer allows the aerosol particles from the inhaler to be slowed and inhaled on each breath. It stops the drug dose from the MDI depositing in mouth or stomach, and allows it to go with inspired air all the way down to the small airways.
- *Dry powder device:* terbutaline sulphate (Bricanyl Turbohaler®), salbutamol (Ventolin Accuhaler®). These can be used in children >5yrs.
- *Propellant metered dose inhaler (PMDI):* these can be used in children >12yrs, although are difficult to use and generally not advised. The device uses a gas propellant to aerosolize the drug.

Inhalation technique

In the clinic you will need to make sure that your patient is getting and taking the medication prescribed. In all children you will need to see that they have the appropriate technique and device for their age.

Child >3yrs

Look for 5-breath tidal volume breathing technique.

- *Stands* to allow full use of the diaphragm.
- *Shake MDI.*
- *Place MDI into spacer.*
- *Place device in mouth.*
- *Firm seal with mouth around mouthpiece.*
- *Breathe in and out tidally:* when good rhythm, activate device (only once).
- *Continue breathing 5 times.*
- *If second dose is needed:* then shake MDI and repeat as above.

Infant

Note that, if the infant is crying, less drug will be inhaled. Make sure that the person giving the medication:

- Tilt the spacer so that the valve is open (in small volume device you do not need to tip as the valve is low resistance).
- Let the infant take at least *five breaths from each dose* actuated.

Asthma: clinic management (1)

The aim of treatment is to allow the child to lead a normal life. In the clinic you will come across children with seemingly distinct clinical patterns of their chronic asthma. Patients with frequent or persistent asthma should be seen in a specialist clinic. Nebulized treatment is used in severe acute asthma. It is not recommended in mild to moderate severity asthma. Instead, use multidosing (up to 10 puffs) bronchodilator.

Infrequent episodic asthma

Characteristics
- 75% of asthmatics.
- <4 episodes per year.
- Symptom-free between acute episodes.
- No regular treatment needed.

Management strategy
- Treat acute episodes with β_2-bronchodilators.
- Use nebulized bronchodilators and short-course prednisolone in more severe episodes (i.e. prednisolone 3 days, given once daily in the morning after breakfast with no need to taper treatment).

Frequent episodic asthma

Characteristics
- 20% of asthmatics.
- Episodes every 2–4 weeks.
- Regular treatment is needed.

Management strategy
- Use β_2-bronchodilator as required.
- Use regular, low-dose inhaled steroid.

Persistent asthma

Characteristics
- Less than 5% of asthmatics.
- ≥3 episodes/wk, with cough at night/morning.
- Regular treatment is needed.

Management strategy
- Use prophylactic inhaled steroids.
- Long-acting β_2-bronchodilator may be helpful.
- Oral steroids may be needed.
- Oral leukotriene inhibitors may enable reduction in steroid usage.

Exercise-induced asthma

Management strategy
- Mild: use β_2-bronchodilator before exercise.
- Severe: low-dose inhaled steroid.

Escalating therapy

Having reviewed the history and categorized your patient in terms of clinical pattern and severity, use a logical, stepwise approach to escalating therapy (see Box 9.1).

Box 9.1 The stepwise approach to drugs

Before altering a treatment, ensure that treatment is being taken in an effective manner

Step 1: occasional use of relief bronchodilators
Short-acting β_2-bronchodilator for relief of symptoms

Step 2: regular inhaled preventer therapy
Short-acting β_2-bronchodilator as required + low-dose inhaled steroid (200–400micrograms/day)

Step 3: add-on therapy
- Short-acting β_2-bronchodilator as required + high-dose inhaled steroid *or*
- Low-dose inhaled steroid +/– long-acting bronchodilator

If control is still inadequate use a trial of other therapies, e.g. leukotriene receptor antagonist or slow release theophylline

Step 4: persistent poor control
- Short-acting β_2-bronchodilator as required + high-dose inhaled steroid (up to 800micrograms/day) + long-acting bronchodilator *or*
- Theophyllines or ipratropium +/– alternate day steroid

Step 5: continuous or frequent use of oral steroid
- Use daily steroid tablet in lowest dose
- Maintain high-dose inhaled steroid at 800micrograms/day
- Refer to respiratory specialist

Asthma: clinic management (2)

0–2yrs

In this age group, a spacer device with an appropriate face mask is used, e.g. a small volume Aerochamber® or Ablespacer® which can take any inhaler; or a large volume Volumatic® or Nebuhaler®, which only fit certain inhalers. Prophylactic therapy with inhaled steroids is more effective than cromoglicate.

Acute treatment

- Salbutamol via Volumatic®: <2400micrograms/day (in 6 doses).
- Terbutaline via Nebuhaler®: <6000micrograms/day (in 6 doses).
- Ipratropium via Volumatic®: <480micrograms/day (in 4 doses).

Prophylactic treatment

- Budesonide via Nebuhaler®: 100–400micrograms/day.
- Beclometasone via Volumatic®: 100–400micrograms/day.

3–5yrs

Acute treatment

- Salbutamol via Volumatic®: <3600micrograms/day (in 6 doses).
- Terbutaline via Nebuhaler®: <6000micrograms/day (in 6 doses).

Prophylactic treatment

- Budesonide via Nebuhaler®: 100–800micrograms/day.
- Beclomethasone via Volumatic®: 100–800micrograms/day.
- Fluticasone via Volumatic®: (>4yrs) 100–200micrograms/day..
- Salmeterol via Volumatic®: (>4yrs) 50micrograms/day. Must never be given alone and only when the child is also taking an inhaled steroid.
- *Combination inhaler:* Seretide® (contains fixed doses of fluticasone and salmeterol).

5–12yrs

Acute treatment

- Salbutamol Accuhaler®: <7200micrograms/day (in 6 doses).
- Salbutamol inhaler: (>12 years) <7200micrograms/day (in 6 doses).
- Terbutaline inhaler: (>12 years) <7200micrograms/day (in 6 doses).

Prophylactic treatment

- Budesonide Turbohaler®: 100–800micrograms/day.
- Beclometasone via Accuhaler®: 100–800micrograms/day.
- Fluticasone via Volumatic®: 100–400micrograms/day.
- Combination inhaler – Seretide® (contains fixed doses of fluticasone and salmeterol); or Symbicort turbohaler® (fixed doses of budesonide and formoterol).

Useful clinic guides

Steroids
- Fluticasone and budesonide are preferable since they have fewer side-effects than beclometasone
- Patients on doses of steroids greater than fluticasone 500micrograms/day, budesonide 800micrograms/day, beclometasone 800micrograms/day should be under the supervision of a specialist clinic

Long-acting β₂-agonists
- Salmeterol may be of value for night-time symptoms or daytime activity
- Should be used as a prophylactic agent
- Consider in patients on inhaled beclometasone or budesonide 400micrograms/day, or fluticasone 200micrograms/day

Allergen avoidance
- Removal of feather or woollen bedding
- Wrapping of mattress in plastic
- Cleaning of carpets and furniture
- No pets in the house if the child is allergic to them

Passive smoking
- No smoking in the house or car.
- Parents/carers must be strongly encouraged to stop smoking completely.

Education
Older patients will need to learn more about their condition and how it is best treated. For example:
- Which medication to use and when
- Best inhaler technique
- What to do if asthma is getting worse
- Not to smoke
- Gargle after steroid inhaler use so as to avoid oral thrush

Cystic fibrosis

Cystic fibrosis (CF) is an autosomal recessive genetic disorder leading to a defect in the CF transmembrane receptor (CFTR) protein, which results in defective ion transport in exocrine glands. In the lung abnormal sodium and chloride ion transport causes thickening of respiratory mucus. The lung is therefore prone to inadequate mucociliary clearance, chronic bacterial infection, and lung injury. There are also similar effects—although not with superadded infection—in other organs that lead to pancreatic insufficiency, liver disease, and, in the male, infertility. There are over 1500 mutations in the CFTR gene; the most common is the ΔF508 deletion. CF is the most common genetic disease in Caucasions (1/2500).

Diagnosis

Screening

Since 2007 in the UK all newborn babies are screened for cystic fibrosis looking for an abnormally raised immunoreactive trypsinogen (IRT) and 29 CFTR gene mutations from blood-spot analysis on the Guthrie card.

History

Give particular attention to:
- Cough and wheeze.
- Shortness of breath.
- Sputum production.
- Haemoptysis.
- Stool type (e.g. fatty, oily, pale) and frequency.
- Weight loss or poor weight gain.

About 10–20% of CF patients present in the neonatal period with meconium ileus. However, most children with CF present with:
- malabsorption;
- failure to thrive;
- recurrent chest infection.

Examination

Full assessment of:
- respiratory system;
- liver and GI system;
- growth and development.

Investigations

- Sweat test showing increased chloride levels (>60mmol/L).
- *CXR:* hyperinflation, increased antero-posterior diameter, bronchial dilatation, cysts, linear shadows, and infiltrates.
- *Lung function:* obstructive pattern with decreased FVC and increased lung volumes.

Cystic fibrosis: problems

Lifelong therapy and supervision are required in CF. There is a variety of problems that can be expected at different ages.

Infancy
- Meconium ileus (📖 p.862).
- Neonatal jaundice (prolonged).
- Hypoproteinaemia and oedema.

Childhood
- Recurrent lower respiratory tract infections.
- Bronchiectasis (occasionally)
- Poor appetite.
- Rectal prolapse (📖 p.871).
- Nasal polyps.
- Sinusitis (rare to have symptoms).

Adolescence
- Bronchiectasis.
- Diabetes mellitus (📖 p.406).
- Cirrhosis and portal hypertension.
- Distal intestinal obstruction (📖 p.274).
- Pneumothorax.
- Haemoptysis.
- Allergic bronchopulmonary aspergillosis.
- Male infertility.
- Arthropathy.
- Psychological problems.

Cystic fibrosis: management (1)

The management of the child with CF requires close co-operation between local hospitals and regional centres. Patients and their families gain much from expert clinics, and from other patients and their families. Effective management requires a multidisciplinary team approach, which should include:

- paediatric pulmonologist;
- physiotherapist;
- dietician;
- nurse liaison or practitioner in CF;
- primary care team;
- teacher;
- psychologist.

All patients with CF should have a thorough annual multisystem review. Table 9.1 summarizes the range of information that is needed. You will find following these parameters helpful when assessing progression, deterioration, and need for supraregional referral for heart–lung transplantation.

Table 9.1 Information needed for the annual multisystem review of a CF patient

Blood tests	
Haematology	FBC, clotting (APTT, PTT)
Biochemistry	Cr, U, Na, K, Cl, HCO3 (Mg, Ca if on IV colistin), iron studies, vitamin A, D & E levels
Liver function	ALP, alanine transferase (ALT), bilirubin, albumin, protein
Glucose control	Random glucose, HbA1c, oral glucose tolerance test (>10yrs)
Immunology	IgE, IgG, RAST to aspergillus, pseudomonas precipitins
Radiology	
X-rays	Chest
US	Liver and bowel
Dual-energy X-ray absorptiometry (DEXA) scan	Consider in children >10yrs, or those on increasing doses of steroids, or those who have increasing fractures
Lung function	
Measurements	FEV$_1$, FVC, PEFR, residual volume (RV), TLC
Oximetry	esting SpO$_2$
Bacteriology	
Sputum/cough swab	Cultures including Burkholderia cepacia, acid-fast bacilli
Morbidity	
Hospital	Number of admissions and days in hospital
Chest	Number of courses of IV antibiotics
Reviews	
Medications	Requirements (dose)
Physiotherapy	Technique, education, equipment
Nutrition	Education, enzymes, supplements
Social	Family support, genetics, housing, school, statement of special needs
Psychology	Is an assessment needed?

Cystic fibrosis: management (2)

Pulmonary care

Physiotherapy

All children with CF should have physiotherapy at least twice a day. Parents and older children are taught how to do some of the following:
- chest percussion;
- postural drainage;
- self-percussion;
- deep breathing exercises;
- use of flutter or acapello device.

Antimicrobial therapy

Most experts recommend antibiotic therapy.
- Oral during periods when well: against *Staphylococcus aureus* and *Haemophilus influenzae*.
- IV for acute exacerbations: initially courses of antibiotics can be administered via an indwelling long-line that should last a number of weeks if needed. However, as infections become more frequent, a permanent form of IV access (such as an indwelling Portacath) will help.
- Nebulized for those chronically infected with *Pseudomonas aeruginosa*.

Other therapies
- Annual influenza immunization.
- Bronchodilators for those with reversible airway obstruction.
- *Mucolytics:* recombinant DNAase 2hr before physiotherapy; or inhaled hypertonic (7%) saline used before physiotherapy.
- Oral azithromycin (long-term anti-inflammatory).

Gastrointestinal management

Distal intestinal obstruction (meconium ileus equivalent)
- *Lactulose:* 1mL/kg/day.
- *Oral acetylcysteine solution:* prophylaxis 15mL of 10%/day in <7-yr-olds and 30mL in >7-yr-olds. Treatment doses are double to three times this amount.
- *Gastrografin®:* oral dose can be used as a single treatment dose (50mL for children 15–25kg, and 100mL for those >25kg). Fluid intake should be encouraged for 3hr after administering the Gastrografin®.

Nutrition
- *Pancreatic insufficiency:* treated with oral enteric-coated pancreatic supplements (Creon®) taken with all meals and snacks. Ranitidine or omeprazole may be useful if the response to enzymes is unsatisfactory.
- *High-calorie diet:* children with CF require 120–150% of normal energy intake.
- *Salt supplements:* salt depletion is a risk in CF patients during the first year of life, and in the summer months in older patients. In exceptionally hot weather supplements include 500mg/day during the first year, 1g/day in <7-yr-olds, and 2–4g/day in >7-yr-olds.

Fat-soluble vitamin supplements
- *Multivitamins:* Dalivit® drops 1mL/day or multivitamin tablets.
- *Vitamin E:* 50mg/day if <1yr; 100mg/day 1–16yrs.
- *Vitamin K:* if there is evidence of liver disease (hepatosplenomegaly or abnormal clotting).

Chronic lung disease of prematurity

See also 📖 pp.166–167.

As the quality and outcome of neonatal intensive care for premature babies has improved, more and more infants with chronic lung disease (CLD) are being seen. There are a variety of lung conditions that affect premature babies and necessitate mechanical ventilation; these are discussed in Chapter 6, 📖 p.107.

- Respiratory distress syndrome (📖 p.150).
- Neonatal pneumonia (📖 p.152).

The following can affect newborn of any gestational age:
- Meconium aspiration (📖 p.152).
- Diaphragmatic hernia (📖 p.852).
- Pulmonary hypoplasia.
- Alveolar capillary membrane dysplasia.
- Interstitial lung disease.
- Surfactant protein deficiency.

On follow-up in the paediatric clinic you may see oxygen-dependency due to any of these conditions. CLD in this context is defined as abnormal CXR and use of supplementary oxygen beyond 28 days.

Management

In many respects the approach to managing oxygen-dependent infants with compromised lung function is very similar to caring for infants with CF. A multisystem and multidisciplinary team approach is needed. This should include home and community liaison—the neonatal unit nurse specialist and health visitor are particularly helpful.

Nutritional support and therapy
- *Weight gain and growth:* these should be monitored and, if there is a problem with inadequate intake, consult a dietician for advice.
- *Gastrostomy:* procedure sometimes required to enable full feeding.
- *Gastro-oesophageal reflux (GOR):* the 'flat' position of the diaphragm, lung hyperinflation, and tachypnoea promote the development of vomiting and GOR. The lungs need to be protected and adequate feeding needs to be ensured. Initially try medical therapy (see Chapter 10, 📖 p.326). If these measures fail, fundoplication and gastrostomy feeds are required.
- *Vitamins:* appropriate vitamin supplements are used until the child is thriving well (i.e. vitamin compound drops, folic acid, iron).

Antimicrobial therapy
- *Vaccination:* all immunizations should be up-to-date. Children on steroids may be at risk if given live or attenuated immunization (e.g. BCG, mumps, measles, and rubella (MMR)).
- *Antibiotics:* viral illness may result in significant deterioration in CLD. Take sputum, throat swab, and nasopharyngeal aspirate for viral and bacterial cultures. Have a low threshold for using antibiotics.

- *Antivirals:* aerosolized ribavirin may be required for severe respiratory syncytial virus bronchiolitis although its benefit is controversial. Patients should have had prophylaxis (see 📖 p.288).

Obstructive airway disease

Wheeze is a common symptom in infants with CLD. Asthma treatments are often used in these children.

Oxygen therapy

The ultimate aim of supervision of these patients is to withdraw oxygen in a safe and timely manner. The target oxygen saturation (SpO_2) in patients on supplemental oxygen via nasal cannulae is ≥92%. Withdrawal is appropriate when the infant is clinically well, gaining weight, and has an SpO_2 consistently above 92% with an oxygen requirement ≤0.1L/min. Children can be weaned from continuous low flow oxygen to night-time and naps only, or remain in continuous oxygen throughout the 24hr until the child has no requirement at all. Oxygen equipment should be left in the home for at least 3mths after the child has stopped using it. If this is in a winter period, it is usually left until the end of winter.

Congenital respiratory tract disorders

The following congenital abnormalities of the upper and lower airway are discussed in Chapter 23, 📖 p.843.

Congenital abnormalities of the upper airway

- Choanal atresia (📖 p.846).
- Laryngeal atresia (📖 p.846).
- Cleft lip and palate (📖 p.846).
- Pierre–Robin sequence (📖 p.847).
- Tracheo-oesophageal fistula (📖 pp.848–849).

Congenital abnormalities of the lower airways

- Congenital cystic adenomatoid malformation (📖 p.851).
- Sequestration (📖 p.851).
- Congenital lobar emphysema (📖 p.851).
- Congenital diaphragmatic hernia (📖 p.852).
- Hiatus hernia (📖 p.852).

Sleep apnoea

Apnoea is defined as a lack of breathing. Obstructive apnoea refers to a lack of airflow in the face of respiratory effort. It is most often associated with sleep. The obstructive sleep apnoea syndrome (OSAS) may be due to tonsillar/adenoidal hypetrophy, macroglossia, or micrognathia.

Diagnosis

History
- Snoring and sleep disturbance.
- Daytime sleepiness or inattention.
- Eneuresis.
- Only about 15% of snoring children have significant airway obstruction.

Examination (see also 📖 p.31)
A thorough examination is needed:
- Symptoms of upper airway obstruction and OSAS are more likely to be due to adenoidal hypertrophy, rather than just tonsillar hypertrophy.
- *Middle ear infection and chronic effusion:* these are features associated with adenoidal hypertrophy.
- Mouth breathing leading to dry mouth and cracked lips.

Investigation
A thorough history and examination should identify children who need further treatment. However, there is a place for the following as part of an assessment.
- *Sleep study:* this could include just overnight pulse oximetry, but to diagnose impaired gas exchange transcutaneous CO_2 measurement is necessary as well. Sometimes more extensive polysomnography may be needed, mainly to differentiate obstructive from central causes of sleep apnoea..
- *Chest X-ray and ECG:* to examine for 2° right heart cardiac consequences of airway obstruction.

Treatment Surgery is indicated when the following criteria are met.

Tonsillectomy
Any of:
- Airway obstruction (usually performed with adenoidectomy).
- History of recurrent tonsillitis (>7 episodes in 1yr, or >10 episodes in 2yrs).
- History of two episodes of peritonsillar abscess.

Adenoidectomy
Any of:
- Airway obstruction.
- Recurrent or chronic middle ear infection.
- Recurrent or chronic nasopharyngitis.
- Chronic mouth breathing.

Allergic rhinitis

Up to 20% of the population have symptoms of allergic rhinitis, which include nasal congestion, itching, sneezing, and discharge.

Diagnosis

History
- Identify seasonality of the symptoms and history of atopy.
- Take a history of environmental exposures such as parental smoking, pets, dust mite, stuffed toys, carpet, bedding, etc.

Examination
Check for:
- mouth breathing;
- postnasal drip;
- cough;
- nose rubbing;
- suborbital venous congestion;
- watery-red eyes.

Investigation
- Skin tests for specific antigens.
- Specific serum IgE measurements.

Treatment

Allergen avoidance
- Dust covers on bedding.
- Avoid stuffed toys.

Symptom relief
- Antihistamines.
- Montelukast.
- Intranasal steroids.

Upper airway infections

Ear, sinus, nose, and throat infections account for 80% of respiratory infections. The diagnosis URTI may mean any of the following.

- *Common cold (coryza):* commonly due to rhinoviruses, coronaviruses, and respiratory syncytial virus (although latter more often causes acute bronchiolitis).
- *Sore throat (pharyngitis and tonsillitis):* pharyngitis is usually due to viral infection with adenovirus, enterovirus, and rhinovirus. Bacterial infection with group A β-haemolytic streptococcus may be present in the older child. Tonsillitis associated with purulent exudates may be due to group A β-haemolytic streptococcus or the Epstein–Barr virus (EBV) (see also 📖 pp.707, 711).
- *Ear infection (acute otitis media):* common pathogens include viruses, pneumococcus, group A β-haemolytic streptococcus, *Haemophilus influenzae*, and *Moraxella catarrhalis* (see also 📖 p.900).
- *Sinusitis* may occur with viral or bacterial infection.

Diagnosis

History

Children often present with a combination of:
- *Painful throat.*
- *Fever* (which may even induce febrile convulsions).
- *Blocked nose* (which may lead to feeding difficulty in infants).
- *Nasal discharge.*
- *Earache.*
- *Wheeze* (in children with asthma there may be an exacerbation).

Examination

A thorough examination is needed. In infants you will need to make sure that there is not a serious infection and, in those with difficulty feeding because of blocked nose, that feeding will be adequate. In older children you will need to check for possible bacterial infection and give antibiotics when the following are identified.

- *Ears:* think of otitis media if there is discharge, if the tympanic membrane is not intact, if the eardrums are bright red and bulging with loss of normal light reflection.
- *Neck:* think of bacterial throat infection if there is tender cervical lymphadenopathy.
- *Pharynx:* think of tonsillitis if there are purulent exudates on inflamed tonsils.

Treatment

Symptom relief

- *Fever:* use paracetamol or ibuprofen.
- *Earache:* use paracetamol or ibuprofen.

Antibiotics

Virus infection causes the majority of URTIs and antibiotics should not be prescribed. However, if bacterial tonsillitis, or pharyngitis due to group A β-haemolytic streptococcus, or acute otitis media is suspected, then they should be given after a throat swab has been taken for bacterial culture. A positive culture will mean that a 10-day course of antibiotics is required.

- *Tonsillitis and pharyngitis:* avoid amoxicillin because it may cause maculopapular rash in cases of EBV infection. Use penicillin V, or erythromycin in allergic patients, for 10 days.
- *Acute otitis media:* co-amoxiclav will cover the common causes of otitis media and be effective against β-lactamase-producing *H. influenzae* and *M. catarrhalis*.

Laryngeal and tracheal inflammation

There are a number of laryngeal and tracheal causes of inflammation and airway obstruction. In the acute setting you will be concerned with three common conditions.

- *Viral laryngotracheobronchitis (croup):* mucosal inflammation affecting anywhere from the nose to the lower airway that is commonly due to parainfluenza, influenza, and respiratory syncytial virus in children aged 6mths to 6yrs.
- *Spasmodic or recurrent croup:* barking cough and hyperreactive upper airways with no apparent respiratory tract symptoms.
- *Acute epiglottitis:* life-threatening swelling of the epiglottis and septicaemia due to *Haemophilus influenzae* type b infection—most commonly in children aged 1–6yrs. This is now rare since routine HiB immunization.

Diagnosis

History In practice the two main conditions that require differentiating are viral croup and acute epiglottitis. The history may help in this process (see Table 9.2).

Examination

Do not examine the throat. Take a careful assessment of severity including:
- Degree of stridor and subcostal recession.
- Respiratory rate.
- HR.
- LOC (drowsiness), tiredness, and exhaustion.
- Pulse oximetry.

Table 9.2 Differentiating between viral croup and acute epiglottitis

	Croup	Epiglottitis
Time course	Days	Hours
Prodrome	Coryza	None
Cough	Barking	Slight if any
Feeding	Can drink	No
Mouth	Closed	Drooling saliva
Toxic	No	Yes
Fever	<38.5°C	>38.5°C
Stridor	Rasping	Soft
Voice	Hoarse	Weak or silent

Treatment

Priority

The main priority in the emergency setting is to differentiate between acute epiglottitis and viral croup (see Table 9.2). If you are unsure, stabilize the child and ensure that nothing precipitates distress and possible airway obstruction. Try and keep the child, family, and staff calm. Alert emergency otolaryngologist and anaesthetist to the possibility of a need for emergency airway support.

Viral croup

Children with mild illness can be managed at home, but advise parents that if there is recession and stridor at rest then they will need to return to hospital. Infants <12mths may need closer attention. Treatments include the following.

- *Moist or humidified air:* although widely used to ease breathing the benefit of these physical measures is unproven.
- *Steroids:* oral prednisolone (2mg/kg for 3 days) or oral dexamethasone (0.15mg/kg stat dose) or nebulized budesonide (2mg stat dose) reduces the severity and duration of croup. They are also likely to reduce the need for endotracheal intubation.
- *Nebulized adrenaline (epinephrine):* can provide transient relief of symptoms.

In cases that require endotracheal intubation steroids should be given and, if there is evidence of secondary bacterial infection or bacterial tracheitis, antibiotics should be added.

Acute epiglottitis

The child with acute epiglottitis will need to be managed in the intensive care unit after endotracheal intubation. Once this procedure has been completed take blood cultures and start IV antibiotics.

- *2nd or 3rd generation cephalosporin* (e.g. cefuroxime, ceftriaxome, or cefotaxime) IV for 7–10 days.
- *Rifampicin prophylaxis* to close contacts.

Bronchial disease

The main symptoms of acute bronchitis in children are cough and fever. Two infections—*Bordetella pertussis* and *Mycoplasma pneumoniae*—may produce symptoms that persist for a number of weeks. Another condition often diagnosed in infants without fever or distress is 'wheezy bronchitis', or 'recurrent bronchitis'. This condition has been the topic of much debate over the years as to whether these infants have asthma or not, and whether they should be treated as such.

Whooping cough

Bordetella pertussis infection typically induces three stages of illness:
- *Catarrhal (1–2wks):* mild symptoms with fever, cough, and coryza.
- *Paroxysmal (2–6wks):* severe paroxysmal cough, followed by inspiratory whoop and vomiting.
- *Convalescent (2–4wks):* lessening symptoms that may take a whole month to resolve.

A whooping cough-like syndrome may be caused by *Bordetella parapertussis*, *Mycoplasma pneumoniae*, *Chlamydia*, or adenovirus.

History
There may be a typical history. In young infants, however, whoop is often absent, and apnoea is a more common finding. In older children, and parents, there may be a history of persistent and irritating cough.

Examination and investigation
A thorough examination is needed. In infants you will need to make sure that the problem is not pneumonia. Also, check the following:
- *Eyes:* subconjunctival haemorrhages are common.
- *CXR.*
- *Blood count:* leucocytosis and lymphocytosis.
- *Pernasal swab:* culture of *Bordetella pertussis*.

Treatment
Hospital care
- *Infants:* admission is required for those with a history of apnoea, cyanosis, or significant paroxysms. Close monitoring is required particularly in infants since there is a risk of seizures, encephalopathy, and death.
- *Isolation:* patients should be isolated for 5 days after starting treatment with antibiotics.

Contacts
- *Immunization:* recommended for children <7yrs who have been in close contact if they are not protected. Immunization reduces the risk of an individual developing infection by 90%, but the level of protection declines steadily through childhood.
- *Prophylactic antibiotics:* should be given to close contacts.

Antibiotics Erythromycin for 14 days (or clarithromycin for 7 days) to reduce infectivity but this may have minimal effect on the cough.

Bronchiolitis

Bronchiolitis, most commonly due to respiratory syncytial virus (RSV), affects everyone by the age of 2yrs. Whether you meet this infection in your first winter, or your second, determines how ill you will be. RSV invades the nasopharyngeal epithelium and spreads to the lower airways where it causes increased mucus production, desquamation, and then bronchiolar obstruction. The net effect is pulmonary hyperinflation and atelectasis. The other causes of bronchiolitis include infection with para-influenza, influenza, adenovirus, rhinovirus, metapneumovirus, chlamydia, and *Mycoplasma pneumoniae*.

There is an increased risk of severe infection in infants with CHD, CLD of prematurity, immunodeficiency, and other lung disease.

Diagnosis

History

In winter months infants with a typical history will have had coryza, followed by a dry cough, followed by worsening breathlessness. Other features in the history include:
- wheeze;
- feeding difficulty;
- episodes of apnoea.

Rarely, other presenting histories in babies include:
- encephalopathy with seizures due to hyponatraemia;
- apnoea and near miss sudden infant death.

Examination and investigation

A thorough examination is needed in order to assess the degree of respiratory distress:
- cyanosis or pallor;
- dry cough;
- tachypnoea;
- subcostal and intercostal recession;
- chest hyperinflation;
- prolonged expiration;
- pauses in breathing or apnoea;
- wheeze and crackles.

Key investigations include:
- *Pulse oximetry:* to assess oxygenation.
- *CXR:* to assess hyperinflation, atelectasis, and consolidation.
- *Nasopharyngeal swab:* immunofluorescent antibody testing for RSV binding.

Hospital treatment

The treatment of RSV bronchiolitis is mainly supportive and includes:

- Oxygen to achieve pulse oximetry saturation >92%.
- If tachypnoea, limit oral feeds and use a NGT.
- *Bronchodilators for wheeze:* nebulized salbutamol, ipratropium, and adrenaline have all been used in studies. The best evidence is for nebulized adrenaline.
- Mechanical ventilation for severe respiratory distress or apnoea.

Antiviral therapy with ribavirin should be reserved for immunodeficient patients and those with underlying heart or lung disease, although its benefit is uncertain.

Prophylaxis

Palivizumab is a monoclonal antibody to RSV and can be used as prophylaxis. Preterm babies and oxygen-dependent infants at risk of RSV infection can receive a monthly IM injection (for 5mths starting in October) to reduce risk of hospitalization and the need for mechanical ventilation.

Follow-up

Recurrent cough, wheeze, and tachypnoea may occur after RSV infection. These may require treatment and are best assessed in outpatients. Daily oral montelukast granules can sometimes help reduce the symptoms. A proportion of patients may develop asthma—they may have been predisposed to develop this problem irrespective of RSV in early infancy.

Pneumonia

Pneumonia is an infection of the lower respiratory tract and lung parenchyma that leads to consolidation. Viruses alone account for 14–35% of all community acquired pneumonia in childhood. In 20–60% of children a pathogen is not found. Common infecting bacterial agents by age are:

- *Neonates:* group B streptococcus, *Escherichia coli, Klebsiella, Staphylococcus aureus.*
- *Infants:* Streptoccus pneumoniae, Chlamydia.
- *School age:* Streptococcus pneumoniae, Staphylococcus aureus, group A streptococcus, Bordetella pertussis, Mycoplasma pneumoniae.

Certain groups of children are at risk of pneumonia, e.g. those with:

- congenital lung cysts;
- chronic lung disease (🕮 p.276);
- immunodeficiency (🕮 pp.295, 724);
- cystic fibrosis (🕮 p.270);
- sickle cell disease (🕮 p.620);
- tracheostomy *in situ.*

Diagnosis

History

The patient may have had a recent URTI and may also be complaining of pleuritic chest pain or abdominal pain. The typical history will have:

- temperature ≥38.5°C;
- shortness of breath;
- cough; with sputum production in older children (>7yrs).

Examination

Check for the following:

- *Signs of respiratory distress:* tachypnoea; grunting; intercostal recession; use of accessory muscles for breathing. A resting respiratory rate of 70breaths/min in infants or >50breaths/min in children indicates severe illness.
- *Desaturation and cyanosis:* pulse oximetry should be performed in every child admitted to hospital with pneumonia. SpO_2 ≤92% in room air indicates severe illness.
- *General health and lethargy.*
- *Auscultation signs of lobar pneumonia:* dullness to percussion; crackles; decreased breath sounds; tactile vocal fremitus; bronchial breathing.

Investigations

The investigations that help in diagnosis include:

- *Sputum:* culture may be of limited value.
- *Nasopharyngeal aspirate:* viral immunofluorescence in infants.
- *Blood:* culture should be done in all children with severe bacterial pneumonia (not necessary in community-acquired pneumonia).
- *CXR:* not as routine (see 🕮 p.291).
- *Pleural fluid:* when there is a significant pleural effusion, an aspirated sample should be sent for culture and antigen testing once a drain is inserted.

- *Viral titres:* save a sample of blood for acute titre testing, which can be assayed the same time as the convalescent sample if a microbiological diagnosis is not made.

See Box 9.2 for summary of investigations.

Chest X-ray
There are a variety of changes ranging from lobar consolidation to the mere presence of patchy bilateral infiltrates. In general, routine CXR is not needed in children with mild uncomplicated LRTI. In other cases, look for pleural effusions, fluid levels, apparent round pneumonia, cavitation, hilar adenopathy, and any calcification. At follow-up, patients with history of significant acute X-ray change (e.g. lobar collapse, apparent round pneumonia, empyema) or continuing symptoms will require repeat X-ray.

Box 9.2 Investigations to consider in children with chronic or recurrent pneumonia

Step 1: initial blood tests
- *Haematology:* FBC, complement screen, ESR
- *Immunology:* IgA, IgE (and aspergillus RAST), IgG, IgM, antibody response to immunizations (tetanus and pneumococcus), rheumatoid factor
- *Antibodies:* aspergillus precipitins, antinuclear antibodies
- *Genetics:* CF genotype

Step 2: other tests
- *Sweat test*
- *Microbiology:* sputum culture
- *Lung function:* spirometry, lung volumes, and reversibility
- *Radiology:* CXR, barium swallow for vascular ring, sinus radiography

Step 3: further investigations
- *Haematology:* neutrophil and monocyte function, lymphocyte subsets, and cellular immune function
- *Imaging:* high resolution CT scan of the chest
- *pH study:* for gastro-oesophageal reflux
- *Video fluoroscopy:* for silent aspiration
- *Nasal ciliary biopsy:* microscopy and function (may be unnecessary if there is a normal nasal nitric oxide)
- *Bronchoscopy:* visualization of dynamic airway function, as well as microbiological sample collection

Pneumonia: treatment

Oral antibiotics are safe and effective in the treatment of community-acquired pneumonia. IV antibiotics are used in children who cannot absorb oral antibiotics or in those with severe symptoms. The specific choice of antibiotic is based on the following:

- Age of the child.
- Host factors.
- Severity of illness.
- Information about cultures if known.
- CXR findings if known.

Antibiotic therapy for pneumonia

Under 5yrs

Streptococcus pneumoniae is the most likely pathogen. The causes of atypical pneumonia are *Mycoplasma pneumoniae* and *Chlamydia trachomatis*

- *First-line treatment:* amoxicillin
- *Alternatives:* co-amoxiclav or cefaclor for typical pneumonia; erythromycin, clarithromycin, or azithromycin for atypical pneumonia

Over 5yrs

Mycoplasma pneumoniae is more common in this age group

- *First-line treatment:* amoxicillin is effective against the majority of pathogens, but consider macrolide antibiotics if mycoplasma or chlamydia is suspected
- *Alternatives:* if *Staphylococcus aureus* is suspected consider using a macrolide, or a combination of flucloxacillin with amoxicillin

Severe pneumonia

Co-amoxiclav, cefotaxime, or cefuroxime IV

Supportive therapies

Consider whether any of the following are needed:

- *Antipyretics* for fever.
- *IV fluids:* consider if dehydrated or not drinking.
- *Supplemental oxygen:* administer oxygen via headbox or nasal cannulae so that SpO_2 is maintained >92% (📖 p.46).
- *Chest drain:* for fluid or pus collections in the chest, as in empyema.

Physiotherapy

Chest physiotherapy is generally not beneficial in children with pneumonia and should not be performed.

Pneumonia: effusion, empyema

The presence, in association with pneumonia, of a small effusion that does not cause any respiratory distress can be managed conservatively without the need for aspirating a sample. A fluid sample, however, is needed if there is:

* a large effusion;
* no clear underlying diagnosis;
* respiratory distress;
* persistent fever despite antibiotic treatment;
* long history (>14 days).

Fluid sample

After US of the chest and checking blood-clotting studies, a small chest drain (or pigtail drain) should be inserted into the pleural fluid unless effusion is small. Samples should be sent for the following:

* *Microbiology:* bacterial culture and sensitivity, acidfast bacilli.
* *Cytology:* presence of pus cells and microscopic assessment of aberrant cell types. Cytology for lymphoma may give false −ve result in up to 10% of cases.

Diagnosis of empyema

The diagnosis of empyema can be based on the presence of:

* *Fluid:* pH < 7.2, glucose <3.3mmol/L, protein >3g/L, pus cells.
* *US scan:* loculation or fibrin strands seen.

Fluid drainage

After inserting the small-bore drain or pigtail catheter, fluid should be allowed to drain into standard commercially available systems (e.g. water-seal two-bottle system). The drain can be removed if draining <50mL in 24hrs.

Urokinase for empyema

In empyema, as opposed to simple pleural effusion, instillation of urokinase via the chest drain is recommended.

* *Dose:* 40,000U urokinase in 40mL (10,000U in 10mL if <1yr) given 12-hourly for 3 days.
* *Method:* instil via the chest drain and then clamp the drain and encourage the patient to move and roll around over the next 4hr.
* *Suction:* use a low pressure suction device (e.g. Robert's pump) to maintain suction of 20cmH₂O between doses.
* *Local anaesthetic:* bupivacaine around the drain site may control pleural pain. Consult the pain control team.

Surgical referral

If the effusion or empyema fails to resolve over a period of 7 days then a surgical opinion may be sought. Sometimes a chest CT scan is needed . A definitive surgical procedure or large bore drain and manual disruption of loculation may be needed.

Pulmonary tuberculosis

Worldwide, tuberculosis of the lung is a major health problem. TB should always be considered in children from endemic areas, as well as those at risk of immunodeficiency or taking immunosuppressive agents. Once diagnosed, TB is a notifiable disease and contact tracing is required so that those exposed to the patient undergo tuberculin testing and CXR screening. BCG vaccination appears to be protective against miliary spread, but is no longer routinely given.

Mycobacterium tuberculosis is spread from person to person by droplet infection. Once inhaled, some bacilli remain at the site of entry and the rest are carried to regional lymph nodes. The bacilli multiply at both sites; the primary focus along with the regional lymph nodes are collectively described as the primary focus. Organisms can then spread via the blood and lymphatics. The pathological sequence after infection is as follows.

- *4–8wks:*
  - febrile illness;
  - erythema nodosum;
  - phlyctenular conjunctivitis.
- *6–9mths:*
  - in most cases progressive healing of primary complex;
  - effusion: focus may rupture into pleural space;
  - cavitation: focus may rupture into bronchus;
  - coin lesion on CXR: focus may enlarge;
  - regional lymph nodes may obstruct bronchi;
  - regional lymph nodes may erode into bronchus or pericardial sac;
  - miliary spread.

Drug management See also 📖 p.722

Pulmonary
- *2mths:* isoniazid, rifampicin, and pyrazinamide. Often ethambutol added as a 4th drug.
- *Then 4mths:* isoniazid and rifampicin.

Miliary spread
- *3mths:* isoniazid, rifampicin, ethambutol and pyrazinamide.
- *Then 12–18mths:* isoniazid and rifampicin.

Other disorders

Aspiration syndromes

* *Acute aspiration* of fluid or particulate matter into the lungs may occur at any age and the typical presentation is choking and coughing. In infants, some aspiration episodes may go unrecognized in the acute phase. These babies may present later with consolidation that fails to improve.
* *Chronic aspiration* may present with recurrent pneumonia—different lobes at different times. Airway anomalies should be sought as an underlying cause (see 📖 pp.846–849). Also swallowing abnormalities need to be excluded with a video fluoroscopy done by an experienced speech and language therapist.

Interstitial lung disease

A rare group of disorders in childhood and children (usually infants) present with progressive tachypnoea and hypoxia. The CXR shows widespread reticular shadowing but a high resolution CT scan is needed for diagnosis. Treatment should be undertaken in specialist centres as these children will require lung biopsy and may need treatment with steroids or chloroquine. A requirement for supplemental oxygen is common.

Lymphoid interstitial pneumonitis (LIP)

See also 📖 p.726. LIP has the appearance of fibrosing alveolitis, but it is a pulmonary feature of HIV infection that responds to steroids.

Immunodeficiency

See also 📖 pp.724–727. Recurrent infection of the lower airway is common in patients with immunodeficiency such as:

* IgA deficiency.
* IgG subclass deficiency.
* Defective cell-mediated immunity: viral or fungal infection.

Gastroenterology and nutrition

Healthy eating for children

Infants
- See also 📖 p.142.
- Breast milk is the ideal feed for almost all infants.
- Solids are not recommended until age 6mths (↓ food allergies).
- Initial solids should be based on baby rice, fruit, and vegetables.
- Gluten is acceptable from age 6mths.
- Following introduction of solids, infants should experience and progress through a wide variety of tastes and appropriate textures.
- Finger foods should be introduced from age 7mths.
- Continue complementary breast or formula feeds until age 1yr. Normal full fat cow's milk can then be introduced as the main drink.
- Avoid addition of salt and sugar to food.
- Low fat products are not suitable for infants.
- Supplemental vitamins A, C, and D are recommended until age 5yrs.

Age 1–5yrs
A well balanced diet in early childhood is important to establish a lifetime pattern of healthy eating. The key recommendations for healthy eating to be achieved by age 5yrs are the following:
- Decrease fat to 35% energy intake by avoiding excess high fat foods and changing milk to semi-skimmed at age 2yrs, and skimmed at age 5yrs.
- Include whole grain cereals and 5 portions per day of fruits and vegetables to increase fibre intake.
- Monitor for (accelerating weight velocity) and avoid obesity.
- Moderate salt intake, e.g. not adding salt to cooking or at the table.
- Avoid iron deficiency anaemia by restricting milk intake to 1 pint per day and including foods rich in iron (red meat, cereals, beans, pulses, egg yolk, dark green vegetables, and dried fruit). Add vitamin C as fruit juice at a meal to increase iron absorption. Drinking tea with meals decreases iron absorption.
- Excessive consumption of fruit juices or squashes can contribute to chronic non-specific diarrhoea of childhood (toddler diarrhoea) and contribute to feeding problems.

Older children
Schoolchildren should eat a diet based on a wide variety of foods. Nutritional guidelines relating to school meals have been set out by many UK local authorities and healthy eating forms part of the UK national curriculum. A healthy diet should include:
- At least one starchy food at each meal time, e.g. whole meal bread, potatoes, pasta, and rice.
- Five portions per day of fruit and vegetables.
- Two servings of meat or alternatives each day.
- Two to three portions a day of skimmed milk, low-fat yoghurt, fromage frais, or cheese (a portion = 1 yoghurt, 1/3 pint milk, 30g cheese).
- Only small and occasional amounts of sugar and fats.

Vomiting

A common symptom in childhood.
  Three clinical scenarios are recognized (see Box 10.1):
- *Acute:* discrete episode of moderate to high intensity. Most common and usually associated with an acute illness.
- *Chronic:* low-grade daily pattern, frequently with mild illness.
- *Cyclic:* severe, discrete episodes associated with pallor, lethargy +/– abdominal pain. The child is well in between episodes. Often there is a family history of migraine or vomiting.

Causes
- *Acute:* GI infection; non-GI infection (e.g. urinary tract infection); GI obstruction (congenital or acquired e.g. pyloric stenosis); adverse food reaction; poisoning; raised intracranial pressure; endocrine/metabolic disease (e.g. diabetic ketoacidosis).
- *Chronic (usually GI):* peptic ulcer disease; gastro-oesophageal reflux; chronic infection; gastritis; gastroparesis; food allergy; psychogenic (see Psychogenic vomiting); bulimia; pregnancy.
- *Cyclic (usually non-GI cause):* idiopathic; CNS disease; abdominal migraine; endocrine (e.g. Addison's disease); metabolic (e.g. acute intermittent porphyria); intermittent GI obstruction; fabricated illness.

Management
- *Full history:* e.g. early morning vomiting with CNS tumour, or family members with similar illness.
- *Full examination:* including ear, nose, and throat (ENT) and growth. Assess for dehydration.

Treatment
- *Supportive treatment as needed:* e.g. oral or IV fluids.
- *Treat cause:* e.g. pyloromyotomy for hypertrophic pyloric stenosis.
- *Pharmacological:* antihistamines; phenothiazines (side-effects: extrapyramidal reactions); prokinetic drugs, e.g. domperidone. 5-HT$_3$ antagonists, e.g. ondansetron, are increasingly being used for treating post-operative or chemotherapy induced vomiting. 5-HT$_{1D}$ agonists, e.g. pizotifen, are useful as prophylaxis and treatment for cyclic vomiting syndrome.

Complications
Dehydration, plasma electrolyte disturbance (e.g. ↓ K$^+$, ↓ Cl$^-$, alkalosis with pyloric stenosis), acute or chronic GI bleeding (e.g. Mallory–Weiss tear), oesophageal stricture, Barrett's metaplasia, broncho-pulmonary aspiration, faltering growth, iron deficiency anaemia.

Psychogenic vomiting
- *Causes:* anxiety; manipulative behaviour; disordered family dynamics. A family history of vomiting is common.
- *Management:* exclude organic disease. Refer to child psychologist.

Box 10.1 Investigations for vomiting

Acute (if severe)
- FBC
- U&E
- Creatinine
- Stool for culture and virology
- AXR
- Surgical opinion if obstruction or acute abdomen possible
- Exclude systemic disease

Chronic
- FBC
- ESR/CRP
- U&E
- LFT
- *Helicobacter pylori* serology
- Urinalysis
- Abdominal US
- Small bowel enema
- Sinus X-rays
- Test feed or abdominal ultrasound for pyloric stenosis
- Brain imaging (CNS tumour)
- Consider urine pregnancy testing in teenage girls
- Upper GI endoscopy

Cyclic
As for chronic vomiting, plus the following:
- Serum amylase
- Serum lipase
- Blood glucose
- Serum ammonia

Acute diarrhoea

Normal stool frequency and consistency vary, e.g. breastfed infants may pass 10–12 stools per day, primary school children may pass stool from three times a day to once every three days. Diarrhoea is a change in consistency and frequency of stools with enough loss of fluid and electrolytes to cause illness. It kills 3 million children per year worldwide.

Acute diarrhoea

Causes
- Infective gastroenteritis. Most common cause (📖 p.338).
- Non-enteric infections, e.g. respiratory tract.
- Food hypersensitivity reactions (📖 p.316).
- NEC (📖 p.178).
- Drugs, e.g. antibiotics.
- Henoch–Schönlein purpura (HSP) (📖 p.788).
- Intussusception (<4yrs) (📖 p.860).
- Haemolytic–uraemic syndrome (📖 p.376).
- Pseudomembranous enterocolitis.

Presentation
- Fever +/– vomiting (infectious gastroenteritis).
- Diarrhoea +/– bloody stools (colitis—infectious or non-infectious).
- Dehydration and ↓ consciousness.

Management
- Assess hydration and vital signs, pallor (blood loss), abdominal tenderness, signs of associated illness (e.g. petechial rash in HSP).
- *Mild/moderate dehydration:*
  - no tests necessary;
  - replace fluid and electrolyte losses with oral glucose–electrolyte based rehydration fluid, e.g. Dioralyte® (UK).
- *Severe/shock dehydration:*
  - U&E, creatinine, FBC, blood gas, stool M,C&S/virology, tests for specific disease (e.g. US in suspected intussuseption);
  - IV fluid and electrolyte replacement (see 📖 pp.65, 89–93).
- Anti-motility drug treatment is not recommended; it can be harmful, particularly in acute infection/inflammation.
- Antibiotics are not indicated unless cause is proven, e.g. *Yersinia* or *Campylobacter* infection, parasitic infection, NEC, or proven bacteraemia/systemic infection.
- Other treatment is disease specific. Some diarrhoeal processes require removal of the offending agent, such as in lactose intolerance or coeliac disease or allergic gastroenteritis. Others may require bowel rest or surgery, e.g. NEC or intussusception.
- Once rehydrated, resume normal diet. Replace on going losses. Continue breast feeding. There is no evidence that prolonged starvation is beneficial in infective gastroenteritis.

- Prevent cross-infection with strict hand washing and barrier nursing. In the less developed world, breastfeeding, provision of clean water, and adequate sanitation are also important to reduce risk of infection.

Investigations See 📖 p.301.

Prognosis
The majority of cases, particularly if caused by infective gastroenteritis, make a complete recovery with appropriate treatment.

Chronic diarrhoea

Chronic diarrhoea

Defined as diarrhoea persisting for >14 days. Many of the diseases that cause acute diarrhoea can lead on to chronic diarrhoea.

The pathophysiology may involve:

- Reduced GI absorptive capacity, e.g. coeliac disease.
- Osmotic diarrhoea, e.g. lactase deficiency.
- Inflammatory, e.g. ulcerative colitis.
- Secretory diarrhoea (rare), e.g. vasoactive intestinal peptide producing tumour.

Causes

Age 0–24mths

- Malabsorption (see 🕮 p.334), e.g. post-infective gastroenteritis syndrome, lactose intolerance, cystic fibrosis, coeliac disease.
- Food hypersensitivity, e.g. to cow's milk protein.
- Chronic non-specific diarrhoea (toddler diarrhoea); child is usually thriving (🕮 p.305).
- Excessive fluid intake.
- Protracted infectious gastroenteritis.
- Immuno-deficiencies, including HIV.
- Hirschsprung's disease (🕮 p.870).
- Rarer causes (intractable diarrhoea) include congenital mucosal transport defects and autoimmune enteropathy.
- Tumours (secretory diarrhoea).
- Fabricated induced illness.

Older children

- Inflammatory bowel disease (IBD).
- Constipation (spurious diarrhoea).
- Malabsorption—see Causes.
- Irritable bowel syndrome (IBS).
- Chronic infections, including giardiasis, bacterial overgrowth, and pseudomembranous colitis.
- Laxative abuse.
- Excessive fluid intake.
- Fabricated induced illness.

History

Nature and frequency of stool, presence of undigested food, relationship to diet changes (e.g. weaning) or travel, stool blood, or mucus, weight loss.

Examination

Features of malnutrition or other illness, e.g. peri-anal disease in inflammatory bowel disease, or finger clubbing in cystic fibrosis.

Investigations
- *Stool:* inspection; microscopy for bacteria or parasites, leucocytes, fat globules (pancreatic diseases), fatty acid crystals (diffuse mucosal defects); culture; pH (<5.5 = carbohydrate malabsorption); reducing substances (>0.5% = carbohydrate malabsorption); faecal occult blood (colitis); electrolytes ($\uparrow$ Na^+ and K^+ = secretory diarrhoea; $\uparrow$ Cl^- = congenital chloridorrhoea).
- *Blood:* U&E; FBC ($\downarrow$ Hb = haematinic deficiency or blood loss; $\uparrow$ eosinophil = food hypersensitivity or parasites); $\uparrow$ CRP/ESR (inflammatory); blood gas; radioallergosorbent test (RAST) (food allergy); hormone level (vanillylmandelic acid (VMA), catecholamines, vasoactive intestinal polypeptide (VIP)) for secretory tumours.
- *Radiology:* AXR, ultrasound, barium meal and follow through.
- *Other:* breath hydrogen test (lactose malabsorption or bacterial overgrowth); GI endoscopy biopsy (e.g. upper for coeliac disease, upper and lower for suspected IBD); sweat test/genetic testing (CF); rectal biopsy (Hirschsprung's disease).

Treatment
- Treat underlying cause.
- Nutritional intervention if deficiencies are present.
- Antibiotics are only useful if systemic illness or prolonged infection is present, e.g. *Salmonella*, *Campylobacter*, giardiasis, or amoebiasis.
- Rarely, other drug treatment may be useful, e.g. loperamide or cholestyramine.

Chronic non-specific diarrhoea (toddler diarrhoea)
- Occurs from 6mths to 5yrs.
- Presents with colicky intestinal pain, $\uparrow$ flatus, abdominal distension, loose stools with undigested food ('peas and carrots' stools).
- Child is otherwise well and thriving.
- Examination and investigations are normal.

Treatment Reassurance; dietary ($\uparrow$ fat intake; normalize fibre intake; $\downarrow$ milk, fruit juice, and sugary drink intake); loperamide occasionally may be necessary.

Encopresis
- Voluntary defaecation in unacceptable places, including the child's pants in older children.
- No organic abnormality is present; it is a symptom of an emotional disorder.
- It is three times more common in boys.
- Once organic disease or spurious diarrhoea secondary to constipation with loading are excluded (see 📖 pp.306–307), consider behavioural problems and referral to a child and adolescent psychiatrist.

Constipation

Defined as infrequent passage of stool associated with pain and difficulty, or delay in defaecation.
- 95% of infants pass ≥1 stool/day.
- 95% of school children pass ≥3 stools/wk.
- Constipation is common in childhood.
- Approximately 5% of school children suffer significant constipation, usually functional.
- Organic cause more likely if: delayed passage of meconium beyond 24hr of age; onset in infancy; severe; associated with faltering growth or abnormal physical signs (include per anal examination).

Causes

Idiopathic
Commonest due to a combination of:
- Low fibre diet.
- Lack of mobility and exercise.
- Poor colonic motility (55% have a positive family history).

Gastrointestinal
- Hirschsprung's disease.
- Anal disease (infection, stenosis, ectopic, fissure, hypertonic sphincter).
- Partial intestinal obstruction.
- Food hypersensitivity.
- Coeliac disease.

Non-gastrointestinal
- Hypothyroidism.
- Hypercalcaemia.
- Neurological disease, e.g. spinal disease.
- Chronic dehydration, e.g. diabetes insipidus.
- Drugs, e.g. opiates and anticholinergics.
- Sexual abuse.

Presentation

- Straining and/or infrequent stools.
- Anal pain on defaecation.
- Fresh rectal bleeding (anal fissure).
- Abdominal pain.
- Anorexia.
- Involuntary soiling or spurious diarrhoea (liquid faeces passes around solid impaction).
- Flatulence.
- ↓ Growth.
- Abdominal distension.
- Palpable abdominal or rectal faecal masses, usually indentible.
- Anal fissure.
- Abnormal anal tone. A rectal examination is normally unnecessary unless child fails to responds to initiation of simple treatment, except in infancy when anal stenosis should be considered.

Management (See Box 10.2)

Investigations are usually not necessary. If an organic cause is suspected consider: FBC; coeliac antibody screen; thyroid function tests; serum Ca^{2+}; RAST testing; AXR; bowel transit studies (older child); rectal biopsy (for Hirschsprung's disease); anal manometry; spinal imaging (neurological cause).

Box 10.2 Treat in a stepwise manner

- Treat any underlying organic cause
- *Dietary:* ↑ oral fluid and fibre intake, natural laxatives, e.g. fruit juice
- *Behavioural measures:* toilet footrests; regular 5min toilet time after meals; star charts and rewards for child passing stool; reassure parents and encourage them not to show concern to the child

The aim of medication is to achieve disimpaction and then maintainance.
- Emphasize the need for consistency and adherence
- Poor adherence and failure to evacuate faecal masses preclude improvement
- Treat for at least 3mths. It is important not to wean therapy too soon
- Regular oral faecal softeners, e.g. Movicol®, lactulose, or sodium docusate, will aid disimpaction
- Oral stimulant laxatives, e.g. senna, sodium picosulphate, may be required
- Consider treatment of any anal fissure with topical anaesthetic (2% lidocaine ointment) to reduce pain and remove voluntary inhibition to defaecate
- Oral magnesium citrate, magnesium phosphate or large volume polyethylene glycol (PEG) electrolyte solution bowel clean out (may require nasogastric administration for rapid infusion)
- Enemas, e.g. Micralax® or phosphate enemas, only if no response to intensive treatment with above
- Hospital admission may be required for the most severe for either manual evacuation under sedation or general anaesthesia, or oral PEG

Prognosis

The vast majority of children can be 'cured' by an enthusiastic and sympathetic paediatrician with complete evacuation of any stool masses, maintaining soft stools, and defaecation training. Many children need long term therapy. Do not underestimate the misery that this condition can inflict on both the child and family.

Faltering growth (failure to thrive)

Faltering growth, also known as failure to thrive (FTT), is when there is a failure to grow at the expected rate (i.e. growth 'falls away' from standardized weight or height centile). Weight is the most sensitive indicator in infants and young children, whilst height is a better in the older child. Under stress, head circumference growth is more preserved than linear growth, which in turn, is more than weight gain.

In infancy, birth weight reflects the intrauterine environment. It is a poor guide to the child's correct 'genetic potential' and weight may naturally fall until the correct 'level' is attained. In a well, happy child consider constitutional small stature (characterized by normal growth velocity in a healthy child of small stature parents).

Causes

95% of true FTT is due to not enough food being offered or taken. In developing countries poverty is the main cause. In the UK, causes include socioeconomic difficulties, emotional deprivation, unskilled feeding, or a particular belief system regarding appropriate nutrition.

Organic causes include:

- Decreased appetite, e.g. psychological or secondary to chronic illness.
- Inability to ingest, e.g. GI structural or neurological problems.
- Excessive food loss, e.g. severe vomiting (gastro-oesophageal reflux disease (GORD), pyloric stenosis, dysmotility), diabetes mellitus (urine).
- Malabsorption (see 📖 p.334).
- Increased energy requirements, e.g. congenital heart disease, cystic fibrosis, malignancy, sepsis.
- Impaired utilization, e.g. various syndromes, IEM, endocrinopathies.

Causes may overlap, e.g. in cystic fibrosis there is simultaneous malabsorption, increased energy requirements, anorexia, and chronic infection.

Management

- *Detailed history:* including age of onset of FTT, and timing of weaning. Consider asking paediatric dietitian to perform detailed dietary history.
- *Full examination:* including accurate measurement of growth.
- *If organic disease possible:* basic investigations should include:
  - FBC, ESR/CRP, U&E, creatinine, total protein and albumin, Ca^{2+}, PO_4^{3-}, LFT;
  - immunoglobulins;
  - coeliac antibody screen;
  - urinalysis, including M, C&S.
- *Further investigations:* are indicated if there are suggestive symptoms or the faltering growth is severe, and include: IEM screen; karyotype; serum lead (pica); sweat test; upper endoscopy and small intestinal biopsy; CXR; bone age, skeletal survey (NAI); abdominal US; head CT/MRI; oesophageal pH monitoring; ECG; faecal occult blood.
- *If non-organic disease:* is likely, seek dietary advice, preferably by a paediatric dietitian:

- If FTT resolves in the next few weeks, give positive reinforcement and supervise subsequent growth as an outpatient.
- If FTT persists, admit to hospital for basic investigations and observe the response to supervised adequate dietary input. Adequate growth in hospital suggests a non-organic cause; explore and support family dynamics.
- Should FTT occur again at home after improvement in hospital, and then refer to social services for family assessment and appropriate intervention.
- If FTT continues in hospital despite adequate dietary input, occult organic disease is most likely and requires extensive investigation as above.
- Provide dietetic input, whatever the cause, to support nutritional correction and education.
- Identify and correct associated comorbidities, e.g. developmental delay or early presentation of neurological disorder such as cerebral palsy; fall off in head growth is suggestive.

Prognosis

The prognosis depends on the severity of FTT. It is good if mild. Severe FTT, whatever the cause, may be associated with later developmental and behavioural impairment.

Recurrent abdominal pain

- Defined as more than two discrete episodes in a 3mth period interfering with school and/or usual activities.
- *Incidence:* 10–15% in school age children.

Causes

No organic cause is found in 90%. Organic causes include: constipation; dietary indiscretion; food intolerance (lactose or fructose); irritable bowel syndrome; psychogenic pain; peptic ulcer (H. pylori); coeliac disease; abdominal migraine (cyclic vomiting syndrome); gallbladder disease; renal colic; dysmenorrhoea; UTI; mittleschmerz; and physical or sexual abuse.

Presentation

Non-organic disease

This form occurs in a thriving, generally well child; with short episodes of peri-umbilical pain, good appetite, no other GI symptoms, no family history of migraine or coeliac disease, and normal examination. Co-existent symptoms such as headache and fatigue are common and this is often referred to as recurrent abdominal pain syndrome.

Organic cause

Likely if presentation is different to above or child <2yrs. 'Red flag' symptoms include weight loss, diarrhoea, blood per rectum, joint symptoms, skin rashes, family history of inflammatory bowel disease, or coeliac disease.

Management

History

Ethnic origin (lactase deficiency occurs in dark skinned races), atopy, relationship to eating, precipitating events (e.g. cow's milk introduction in milk protein enteropathy), social history (e.g. start of school, parental separation), and family history.

Full examination

Investigation
- *If non-organic disease is likely:* no or very little investigation is needed, e.g. FBC, ESR/CRP, U&E, LFT, coeliac antibody screen, urine M, C&S, faecal M, C&S (if there is a recent history of foreign travel).
- *If organic disease is likely:* investigate as above, plus consider hydrogen breath test (lactose intolerance); C^{13} breath test (*Helicobactor pylori*); US; barium radiology; upper and lower GI endoscopy.

Treatment

Non-organic disease

Confident reassurance; education that condition is common and pain is genuine (just like headaches); personal support; avoidance of associated stressful events (e.g. bullying); acknowledgement of symptom, whilst at same time down playing pain; minimize secondary gains from abdominal pain, e.g. school avoidance; increased dietary fibre intake may be beneficial;

formal psychotherapy in complex and resistant cases. Multidisciplinary support and engagement of the family is essential.

Organic disease: Treat the underlying cause.

Prognosis

Approximately 25% of children with functional recurrent abdominal pain continue to have pain or headaches in adulthood. Functional sequelae are common.

Abdominal migraine

Abdominal pain is associated with pallor, headaches, anorexia, nausea, +/− vomiting. The condition overlaps with periodic syndrome and cyclic vomiting syndrome. There is usually a strong family history of migraine.

Treatment

- *Dietary:* avoid citrus fruits, chocolate, caffeine-containing drinks (e.g. cola), solid cheeses.
- *Pharmacological:* pizotifen, sumatriptan, gabapentin, or amitriptyline may be helpful.

Gastrointestinal haemorrhage

This condition is relatively rare in childhood. Upper GI tract bleeding may present as haematemesis (vomiting of frank blood or 'coffee grounds') or melaena (black, tarry, foul-smelling stools). Haematochezia (bright or dark red blood PR) indicates lower GI tract bleeding.

Beware of spurious haemorrhage, e.g. black stools after bismuth/iron ingestion, red vomit after beetroot, urate crystals in nappies, or normal pseudomenstruation in newborns. Use Dipstix test or laboratory testing to confirm blood you are if unsure.

Causes

Neonates
- Swallowed maternal blood, i.e. not GI haemorrhage.
- NEC.
- Dietary protein intolerance.
- Coagulopathy.
- Stress ulcers.
- Gastritis, vascular.
- Malformations.
- Duplication cyst.
- Infectious colitis, including pseudomembranous colitis.
- Inflammatory colitis.

Infants
Most of the above plus:
- Oesophagitis.
- Swallowed blood from upper airway, e.g. epistaxis.
- Anal fissure.
- Intussusception (📖 p.860).
- Meckel's diverticulum (often presents as a massive painless rectal bleed; 📖 p.865).

Older children
Most of the above plus:
- Peptic ulcer disease.
- Mallory–Weiss tear.
- Oesophageal varices.
- Nonsteroidal anti-inflammatory drugs (NSAIDs).
- Intestinal polyps.
- IBD (📖 p.332).
- GI infection, e.g. dysentery.
- HSP (📖 p.788).
- HUS (📖 p.376).

Management See Box 10.3

- *Detailed history:* e.g. is there associated abdominal pain?
- *Examination:* specifically, vital signs; skin (pallor, abnormal blood vessels); hepatic stigmata; ENT examination (e.g. epistaxis); organomegaly; abdominal tenderness; anal inspection (e.g. fissure or fistula); rectal examination. Examine vomit or stool to confirm nature of bleed.
- *Supportive treatment:* fluids; blood product transfusion; airway protection with NGT or ETT as necessary.
- *Drug treatment:* somatostatin or vasopressin reduces splanchnic blood flow and, thereby, upper GI bleeding.
- *Therapeutic endoscopy:* in severe bleeds, e.g. balloon tamponade, electrocautery, bleeding vessel ligation, paravariceal injection.
- *Treat underlying cause:* e.g. surgical removal of Meckel's diverticulum.

Box 10.3 Investigations for GI haemorrhage

Guided by findings from examination and history, these may include:
- FBC
- U&E
- Coagulation studies
- LFT
- Albumin
- Protein
- ESR/CRP
- Apt's test in newborns (confirms swallowed maternal blood by distinguishing adult from foetal Hb)
- Stool M,C&S
- Stool *Clostridia difficile* toxin assay (pseudomembranous colitis)
- Formal ENT examination
- Abdominal US (e.g. intussusception or portal hypertension)
- Upper GI barium meal
- Nuclear medicine scan (Meckel's diverticulum)
- Labelled RBC scan (occult bleeding)
- CXR (in case haemoptysis is true cause)
- Endoscopy (oesophago-gastro-duodenoscopy if melaena or haematemesis; flexible sigmoidoscopy or colonoscopy if haematochezia)

Jaundice

See also ☐ pp.130–131. Jaundice occurs when serum bilirubin >25–30mmol/L. It is rare outside neonatal period. First determine the SBR and conjugated (direct) fraction. Unconjugated jaundice is rarely due to liver disease. Conjugated jaundice (>20mmol/L) is due to liver disease and requires investigation.

Unconjugated jaundice

Due to excess bilirubin production, impaired liver uptake, or conjugation.

Causes

• Haemolysis (spherocytosis, G6PD deficiency, sickle cell anaemia, thalassaemia, HUS).
• Defective bilirubin conjugation (Gilbert syndrome, Crigler–Najjar syndrome).

Intrahepatic cholestasis

Here, jaundice is due to hepatocyte damage +/– cholestasis. There is unconjugated +/– conjugated hyperbilirubinaemia.

Causes

Infectious
• Viral hepatitis, including chronic hepatitis.
• Bacterial hepatitis (leptospirosis [Weil's disease], septicaemia, *Mycoplasma*, liver abscess).
• *Toxoplasma gondii.*

Toxic
• Drugs or poisons, e.g. paracetamol overdose, sodium valproate, anti-TB drugs, cytotoxic drugs.
• Fungi (*Amanita phalloides*).

Metabolic
• Galactosaemia, hereditary fructose intolerance.
• Tyrosinaemia type 1.
• Wilson's disease.
• α_1-antitrypsin deficiency.
• Hypothyroidism.
• Peroxisomal disorders, e.g. Zellweger syndrome.
• Dubin–Johnson syndrome, Rotor syndrome.

Biliary hypoplasia
• Non-syndromic.
• Syndromic, e.g. Alagille syndrome.

Cardiovascular
• Budd–Chiari syndrome.
• Right heart failure.

Autoimmune hepatitis Autoimmune hepatitis.

Cholestatic (obstructive) jaundice
Conjugated hyperbilirubinaemia is due to bile tract obstruction.

Causes
- Biliary atresia.
- Choledochal cyst.
- Caroli's disease.
- Primary sclerosing cholangitis (commonly associated with IBD).
- Cholelithiasis (may be secondary to chronic haemolysis).
- Cholecystitis.
- Cystic fibrosis.
- Obstructive tumours or cysts.

Management of jaundice
Full history e.g. medications, family history, overseas travel, past blood transfusions, jaundice contacts, pale stools, or dark urine (cholestasis).

Examination Vital signs; conscious level (hepatic coma); hepatic stigmata (= chronic liver disease); pallor (haemolysis); hepatomegaly; splenomegaly; ascites; peripheral oedema.

Investigations
Depending on which of the above pattern presents these may include:
- FBC, blood film, reticulocyte count.
- Coagulation studies.
- U&E, SBR (total and conjugated), LFT, albumin, total protein, TFT.
- Viral serology (hepatitis A, B, C, EBV, CMV), blood culture, leptospira and toxoplasma antibody titres.
- IEM screen, ammonia, copper studies (serum copper ↑, ↓, or ↔, serum caeruloplasmin ↓ in Wilson's disease), blood glucose, α_1-antitrypsin level, galactose-1-uridyl-phosphatase level.
- Immunoglobulins, anti-nuclear antibody, smooth muscle and liver/kidney antibodies (autoimmune hepatitis);
- Abdominal US, abdominal CT/MRI, biliary scintigraphy, e.g. hepatoiminodiacetic acid [HIDA] scan).
- Liver biopsy.

Treatment
- Remove or treat underlying cause.
- Correct blood glucose if it is low.
- Correct any clotting abnormalities.
- Phototherapy may be helpful only if jaundice has a significant unconjugated component, e.g. Crigler–Najjar syndrome.
- Treat any associated anaemia if due to haemolysis.
- Treat liver failure as appropriate.

Adverse reactions to food

Food allergy

Defined as an abnormal immunological response to food (incidence is 6–8% in children aged <3yrs).
- Immediate allergic reactions involve production of food-specific IgE antibodies.
- 70% of cases have a family history of atopy.
- Allergy becomes less common as age increases.
- The commonest food allergens are cow's milk proteins, eggs, peanuts, wheat, soya, fish, shellfish, and tree nuts.

Presentation
- Diarrhoea +/− blood/mucus.
- Vomiting.
- Dysphagia, gastro-oesophageal reflux symptoms.
- Abdominal pain.
- Faltering growth (FTT).
- Eczema.
- Urticaria.
- Erythematous rash, particularly peri-oral.
- Asthma symptoms.
- Food induced anaphylaxis.

Food intolerance

Intolerance involves adverse reactions to food that are mediated by non-immunological responses. This condition is more common than food allergy. Its presentation is similar to that of food allergy. Fructose intolerance is very common due to usage of high-fructose corn syrup in prepared foods and beverages. Other food intolerances may be due to:
- GI enzyme deficiency, e.g. lactose intolerance (📖 p.317), congenital sucrase-isomaltase deficiency.
- Pharmacological reactions to agents contained in food, e.g. caffeine, histamine, tyramine, tartrazine, acetylsalicylic acid.
- Reactions to food toxins or microbes, e.g. haemagglutinins in soy or mycotoxin present in mould-contaminated cereals.

Management of suspected food allergy or intolerance

See Box 10.4 for clinical approach.

Treatment
- *Dietary treatment:* exclusion of offending food(s) from diet, e.g. milk free, soya free, egg-free diet.
  - Involve a paediatric dietitian in the diagnosis and management.
  - Extensively hydrolysed or amino acid based milks can be used.
  - Dietary exclusion in the mother should be considered if breast feeding.
- *Drug treatment:* regular therapy may have a role, e.g. oral sodium cromoglicate, corticosteroids, and antihistamines.

- IM adrenaline is used by the child or parents for emergency treatment of anaphylactic reactions, particularly if IgE mediated and there are respiratory or systemic symptoms and signs.
- After at least 6–12mths of being symptom-free on exclusion diet, consider food challenge if there is a food allergy. If the previous reaction was severe, this should only be done in hospital with full resuscitation facilities available in the event of a serious adverse reaction.

Prophylaxis
Data are not clear. In newborns with a first degree relative with confirmed food allergy, exclusive breastfeeding to at least age 1yr reduces risk of allergy. If this is not possible then a hydrolysed milk formula can be used. After weaning temporary avoidance of at risk foods may also reduce risk.

Box 10.4 Approach to adverse food reaction

History
Including diet history and examination. A food diary may be helpful.

Investigations
These may include: RAST or enzyme-linked immunosorbent assay (ELISA) test to detect specific food IgE antibodies; serum ↑ total IgE or eosinophils; favourable response to dietary elimination of specific suspected food protein and then recurrence after challenge; allergen prick or patch skin testing. If the diagnosis is still in doubt, a double-blind, controlled food antigen challenge, or upper and lower gastrointestinal endoscopy (non-specific inflammatory infiltrate) may be helpful in children with predominantly gut symptoms.

In severe cases when allergen(s) cannot be identified, start a full elimination diet in which only a few hypoallergenic foods are given for 1–2wks, e.g. lamb, rice, water, pears, followed by a gradual reintroduction of increasingly allergenic foods until a food reaction(s) is detected.

Prognosis of food allergy or intolerance
The prognosis depends on the cause. The majority of infantile food allergic reactions resolve by 2yrs. The exception is peanut allergy that tends to persist. Allergies that develop in older children may become chronic.

Lactose intolerance
- This is most commonly due to post-viral gastroenteritis lactase deficiency, e.g. rotavirus. Most cases are transient and short lasting (<4–6wks).
- In older healthy children and adults, lactase levels commonly decline with subsequent variable severity intolerance (especially in certain populations, e.g. South-east Asian and Afro-Caribbean).
- Rarely due to genetic congenital lactase deficiency (primary). Infants present with severe diarrhoea after lactose exposure (present in high quantities in breast milk).
- *Presentation:* diarrhoea; excessive flatus; colic; peri-anal excoriation; stool pH <5.

- *Treatment:* lactose-free formula milk (soya milk not recommended in children under 6/12).

Cow's milk protein allergy

- Commonest food allergy in infancy.
- Symptoms depend on where the allergic inflammation is.
  - *Upper GI tract*—vomiting, feeding aversion, pain.
  - *Small intestine*—diarrhoea, abdominal pain, protein-losing
  - enteropathy, FTT.
  - *Large intestine*—diarrhoea, acute colitis with blood and mucus in
- stools, rarely, chronic constipation.
- Limited use for RAST or skin testing in infants.
- May occur in breast-fed infants, the reaction is to cow's milk protein secreted into breast milk following maternal ingestion. Usually presents as allergic colitis in an otherwise healthy happy infant.
- In infants, first treat by limiting cow's milk protein intake (and commonly soy protein):
  - In exclusively breast-fed infants, this is achieved by a maternal exclusion diet to these proteins.
  - In formula fed infants feed with a hydrolysed formula (short peptides).
- If symptoms severe, or unresponsive to hydrolysed formula, then an elemental (amino acid) formula may be required.
- Anti-inflammatory medications are very rarely needed.
- Avoid using goat's or sheep's milk as a cow's milk substitute, as 25% will also develop allergy to these milks (cross-reactivity). Similar cross-reactivity also often occurs with soya milk. Use of soya milk is not recommended under age 6mths.
- After weaning, introduce a cow's milk protein free diet (supplement with oral calcium if required).
- Consider a cow's milk protein challenge after 6–12mths (see 📖 p.317).

Nutritional disorders

Malnutrition is a common cause of child mortality and morbidity. There is a wide spectrum of nutritional disorders, varying from protein-energy malnutrition to micronutrient nutritional deficiencies to morbid obesity (see Table 10.1). In non-industrialized nations malnutrition and associated infection are leading causes of child death.

Causes
- Diets low in protein, energy, or specific nutrients.
- Strict fad or vegetarian diets.
- Diseases causing malabsorption (e.g. coeliac disease, cystic fibrosis, Crohn's disease), severe GORD, immunodeficiency, chronic infection.
- Eating disorders, e.g. anorexia nervosa (see 🕮 Chapter 16).

Assessment of nutritional status
Refer to a paediatric dietician and review the following:
- Recent weight loss (≥10% over 3mths is suggestive of impaired nutritional status).
- Accurately plot serial height and weight (falling across 2 centile lines or below 3rd centile may indicate nutritional impairment).
- Percentage weight for height (= [actual weight/expected weight for height centile] × 100; a value of ≤90% may indicate impairment.
- Body mass index (BMI) = weight (kg)/height (m)^2.
- Mid-arm circumference divided by head circumference (malnutrition if <0.31).
- Detailed dietary assessment of 5–7-day food diary.
- Serum albumin.

Protein–energy malnutrition
Kwashiorkor and marasmus usually occur together. Because of oedema, mid-upper arm circumference is a better guide to malnutrition than weight. *Kwashiorkor* is due to severe deficiency of protein/essential amino acids.
- *Clinical features:* growth retardation; diarrhoea; apathy; anorexia;
- oedema; skin/hair depigmentation; abdominal distension with fatty
- liver.
- *Investigations:* hypoalbuniaemia, normo- and microcytic anaemia, ↓ Ca^{2+}, ↓ Mg^{2+}, ↓ PO_4^{3-}, and ↓ glucose.
- *Marasmus:* is due to severe energy (calories) deficiency.
- *Clinical features:* height is relatively preserved compared to weight; wasted appearance; muscle atrophy; listless; diarrhoea; constipation.
- *Investigations:* ↓ Serum albumin, Hb, U&E, Ca^{2+}, Mg^{2+}, PO_4^{3-}, and glucose; stool M,C&S for intestinal ova, cysts, and parasites.

Treatment
- Correct dehydration and electrolyte imbalance (IV if required).
- Treat underlying infection and/or parasitic infections.
- Treat concurrent/causative disease.
- Treat specific nutritional deficiencies.
- Orally refeed slowly- watch out for refeeding syndrome (🕮 p.322).

Table 10.1 Specific nutritional deficiencies

Name	Causes	Presentation	Treatment
Vitamin A	Fat malabsorption states, e.g. cystic fibrosis; deficient indigenous diet.	↑ Morbidity and mortality from infections, follicular hyperkeratosis, xerophthalmia, night blindness. Plasma retinol <0.7mmol/l.	Oral vitamin A supplementation.
Vitamin D	Dietary deficiency; low UV light; fat malabsorption, hepatic or renal failure.	Rickets (limb x-rays: distal bony cupping and fraying), ↓ serum Ca^{2+} and PO_4^{3-}, ↑ alkaline phosphatase, plasma 25-hydroxy cholecalciferol <25nmol/l.	Oral 40–125 micrograms/day vitamin D, Ca^{2+} and PO_4^{3-} supplements.
Vitamin K	Congenital, fat malabsorption states, small bowel bacterial overgrowth.	Bleeding, including haemorrhagic disease of the newborn.	IV 1mg vitamin K_1.
Vitamin B1	Dietary deficiency (particularly when polished rice staple diet).	Beri-beri (muscle weakness, oedema, heart failure), Wernicke's encephalopathy. Red cell thiamine pyrophosphate <150nmol/l.	Oral 5mg vitamin B_1 daily.
Vitamin B12	Vegan diets, distal small bowel disease (e.g. Crohn's disease), pernicious anaemia.	Macrocytic megaloblastic anaemia, peripheral neuropathy, motor weakness. Vitamin B_{12} level <75pmol/l, Schilling test of B_{12} absorption.	IM vitamin B_{12} 1mg every 1–3mths.
Vitamin C	Lack of fresh fruit and vegetables.	Scurvy: petechiae, ecchymosis, bleeding gums, painful sub-periosteal bleeding of legs, motor weakness. Plasma vitamin C level <6–11μmol/l.	Oral vitamin C 25mg QDS for 4 days then BD.
Vitamin E	Prematurity, fat malabsorption.	Haemolytic anaemia. Serum vitamin E level <5mg/l.	Oral 75–100mg vitamin E daily.
Folic acid	Small bowel disease, malignancy, drugs (anticonvulsants, cytotoxics).	Macrocytic megaloblastic anaemia, irritability, failure to thrive, thrombocytopenia. Red cell folate <160ng/ml.	Oral 0.5–1mg folic acid daily.
Iron	Low dietary intake, chronic blood loss (e.g. intestinal parasites or malaria), prematurity.	Common (~10% in UK children). Microcytic hypochromic anaemia, developmental delay, angular stomatitis, koilonychia, serum ferritin <7mg/l, serum iron <5nmol/l, total iron binding capacity >90mmol/l.	Oral 4–6 mg/kg/day iron.
Zinc	Prematurity, dietary insufficiency, intestinal disease or chronic diarrhoea, acrodermatitis enteropathica (inborn error of zinc absorption).	Peri-orificial and anal dermatitis, diarrhoea, alopecia, failure to thrive, neurological dysfunction. Serum zinc <11μmol/l.	Infants oral 1mg/kg/day zinc, children 1–5yrs 5mg/day, >10yrs 10mg/day.
Iodine	Dietary deficiency. Endemic in some regions.	Hypothyroidism and retarded development. Low urine iodine: creatinine ratio.	Oral 100–300 micrograms/day iodine and oral levothyroxine replacement.

Nutritional support

Nutritional support can be either enteral or parenteral. Enteral nutrition, when possible, is preferred as it is cheaper, technically less demanding, more physiological, and associated with fewer complications.

- Involve a paediatric dietitian to assess nutritional status, requirements, and support.
- Beware of 'refeeding syndrome' (potentially fatal respiratory and cardiac failure induced by electrolyte disturbance following overzealous nutritional therapy in severe malnutrition) and be prepared to use PN in severe cases.

Indications

- Severely ill patients, e.g. ill preterm infants.
- Nutritional supplementation is required, e.g. FTT, cystic fibrosis.
- Swallowing difficulty, e.g. severe cerebral palsy.
- Metabolic diseases, e.g. phenylketonuria.
- Gastrointestinal failure, e.g. malabsorption, short bowel syndrome.
- Other primary disease state, e.g. chronic renal failure.

Oral supplementation Includes high energy milks, mineral/vitamin supplementation.

Specialized foods Huge range of specialized milk and feeds exist for many different conditions, (modular elemental diets for IBD, hypoallergenic milk for milk protein allergy).

Enteral tube feeding

- Can be orogastric, NG, nasojejunal, and gastrostomy.
- Liquid feeds are given as boluses or continuously, e.g. overnight.
- *Indications:* swallowing problems (e.g. severe cerebral palsy, prematurity), cardiorespiratory compromise, GORD, anorexia, generalized debilitation, e.g. trauma.
- *Feeds:* standard polymeric diets (e.g. ready to feed nutritionally complete whole protein products); elemental diets and semi-elemental diets requiring little or no digestion; or disease-specific formulations.
- Gastrostomy reduces orofacial complications/discomfort, but complications include: Gastric leakage; localized skin infection or
- inflammation; GI perforation/trauma/haemorrhage.

Trophic feeding

- *Synonyms:* minimal enteral feeding, gut priming.
- *Indications:* during PN in newborn infants, particularly if preterm.
- *Rationale:* prolongation of enteral starvation leads to loss of normal GI structure and function despite PN-induced anabolic body state. Small milk volumes appear to prevent this. Also promotes GI development in newborn infants.
- Typically 0.5–1mL/kg/h milk is fed within 2–3 days of birth.
- *Evidence of beneficial effects (in newborns) includes:* fewer episodes of sepsis; fewer days of PN; improved growth; improved gut function.

Parenteral nutrition

IV parenteral nutrition may be supplemental or provide TPN. Parents can be trained to give prolonged PN at home to children.

Indications

- Post-operative, e.g. abdominal or cardiothoracic.
- Treatment of IBD.
- After severe trauma or burns.
- Acute pancreatitis.
- Oral feeds are contraindicated, e.g. NEC.
- Intestinal failure, e.g. short bowel syndrome, congential enteropathy.
- Protracted vomiting or diarrhoea.
- GI obstruction, e.g. chronic intestinal pseudo-obstruction.
- Very preterm infants.
- Oncology patients, e.g. severe mucositis, graft versus host disease.

Administration

- A multidisciplinary team of clinician, pharmacist, and paediatric dietitian should be involved in supervising PN.
- Follow unit/hospital dietetic/pharmacy guidelines for individual needs.
- Allowance should be made of body weight (you may need to estimate a working weight, e.g. if oedematous or gross ascites), recent weight trends, clinical condition, fluid and nutritional requirements, additional infused fluids.

Method

Once requirements are calculated, sterile pharmacy-prepared solutions are given via central (preferable) or peripheral venous lines. Rapid commencement of PN may risk 'refeeding syndrome' in chronically undernourished patients (see 📖 p.320). When significant malnutrition exists, measure and correct electrolyte abnormalities before commencing PN and introduce slowly.

PN is usually supplied and administered as two components.

- *Lipid component:* contains fat (triglyceride emulsion, e.g. *Intralipid* 20%) and fat soluble vitamins. Usually infused over 20hr.
- *Aqueous component:* contains carbohydrate (glucose solution), protein (crystalline L-amino acid solution), electrolytes, water soluble vitamins, minerals, trace elements (zinc, copper, manganese, selenium, +/– iron). Usually infused over 24hr.

Monitoring

Serious, unexpected biochemical disturbances occur rarely as a result of PN. An appropriate monitoring regimen is suggested in Table 10.2.

Weaning

PN should be weaned slowly so that hypoglycaemia is avoided. This also allows GI mucosal recovery as enteral feeding is increased. When weaning is protracted parenteral nutrition can be administered over shortened periods. A paediatric dietitian should assess the contribution of both enteral and parenteral feeds to ensure nutritional adequacy.

Complications/problems

- *Sepsis*: usually S. epidermidis, S. aureus, Candida, Pseudomonas, E. coli.
- *Demanding*: in expertise, cost, etc.
- *Central-line*: occlusion, breakage, displacement.
- *Electrolyte/metabolic disturbances*: e.g. glucose ↑ or ↓.
- *Vascular*: thrombophlebitis, thromboembolism, extravasation injuries.
- *Cardiac tamponade*: avoid by placing IV line tip proximal to right atrium.
- *From amino acids*: PN-associated liver disease, including, steatosis, cholestasis, or, rarely cirrhosis or portal hypertension.
- *From lipids*: platelet dysfunction, hyperlipidaemia, fatty liver, pulmonary hypertension.
- *Metabolic bone disease*: due to insufficient Ca^{2+} and PO_4^{3-}.

Table 10.2 Guidelines for monitoring stable patients during short-term PN

Measurements	Pre-PN	During		
		1st week	2nd week	3rd and subsequent weeks
Creatinine, urea, Na, K	✓	×2	×2	×2
Calcium	✓	×1	×1	×2
Magnesium	✓	×1	×1	Mthly
Phosphate	✓	×2	×1	×2
ALP, ALT, bilirubin, albumin	✓	×1	×1	×2
Glucose	✓	Daily blood glucose	Urine dipstick daily	Urine dipstick daily
Cu, Zn, Se	—	—	—	Mthly
FBC	—	—	×1	×1
Triglycerides	✓	×1	×1	×1
Weight	✓	Daily	Daily	Daily

Oesophageal disorders

See also 📖 pp.276, 295.

Gastro-oesophageal reflux (GORD)

Gastro-oesophageal reflux occurs when there is inappropriate effortless passage of gastric contents into the oesophagus. GORD exists when reflux is repeated and severe enough to cause harm. Reflux is very common in infancy and is associated with slow gastric emptying, liquid diet (milk), horizontal posture, and low resting lower oesophageal sphincter (LOS) pressure.

Other causes in infancy and in older children include: LOS dysfunction (e.g. hiatus hernia); ↑ gastric pressure (e.g. delayed gastric emptying); external gastric pressure; gastric hypersecretion (e.g. acid); food allergy; and CNS disorders (e.g. cerebral palsy).

Presentation of GORD

- *Gastrointestinal:* regurgitation, non-specific irritability, rumination, oesophagitis (heartburn, difficult feeding with crying, painful swallowing, haematemesis), faltering growth (calorie deficiency due to profuse reflux of ingested calories).
- *Respiratory:* apnoea, hoarseness, cough, stridor, lower respiratory disease (aspiration pneumonia, asthma, BPD).
- *Neurobehavioural symptoms:* e.g. Sandifer's syndrome (bizarre extension and lateral turning of head, dystonic postures).
- *Complications:*
  - oesophageal stricture (dysphagia);
  - barrett's oesophagus (premalignant intestinal metaplasia);
  - faltering growth;
  - anaemia (chronic blood loss);
  - lower respiratory disease.

Management of GORD

- *History:* e.g. effortless regurgitation, relationship to feeds.
- *Examination:* including growth, possible anaemia, respiratory.
- *Investigations* (appropriate when diagnosis is uncertain, there is a poor response to treatment, or complications occur) may include: upper GI endoscopy; oesophageal biopsy; 24hr oesophageal pH probe; barium swallow with fluoroscopy; radioisotope 'milk' scan (aspiration); oesophageal manometry (oesophageal dysmotility); and CXR (associated respiratory disease).

Treatment

Treatment is carried out in a stepwise fashion.

- *Positioning:* nurse infants on head-up slope of 30° ± prone.
- *Dietary:* thickened milk feeds (infants); small frequent meals; avoid food before sleep; avoid fatty foods, citrus juices, caffeine, carbonated drinks, 'alcohol and smoking'.
- *Drugs:* gastric acid reducing drugs, e.g. ranitidine or omeprazole (if oesophagitis); Gaviscon® (contains antacids and an alginate that forms

viscous surface layer to reduce reflux); prokinetic drugs, e.g. domperidone; mucosal protectors, e.g. sucralfate; corticosteroids (allergic oesophagitis).
- *Surgery:* usually Nissen's fundoplication is performed when medical treatment has failed:
  - Indications for surgery are failed intense medical treatment; oesophageal stricture; Barrett's oesophagus; severe oesophagitis; recurrent apnoea; lower respiratory disease; faltering growth (FTT).
  - Complications of surgery include: 'gas bloating' syndrome; dysphagia; profuse retching; 'dumping' syndrome.

Prognosis
Vast majority of infants outgrow symptoms by 1yr. In older children, 50% develop a chronic, relapsing course.

Oesophageal foreign body
See also 📖 pp.856–857. This usually occurs in toddlers or older children with neurological or psychiatric conditions. If the object reaches the stomach 90% will pass spontaneously. Confirm position with AP and lateral CXR. Remove endoscopically if:
- Dysphagia or drooling persists.
- Object is still in the oesophagus for >12hr.
- Object is sharp (risk of perforation).
- Object is hazardous, e.g. mercuric oxide disc batteries.

Upper oesophageal dysfunction
This disorder is usually due to diffuse CNS dysfunction.
- *Presentation:* choking, cough, drooling, dysphagia, nasal regurgitation.
- *Diagnosis:* barium swallow with video-fluoroscopy or oesophageal manometry.
- *Treatment:* treat primary underlying disorder. Rarely, cricopharyngeal myotomy is helpful.

Achalasia
This rare, idiopathic, condition of obstruction is due to failure of lower oesophageal sphincter relaxation.
- *Presentation:* vomiting, dysphagia with solids or liquids; FTT; aspiration.
- *Diagnosis:* barium swallow (dilated tapering lower oesophagus) or oesophageal manometry.
- *Treatment:* nifedipine (short-term); endoscopic balloon dilatation; Heller's cardiomyotomy.

Benign oesophageal stricture
Causes include severe GORD; caustic ingestion; and radiotherapy.

Treatment
Treat the underlying cause, e.g. reduce gastric acid production in GORD; perform balloon endoscopic dilatation.

Pancreatitis

Acute pancreatitis

This rare disorder consists of acute pancreatic inflammation with variable involvement of local tissues and remote organ systems.

Causes
- *Blunt abdominal trauma:* e.g. road traffic accident.
- *Viral infection:* e.g. mumps, hepatitis A, coxsackie B.
- *Multisystem disease:* e.g. SLE, Kawasaki disease, haemolytic–uraemic syndrome, IBD, hyperlipidaemia.
- *Drugs and toxins:* e.g. thiopurines, metronidazole, cytotoxic drugs.
- *Pancreatic duct obstruction:* e.g. cystic fibrosis, choledochal cyst,
- tumours.

Presentation
Abdominal pain involving the upper central abdomen, radiating to back, chest, or lower abdomen, vomiting, fever, abdominal tenderness.
Severe cases also exhibit:
- hypotension;
- abdominal distension;
- Cullen's or grey–Turner's sign (bruising of peri-umbilical area and flanks, respectively);
- ascites;
- pleural effusion;
- jaundice;
- multi-organ failure.

Investigations
- *Blood:* amylase (↑↑); lipase (↑); Ca^{2+} (↓); ESR/CRP (↑); deranged LFT.
- *Radiology:* abdominal US or CT; endoscopic retrograde cholangiopancreatography (ERCP) if structural or obstructive cause.

Treatment
Mild
- Supportive only, e.g. NGT, analgesia.
- Start short period of nil by mouth to 'rest' pancreas.

Severe
Treat as for the mild form, plus:
- Admit to intensive care unit.
- Correct hypotension.
- Treat multi-organ failure.
- Surgery if significant pancreatic necrosis, major ductal rupture (trauma), gallstones (cholecystectomy), presence of pseudocyst.
- Endoscopy (ERCP) may be therapeutic if structural obstructive cause.

Prognosis
- Complete recovery is likely if there is minimal organ dysfunction.
- 20% mortality if there is severe disease or organ failure present, or if local complications develop (e.g. pancreatic pseudocyst).
- Most children have only a single acute episode.

Chronic pancreatitis

This very rare condition follows acute pancreatitis with continuing inflammation, destruction of pancreatic tissue, and fibrosis, leading to permanent exocrine or endocrine pancreatic failure. It is usually caused by cystic fibrosis, congenital ductal anomalies, sclerosing cholangitis (IBD), hyperlipidaemia, or hypercalcaemia.

Presentation
- Repeated episodes of acute pancreatitis are separated by good health.
- Eventually, features of pancreatic exocrine failure or diabetes mellitus become apparent.

Investigations
- Abdominal US or CT scan confirms chronic pancreatitis.
- Pancreatic function tests may be useful, e.g. stool chymotrypsin (↑), pancreozymin-secretin test, 72hr faecal fat measurement (↑).

Treatment
- Treat acute exacerbations as for acute pancreatitis.
- Give pancreatic enzyme replacement and nutritional supplementation (well-balanced diet with moderated fat intake and fat soluble vitamins—involve a paediatric dietician).
- Relieve any ductal obstruction by endoscopy or surgery.

Prognosis
Recovery or risk of developing long-term pancreatic exocrine and/or endocrine failure is dependent on cause and severity.

Intestinal disorders

Gastritis and peptic ulcer disease
This disease is rare in children. It most commonly affects the duodenum.

Causes
- *Helicobactor pylori* infection (strong familial link, associated with increased risk of adult gastric cancer).
- Stress ulcers, e.g. post-trauma, HIE.
- Drug-related, e.g. NSAIDs.
- Increased acid secretion (Zollinger–Ellison syndrome, multiple endocrine neoplasia type I, hyperparathyroidism).
- Crohn's disease.
- Eosinophilic gastroenteritis.
- Hypertrophic gastritis.
- Autoimmune gastritis.

Presentation
- Often asymptomatic.
- Chronic abdominal and epigastric pain.
- Nausea +/– vomiting.
- GI haemorrhage.
- FTT +/– anorexia.
- Iron deficiency anaemia.
- Perforation (very rare).

Investigation
- C^{14} urea breath test (*H. pylori*).
- Upper GI endoscopy and biopsy (*H. pylori* histology and culture).

Treatment
- Treat underlying cause, e.g. eradicate *H. pylori* with 7–10 days oral amoxycillin (clarithromycin), bismuth, metronidazole +/– omeprazole (quadruple therapy).
- ↓ gastric acid production, e.g. proton pump inhibitors (PPI), H_2 antagonists; sucralfate (cytoprotective).
- Antacids, e.g. aluminium hydroxide.

Protein-losing enteropathy
This disorder is characterized by chronic intestinal protein loss.

Causes
- GI infection, e.g. giardiasis.
- Severe food hypersensitivity.
- Coeliac disease or IBD.
- Severe cardiac failure.
- SLE; graft vs. host disease.
- Polyposis or lymphatic obstruction.

Presentation There is hypoalbuminaemia +/– diarrhoea or abdominal pain. Increased faecal α_1-antitrypsin confirms the condition.

Treatment Treat the underlying disease; give nutritonal support and albumin infusions as required.

Short bowel syndrome

Is due to severe intestinal disease or the surgical removal of a large portion of the small intestine. The condition manifests as malabsorption, fluid and electrolyte loss, and malnutrition.

Presentation
- Diarrhoea, steatorrhoea.
- FTT.
- Dehydration, electrolyte loss (Na, K, Mg, Ca).
- Cholestasis (bile salt loss).
- Peptic ulcer disease (due to increased gastrin).
- Specific (e.g. vitamin B_{12}) +/- generalized malnutritional disorders.
- Renal stones (oxalate).

Treatment
- Correct fluid and electrolyte disturbance.
- Specific nutritional supplements; hydrolysed protein/elemental diets.
- PN.
- Gastric acid reducing drugs, e.g. PPI or H_2 antagonists.
- Anti-diarrhoeal drugs, e.g. loperamide.
- Cholestyramine (chelates bile salts).
- Parenteral somatostatin.
- Oral antibiotics to reduce bacterial overgrowth.
- Surgery to reduce GI motility or small bowel transplant.

Prognosis is improving, with 90% 5yr survival. Retention of ileo-caecal valve significantly improves prognosis.

Intestinal polyps

Most juvenile polyps are hamartomas, single, and located in the distal colon. Polyposis (multiple polyps) syndromes include:
- Peutz–Jegher's syndrome (mucocutaneous pigmentation).
- Familial polyposis coli.
- Gardner's syndrome (GI polyps, osteomas and soft tissue tumours).

Presentation
- Often asymptomatic.
- Haematochezia.
- Rectal polyp prolapse.
- Protein-losing enteropathy.
- Intussusception.
- Mucoid diarrhoea.

Investigation Gastroscopy and ileo-colonoscopy, barium radiology.

Treatment
- Endoscopic or surgical removal.
- Periodic colonoscopy surveillance is required in polyposis syndromes because of significant risk of neoplasia.

Inflammatory bowel disease

Includes Crohn's disease (CD) and ulcerative colitis (UC). UK incidence is ~5.2/100,000/yr. CD is twice as common as UC. The cause is unknown, although there is a recognized genetic disposition.

Ulcerative colitis

- Involves colon only.
- Rectal (proctitis) is most common or may extend continuously up to involving the entire colon (pancolitis).
- Terminal ileum may be affected by 'backwash ileitis'.

Crohn's disease

- May affect any part of GI tract, but terminal ileum and proximal colon are commonest sites of involvement.
- Unlike UC, bowel involvement is non-continuous ('skip' lesions).

Presentation

Symptoms

- Anorexia, weight loss, lethargy.
- Abdominal cramps.
- Diarrhoea +/− blood/mucus, urgency and tenesmus (proctitis).
- Fever.

GI signs

- Aphthous oral ulcers.
- Abdominal tenderness.
- Abdominal distension (UC > CD), right iliac fossa (RIF) mass (CD).
- Peri-anal disease (CD), i.e. abscess, sinus, fistula, skin tags, fissure, stricture.

Non-GI signs and associations

- Fever.
- Finger clubbing.
- Anaemia.
- *Skin:* erythema nodosum; pyoderma gangrenosum.
- *Joints:* arthritis; ankylosing spondylitis.
- *Eyes:* iritis; conjunctivitis; episcleritis.
- Poor growth.
- Delayed puberty.
- Sclerosing cholangitis.
- Renal stones.
- Nutritional deficiencies, e.g. vitamin B_{12}.

Complications

- 'Toxic' colon dilatation (UC > CD).
- GI perforation or strictures.
- Pseudopolyps (apparent "polyps" resulting from inflammation).
- Massive GI haemorrhage.
- Colon carcinoma (UC: 50% risk after 10–20yrs disease).
- Fistula involving bowel only or bowel and skin, vagina, or bladder (CD).
- Abscesses (CD).

Investigations

- *Blood:* FBC; ESR/CRP (↑); U&E; LFT; albumin (↓); blood culture; serum iron (↓); vitamin B_{12} and folate (↓).
- *Serum serological markers:* ASCA (anti-*Saccharomyces cerevisiae* antibodies, better for CD); p-ANCA (perinuclear antineutrophil cytoplasmic antibody, better for UC).
- *Stool M,C&S:* (infectious colitis can mimic CD/UC).
- *Endoscopy:* colonoscopy to determine extent and pattern of abnormal mucosa and intestinal biopsy (UC histology: crypt abscesses, mucosal inflammation only, goblet cell depletion; CD: crypt abscesses granulomas, transmural inflammation); upper GI endoscopy (CD).
- *Radiology:* barium radiology/ultrasound (CD: mucosal 'cobblestone' appearance, ulceration, dilatation, narrowed segments, fistula, 'skip' lesions; UC: mucosal ulceration, haustration loss, colonic narrowing +/– shortening).

Treatment

Supportive treatment If severe, e.g. bowel rest, IV hydration, PN.

Drug treatment

- *Mild to moderate disease:* oral 5-aminosalicylic acid (ASA) dimers, e.g. mesalazine, may be useful to induce and maintain colonic disease remission in UC. ASA or corticosteroid enemas are effective for treating rectal disease. Dietary treatment may be useful to induce remission (see Dietary treatment).
- *Moderate to severe disease:* induce remission with oral prednisolone or IV methylprednisolone, 1–2mg/kg/day until condition improved (<2wks) then wean over 6–8wks.
- *Antibiotics:* e.g. ciprofloxacin or metronidazole, may also be useful.
- *Maintenance treatment, or to treat resistant active disease:* immunomodifiers, e.g. azathioprine, ciclosporin, tacrolimus, methotrexate, or infliximab (anti-TNF antibody).

Dietary treatment

Polymeric/elemental diets are useful to induce remission (CD>UC), but the relapse rate is high. Dietary supplementation often required to minimize poor growth and correct specific nutritional deficiencies, e.g. vitamin and mineral supplements. Involve a paediatric dietitian.

Surgery

- *UC:* total colectomy and ileostomy, and later pouch creation and anal anastomosis, cures UC. There is 10–20% complication rate, e.g. pouchitis.
- *CD:* local surgical resection for severe localized disease, e.g. strictures, fistula, may be indicated, but there is a high re-operation rate as inflammation recurrence is universal.

Prognosis

UC and CD are marked by relapse and remission. Patients can have very good quality of life with current therapy. Poor prognostic factors include extensive disease, frequent remissions, and young age at diagnosis.

Malabsorption

Defined as subnormal intestinal absorption of dietary constituents with excessive faecal nutrient loss. The prognosis depends on the cause. Reduced adult height, teeth enamel defects, and osteoporosis may result from long-term malabsorption. Causes are listed in Box 10.5.

Presentation

- Diarrhoea.
- Steatorrhoea.
- Flatulence.
- FTT/weight loss.
- Muscle wasting.
- Abdominal distension.
- Peri-anal excoriation.
- Delayed puberty.
- Features of underlying illness, e.g. abdominal pain in Crohn's disease.
- Signs of nutritional deficiency states, e.g. ascites due to hypoalbuminaemia.

Investigations

Initial screening tests should include: FBC; U&E; creatinine; albumin; total protein; Ca^{2+}; PO_4^{3-}; LFT; iron status, coeliac antibody screen; coagulation screen, stool M,C&S.

   If diagnosis still unclear, consider:

- Upper GI endoscopy with biopsy to look for an enteropathy, ileo-colonoscopy if features suggest colitis (ensure clotting screen normal before procedure).
- Sweat test.
- Immune function tests.
- Faecal fat measurement.
- Faecal elastase.
- Faecal α_1-antitrypsin.
- Exocrine pancreatic function tests.

Treatment

- Treat underlying disease, e.g. metronidazole for giardiasis, gluten-free diet for coeliac disease.
- Supplemental digestive enzymes, e.g. pancreatic enzymes in cystic fibrosis.
- Nutritional supplements to correct deficiencies.
- PN if malabsorption severe or slow to recover.

Box 10.5 Causes of malabsorption

Intraluminal digestive defect
- Carbohydrate intolerance (most commonly lactose intolerance)
- Protein–energy malnutrition
- Cystic fibrosis
- Shwachman–Diamond syndrome (📖 p.627)
- Chronic pancreatitis
- Cholestasis
- Pernicious anaemia
- Specific digestive enzyme deficiency, e.g. lipase

Mucosal abnormality
- Coeliac disease
- Short bowel syndrome
- Dietary protein intolerance, e.g. milk protein allergy
- Intestinal infection or parasites, e.g. giardiasis
- IBD
- Abetalipoproteinaemia (disorder of lipid metabolism—FTT, steatorrhoea, progressive ataxia, retinitis pigmentosa, acanthocytes on FBC)
- Protein–energy malnutrition; intestinal venous or lymphatic obstruction, e.g. congestive cardiac failure, intestinal lymphangiectasia

Miscellaneous
- Immunodeficiency syndromes, e.g. HIV
- Drug reaction, e.g. cytotoxics, post-radiation
- Bacterial overgrowth, e.g. pseudo-obstruction

Coeliac disease

Coeliac disease is an enteropathy due to lifelong intolerance to gluten protein (present in wheat, barley, rye, and oats by cross contamination).

Prevalence is approximately 1% when populations are screened. It is associated with:
- A positive family history.
- Type 1 diabetes.
- Down syndrome.
- IgA deficiency.

Presentation

The condition may present at any age after starting solids containing gluten.

The 'classic' initial features include:
- Pallor.
- Diarrhoea.
- Pale, bulky floating stools.
- Anorexia.
- FTT.
- Irritability.

Later, there is:
- Apathy.
- Gross motor developmental delay.
- Ascites.
- Peripheral oedema.
- Anaemia.
- Delayed puberty.
- Arthralgia.
- Hypotonia, muscle wasting.
- Specific nutritional disorders.

Increased recognition, and the widespread practice of antibody screening of children at high risk, has changed considerably the clinical spectrum of cases seen, with less classical and severe symptoms now more common at time of initial diagnosis.

There are three settings in which the diagnosis of coeliac disease should be considered and screened for:
- Children with frank gut symptoms.
- Children with the non-gastrointestinal manifestations described here.
- Asymptomatic individuals with conditions that are associated with coeliac disease.

Coeliac crisis

Life-threatening dehydration due to diarrhoea accompanying malabsorption. This condition is now very rare except in the less-developed world.

Investigations

- Measurement of serum tissue transglutaminase IgA antibody (TTG) is recommended for initial testing for coeliac disease. IgA sensitivity and specificity approach 100%, although false positives are occasionally seen. Anti-endomysium IgA antibody is observer-dependent and expensive. Anti-gliadin antibody tests are less accurate and are now not advised. It is important to exclude IgA deficiency as a cause of falsely negative serology.
- Endoscopic small bowel biopsy of the third part of the duodenum shows diffuse, subtotal villus atrophy, increased intraepithelial lymphocytes, and crypt hyperplasia. The villi return to normal on a gluten-free diet.

Most clinicians consider positive mucosal histology and full clinical recovery on gluten-free diet +/– positive IgA antibodies sufficient to make a diagnosis. Antibody levels should return to normal on treatment and negative serology is a marker of compliance. Avoid gluten challenge (>10g oral gluten per day for 3–4mths and re-biopsy) unless diagnosis is in doubt, e.g. initial biopsy is inadequate or not typical, or alternative diagnosis is possible, e.g. transient gluten intolerance may occur after gastroenteritis, giardiasis, or cow's milk protein intolerance.

Treatment

- Gluten-free diet under the supervision of a paediatric dietitian.
- Gluten-free foods are prescribable in UK.
- Gluten avoidance should be life-long if coeliac disease is confirmed.
- Nutritional supplements may be required.

Prognosis

Excellent if patient is compliant with strict, life-long gluten-free diet. There is a possible increased risk of intestinal lymphoma if gluten is ingested, even in asymptomatic coeliac disease.

Gastrointestinal infections

GI infections are the second commonest cause of primary care consultation after the common cold. These infections also cause over 3 million children deaths per year (mostly in developing world) (see also 📖 pp.1022–1023).

Viral gastroenteritis

Transmission is by the faecal–oral route, including contaminated water. Epidemics are frequent and usually occur during winter. Breastfeeding is protective. Severity is increased in malnourished children.

Causes
- Rotavirus (most common).
- Small round structural virus, e.g. winter vomiting disease caused by 'Norwalk agent'.
- Enteric adenovirus.
- Astrovirus.
- CMV (in immune-comprised patients).

Presentation
- Watery diarrhoea (rarely bloody).
- Vomiting.
- Cramping abdominal pain.
- Fever.
- Dehydration.
- Electrolyte disturbance.
- Upper respiratory tract signs common with rotavirus.
- Vomiting predominates with Norwalk virus.

Investigation Is rarely necessary (see 📖 p.302). Stool electron microscopy or immunoassay can sometimes be useful.

Treatment
Give supportive rehydration orally or with a nasogastric tube, or IV glucose and electrolyte solution. Hospitalization is rarely needed (e.g. ≥10% dehydration, or unable to tolerate oral fluids).

Prognosis
Symptoms generally last <7 days, except in enteric adenovirus, when diarrhoea frequently goes on beyond 14 days. The child may develop temporary secondary lactose intolerance.

Prevention Rotavirus immunization is now available and effective.

Bacterial gastroenteritis

Causes secretory and inflammatory diarrhoea. It is most common under 2yrs of age. Commonest causative organisms include:
* *Salmonella* spp.;
* *Campylobacter jejuni*;
* *Shigella* spp.;
* *Yersinia enterocolitica*;
* *Escherichia coli*;
* *Clostridium difficile*;
* *Bacillus cereus*;
* *Vibrio cholerae*.

Sources of infection include contaminated water, poor food hygiene (meat, fresh produce, chicken, eggs, previously cooked rice), faecal–oral route.

Presentation
As for viral gastroenteritis plus:
* malaise;
* dysentery (bloody and mucous diarrhoea);
* abdominal pain may mimic appendicitis or IBD;
* tenesmus.

Complications
* Bacteraemia.
* Secondary infections (particularly *Salmonella*, *Campylobacter*), e.g. pneumonia, osteomyelitis, meningitis.
* Reiter's syndrome (*Shigella*, *Campylobacter*).
* Haemolytic–uraemic syndrome (*E. coli* 0157, *Shigella*).
* Guillain–Barré syndrome (*Campylobacter*).
* Reactive arthropathy (*Yersinia*).
* Haemorrhagic colitis.

Investigation
* Stool +/– blood culture (some organisms need specific culture medium).
* Stool *Clostridium difficile* toxin.
* Sigmoidoscopy if inflammatory bowel disease or colitis.

Treatment
* Rehydration as for viral gastroenteritis.
* Antibiotics are not indicated, as the duration of symptoms is not altered and may increase chronic carrier status, unless there is high risk of disseminated disease, presence of artificial implants (e.g. V-P shunt), severe colitis, severe systemic illness, age <6mths, enteric fever, cholera or *E. coli* 0157. Most organisms are sensitive to ampicillin, co-trimoxazole, or third generation cephalosporins.
* *Consider:*
    * erythromycin if *Campylobacter*;
    * oral vancomycin or metronidazole if *Clostridium difficile* (causes pseudomembranous colitis).

Intestinal parasites

Infection is usually via the faecal–oral route. Pets and livestock can be hosts. Parasitic infection can mimic IBD (📖 p.332), hepatitis (📖 p.342), sclerosing cholangitis, peptic ulcer disease, and coeliac disease (📖 p.336).

Presentation
- Abdominal pain.
- Diarrhoea; dysentery; flatulence.
- Malabsorption and FTT.
- Abdominal distension.
- Intestinal obstruction.
- Biliary obstruction; liver disease.
- Pancreatitis.
- Fever.

Investigations
- Stool M,C&S for ova, cysts, parasites, and leukocytes.
- Specific stool staining for cryptosporidiosis.
- Stool ELISA for giardiasis and cryptosporidiosis.
- Blood specific serology, e.g. *Entamoeba histolytica*.
- Duodenal fluid aspiration for M,C&S.
- Duodenal villus biopsy, e.g. giardiasis.

Protozoa

Giardia lamblia
- Very common.
- Swallowed cysts develop into trophozoites that attach to the small intestinal villi, causing mucosal damage.

Presentation
- Diarrhoea, flatulence, abdominal discomfort.
- Sometimes FTT.

Treatment Metronidazole.

Entamoeba histolytica
Symptoms are usually mild, but may cause:
- Fulminating colitis (amoebic dystentery can mimic ulcerative colitis).
- Intestinal obstruction due to chronic localized lesion (an 'amoeboma').
- Amoebic hepatitis.
- Liver abscess (right upper quadrant pain, fever, hepatomegaly).

Treatment Metronidazole.

Cryptosporidium
This organism causes a mild self-limiting illness except in immune-compromised patients, where it can cause:
- Severe chronic watery diarrhoea, flatulence.
- Malaise.
- Abdominal pain.
- Weight loss.

Treatment Erythromycin, metronidazole, or spiramycin.

Nematodes
Ascaris lumbricoides
The most common parasitic worm infection in humans, with up to 25% of the world's population infected (rare in industrialized countries). They look like earthworms and can cause Loeffler's syndrome (an eosinophilic pneumonia, that can mimic asthma, also caused by the parasites *Strongyloides stercoralis,* and the hookworms *Ancylostoma duodenale* and *Necator americanus.* Heavy infestation can cause specific nutritional deficiencies or bowel obstruction. Infection occurs by faecal-oral transmission of eggs.

Treatment Mebendazole, albendazole, pyrantel pamoate.

Trichuris trichiura (whip worm) Lives in the colon and causes diarrhoea, abdominal pain, and weight loss.

Treatment Mebendazole or albendazole.

Hookworms (Necator americanus, Ancylostoma duodenale)
Infection is by larvae penetrating the skin, e.g. bare feet. The adult worms live in the intestine voraciously sucking blood leading to anaemia and hypoproteinaemia.

Treatment Mebendazole.

Strongyloides stercoralis
• Penetrates the skin and migrates to the lungs. Then coughed up and ingested into the gut.
• Causes bloating, heartburn, and malabsorption.

Treatment Mebendazole, albendazole, or thiabendazole.

Enterobius vermicularis (thread or pinworm)
• Very common and causes anal pruritis as females emerge and lay eggs in peri-anal region.
• *Infection:* occurs by faecal-oral transmission of eggs.
• *Diagnosis:* is confirmed by direct visualization of worms on peri-anal area or in stool, or microscopy of sellotape previously applied to the anus.

Treatment Mebendazole.

Cestodes (tapeworms)
• *Infection:* results from ingesting undercooked contaminated pork (*Taenia solium*), beef (*Taenia saginata*), or fish (*Diphyllobothrium latum*).
• *Diagnosis:* is by microscopy of eggs or proglottides in stool.

Treatment Praziquantel.

Acute hepatitis

Viral causes

Hepatitis A (HAV) incubation 2–6wks, faecal–oral transmission.

Hepatitis B (HBV) incubation 6wks to 6mths. Endemic in the Far East and Africa. Infection may be transmitted from:
- Blood products.
- IV drug abuse, contaminated needles, or syringes.
- Sexual intercourse.
- Close direct contact (e.g. intrafamilial, health workers).
- Vertical (may cause fulminant hepatitis).

Hepatitis C (HCV) incubation 2wks to 6mths. Transmission is as for HBV. Usually causes a mild severity acute illness or is asymptomatic. HCV rarely causes acute hepatitis.

Hepatitis E faecal–oral transmission, endemic in India.

Hepatitis D requires previous HBV infection.

Hepatitis G parenteral transmission.

Other organisms can cause hepatitis as part of systemic infection: Epstein–Barr virus (EBV, common in adolescents, only 40% have hepatitis); TORCH organisms (neonatal hepatitis); HIV; CMV (immune-compromised); *Listeria*.

Other causes
- *Poisons and drugs:* e.g. paracetamol, isoniazid, halothane.
- *Metabolic disease:* e.g. Wilson's disease, tyrosinaemia type I.
- *Autoimmune hepatitis:* May present with acute hepatitis.
- *Reye's syndrome:* a rare, acute encephalopathic illness associated with aspirin therapy and microvesicular fatty infiltration of the liver.
  - *Prodrome:* (nausea, vomiting, hypoglycaemia, abdominal pain) occurs 2–3 days before onset of jaundice or abnormal LFT (see also 📖 pp.343, 960, 970).

Presentation
Acute fulminant hepatic failure (encephalopathy and coagulopathy) may rarely occur. Many infections are asymptomatic, particularly HAV and HCV. There are many presentations which include:
- fever;
- fatigue;
- malaise;
- anorexia;
- nausea;
- arthralgia;
- right upper quadrant abdominal pain;
- jaundice +/– hepatomegaly;
- splenomegaly;
- adenopathy;
- urticaria.

Investigations
- LFT: ↑ bilirubin >20mg/L; ↑ AST/ALT (× 2–100).
- ↓ Blood glucose (especially in Reye's syndrome).
- Viral serology (IgM antibodies), viral PCR (HCV), EBV heterophil antibodies (Monospot or Paul–Bunnell). Blood culture if appropriate.
- Paracetamol level or halothane antibodies, if relevant.
- Serum immunoglobulin, complement (C3, C4), positive autoimmune antibodies (anti-smooth muscle, anti-mitochondrial, and/or anti-liver and kidney microsomal) in autoimmune hepatitis.
- Serum copper/caeruloplasmin, 24hr urinary copper (Wilson's disease).
- Urinary succinylacetone (tyrosinaemia type I).

Management
Usually none is required, except support and rest.
- Alcohol avoidance in teenagers.
- There is no place for antivirals unless the child is immune-compromised.
- Fulminant hepatitis requires referral to a specialist unit for intensive care management and possible liver transplantation.
- *Reye's syndrome:* maintain blood glucose >4mmol/L; prevent sepsis; provide intensive care support.

Prognosis
- Acute hepatitis is usually self-limiting.
- Mortality after fulminant hepatitis is ~30% if both cerebral oedema and renal failure are absent, ~70% if both are present without liver transplant.
- There is a long-term risk of:
  - chronic hepatitis (HAV 0%; HBV 5–10%; HCV ~85%);
  - cirrhosis;
  - hepatocellular carcinoma (HBV and HCV);
  - glomerulonephritis (circulating immune-complexes).

Prevention
Active immunization exists for both HAV and HBV. Within 24hr after an infectious contact, infection may be prevented by giving pooled serum immunoglobulin for HAV and CMV, or specific HBV serum immunoglobulin for HBV.

Chronic liver failure

Causes
- Chronic hepatitis (after viral hepatitis B or C).
- Biliary tree disease, e.g. biliary atresia.
- Toxin-induced, e.g. paracetamol, alcohol.
- α_1-antitrypsin deficiency.
- Autoimmune hepatitis.
- Wilson's disease (age >3yrs).
- Cystic fibrosis.
- Alagille syndrome or non-syndromic paucity of bile ducts.
- Tyrosinaemia.
- Primary sclerosing cholangitis.
- PN-induced.
- Budd–Chiari syndrome.

Presentation
- Jaundice (not always).
- GI haemorrhage (portal hypertension and variceal bleeding).
- Pruritis.
- FTT.
- Anaemia.
- Enlarged hard liver (though liver often small in cirrhosis).
- Non-tender splenomegaly.
- Hepatic stigmata, e.g. spider naevi.
- Peripheral oedema and/or ascites.
- Nutritional disorders, e.g. rickets.
- Developmental delay or deterioration in school performance.
- Chronic encephalopathy.

Investigations
Blood tests
- LFT ($\uparrow$ or $\leftrightarrow$ bilirubin, $\uparrow$ AST/ALT ($\times$ 2–10), albumin <35g/L).
- FBC ($\downarrow$ Hb if GI bleeding); $\downarrow$ WCC and platelets (hypersplenism).
- Coagulation (prothrombin time $\uparrow$ if vitamin K deficiency).
- $\downarrow$ or $\leftrightarrow$ blood glucose.
- U&E ($\downarrow$ Na$^+$, $\downarrow$ Ca2$^+$, $\uparrow$ PO$_4^{3-}$, $\uparrow$ alkaline phosphatase if biochemical rickets).
- Viral serology or PCR for hepatitis B and C.
- $\uparrow$ IgG, $\downarrow$ complement (C3, C4), autoimmune antibodies (see 📖 p.343).

Metabolic studies
- Sweat test (cystic fibrosis); α_1-antitrypsin level and phenotype.
- $\downarrow$ Serum copper and caeruloplasmin (Wilson's disease).
- $\uparrow$ 24hr urinary copper (Wilson's disease).

Abdominal US
- Hepatomegaly.
- Echogenic liver.
- Splenomegaly.
- Ascites.

Upper GI endoscopy
- Oesophageal or gastric varices.
- Portal hypertension related gastritis.

EEG To confirm chronic encephalopathy if suspected.

Liver biopsy Histology; enzymes; electron microscopy.

Management
- Treat the underlying cause and give nutritional support.
- Lower protein, increased energy, higher carbohydrate diet.
- Vitamin supplementation, particularly fat soluble vitamins A, D, E, K. Involve a paediatric dietitian.

Drug therapy
- Prednisolone +/– azathioprine for autoimmune hepatitis.
- Interferon-α +/– ribavirin for chronic viral hepatitis.
- Penicillamine for Wilson's disease.
- Colestyramine may be useful to control severe pruritis.
- Vitamin K_1 and FFP (10mL/kg) if significant coagulopathy or bleeding.

Oesophageal varices Endoscopy, i.e. sclerotherapy or surgery.

Ascites
- Fluid and Na^+ restriction (2/3 maintenance and 1mmol/kg/day, respectively).
- Spironolactone (1–2mg/kg 12-hourly).
- Consider IV 20% albumin if ascites is resistant to above treatment.

Encephalopathy Reduce GI ammonia absorption using oral or rectal lactulose, neomycin, or soluble fibre pectin.

Liver transplantation See 📖 p.347.

Prognosis
There is up to 50% 5yr mortality without liver transplant. Poor prognostic factors are:
- bilirubin >50μmol/L;
- albumin <30g/L;
- PT >6s;
- ascites;
- encephalopathy;
- malnutrition.

Alpha$_1$-antitrypsin deficiency

Alpha$_1$-antitrypsin is a serum protease inhibitor responsible for controlling inflammatory cascades.

- It is the commonest genetic cause of liver disease in children, with autosomal dominant inheritance. Prevalence is 1:2000 to 1:7000.
- Genetic variants are identified by enzyme electrophoretic mobility as medium (M), slow (S), or very slow (Z). S is associated with ~60% Alpha$_1$-antitrypsin level of normal; Z ~15%. Normal genotype is designated PiMM. Only PiZZ individuals are at risk of liver disease.

Presentation

- Cholestasis in infancy, may progress to liver failure.
- Cirrhosis can occur in late childhood to adult. Chronic liver disease affects 25% of patients in late adulthood.
- Pulmonary emphysema is the commonest presentation in adulthood.

Diagnosis

- Serum α_1-antitrypsin level ↓.
- Phenotyping by enzyme isoelectric focusing (see Alpha$_1$-antitrypsin deficiency).

Treatment

- Supportive treatment of liver complications.
- Strongly advise against smoking.
- Liver transplant for end-stage liver failure.

Wilson's disease

A rare autosomal recessive disorder leading to toxic accumulation of copper in the liver and, subsequently, other tissues especially the brain and eye. See also ☐ p.976.

Presentation

- Kayser–Fleischer rings (copper deposition in Descemet's membrane of the eye) often present (45% with hepatic presentation and 90% with neurological) and are pathognomonic. May require slit-lamp examination to visualize.
- Hepatic problems usually present in childhood (hepatitis, cirrhosis, fulminant hepatic failure).
- Adolescents/young adults usually present with neurological disease.

Investigations

- Serum copper and caeruloplasmin ↓.
- 24hr urinary copper excretion >100microgram (normal <40microgram).
- Molecular genetic testing—Wilson's disease gene (*ATP7B*) mutation.

Treatment

- Lifelong chelation therapy with penicillamine (reverses pre-cirrhotic liver disease, but not neurological damage).
- Liver transplantation if end-stage hepatic failure.

Liver transplantation

Indications for liver transplantation
The commonest underlying conditions leading to irreversible liver failure and transplant are:
- *Fulminant hepatic failure:* e.g. viral, toxic, Wilson's disease.
- Biliary atresia.
- *Chronic end-stage liver disease:* e.g. post-viral hepatitis with cirrhosis.
- *Liver based metabolic conditions:* e.g. Wilson's disease, α_1-antitrypsin deficiency, Crigler–Najjar syndrome, tyrosinaemia.
- *Acute liver failure following a liver transplant:* e.g. primary non-function of transplant or hepatic artery thrombosis.
- Neonatal hepatitis.
- Autoimmune hepatitis.
- *Unresectable tumour confined to the liver:* e.g. hepatoblastoma.

Clinical features requiring consideration for transplantation
- Bleeding varices due to portal hypertension.
- Failure of growth or development.
- Resistant ascites.
- Hepatic encephalopathy.
- *Poor quality of life:* e.g. pruritis, lethargy.
- Coagulopathy (PTT >2 × normal).
- *Multi-organ failure:* e.g. hepatorenal syndrome, hepatopulmonary syndrome.

Preparation for transplant
Requires multidisciplinary evaluation to include the following:
- Nutritional support.
- Development and psychological assessment of child and family.
- Education and counseling.
- Ensure vaccinations are current: e.g. MMR, varicella, hepatitis A and B.
- Cardiac evaluation (ECG, echocardiogram).
- Abdominal US (patency of major hepatic blood vessels).

Post-transplant complications
- Primary non-function of the liver (<5%).
- Hepatic artery thrombosis (10–15%).
- Biliary leaks and strictures (20%).
- Acute rejection (50%).
- Chronic rejection (5–10%).
- Sepsis (main cause of death).

Prognosis
Long-term studies indicate normal psychosocial development and quality of life in survivors. Patients require lifelong immunosuppression drug therapy, e.g. ciclosporin or tacrolimus.
- 1yr survival is 90%.
- 5yr survival is 80%.

Nephrology

Polyuria and frequency

This is often subjective and difficult to assess, particularly in small children. Frequency can be considered to be the inappropriate and frequent passage of small amounts of urine. Polyuria can be quantitatively defined as the passage of greater than 2000mL/1.73m^2 per 24hr period.

Assessment of polyuria and frequency requires a detailed history of urinary frequency habit.

Causes of polyuria

- *Renal disorders:*
  - chronic kidney disease (see 🕮 p.366);
  - post-obstructive uropathy;
  - nephrogenic diabetes insipidus (see 🕮 p.450);
  - Fanconi syndrome (see 🕮 pp.372, 384).
- *Metabolic/endocrine disorders:*
  - diabetes mellitus;
  - cranial diabetes inspidus (see 🕮 p.450);
  - hypoadrenalism.
- Excess and inappropriate water intake: psychogenic polydipsia (see 🕮 p.450).

Causes of urinary frequency

- Urinary tract infection (see 🕮 p.356).
- Bladder irritability and instability.
- All causes of polyuria.
- Small bladder capacity.

Investigations

Baseline screening investigations should include the following.

Urine
- Urinalysis by urine dipstick testing.
- Urine culture.
- Urine osmolality.

Blood
- Urea and electrolytes.
- Plasma osmolality.
- Blood glucose (random or fasting).

Abdominal/renal mass

A rare presentation of urinary tract problems, which needs to be differentiated from other causes of abdominal mass and swelling.

Causes

Intrarenal
- Wilms' tumour (young child with rapidly growing mass). See 📖 p.668.
- Renal venous thrombosis (newborn with haematuria).
- Benign nephroma (rare neonatal problem).
- Horseshoe kidney.
- Pyelonephritis (renal abscess).

Other renal
Hydronephrosis associated with the following.
- Pelviureteric junction (PUJ) obstruction.
- Vescioureteric junction (VUJ) obstruction.
- Large bladder and bladder outlet obstruction: e.g.
  - posterior urethral valves (PUV);
  - prune belly syndrome;
  - neurogenic bladder.
- *Urinoma:* i.e. an encapsulated extrapelvicalyceal collection of urine that forms from urine leakage through a tear in the collecting system or the proximal ureter.
- Single cyst (benign renal cyst).
- Multicystic dysplastic kidney—usually newborn.
- *Polycystic disease:*
  - autosomal recessive;
  - autosomal dominant—rare in children.
- Haematoma (trauma).

Extrarenal
Adrenal mass (e.g. neuroblastoma). See 📖 p.666.

Investigation
- US will distinguish between most of the above.
- Further investigation, depending on likely causes and discussion with radiology and urology colleagues, e.g. CT, MRI.

Haematuria

Blood in the urine (haematuria) may be visible to the naked eye or it may be microscopic and detected only by dipstick testing or by microscopy. The presence on microscopy of 10 or more RBCs per high-power field is abnormal. Urinary dipsticks are very sensitive and can be positive at <5 RBCs per high-power field. Asymptomatic haematuria is found in about 0.5–2% of children.

Presentation
- Episode of macroscopic haematuria (causes alarm to child/family).
- Incidental finding of microscopic haematuria.
- Family screening and routine urinalysis.

Other causes of 'red urine'
The following can usually be distinguished from haematuria by taking a careful history, and with urine dipstick testing and microscopy:
- Haemoglobinuria/myoglobinuria.
- Foods—colouring (e.g. beetroot).
- Drugs (e.g. rifampicin).
- Urate crystals (in young infants, usually 'pink' nappies).
- External source (e.g. menstrual blood losses).
- Fictitious—consider if no cause found.

Causes of haematuria
- *Urinary tract infections:*
  - bacterial;
  - viral (e.g. adenovirus in outbreaks);
  - schistosomiasis (history of foreign travel);
  - tuberculosis.
- *Glomerular:*
  - post-infectious glomerulonephritis;
  - Henoch–Schönlein purpura IgA nephropathy, SLE;
  - hereditary—thin basement membrane, Alport's syndrome.
- *Urinary tract stones:* e.g. due to hypercalciuria.
- Trauma.
- Other renal tract pathology:
  - renal tract tumour;
  - polycystic kidney disease.
- *Vascular:*
  - renal vein thrombosis;
  - arteritis.
- *Haematological:* coagulopathy/sickle cell disease.
- *Drugs:* cyclophosphamide.
- Exercise-induced.

History
- *UTI:* fever/frequency/dysuria.
- *Renal stones:* colicky abdominal pain.

- *Glomerular:* sore throat/rashes.
- *Coagulopathy:* easy bruising.
- *Trauma.*
- *Family history:* haematuria, deafness (Alport's), sickle cell disease.

Examination
- BP.
- *Abdomen:* palpable masses.
- *Skin:* rashes.
- *Joints:* pain/swelling.

Investigations
It is important to identify serious, treatable, and progressive conditions. During an acute illness, exclude UTI by urine culture. Asymptomatic or 'benign haematuria' in children without growth failure, hypertension, oedema, proteinuria, urinary casts, or renal impairment is a frequent finding. Many such children require no immediate investigation but need to be checked in the outpatient clinic to see if the problem persists.
- *Urine:*
  - microscopy (look for casts—suggestive of nephritis) and culture;
  - protein:creatinine ratio (normal, <20mg/mmol);
  - calcium:creatinine ratio (normal, <0.7mmol/mmol).
- *Bloods:*
  - U&E/creatinine/albumin;
  - FBC/clotting;
  - *complement*—C3/C4, ASOT titres;
  - ANA/anti-dsDNA.
- US urinary tract.
- Urinalysis of parents (hereditary causes).
- *Cystoscopy:* rarely indicated in children.

Treatment
- If obvious cause (e.g. UTI), treat.
- If complex diagnosis (impaired renal function, proteinuria, or family
- history) refer to paediatric nephrology unit.
- If no cause found and normal renal function, BP, and no proteinuria,
- monitor until resolves.
- If no resolution after 6mths or change in any of above parameters
- refer to paediatric nephrology unit.

Proteinuria

This is defined as excessive urinary protein excretion. Protein may be found in the urine of healthy children, and does not exceed 0.15g/24hr.

Detection of proteinuria

Urinalysis

Performed by dipstick testing (Table 11.1), this is a cheap, practicable, sensitive method that primarily detects albumin in the urine. It is less sensitive for other forms of proteinuria.

Table 11.1 Urinalysis by dipstick testing

Test result	Equivalent protein estimate (g/L)
+	0.2
++	1.0
+++	3.0
++++	≥ 20

Urinary protein:creatinine ratio (UP:UCr)

Collection of an early morning urine (EMU) specimen for measurement of the urinary protein to creatinine ratio. Normal <20mg/mmol

24hr urinary protein excretion

This is the gold standard test and requires a 24hr collection of urine to estimate urinary protein excretion.
- Normal: <30mg/24hr.
- Microalbuminuria: 30–300mg/24hr.
- Proteinuria: >300mg/24hr.

Causes

Proteinuria may be due to benign or pathological causes.

Non-pathological proteinuria
- Transient.
- Fever.
- Exercise.
- Urinary tract infection (UTI).
- Orthostatic proteinuria (postural proteinuria). This is a common cause of referral in older children. There is usually no history of significance and a normal examination. Investigations reveal a normal UP:UCr ratio in early morning urine with elevated level in afternoon specimen (may require two 12hr collections). This is regarded as a benign finding and requires no treatment.

Pathological (persistent) proteinuria

This may be seen in a number of renal disorders including:
- Nephrotic syndrome (see 📖 p.378);
- Glomerulonephritis (see 📖 p.374);
- Chronic kidney disease (see 📖 p.366);
- Tubular interstitial nephritis.

Investigations

Proteinuria detected on dipstick testing should be confirmed using EMU UP:Ucr ratio. If the proteinuria is combined with haematuria, investigations should be directed at causes of haematuria and nephritis.
- A renal US scan should also be performed.
- Patients with persistent proteinuria detected over a period of 6–12mths should be referred to a paediatric nephrology centre for consideration for biopsy.

Urinary tract infection

Up to 3% of girls and 1% of boys suffer from UTI during childhood. A UTI may be defined in terms of the presence of symptoms (dysuria, frequency, loin pain) plus the detection of a significant culture of organisms in the urine:

- Any growth on culture of suprapubic aspirate.
- >10^5 Organisms/mL in pure growth from a carefully collected urine sample (midstream urine, clean catch urine, or bag urine). Ideally 2 consecutive growths of the same organism with identical sensitivities, but this is not always practical.

Note: Bacteriuria in the absence of symptoms does not necessarily need treatment, but needs to be considered in the clinical context (e.g. previous UTI, predisposing urinary tract abnormalities).

Guidance on the investigation, treatment and management of UTIs have been published.[1]

Clinical features

Presentation varies; symptoms in infants may be non-specific:

- vomiting/diarrhoea;
- poor feeding/failure to thrive;
- prolonged neonatal jaundice.

Examination

- Height and weight: plot on growth chart.
- BP.
- Examination for abdominal masses.
- Examine genitalia and spine for congenital abnormalities.
- Examine lower limbs for evidence of neuropathic bladder.

Diagnosis

Try to distinguish between upper (fever, vomiting, loin pain) vs. lower urinary tract symptoms (dysuria, frequency, mild abdominal pain, enuresis). Differentiation is often not possible in the younger child.

- UTI is a major cause of sepsis in a young infant.
- Ask about urinary stream in boys and family history of vesicoureteric reflux (VUR) or other urinary tract abnormality.
- Dipstick test in the urine. 'Leucocytes' and 'nitrites' strongly suggests UTI. Urine should be sent for microscopy, culture, and sensitivity.

Acute treatment

Antibiotics should be started after urine collection (see Table 11.2).

Table 11.2 Antibiotic regimes

If child is younger than 3mths of age	Treat with parenteral antibiotics
If child 3mths or older with acute pyelonephritis/upper UTI	Treat with oral antibiotics for 7–10 days or IV antibiotics for 2–4 days followed by oral antibiotics for a total duration of 10 days
If child 3mths or older with cystitis/lower UTI	Treat with oral antibiotics for 3 days. If the child is still unwell after 24–48hr, reassess

Chose antibiotic from:
• Trimethoprim 4mg/kg twice daily.
• Cefradine 25mg/kg twice daily.
• Cefalexin 25mg/kg twice daily.
• Co-amoxiclav 125/31 (1–6yrs), 5mL 3 times a day.
• Co-amoxiclav 250/62 (7–12yrs) 5mL 3 times a day.
• IV cefuroxime 25mg/kg 8-hourly; or
• IV gentamicin 2.5mg/kg/dose 8-hourly.

A repeat urine culture should be obtained on completion of antibiotics.

Follow-up and investigations

All children presenting with UTI should be investigated for any renal scarring and predisposing urinary tract abnormalities. Pyelonephritis or recurrent pyrexial UTIs need more comprehensive investigation than those at low risk (single, uncomplicated UTI with lower tract symptoms). Oral antibiotic prophylaxis (see 📖 p.358) may need to be started and continued until investigations are complete.

Recommended imaging tests (Tables 11.3–11.5)

Table 11.3 Infants aged <6mths

Test	Responds well to treatment with 48hr	Atypical UTI or recurrent UTI
US during the acute infection	NO	YES
US within 6wks	YES	NO
DMSA 4–6mths after acute infection	NO	YES
Micturating cystoure-thrography (MCUG)	NO	YES

Table 11.4 Children aged >6mths, but <3yrs

Test	Responds well to treatment with 48hr	Atypical UTI	Recurrent UTI
US during the acute infection	NO	YES	NO
US within 6wks	NO	NO	YES
DMSA 4–6mths after acute infection	NO	YES	YES
MCUG	NO	NO	YES

Table 11.5 Children aged >3yrs

Test	Responds well to treatment with 48hr	Atypical UTI	Recurrent UTI
US during the acute infection	NO	YES	NO
US within 6wks	NO	NO	YES
DMSA 4–6mths after acute infection	NO	NO	YES
MCUG	NO	NO	YES

UTI prevention

Predisposing factors to recurrent UTIs should be avoided:
• Treat and prevent constipation.
• *Hygiene:* clean perineum front to back.
• Avoid nylon underwear and bubble baths.
• Encourage fluid intake and regular toileting with double micturition.

Do not routinely use antibiotic prophylaxis after first-time UTI, but consider it after recurrent UTI.

Oral antibiotic prophylaxis (trimethoprim 2mg/kg at night or nitrofurantoin 1mg/kg) is required if:
• VUR.
• Recurrent UTIs (more than 2–3 episodes).

Reference

1 NICE (2007). Urinary tract infection in children: diagnosis, treatment and long-term infection, Clinical Guideline CG54. Available at: ℘ www.nice.org.uk/nicemedia/pdf/CG54fullguideline.pdf

Vesicoureteric reflux

This is the retrograde flow of urine from the bladder into the upper urinary tract. VUR is usually congenital in origin, but may be acquired (e.g. post-surgery). VUR combined with UTI leads to progressive renal scarring. Such reflux nephropathy may progress to end-stage renal failure if untreated. Incidence of VUR is ~1% in newborn infants. It is observed in 30–45% of young children (<5yrs) presenting with UTI. There is often a strong family history with a 35% incidence rate among siblings of affected children. So called 'congenital reflux' is also now recognized as result of routine antenatal scanning. This can result in small, smooth underdeveloped kidneys in otherwise asymptomatic children.

Grade of VUR

The extent of retrograde reflux from the bladder can be graded according to the International Reflux Study grading system:

- *I:* into ureter only.
- *II:* into ureter, pelvis, and calyces with no dilatation.
- *III:* with mild/moderate dilatation, slight or no blunting of fornices.
- *IV:* with moderate dilatation of ureter and/or renal pelvis and/or tortuosity of ureter, obliteration of sharp angle of fornices.
- *V:* gross dilatation, tortuosity, no papillary impression visible in calyces.

Diagnosis

The diagnosis of VUR is established by radiological techniques.

Micturating cystourethrogram

This technique involves urinary catheterization and the administration of radiocontrast medium into the bladder. Reflux is detected on voiding.

- *Advantages:* grade of reflux seen.
- *Disadvantages:* requires bladder catheterization, radiation dose.

Indirect cystogram

A radionucleotide method. Includes mercaptoacetyltriglycine (MAG-3) and diethylenetriamine pentaacetic acid (DTPA) scans.

- *Advantages:* no catheterization required; lower radiation dose.
- *Disadvantages:* false negatives found; co-operation of child to void is needed.

Follow-up and treatment

The aims are to prevent progressive renal scarring. Prophylactic antibiotics may be used to prevent this and imaging by indirect cystogram (e.g. MAG-3) and DMSA are sometimes used for follow-up. Randomized controlled trials of medical versus surgical treatment show surgery can reduce the incidence of pyelonephritis, but there is no difference in scarring compared with medical treatment.

Medical therapy

Antibiotic prophylaxis therapy (as for UTI – see 📖 previous section).

Surgery

Not routinely recommended. Indications for surgery include failed medical therapy, or poor compliance.

- *'STING' procedure (suburetic Teflon injection):* commonly used.
- Endoscopic injection of materials behind ureter to provide a valve mechanism during bladder filling and emptying. Longevity and need for repeat treatments not fully known.
- *Open surgery:* re-implantation of ureters.

Prognosis

- Spontaneous resolution of VUR often occurs, especially with lower grades of reflux.
- Bilateral reflux (grades IV and V) and reflux into duplex systems is associated with lower probability of resolution.

Acute kidney injury

Acute kidney injury (AKI) is a sudden reduction in glomerular filtration rate resulting in an increase in blood concentration of urea and creatinine and disturbed fluid and electrolyte homeostasis (see also 📖 p.94).

Classification

The causes of AKI (Box 11.1) can be divided into pre-renal, renal, and post-renal. A patient may have more than one cause for their AKI.

Box 11.1 Causes of AKI

Pre-renal
- Hypovolaemia, e.g. s to gastroenteritis, haemorrhage, DKA,
- nephrotic syndrome
- Peripheral vasodilatation, e.g. sepsis
- Impaired cardiac output, e.g. congestive cardiac failure
- Drugs, e.g. ACE inhibitors

Renal
- Acute tubular necrosis (usually following pre-renal)
- Interstitial nephritis (usually drug-induced)
- Glomerulonephritis
- Haemolytic–uraemic syndrome (HUS; see 📖 p.376)
- Cortical necrosis
- Bilateral pyelonephritis
- Nephrotoxic drugs, e.g. aminoglycoside, IV contrast, NSAIDs
- Myoglobinuria, haemoglobinuria
- Tumour lysis syndrome (see 📖 p.684)
- Renal artery/vein thrombosis

Post-renal
- Obstruction
- Post-urethral valves (PUV)
- Neurogenic bladder
- Calculi
- Tumours (rhabdomyosarcoma in infancy)

History

It is important to include the following points:
- History of sore throat/rash (e.g. streptococcal glomerulonephritis).
- Urinary symptoms of:
  • haematuria, frequency, dysuria (e.g. pyelonephritis);
  • poor stream (e.g. PUV).
- Significant antenatal history.
- Drugs.

Examination

It is important to assess and document the following.
- Height and weight (compare with any recent/past measurements).
- Fever.
- *Hydration status:* any evidence of oedema/dehydration?
- Haemodynamic status including BP.
- Presence of any rashes/arthropathy.
- *Abdomen:* tenderness or masses.
- *Neurology:* exclude possible neuropathic bladder.

Investigations

Urine

- Urinalysis with microscopy of fresh urine, e.g. evidence of casts.
- Culture, e.g. pyelonephritis.
- Osmolality, Na, creatinine, fractional excretion of sodium (📖 p.364).
- Protein:creatinine ratio to document proteinuria if dipstick +ve.
- Myoglobin if evidence of rhabdomyolysis.
- Urine calcium/oxalate to creatinine ratios if renal calculi suspected.

Blood investigations

- Urea, electrolytes, creatinine, Ca^{2+}, PO_4^{3-}, albumin, glucose, bicarbonate.
- Plasma osmolality.
- FBC and film.
- Blood cultures, if clinically septic.
- *In suspected nephritis:*
  - complement levels;
  - anti-streptolysin O titre (ASOT), antiDNAaseB;
  - antinuclear antigen (ANA), anti-dsDNA, anti-neutrophil cytoplasmic antibodies (ANCA).
- Uric acid if tumour lysis suspected.
- Creatinine kinase if possible myoglobinuria.
- Clotting if septic or potential need for biopsy or dialysis access.
- Drug levels if relevant (e.g. gentamicin).
- *Escherichia coli* 0157 serology.

Cultures

- Stool culture: *E. coli* 0157 (HUS).
- Throat swab.

Radiology

- *US(+/− Doppler):* kidneys and bladder.
- CXR if evidence of fluid overload.

Acute kidney injury: diagnosis and treatment

Diagnosis
The following urinary indices may be helpful providing no diuretics have been given (Table 11.6).

Table 11.6 Urinary indices indicating AKI

Test	Pre-renal	Renal	Post-renal
Urine osmolality (mosmol/kg)	>400–500	<350	Variable
Urine/plasma Cr ratio	>40	<20	<20
Urine Na (mmol/L)	<20	>40	Variable
FENa	<1%	>2%	Variable

To accurately interpret fractional excretion of sodium (FENa), patients should not have recently received diuretics. FENa is greater than 1% (and usually greater than 3%) with acute tubular necrosis and severe obstruction of the urinary drainage.

$$FENa = [(U_{Na} \times P_{Cr})/(P_{Na} \times U_{Cr})] \times 100$$

where U_{Na} and U_{Cr} are urinary Na and creatinine, respectively, and P_{Na} and P_{Cr} are plasma Na and creatinine, respectively.

Treatment
Liaise with a paediatric nephrology centre early and treat the following.
- Hyperkalaemia (K^+ >6.5mmol/L; see 📖 p.93).
- Metabolic acidosis (see 📖 p.104).
- Hypertension (see 📖 pp.58, 396).
- Shock (see 📖 p.56).
- Fluid overload (see 📖 p.375).
- Hypocalcaemia (see 📖 p.93).
- Hypo/hypernatraemia (see 📖 p.92).

Specific treatment depends on the underlying cause. However, the following general management principles apply:
- *Observations:* daily weight, BP, strict fluid input and output monitoring.
- *Fluids management:* Pre-renal—fluid bolus (10mL/kg of 0.9% saline) and furosemide. Otherwise, restrict to insensible losses (400mL/m^2) + urine output. Consider adding diuretic therapy.
- *Electrolytes:* monitor at least 12-hourly until stable. K^+ and PO_4 restricted diet. Consider adding PO_4 binder.

- *BP:* treat hypertension (see 📖 p.396).
- *Medications:* adjust drug doses according to level of renal impairment.

The patient may require transfer to a paediatric nephrology centre if dialysis looks likely or there is uncertainty about the diagnosis.

Indications for dialysis

The following are indications for urgent dialysis in ARF.

- Severe hyperkalaemia.
- Symptomatic uraemia with vomiting/encephalopathy (usually urea
- >40mmol/L).
- Rapidly rising urea and creatinine.
- Symptomatic fluid overload, especially cardiac failure or pericardial
- effusion.
- Uncontrollable hypertension.
- Symptomatic electrolyte problems or acidosis.
- Encephalopathy or seizures.
- *Prolonged oliguria:* conservative regimen controls ARF, but causes nutritional failure.
- Removal exogenous toxins or metabolite (inborn error).

Note: Patients with haemolytic–uraemic syndrome should be referred as soon as the child becomes oliguric or if urea is raised as current practice is to dialyse early to reduce neurological complications and to allow transfusion.

Acute dialysis—methods

- Peritoneal dialysis (abdominal catheter).
- Haemodialysis (femoral or jugular access).
- Haemofiltration (usually continuous veno-venous haemofiltration).

Chronic kidney disease

Most children with CKD are asymptomatic until approaching chronic renal disease stage 4 (see Table 11.7). CKD should be suspected if:
- failure to thrive;
- polyuria and polydipsia;
- lethargy, lack of energy, poor school concentration;
- other abnormalities such as rickets.

See Box 11.2 for summary of causes.

Table 11.7 Stages of chronic kidney disease

Stage	Description	GFR* (mL/min/1.73m2)
1	Kidney damage with/without increased GFR	>90
2	Kidney damage with mild decrease in GFR	60–89
3	Moderate decrease in GFR	30–59
4	evere decrease in GFR	5–29
5	Kidney failure	<15 (or dialysis)

* GFR, Glomerular filtration rate.

CKD: correcting common misconceptions
- Plasma creatinine can remain normal until GFR reduced to <50%.
- Urine flow rate may not mean a good GFR as many children with renal dysplasia have polyuria and nocturia.
- Other urinary abnormalities such as proteinuria, glycosuria can be an indicator of tubular dysfunction.

The focus is on GFR and not plasma creatinine
- GFR can be formally measured by the Iohexol method or alternatively by ^{51}Cr EDTA or inulin methods clearance,
- In ordinary clinical practice GFR (mL/min/1.73m^2) may be estimated (note: less accurate in children <2yrs or >14yrs):

 GFR (estimated) = 40 × height (cm)/creatinine (µmol/L).

Box 11.2 Causes of CKD

Congenital (55%)
- Renal dysplasia
- Obstructive uropathies
- Vesicoureteric reflux nephropathy

Hereditary (17%)
- Polycystic kidney disease
- Nephronophthisis
- Hereditary nephritis
- Cystinosis
- Oxalosis

Glomerulopathies (10%)
Focal segmental glomerulosclerosis

Multisystem disorders (9%)
- Systemic lupus erythematosus
- Henoch–Schönlein purpura
- Haemolytic–uraemic syndrome

Others
- Wilms' tumour
- Renal vascular disease
- Unknown

Investigations

- Urinalysis.
- *Blood:*
  - FBC + iron studies if anaemic;
  - electrolytes/Ca/PO$_4$/ALP/albumin;
  - pH/bicarbonate;
  - parathyroid hormone (PTH).
- Renal tract US.
- Left hand and wrist X-ray for bone age and renal osteodystrophy score.
- ECG/echocardiography for signs of left ventricular hypertrophy if hypertensive.

Chronic kidney disease: treatment

There should be early liaison with and referral to a regional paediatric nephrology centre.

Urgent life-threatening abnormalities
- High/low plasma K^+.
- Low plasma Na^+/acidosis/low Ca^{2+}/high. PO_4^{3-}.
- High/low BP.

Nutrition
Early involvement of the paediatric dietician is needed.
- Estimated average requirement (EAR) should be worked out.
  - often require supplements to achieve this;
  - NG/gastrostomy feeds.
- Minimum protein intake of EAR for age.
- Vitamin supplements (but not vitamin A).

Fluid and electrolyte balance
- Avoid high K^+-containing foods (e.g. banana, chocolate).
- Many causes of chronic renal failure (CRF) cause polyuria and Na^+ wasting; therefore, Na^+ supplements are needed.
- If clinical fluid overload, Na^+ restriction and diuretics.

Acid–base balance sodium bicarbonate supplements.

Renal osteodystrophy
- Control of plasma PO_4. Restrict dietary intake/PO_4 binders.
- Calcitriol (vitamin D) 15ng/kg/day.
- Monitor PTH.

Anaemia
- Assess iron status: oral iron supplements.
- Subcutaneous erythropoietin.
- Hypertension, see 📖 p.396.

Preservation of renal function
- Control hypertension.
- *Reduce proteinuria:* e.g. angiotensin-converting enzyme (ACE) inhibitor/ angiotensin receptor blocker therapy.
- *'Statin' therapy:* evidence of benefit from adult CRF trials.

Growth

- Optimize nutrition, acid–base balance, electrolyte balance.
- If failing height velocity (HV −2 SD or below) or short stature (Ht −2 SD or below) despite correction of above, treatment with recombinant human growth hormone is indicated.

Education and preparation for dialysis/transplantation

- Information provision.
- Meet team.
- Meet other families.

Dialysis

Peritoneal dialysis (PD)

- Preferred choice is automated peritoneal dialysis (APD) performed in
- patient's home (with mobile machines); therefore minimal disruption.
- Main risks: peritonitis and catheter blockage.
- Needs family and social support.

Haemodialysis (HD)

- Extracorporeal circuit.
- Vascular access by jugular venous catheter.
- Increasingly, long-term vascular access is by AV fistula (wrist or elbow). Therefore, avoid non-dominant arm for venepuncture and IV.
- Usually 4hr session, 3 times/wk in hospital.
- Home HD possible if there is a family member to support this.

Renal transplantation

This is the ultimate goal in CRF.

- Minimum 10kg (or when immunizations complete).
- Deceased donor vs. living-related donor (LRD) source.
- Pre-emptive transplantation before dialysis required is ideal.
- LRD by laparoscopic donor nephrectomy is now standard.
- Graft survival 85% after 2yrs.
- Lifelong immunosuppression is required.

Psychosocial support

- For patient and family this is crucial as CRF is lifelong treatment.
- Focus on prevention of cardiovascular disease, which is a major cause
- of mortality and morbidity in adult life.

Congenital urinary tract anomalies

- Increasingly, urinary tract anomalies are being detected earlier by the use of routine antenatal ultrasound scans.
- Renal anomalies account for about 20% of all significant abnormalities found on detailed scans at 18–20wks gestation.
- Close liaison between obstetricians, paediatrician, and surgeon with regard to counselling the parents and follow-up is vital.
- Centres should have a postnatal investigation protocol as the majority of infants will be asymptomatic.

Amniotic fluid volume

- *Oligohydramnios:* low urine production or obstruction of urine excretion that may lead to pulmonary hypoplasia.
- *Polyhydramnios:* polyuria.

Renal size

- *Enlarged:* cystic kidneys (any cause); hydronephrosis.
- *Small:* dysplasia.

Hydronephrosis

- *Unilateral:* pelviureteric junction (PUJ) or vescioureteric junction (VUJ) obstruction; vescioureteric reflux (VUR).
- *Bilateral:* bladder outlet obstruction, e.g. PUV, VUR, prune belly syndrome.

Renal cysts

- Multicystic dysplastic kidneys (MCDK).
- Polycystic kidney disease (PCKD).
- Cystic dysplasia.

Abnormal renal parenchyma

Echogenic:
- cystic kidneys (any cause);
- congenital nephrotic syndrome (may have polyhydramnios, large
- placenta).

Investigations

If a major problem is suspected (e.g. PUV, bilateral severe hydronephrosis, palpable kidneys), a renal US should be performed after 24hr of age. Otherwise routine postnatal investigation with U/S (at 2–4wks), MCUG (at 4–8wks), and radionuclide scan (at 8–12wks of age).

Clinical management

In the postnatal period, ensure male infants have voided and that a good urinary stream is observed. The initial postnatal US finding guides further management.

- MCUG only routine if strong suspicion of VUR (e.g. dilated ureters/ intermittent dilatation of pelvis). Will need cover with antibiotics (e.g. oral trimethoprim) for the procedure.
- Give antibiotic prophylaxis (e.g. oral trimethoprim) to all babies with suspicion of VUR.
- Radionuclide scan depends upon lesion:
  - DMSA if function of kidney required (e.g. MCDK, VUR);
  - MAG-3 renogram if 'obstruction' being evaluated (e.g. PUJ, VUJ).

Most infants with hydronephrosis can be conservatively managed if they are asymptomatic.

Inherited renal disease

Many renal abnormalities are inherited. Recognition of these is important, not only in terms of diagnosis and treatment of the patient, but also for screening and genetic counselling for the whole family.

- New therapies may become available as gene therapy is researched.
- Ethical considerations are very important in this group in terms of family screening and counselling.
- Databases such as Online Mendelian Inheritance in Man (OMIN) provide comprehensive lists. Below are a few of the more common conditions.

Autosomal dominant inheritance

Polycystic kidney disease (ADPKD). Commonest inherited renal disease (1/400 to 1/1000), which usually only manifests in adult life, but cysts can be seen on US scan in children. Multi-organ involvement (intracranial aneurysms, liver and pancreatic cysts, mitral valve prolapse), abdominal mass, haematuria, pain (rare presentation in neonatal period with abdominal masses and/or high or low BP, renal impairment).

Tuberous sclerosis (see 📖 pp.530, 947)

- *Skin:* 'ash-leaf' macule; adenoma sebaceum; shagreen patch.
- *Neurological:* seizures.
- *Cardiac:* rhabdomyoma.
- *Renal:* cysts; angiomyolipomas; high or low BP; renal impairment.
- *Neurofibromatosis:* neurofibroma, renal artery stenosis; therefore, BP should be monitored (see 📖 pp.561, 986).
- Branchio-oto-renal syndrome Hearing loss, branchial arch defects, renal anomalies.

Autosomal recessive inheritance

Polycystic kidney disease (ARPKD)

- Incidence 1:20 000 to 1:40,000.
- Oligohydramnios and large echogenic kidneys.
- Fusiform dilatation of collecting tubules.
- Prognosis depends on degree of pulmonary involvement.
- This usually presents at an earlier age than ADPKD and progresses to renal failure in a shorter time.
- Liver involvement leads to portal hypertension in later life
- *Bardet–Biedl syndrome:* obesity, polydactyly, mental retardation, retinitis pigmentosa, hypogenitalism, renal anomalies commonly found (📖 p.949).
- *Cystinosis (Fanconi's syndrome):* excess storage of cystine due to defect in transport system of cystine out of cell. Accumulates in various organs (cornea, thyroid, brain, leading to growth failure)—eventual renal failure.
- *Nephronophthisis:* polyuria, polydipsia, tubulopathy and childhood onset renal failure.
- *Primary hyperoxaluria:* see 📖 p.389 (renal calculi).
- *Cystinuria:* recurrent calculi.

X-linked

- *Alport's syndrome:* sensorineural deafness with progressive nephritis.
- Nephrogenic diabetes insipidus.
- *Fabry's disease:* deficiency of alpha-galactosidase A; now treatable (📖 p.968).

Sporadic

- *VATER association:* vertebral, anal, tracheo-oesophageal, radial/renal (see 📖 pp.948, 951); renal problems include agenesis, ectopy, or obstruction.
- *CHARGE association* (📖 pp.846, 950): Coloboma, heart defects, choanal atresia, retarded growth, genital anomalies, ear abnormalities (renal anomalies include dysplasia, agenesis, and ectopy).
- *Turner's (XO):* horseshoe or duplex kidneys (see 📖 pp.469, 948).
- *William's syndrome:* hypertensive, hypercalcaemia (see 📖 pp.237, 941).
- *Bartter's:* metabolic alkalosis, low K^+, high aldosterone with normal BP (📖 p.386).

Glomerulonephritis

A combination of haematuria, oliguria, oedema, and hypertension with variable proteinuria.
- Majority of cases post-infectious.
- Usually presents 1–2wks after a URTI and sore throat.

Causes of acute glomerulonephritis

Post-infectious
- *Bacterial:* streptococcal commonest, *Staphylococcus aureus*,
- *Mycoplasma pneumoniae, Salmonella*
- *Virus:* herpesviruses (EBV, varicella, CMV)
- *Fungi:* candida, aspergillus
- *Parasites:* toxoplasma, malaria, schistosomiasis

Others (less common)
- MPGN
- IgA nephropathy
- Systemic lupus erythematosis
- Subacute bacterial endocarditis
- Shunt nephritis

Investigations
- *Urine:*
  - urinalysis by dipstick: haematuria +/– proteinuria;
  - microscopy—casts (mostly red cell casts).
- *Throat swab:* culture.
- *Bloods:*
  - FBC;
  - U&E, including creatinine, bicarbonate, calcium, phosphate, and
  - albumin;
  - ASOT/antiDNAase B;
  - complement (expect low C3, normal C4);
  - autoantibody screen (include ANA).
- Renal US (urgent).
- CXR (if fluid overload suspected).

Management

Most require admission because of fluid balance, worsening renal function, or hypertension. Treat life-threatening complications first:
- hyperkalaemia (see 📖 p.93);
- hypertension (see 📖 pp.58, 396);
- acidosis (see 📖 p.104);
- seizures (see 📖 p.80);
- hypocalcaemia (see 📖 p.93).

Otherwise supportive treatment.
- *Fluid balance:*
  - weigh daily;
  - no added/restricted salt diet;
  - if oliguric, fluid restrict to insensible losses (400mL/m^2) + urine
  - output;
  - consider furosemide 1–2mg/kg bd if fluid overloaded.
- *Hypertension:*
  - treat fluid overload;
  - α-blockers and calcium channel blocker usual first choice;
  - *Note:* Do not use ACE inhibitor (may worsen renal function).
- *Infection:* 10-day course of penicillin (does not affect natural history, but limits spread of nephritogenic bacterial strains).

When to refer to paediatric nephrology unit

- Patients with life-threatening complications (see Management).
- Those with atypical features, including:
  - worsening renal function;
  - nephrotic state;
  - evidence of systemic vasculitis (e.g. rash);
  - normal C3 complement levels;
  - increased C4 complement levels;
  - +ve ANA;
  - persisting proteinuria at 6wks;
  - persisting low C3 at 3mths.

Prognosis

- 95% with post-streptococcal glomerular nephritis (GN) show complete recovery.
- Microscopic haematuria may persist for 1–2yrs.
- Discharge from follow-up once urinalysis, BP, and creatinine are normal.

Haemolytic–uraemic syndrome

This is the commonest cause of AKI in children in Europe and the USA. It typically has a seasonal variation with peaks in the summer and autumn months. It presents with a triad of:

- microangiopathic haemolytic anaemia;
- thrombocytopenia;
- acute renal failure.

Two forms of HUS are recognized.

- *Atypical/sporadic:*
  - not diarrhoea-associated (D⁻ HUS);
  - often familial.
- *Epidemic form:*
  - diarrhoea-associated (D⁺ HUS);
  - commonly associated with verocytotoxic producing E. coli 0157. H7 type, although other pathogens have also been implicated (e.g. Shigella, Streptococcus pneumoniae).

E. coli are common bacteria, normally found in the gut of warm-blooded animals. There are many types of E. coli, most of which are harmless. However, the enterohaemorrhagic E. coli (EHEC) produce toxins (poisons) that can cause gastroenteritis with blood in the stool. The toxins are called shiga toxins or verotoxins; hence, EHEC is also called STEC or VTEC. VTEC is found in the gut of cattle, and can also be found in the gut of humans without causing illness. The bacteria can be passed on to humans by:

- Eating improperly cooked beef, in particular, ground or mince beef.
- Drinking raw (unpasteurized) milk.
- Close contact with a person who has the bacteria in their faeces.
- Drinking contaminated water.
- Swimming or playing in contaminated water.
- Contact with farm animals.

Clinical features

Acute renal failure

Gut

- Prodrome of bloody diarrhoea.
- Rectal prolapse.
- Haemorrhagic colitis.
- Bowel wall necrosis and perforation.

Pancreas (occurs in <10%)

- Glucose intolerance/insulin-dependent diabetes mellitus.
- Pancreatitis.
- Liver jaundice.
- Neurological Irritability to frank encephalopathy.

Cardiac myocarditis (rare)

Investigations
- FBC + film.
- Blood cultures.
- U&E.
- LFTs.
- *E. coli* polymerase chain reaction (PCR).
- *Stools:* microscopy and culture.

Treatment
Early liaison with a paediatric nephrology unit is required, as early dialysis may be needed. Management is mainly supportive and directed at treating the clinical features of HUS. Antibiotics for underlying *E. coli* infection are not indicated.
- Monitor electrolyte balance.
- Monitor fluid balance.
- Nutrition.
- Blood transfusion (note risks/concerns regarding fluid overload and
- hyperkalaemia).
- Treat hypertension.

Outcome
- Generally good.
- Mortality <5%.
- *Long-term:* up to 30% may develop mild impairment of GFR.

Nephrotic syndrome

This is defined as a combination of:
- Heavy proteinuria (urinary protein to creatinine ratio >200mg/mmol).
- Hypoalbuminaemia (albumin <25g/L).
- Oedema.
- Hyperlipidaemia.

The incidence is approximately 2/100,000 children with a peak age of onset in children aged <6yrs. Boys are more commonly affected than girls (2:1) and there is an increased frequency in certain ethnic groups, e.g. Indian subcontinent. Nephrotic syndrome can be either primary or secondary

Primary
- Congenital.
- Infantile.

Secondary
- *Minimal change disease (MCD):* commonest (85%).
- Focal segmental glomerulosclerosis (FSGS; 10%).
- Membranoproliferative glomerulonephritis (MPGN; 5%).
- Membranous glomerulonephritis (MGN).

Classification

Nephrotic syndrome can be clinically classified as being either steroid-sensitive (SS), steroid dependent or steroid-resistant (SR). The majority of MCD is SS.
- MCD (SS), >95%.
- FSGS (SS), 20%.
- MPGN (SS), 55%.

Clinical features

Most children present with insidious onset of oedema, which is initially perorbital, but becoming generalized with pitting oedema. Perorbital oedema is often most noticeable in morning on rising. Ascites and pleural effusions may subsequently develop.

Examination

This should establish the extent of dependent oedema, e.g. facial, ankle, scrotal, etc. Assessment should also include:
- Height and weight (compare with previous/recent measurements).
- BP.
- Peripheral perfusion.

Investigations

Urine
- *Urinalysis:* protein +++.
- *Microscopy:* haematuria/casts (suggest causes other than MCD).
- *Na⁺:* If <10mmol/L suggests hypovolaemia. (*Note:* If patient has received diuretics this is not accurate.)
- Culture.
- Protein:creatinine ratio (early morning urine specimen).

Bloods
- Serum albumin (reduced, <25g/L).
- U&E/creatinine (decreased sodium and total calcium—with normal ionized calcium).
- C3/C4 (if decreased suggests not MCD).
- Consider ANF, ASOT, ANCA, immunoglobulins if mixed nephritic/nephrotic picture.
- *Lipids:* total cholesterol/low density lipoprotein (LDL)/very low density lipoprotein (VLDL).
- Haemoglobin may be increased or decreased depending on plasma volume.
- Varicella zoster immunity status.

Management
Patients should be admitted, particularly if this is their first episode or if there are concerns regarding complications. Management is initially aimed at fluid restriction and prevention of hypovolaemia. A trial of oral steroid therapy to induce remission is also started. Prophylaxis against bacterial infection (particularly pneumococcal) is also required.

Treatment
- Treat hypovolaemia if present but albumin infusion is not routine.
- Fluid restriction to 800–1000mL/24hr.
- Diuretics if very oedematous and no evidence of hypovolaemia. Furosemide/spironolactone.
- *Steroid therapy:*
  - oral prednisolone 60mg/m²/day for 4wks;
  - followed by 40mg/m²/alternate days for 4wks; then
  - *stop*—slow wean over next 4mths with slow taper, but need to consider side-effects of steroids.

Other measures
- Diet (no added salt and healthy eating—not high protein).
- Prophylactic antibiotics (oral penicillin V) until oedema-free.
- Immunize with pneumococcal vaccine.

Nephrotic syndrome: complications and follow-up

Complications

Complications are 2° to the relative hypovolaemic state and to impaired immunity.

Infection

Predisposition to infection is s to decreased IgG levels, and to impaired opsonization due to steroid immunosuppression. Bacterial peritonitis (especially *Streptococcus pneumoniae*) is an important complication and should be considered in any child with nephrotic syndrome who complains of abdominal pain. Urgent assessment, cultures, and IV antibiotic therapy are required.

Thrombosis

Nephrotic syndrome produces a hypercoagulable state and predisposition to both arterial and venous thrombosis is recognized.

Hypovolaemia

Suggested by development of oliguria and or presence of low BP. Patients may also complain of abdominal pain. If present, administration of an infusion of 20% human albumin solution 1g/kg over 2hr with furosemide (2mg/kg IV) should be given.

Acute renal failure This is pre-renal and 2° to hypovolaemia.

Indications for renal biopsy

The majority of patients will have MCD and will respond to steroids. Biopsy is therefore reserved for those with atypical features:
- Age <12mths or >12yrs.
- Increased BP.
- Macroscopic haematuria.
- Impaired renal function.
- Decreased C3/C4.
- Failure to respond after 1mth of daily steroid therapy.

Follow-up

Prognosis
- 30% single relapse.
- 30% occasional relapses.
- 30% steroid dependence.

Relapse
- Many patients with steroid-sensitive nephrotic syndrome will relapse. A relapse is defined as detection of urine dipstick ++ proteinuria for >3 days.
- Frequent relapse is defined as >2 relapses within 6mths of initial response or 4 or more relapses in any 12mths.

Management of relapses

Each relapse is treated with oral steroids in a similar manner to above. Alternative strategies for frequent relapsers include a trial of therapy with other agents such as:

- Cyclophosphamide.
- Levamisole.
- Ciclosporin A.
- Other agents including the immunosuppressants tacrolimus, mycophenolate mofetil and anti-CD20 monoclonal antibody (rituximab) may be considered.

Renal tubular disorders

The renal tubules are responsible for the regulation of fluid, acid–base, and electrolyte balance. Abnormalities of renal function may occur at any point along the length of the renal tubule system and may lead to a disturbance in the equilibrium of any of the substances handled by it. It is essential to consider these disorders when there are any of the following:
- Glycosuria, amino-aciduria, or impaired ability to concentrate or acidify urine shown on urinalysis.
- *Stones or nephrocalcinosis:* distal tubular acidosis and oxalosis are major causes.
- *Polyhydramnios and failure to thrive in a newborn:* e.g. Bartter syndrome associated with hypokalaemic alkalosis.
- *Failure to thrive with rickets:* cystinosis is commonest cause of Fanconi syndrome.
- *Major rickets with low plasma phosphate levels:* familial hypophosphataemic rickets.
- *Failure to thrive with low urine osmolality:* nephrogenic diabetes insipidus.

Renal tubular acidosis

Renal tubular acidosis (RTA) is a state of systemic hyperchloraemia resulting from impaired urinary acidification. Three types of RTA exist:
- Proximal type.
- Distal type.
- Mineralocorticoid deficiency-associated (see 📖 pp.430–432, 439).

Proximal renal tubular acidosis

See also ☐ pp.104, 385. This type of RTA results from reduced proximal tubular reabsorption of bicarbonate.
• 25% of urinary bicarbonate is lost.
• Plasma bicarbonate level falls until it reaches a threshold when urinary bicarbonate wasting ceases (approximately 15–18mmol/L).
• Urinary acidification to pH values <5.5 is not possible.

Proximal RTA may occur as an isolated disorder with no other abnormalities of tubular function. This form may be transient and is occasionally inherited. Proximal RTA also occurs as a more generalized defect of proximal tubular transport characterized by:
• RTA.
• Excessive urinary loss of glucose, phosphate, amino acids, sodium, potassium, calcium, and uric acid. This generalized form is known as Fanconi syndrome, which may be 1° or 2° to several inherited and acquired disease states (see Box 11.3).

Distal RTA See also ☐ p.385. This is due to deficiency in hydrogen ion secretion by the distal renal tubules and collecting ducts. Urine pH cannot be reduced 5.8. Hyperchloraemia and hypokalaemia are characteristic, but less severe than that found in proximal RTA. Nephrocalcinosis may be present. Distal RTA may be isolated or secondary (see Box 11.3).

Clinical features of RTA Children with isolated forms of proximal and distal RTA usually present with failure to thrive in infancy. Those with the 2° forms of RTA may present in a similar way.

Diagnosis

Other causes of systemic acidosis (e.g. chronic diarrhoea, lactic acidosis, diabetic ketoacidosis) should be excluded. Investigation to establish a diagnosis of RTA should include:
• *Blood:* pH; bicarbonate (low); potassium (low); chloride (high).
• *Urine—early morning sample:*
  • pH < 5.5 suggests proximal RTA;
  • pH ≥ 5.8 suggests distal RTA.

If proximal RTA is detected, blood and urinalysis to establish other tubular defects should be undertaken.

Treatment

The main aims are correction of acidosis and maintenance of normal bicarbonate and potassium. This can be achieved by alkali (citrate or bicarbonate)/potassium-containing solutions.

Box 11.3 Causes of renal tubular acidosis

Proximal
- *Isolated:* sporadic or inherited
- Primary Fanconi syndrome
- *Secondary Fanconi syndrome, inherited:*
  - cystinosis;
  - galactosaemia;
  - Wilson's disease;
  - Lowes syndrome.
- *Secondary Fanconi system, acquired:* vitamin D deficient rickets.
- *Secondary Fanconi system:* hypothyroidism

Distal
- *Isolated:* sporadic or inherited.
- *Secondary to nephritis:*
  - obstructive nephropathy
  - pyelonephritis
- *Secondary to toxins:* amphotericin B
- Lithium

Bartter's syndrome

This is a relatively rare form of renal tubular dysfunction. The condition is best described as a defect in chloride reabsorption in the ascending loop of Henlé, resulting in:
• excessive potassium excretion;
• increased prostaglandin synthesis;
• stimulation of the renin–angiotensin–aldosterone system.

Clinical features

Young children present with:
• failure to thrive;
• poor growth;
• muscle weakness;
• constipation.

Polyuria and polydipsia due to excessive salt and water loss may be evident.

Diagnosis

Characteristic findings include:
• hypokalaemia;
• hypochloraemia;
• raised plasma renin and aldosterone levels;
• normal BP.

Urine potassium and chloride levels are high.

Treatment

Goals are to maintain serum potassium levels >3.5mmol/L and to ensure adequate nutrition. Therapy includes a combination of oral potassium supplement together with a potassium-sparing diuretic (e.g. spironolactone) and indomethacin (prostaglandin inhibitor).

Renal calculi

The incidence of renal calculi varies according to geography and socio-economic conditions around the world. In the UK it affects approximately 1.5/million child population.

Aetiology

Infective

- Commonest cause in children in UK.
- Associated with chronic UTI with Proteus—'staghorn' calculi.
- Also UTI with *Pseudomonas*, *Klebsiella*, *E. coli*.

Associated with urinary stasis

Congenital malformations, e.g.:
- pelviureteric junction obstruction;
- megaureter.

Metabolic

- *Hypercalciuria:* i.e. 24hr urinary Ca >0.1mmol/kg/day or urinary
- Ca:creatinine ratio >0.74mmol/mmol:
  - primary hyperparathyrodism;
  - idiopathic infantile hypercalcaemia;
  - hypervitaminosis D;
  - prolonged immobilization.
- Cystinuria (autosomal recessive condition): typically radiolucent stones.
- *Oxalosis:* primary hyperoxaluria type I (PH1).
- *Uric acid stones:*
  - myeloproliferative disorders following medication/chemotherapy
  - for patients with leukaemia, lymphoma;
  - Lesch–Nyhan syndrome.

Clinical features

Most children will present with either gross or microscopic haematuria. They may be otherwise asymptomatic. The classic symptoms of renal colic are uncommon, e.g. intense pain located in the abdomen or in the loins and back. Symptoms and signs of a UTI may also be present. Some children may describe a sensation of 'having passed gravel' on micturition.

Investigations

Urine

- Dipstick analysis.
- Microscopy (pH, cells, crystals).
- Culture (exclude infection).
- Calcium:creatinine ratio; oxalate:creatinine ratio.
- Amino acid screen.

Blood
- U&E, bicarbonate, creatinine.
- Calcium, phosphate, PTH.
- Liver function tests.
- Uric acid.

Renal tract ultrasound

Other investigations
- *AXR:*
  - radio-opaque stones: calcium/cysteine/infective;
  - radiolucent stones: uric acid/xanthine.
- IV pyelogram or CT scan.
- Renal stone analysis: composition.

Treatment

The acute treatment of renal colic secondary to renal stones is based on the provision of adequate analgesia and hydration. Treat any underlying UTI with antibiotics. If severe renal impairment and urinary tract obstruction is evident refer to the paediatric urology team for consideration for extracorporeal shock-wave lithotripsy. Surgery (e.g. percutaneous nephrolithotomy or open surgery) is now seldom indicated. Long-term management is aimed at preventing further obstruction and bouts of renal colic. The simplest and most effective measures to achieve this are to ensure adequate hydration and diuresis to maintain a good urinary flow and dilute urine. Treatment of any underlying urinary tract infection and metabolic disorder is also required.

Primary hyperoxaluria type 1

This is an autosomal recessive condition. Three forms are recognized.
- *Infantile form:* early nephrocalcinosis and progression to CKD and end-stage renal failure (ESRF/Stage 5 CKD).
- *Child/adolescent form:* recurrent urolithiasis and progression to ESRF.
- *Adult form:* urolithiasis only.

Hypertension: definition

Defined by reference to sex, height centile charts (see Fig. 11.1).
- *Normal:* systolic and diastolic <90th centile.
- *High normal:* systolic or diastolic between 90th and 95th centile.
- *Hypertension:* systolic or diastolic >95th centile.
- *Severe hypertension:* systolic or diastolic >99th centile.

BP measurement should be part of routine examination.

Measurement technique
- Cuff size.
  - *bladder width*—70% of acromion olecranon distance or 40%
  - mid-arm circumference;
  - *bladder length*—should completely encircle arm.
  - *Note:* small cuff area is a common cause of false positive high BP!
- After 5min rest (ideally!).
- Sitting position with arm at level of heart (children).
- Supine position in infants.
- *On auscultation:* 1st and 5th (disappearance) Korotkoff sounds used for systolic and diastolic values, respectively.

Measurement devices
- Manual oscillometric sphygmomanometer (mercury now withdrawn).
- *Doppler:* infants (for systolic pressure).
- *Automatic oscillometry:* not all devices suitable.
- Ambulatory blood pressure monitoring (ABPM) for 24-hr profiles:
  - little normative data in paediatrics;
  - significant hypertension ≥30% readings above 95th centile.
- Intra-arterial (in intensive therapy unit (ITU) setting).

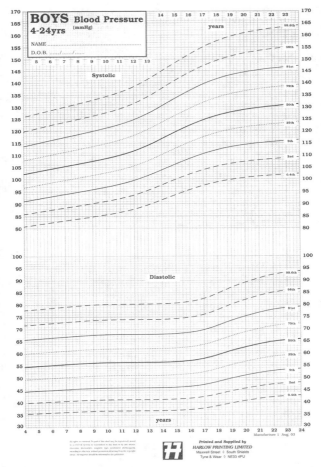

Fig. 11.1 Blood pressure centile figures for girls and boys. Copyright Lisa Jackson and Nandu Thalange.

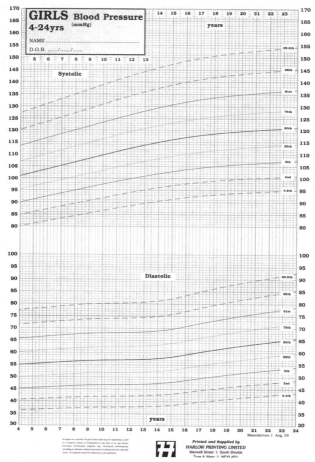

Fig. 11.1 (Contd.)

Hypertension: causes and features

Causes of hypertension

Primary (essential) hypertension
This is a diagnosis of exclusion. High body mass index, excessive salt intake, lack of exercise, and family history may be underlying predisposing factors

Secondary hypertension
* *Renal (commonest cause in hospital referral practice):*
  * chronic renal parenchymal disease (reflux/scarring)
  * polycystic kidney disease
  * obstructive uropathy
  * acute nephritis
  * chronic renal failure
* *Vascular:*
  * umbilical arterial/venous catheters
  * renal artery stenosis
  * renal vein thrombosis
  * coarctation of aorta
  * vasculitis
* *Endocrine:*
  * congenital adrenal hyperplasia
  * hyperthyroidism
  * increased steroids (iatrogenic or endogenous)
  * phaeochromocytoma (BP intermittently raised)
  * hyperaldosteronism
* *Trauma*
* *Neurological:*
  * 2° to pain
  * raised intracranial hypertension
* *Tumours:*
  * neuroblastoma
  * Wilms
* *Medication:*
  * steroids
  * aminophylline/caffeine
  * oral contraceptive pill
  * erythropoietin
  * calcineurin inhibitors; decongestants
  * amphetamines; cocaine
* *Others:*
  * bronchopulmonary dysplasia
  * ECMO
  * 'white-coat' hypertension

Clinical features

Most are asymptomatic.

Infants
- Vomiting.
- Failure to thrive (rare).
- Congestive cardiac failure/respiratory distress (in newborns).

Children
- Headache/nausea and vomiting.
- Visual symptoms.
- Irritable/tired.
- Bell's palsy.
- Epistaxis.
- Growth failure.
- Fits.
- Altered consciousness.

Examination
- Check fundi.
- Feel abdomen for abdominal masses.
- Listen for renal bruits.
- Feel femoral pulses and compare to radial/brachial pulses (to exclude
- coarctation) and check BP in all 4 limbs.
- Examination of the heart.

Investigations

A 2° cause is more likely with severe hypertension. Treatment and investigations may need to proceed together.
- *Urine:*
  - urinalysis, microscopy, and culture;
  - vanillylmandelic acid (VMA):creatinine ratio;
  - steroid profile and toxicology.
- *Blood tests:*
  - FBC;
  - U&E and creatinine;
  - bicarbonate, calcium, phosphate, albumin;
  - plasma renin and aldosterone.
- CXR and ECG.
- ECG.
- US of urinary tract + Doppler if renal artery stenosis suspected.
- Further imaging will depend upon suspected cause and ultrasound
- findings, e.g. DMSA, CT scan, arteriogram.
- Specialized tests, e.g. for phaeochromocytoma (see 📖 p.675).

Hypertension: management

Hypertensive crises

Acute, severe hypertension will require careful monitoring in a paediatric ICU and treatment with drugs shown in Table 11.8.

Maintenance antihypertensive therapy

Dosing schedules of many hypertensive drugs have not been evaluated in children. The favoured combination is a beta-adrenergic blocker with a vasodilator. A diuretic can be used if BP is still not controlled. ACE inhibitors should be avoided if renal artery stenosis is suspected but are useful for renin-mediated hypertension. Phentolamine is used if catecholamine-induced hypertension is suspected, e.g. phaeochromocytoma.

Table 11.9 gives dosing schedules for various hypertensive drugs.

Table 11.8 Emergency treatment of hypertensive crisis (see also 📖 pp.58, 397)*

Drug	Administration	Onset of effect	Side-effects
Nifedipine	Sublingual hourly prn 200–500micrograms/kg	Minutes	Headaches, tachycardia
Sodium nitroprusside	0.5–10micrograms/kg/ min as infusion	Seconds to minutes	Very rapid effect; titrate dose; cyanide accumulates after 48hr of use
Labetalol	1–3mg/kg/hr	10–30min	Postural hypotension
Hydralazine	Slow IV 100–500-micrograms/kg	10–30min	Tachycardia, flushes, headache
Phentolamine	10–100micrograms/kg	Minutes	Use in catecholamine excess states

* The aim is to reduce systolic and diastolic BP to <95th centile for age and sex but, if severely hypertensive, only one-third of desired BP reduction should occur in the first 6hr. Aim for controlled reduction in BP over 72hr.

Table 11.9 Maintenance oral therapy for treatment of hypertension

Drug	Administration	Dose
Vasodilators		
Nifedipine	0.25–2mg/kg/24hr	2 divided doses
Hydralazine	1–7.5mg/kg/24hr	2–3 divided doses
Prazosin	50–500micrograms/kg/24hr	2–3 divided doses
Minoxidil	200–1000micrograms/kg/24hr	Single dose
Beta-blockers		
Propranolol	1–6mg/kg/24hr	2–3 divided doses
Atenolol	1–4mg/kg/24hr	Once a day if adequate renal function
Diuretics		
Furosemide	1–5mg/kg/24hr	1–2 divided doses
Spironolactone	1–3mg/kg/24hr	1–2 divided doses
ACE inhibitors		
Captopril	0. 3–6mg/kg/24hr	2–3 divided doses
Enalapril	0.1–1mg/kg/24hr	Single dose

Endocrinology and diabetes

Obesity

This has become an important public health problem, which has achieved epidemic levels in the developed world. In the UK approximately 20% of children and adolescents are either overweight or obese. Obesity in childhood strongly predicts obesity in adulthood. Obesity is an important risk factor for the development of life-threatening disease in later life, including type 2 diabetes mellitus (T2DM), hypertension, cardiovascular disease, and cancer.

Definition and diagnosis

Obesity implies increased central (abdominal) fat mass, and can be quantified using a number of clinical surrogate markers. BMI is the most convenient indicator of body fat mass (see Fig. 12.1).

> BMI = weight (kg)/[height (m)]^2
> * *Overweight*: BMI >91st centile, wt <98th centile
> * *Obese*: BMI >98th centile

Other measures of obesity include:
* waist circumference;
* waist:hip ratio.

Epidemiology

The worldwide increase in incidence in obesity has been mainly observed in Western countries and in other developed societies. Risk factors for the development of obesity include the following:
* Parental/family history of obesity.
* Afro-Caribbean/Indian–Asian ethnic origins.
* *Catch-up growth (weight) in early childhood (0–2yrs)*: infants born small for gestational age who demonstrate significant weight catch up (>2SDs) in first 2yrs of life.

Causes

So-called idiopathic (or 'simple') obesity is by far the commonest cause of obesity accounting for up to 95% of cases. It is multifactorial in origin and represents an imbalance in normal nutritional–environmental–gene interaction, whereby daily calorie (energy) intake exceeds the amount of calories (energy) expended:
* genetic predisposition (energy conservation);
* increasingly sedentary lifestyle (energy expenditure);
* increasing consumption and availability of high energy foods.

Obesity may be associated with other identifiable underlying pathological conditions.

Endocrine (rare)
- Hypothyroidism (see 📖 p.424).
- Cushing's syndrome/disease (see 📖 p.434).
- Growth hormone deficiency (see 📖 pp.470–473).
- Pseudohypoparathyroidism (see 📖 p.443).
- Polycystic ovarian syndrome.
- Acquired hypothalamic injury (see 📖 p.430), i.e. CNS tumours and/ or surgery resulting in disruption to the neuroendocrine pathways regulating appetite and satiety.

Genetic
Obesity is a recognized feature characterizing the phenotype of a number of genetic syndromes.
- Prader–Willi syndrome (see 📖 p.949).
- Bardet–Biedl syndrome (see 📖 p.949).
- Monogenic causes: leptin deficiency (rare); melanocortin 4 receptor gene (5–6% of all causes).

BOYS BMI CHART

(BIRTH - 20 YEARS): United Kingdom cross-sectional reference: 2002/1

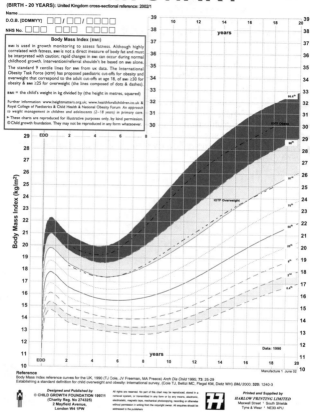

Body Mass Index (BMI)

BMI is used in growth monitoring to assess fatness. Although highly correlated with fatness, BMI is not a direct measure of body fat and must be interpreted with caution; rapid changes in BMI can occur during normal childhood growth. Intervention/referral shouldn't be based on BMI alone.

The standard 9 centile lines for BMI from UK data. The International Obesity Task Force (IOTF) has proposed paediatric cut-offs for obesity and overweight that correspond to the adult cut-offs at age 18, of BMI ≥30 for obesity & BMI ≥25 for overweight (the lines composed of dots & dashes).

BMI = the child's weight in kg divided by (the height in metres, squared)

Further information: www.heightmatters.org.uk; www.healthforallchildren.co.uk & Royal College of Paediatrics & Child Health & National Obesity Forum *An approach to weight management in children and adolescents (2–18 years)* in primary care.

► These charts are reproduced for illustrative purposes only, by kind permission. © Child growth foundation. They may not be reproduced in any form whatsoever.

Reference
Body Mass Index reference curves for the UK, 1990 (TJ Cole, JV Freeman, MA Preece) *Arch Dis Child* 1995; **73**: 25-29
Establishing a standard definition for child overweight and obesity: international survey, (Cole TJ, Bellizi MC, Flegal KM, Dietz WH) *BMJ* 2000; **320**: 1240-3

Designed and Published by
© CHILD GROWTH FOUNDATION 1997/1
(Charity Reg. No 274325)
2 Mayfield Avenue,
London W4 1PW

Printed and Supplied by
HARLOW PRINTING LIMITED
Maxwell Street ' South Shields
Tyne & Wear ' NE33 4PU

Fig. 12.1 BMI Centile Charts. © Child Growth Foundation.

GIRLS BMI CHART

(BIRTH - 20 YEARS): United Kingdom cross-sectional reference: 2002/1

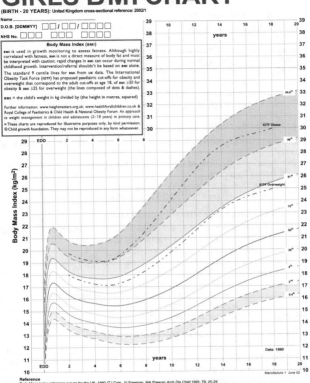

Name ....

D.O.B. [DDMMYY] ☐☐ / ☐☐ / ☐☐☐☐

NHS No. ☐☐☐ ☐☐☐ ☐☐☐☐

Body Mass Index (BMI)

BMI is used in growth monitoring to assess fatness. Although highly correlated with fatness, BMI is not a direct measure of body fat and must be interpreted with caution; rapid changes in BMI can occur during normal childhood growth. Intervention/referral shouldn't be based on BMI alone.

The standard 9 centile lines for BMI from UK data. The International Obesity Task Force (IOTF) has proposed paediatric cut-offs for obesity and overweight that correspond to the adult cut-offs at age 18, of BMI ≥30 for obesity & BMI ≥25 for overweight (the lines composed of dots & dashes).

BMI = the child's weight in kg divided by (the height in metres, squared)

Further information: www.heightmatters.org.uk; www.healthforallchildren.co.uk & Royal College of Paediatrics & Child Health & National Obesity Forum An approach to weight management in children and adolescents (2–18 years) in primary care.
► These charts are reproduced for illustrative purposes only, by kind permission.
© Child Growth Foundation. They may not be reproduced in any form whatsoever.

Reference
Body Mass Index reference curves for the UK, 1990 (TJ Cole, JV Freeman, MA Preece) *Arch Dis Child* 1995; 73: 25-29
Establishing a standard definition for child overweight and obesity: international survey (Cole TJ, Bellizi MC Flegal KM, Dietz WH) *BMJ* 2000; 320: 1240-3

Designed and Published by
© CHILD GROWTH FOUNDATION 1997/1
(Charity Reg. No 274325)
2 Mayfield Avenue,
London W4 1PW

Printed and Supplied by
HARLOW PRINTING LIMITED
Maxwell Street ' South Shields
Tyne & Wear ' NE33 4PU

Fig. 12.1 (Contd.)

Obesity: management

Evaluation and investigations

This includes taking a detailed clinical and family history.
- Birth weight (note: small for gestational age).
- Feeding habits and behaviour: particularly infancy/early childhood. Hyperphagia: may suggest genetic cause.
- Weight gain/growth pattern (check previous health records).
- Physical activity.
- Neurodevelopment and school performance.
- Screen for comorbid factors (see Complications and comorbid conditions).
- Family history: obesity; T2DM; cardiovascular disease.

Laboratory investigations are directed at excluding secondary causes of obesity:
- *Blood biochemistry:* thyroid function test; serum cortisol; liver function test; fasting lipid profile.
- Genetic studies (e.g. Prader–Willi syndrome).
- Oral glucose tolerance test (OGTT; see Box 12.1).

Complications and comorbid conditions

Severe obesity is associated with the following comorbid conditions, which should be screened for at the time of assessment.
- *Pyschological:* low self-esteem; depression.
- *ENT/respiratory:* obstructive sleep apnoea; obesity–hypoventilation syndrome; pulmonary hypertension.
- *Orthopaedic:* bowing of legs; slipped femoral epiphysis; osteoarthritis.
- *Metabolic:* impaired glucose tolerance/type 2 diabetes; hypertension; dyslipidaemia; polycystic ovarian syndrome.
- *Hepatic:* non-alcoholic steatohepatitis.

Obesity and oral glucose tolerance testing

In children and adolescents with obesity the prevalences of impaired glucose tolerance (IGT) and T2DM have been estimated to be in the region of 20–25% and 4%, respectively.

An oral glucose tolerance test should be considered when one or more of the following risk factors are present.
- *Severe obesity:* BMI >98th centile
- *Acanthosis* nigricans.
- Positive family history of T2DM.
- *Ethnic origin:* Asian/Afro-Caribbean/African-American.
- Polycystic ovarian syndrome.
- Hypertension.

Box 12.1 Oral glucose tolerance testing

Conditions Performed in the morning after 8–10hr fast

Dose Glucose 1.75g/kg to a maximum of 75g, drunk within 5–10min

Sampling Blood glucose at 0 min and at 30min intervals thereafter for 120min

Interpretation See table below

	Blood glucose (mmol/L)	
	At 0 min	At 120 min
Normal	<6.0	<7.8
IGT	6.0–7.0	7.8–11.1
DM	>7.0	>11.1

Management

There is currently no consensus on the best approach to treating childhood obesity. Treatment requires a multidisciplinary approach.
- Nutrition and lifestyle education/counselling: important.
- Decreasing calorie intake/increasing exercise.
- Behaviour modification and family therapy strategies.
- Drug therapies (currently limited, not licensed for children).
- Obesity (bariatric) surgery (rarely).

Population-based intervention and prevention strategies may be more effective than approaches targeted at the obese individual.

Type 1 diabetes mellitus

This is the most common form of diabetes mellitus in children and adolescents (90% of cases). It is an autoimmune disorder characterized by T-cell mediated destruction and progressive loss of pancreatic β-cells leading to eventual insulin deficiency and hyperglycaemia.

Epidemiology The incidence of Type 1 diabetes mellitus (T1DM) has been increasing, but shows marked geographical variation. In Europe the highest incidence rates are seen in the Nordic countries (Finland, Sweden). During childhood there are two peaks in presentation, one between ages 5 and 7yrs and the other, larger peak, just before or at the onset of puberty. Seasonal variation in presentation of T1DM is also observed with a peak seen in the winter months.

Aetiology

The cause of T1DM involves both genetic and environmental factors. Over 20 different T1DM susceptibility genes have been identified. The insulin-dependent diabetes mellitus (*IDDM1*) gene locus, which represents the human leukocyte antigen (HLA) DR/DQ locus on the major histocompatibility complex, accounts for the greatest susceptibility.

The role of various environmental interactions and triggers is controversial.

Pathophysiology

T1DM is a chronic autoimmune condition.
- Immune tolerance is broken and antibodies against specific β-cell autoantigens are generated (e.g. anti-islet cell; anti-insulin; anti-GluAD; anti-IA2 antibodies).
- T-cell activation leads to β-cell inflammation ('insulitis') and to subsequent cell loss through apotosis.
- The rate of β-cell loss varies (months–years) and the timing and presentation of symptomatic diabetes may depend on factors that increase insulin requirements (e.g. puberty).

Clinical presentation

The onset of symptoms evolves over a period of weeks. Symptoms are a reflection of insulin deficiency resulting in increased catabolism and hyperglycaemia. In the majority, first presentation is usually made in the early symptomatic phase with:
- weight loss;
- polyuria/polydipsia;
- nocturia/nocturnal enuresis.

Other less common symptoms include:
- candida infection (e.g. oral thrush, balanitis, vulvovaginitis);
- skin infections.

Failure to recognize these symptoms will result in delayed or late diagnosis of T1DM and possible presentation with DKA (see 📖 pp.98–101, 413). The risk of first presentation of T1DM with DKA is increased when non-specific symptoms of diabetes may go unrecognized:

• intercurrent/febrile illness;
• infants and preschool age child.

Assessment of new patient

Emphasis should be put on:

• *History:* duration of symptoms.
• *Family history:* of diabetes/other autoimmune disease.
• *Examination:* weight/BMI; signs of DKA (see 📖 pp.98–101, 413).

Diagnosis and investigations

The diagnosis is readily established in a symptomatic child with a random blood glucose level >11.1mmol/L. Other investigations:

• U&E.
• Blood pH (to exclude DKA).
• Diabetes-related autoantibodies: islet cell antibody (ICA)/anti-insulin antibody (IAA)/anti-GluAD antibody (GluAD)/anti-IA-2.
• Other autoimmune disease screen: thyroid function test/thyroid antibodies; coeliac disease antibody screen.

Type 1 diabetes mellitus: management

The initial care and subsequent long-term management of patients with T1DM should be delivered by a specialist paediatric diabetes team. All newly diagnosed patients must start insulin therapy as soon as possible. An intensive programme of education and support is needed for the child and parents. The aims of management of T1DM are:
- education of child and family about diabetes;
- insulin therapy;
- nutritional management;
- monitoring of glycaemic control;
- avoidance and management of hypoglycaemia;
- management of acute illness and avoidance of DKA;
- screening for development of associated illness;
- screening for diabetes-related microvascular complications;
- prevention and treatment of microvascular complications.

Education, counselling, and support

An intensive programme of education and counselling is needed in the first few days/weeks to cover the fundamental principles about T1DM and its management.
- Basic pathophyisology of T1DM.
- *Insulin therapy:*
  - actions of insulin;
  - SC injection techniques;
  - dose adjustment principles, including carbohydrate counting techniques.
- Home/self blood glucose monitoring.
- *Acute complications:*
  - avoidance, symptom recognition, and treatment of hypoglycaemia and diabetic ketoacidosis (see 📖 pp.412–413).
  - 'sick day rules' during illness to prevent DKA (see 📖 p.412).
- *Diet:*
  - healthy, low-fat;
  - high complex carbohydrate.
- *Long-term complications:* risk factors and avoidance.
- Psychological issues.

A considerable amount of time and need for repetition is required to deliver this information. The process of education and support is a continual one with a need for regular review and updates of knowledge.

Nutritional management

Diet and insulin regimen need to be matched to optimize glycaemic control. Instruction on and application of carbohydrate counting techniques are required. A healthy diet is recommended with a high complex carbohydrate and relatively low fat content.

Daily dietary balance for a healthy diet

- 50–60% carbohydrate (complex/high fibre)
- <30% fat (<10% in form of saturated fat)
- 15–20% protein
- Refined sugars limited to <25g/day

Blood glucose monitoring

- Regular daily blood glucose monitoring and testing when blood levels are suspected to be low or high is recommended.
- Home blood glucose monitoring is normally carried out using a portable glucose meter and finger-pricking device.
- Regular testing is required to assist with insulin dose-adjustment decisions, and to learn and predict how changes in lifestyle, food, and exercise affect glycaemic control.
- A minimal testing frequency of 4 times per day should be encouraged.
- SC continuous glucose monitoring (CGM) devices are also now available and in certain select situations may offer some advantages and benefits to patients.

Type 1 diabetes mellitus: insulin therapy

Table 12.1 describes the various insulin analogue preparations (created by minor amino acid substitutions to the 'native' human insulin molecule).

Table 12.1 Characteristics of various insulin analogue preparations

Type	Example	Onset	Peak	Duration
Short-acting	Regular/soluble	30–60min	1.5–3hr	4–6hr
Rapid (analogue)	Insulin lispro	5–30min	30–90min	3–5hr
	Insulin aspart	15–30min	1–3hr	3–5hr
Intermediate acti g	NPH	1–4hr	–10hr	10–16hr
	Lente	3–4hr	6–12hr	12–18hr
Long-acting	Ultralente	1–4hr	8–16hr	18–22hr
Long-acting (analogue)	Insulin detemir	2–4hr	None	12–20hr
	Insulin glargine	–2hr	None	20–24hr

The daily requirement for insulin varies with age:
- at diagnosis, 0.5U/kg/day;
- childhood/prepubertal, 0.5–1.0U/kg/day;
- puberty, 1.2–2.0U/kg/day;
- post-puberty, 0.7–1.2U/kg/day.

Insulin is administered SC, usually as a bolus injection. A number of patients receive insulin in the form of a continuous SC insulin infusion (CSII) delivered by a pump device. Insulin injection sites include the SC tissues of the upper arm, the anterior and lateral thigh, the abdomen, and buttocks.

There is a variety of different daily insulin injection therapy regimens. The choice of regime is a compromise between achieving optimal therapy and minimizing psychosocial development. The patient and family must have input into the choice.

Insulin regimens

Two dose regimen

The simplest regimen. Two injections per day. Each injection is a mix of short/rapid-acting insulin *plus* an intermediate-acting insulin. Traditionally 2/3 of the total daily dose is given at breakfast and 1/3 given before/at the evening meal.

Disadvantages
- Need to mix insulins.
- Peak action of insulin does not correspond with timing of main meals.
- Increased frequency of between meal and nocturnal hypoglycaemia.
- Between meal snacks required to minimize hypoglycaemia.

Note: Less hypoglycaemia with rapid analogue insulin use.

Three-dose regimen Improvement and intensification of the two-dose regimen:
- *At breakfast:* mix of short or rapid acting insulin *plus* an intermediate-acting insulin.
- *Before/at evening meal:* short- or rapid-acting insulin only.
- *At bedtime:* intermediate-acting insulin only.

Advantages Delayed evening intermediate-acting insulin results in reduced frequency of nocturnal hypoglycaemia.

Basal bolus regimen This regimen attempts to mimic physiological secretion. Low level, background, basal insulin provides for fasting and between meal insulin requirements and larger acute doses of fast-acting insulin are given to provide for prandial requirements.
- *Basal insulin:* once a day intermediate- or long-acting insulin (traditionally at bedtime).
- *Fast-acting insulin:* At meal times (i.e. 3 per day) and with between meal snacks.

Advantages
- Increased flexibility with meal times/exercise planning.
- Insulin dose adjustment— carbohydrate (CHO) counting.

Disadvantages
- Need for more injections.
- Need more frequent blood glucose monitoring.

CSII Current insulin infusion pumps are reliable and portable. CSII therapy can be used in children of all ages. Short/rapid-acting insulin is administered as a continuous insulin infusion. Meal time boluses and 'blood glucose correction' boluses are administered when required.

Advantages
- No bolus injections/reduced injection frequency.
- Increased flexibility meal times/exercise planning.
- Insulin dose adjustment—CHO counting.
- Reduced frequency hypoglycaemia.

Disadvantages
- No long-acting insulin. Infusion interruption: risk of rapid DKA.
- Need more frequent blood glucose monitoring.
- Greater management expertise required.

Insulin requirements and dose adjustment Insulin doses are adjusted based on home blood glucose monitoring. Generally it is best not to alter the basic insulin regimen every time the blood glucose levels are outside the target range (4–10mmol/L). Rather, recorded blood glucose levels should be reviewed and insulin adjustments should be made to correct recurrent profiles that are either too low or high. Insulin doses are adjusted by 5–10% at a time.

CHO counting: insulin dose adjustment system Applies the principle that the amounts of fasting/rapid acting insulin given at mealtimes are adjusted and matched according to the amount of CHO consumed.

Acute complications of Type 1 diabetes mellitus

Hypoglycaemia

All children with T1DM will experience an episode of hypoglycaemia. Symptoms develop when blood glucose <3.5mmol/L. The frequency of hypoglycaemia is higher with more intensive insulin regimens and in young children. Symptoms and signs include:
- feeling of hunger;
- sweatiness;
- feeling faint/dizzy;
- 'wobbly feeling';
- irritability/confusion/misbehaviour;
- pallor.

Hypoglycaemia unawareness

Occasionally, sudden onset of hypoglycaemia may result in unconsciousness and seizures. Children experiencing frequent episodes of hypoglycaemia may fail to develop the typical (i.e. counter-regulatory/adrenergic) symptoms of hypoglycaemia. Avoidance of hypoglycaemia usually results in restoration of warning symptoms.

Nocturnal hypoglycaemia

The frequency is thought to be high in T1DM (up to 50%). Nocturnal hypoglycaemia should be suspected when fasting early morning blood sugars are repeatedly high, despite seemingly adequate overnight insulin cover (secondary to hypoglycaemia counter-regulation). Detection and confirmation of nocturnal hypoglycaemia can be achieved by utilizing a SC continuous glucose monitoring system (CGMS) device.

Hypoglycaemia: management

Acute episodes of mild to moderate symptomatic hypoglycaemia can be managed with oral glucose (glucose tablets or sugary drink). Oral glucose gels applied to the buccal mucosa can be used in the child who is unwilling or unable to cooperate to eat. Severe hypoglycaemia can be managed in the home with an intramuscular injection of glucagon (1.0mg). This is available as a specific injection kit.

Sick day management

During illness and other physiological stresses (e.g. following injury) insulin requirements dramatically increase in response to the body's increased catabolic state. Blood glucose should be monitored more frequently than usual and insulin doses may need to be increased. Insulin must be continued at all times, even though oral intake of food and fluids may be decreased. Urine or plasma ketones must be monitored and, if elevated, are a sign of increased insulin needs and possible impending DKA.
- In the presence of moderate to high ketone levels doses of soluble/regular insulin must be increased (by 25–50%) and supplemental doses may need to be given.

- Carbohydrate and fluid intake should be maintained as much possible to avoid hypoglycaemia and dehydration.

If the child is unable to maintain hydration (e.g. due to excessive vomiting) or cannot take in adequate carbohydrate to avoid hypoglycaemia then the child should be evaluated by the diabetes or other medical team and consideration given to treatment with IV fluids and insulin infusions (see DKA).

Diabetic ketoacidosis

See also 📖 pp.98–101. DKA is caused by a decrease in effective circulating insulin associated with elevations in counter-regulatory hormones (glucagon, catecholamines, cortisol, GH). This leads to increased glucose production by the liver and kidney and impaired peripheral glucose utilization with resultant hyperglycaemia and hyperosmolality. Increased lipolysis, with ketone body (beta-hydroxybutyrate, acetoacetate) production causes ketonaemia and metabolic acidosis. Hyperglycaemia and acidosis result in osmotic diuresis, dehydration, and obligate loss of electrolytes. Ketoacid accumulation also induces an ileus, resulting in nausea and vomiting and an exacerbation of the dehydration.

DKA frequency

The frequency of DKA occurring at T1DM onset, or diagnosis, is 10/100 000 children and is more common in children <4yrs of age. In established T1DM the frequency of DKA is approximately 1–10% per patient per year. The risk of DKA is increased in children with: poor metabolic control; previous episodes of DKA; peripubertal and adolescent girls; children with psychiatric disorders, including those with eating disorders; and those with difficult family circumstances.

DKA mortality and morbidity

Mortality rates for DKA are 0.15–0.31%. Cerebral oedema (CeO) accounts for 57–87% of all DKA-related deaths. The incidence of DKA-associated CeO is 0.46–0.87%. Reported mortality from CeO is high (21–25%) and significant morbidity is evident in 10–26% of all CeO survivors.

Type 1 diabetes mellitus: long-term complications

The risk of developing microvascular or macrovascular complications is related to the duration of diabetes and to the degree of glycaemic control achieved over time. Patients who achieve and maintain good glycaemic control (i.e. HbA1c 7.0% or less) have a lower risk. Genetic factors may also influence the risk of complications. The conditions outlined in Box 12.2 require screening.

> **Box 12.2 Long-term complications of T1DM** (see 📖 p.415)
>
> **Microvascular complications**
> - *Renal:* microalbuminuria, diabetic nephropathy
> - *Eyes:* retinopathy
> - *Nervous:* peripheral neuropathy, autonomic neuropathy
>
> **Macrovascular**
> - Hypertension
> - CHD

- *Macrovascular* complications are almost never seen in children and adolescents.
- *Microvascular* complications may be seen during the childhood and adolescent years of T1DM. The incidence and frequency is low before puberty. Risk factors for the development of early microvasular disease are duration of diabetes, glycaemic control (long-term), and the onset of puberty.

Microalbuminuria (MA)
- Rare before puberty.
- May be intermittent and transient.
- May be associated with increased BP.
- May require treatment with ACE inhibitor if MA persists (+/– hypertension).

Retinopathy
Significant changes are rare before onset of puberty. Background retinopathy (microaneurysms, retinal haemorrhages, soft and hard exudates) may be seen. Pre-proliferative/proliferative retinopathy rare (📖 p.920).

Both the conditions should be screened for annually from age 11yrs (or from 9yrs if duration of DM >5yrs). MA screening by EMU estimation of urinary albumin: creatinine ratio. Retinopathy screening by digital retinal photography.

Type 1 diabetes mellitus: associated illnesses

Patients with T1DM are at increased risk for a number of other autoimmune disorders.

The most important of these are the following:

- *Autoimmune thyroiditis:* up to 5% develop hypothyroidism.
- *Coeliac disease:*
  - prevalence rate 5–10%;
  - usually atypical symptoms or asymptomatic.
- *Adrenal insufficiency: uncommon.*

Testing for thyroid autoantibodies, thyroid function tests (TSH and free T4), together with a coeliac disease antibody screen (transglutaminase or endomysial antibodies), should be carried out on an annual basis for the early detection and treatment of these disorders.

Screening and long-term monitoring

Glycaemic control Glycated haemoglobin index (HbA1c) measured every 3–4mths.

Growth and development
- Height/weight/BMI (regularly at clinic).
- Puberty stage (annual).

Microvascular complications
- Microalbuminuria screening:
  - urine dipstick test (regularly at clinic);
  - 3 early morning urinary albumin/creatinine ratio (annual screening).
- Retinopathy screening: retinal photography (annual screening).
- Neuropathy (rare).
- Associated autoimmune disease:
  - thyroid disease (annual);
  - coeliac disease (annual).

Type 2 diabetes mellitus

T2DM is a multifactorial and heterogeneous condition in which the balance between insulin sensitivity and insulin secretion is impaired. The condition is characterized by hyperinsulinaemia; however, there is relative insulin insufficiency to overcome underlying concomitant tissue insulin resistance.

Epidemiology

T2DM is emerging as a significant health problem with increasing incidence in most developing countries. The increasing frequency of T2DM parallels the upward trend in childhood obesity in these populations. In the USA, T2DM now accounts for up to 45% of the new cases of diabetes diagnosed in childhood.

Aetiology

T2DM is not an autoimmune disease. There is no association with HLA-linked genes; however, there is a strong genetic basis, which is thought to be polygenic. The known risk factors for the development of T2DM are as follows.

- Obesity.
- Family history of T2DM.
- *Ethnic origin:*
  - Asian;
  - African-American;
  - Afro-Caribbean;
  - Pacific-Islander;
  - Mexican-American;
  - Native American.
- Polycystic ovarian syndrome.
- Small for gestational age (SGA).

Clinical features

Clinical presentation ranges from mild incidental hyperglycaemia to the typical manifestations of insulin deficiency. Presentation with DKA may occasionally be seen. Frequent clinical findings include evidence of obesity and acanthosis nigricans.

Diagnosis

Current diagnostic prerequisites for T2DM are:
- presence of T2DM risk factors (see list in 📖 'Aetiology' above);
- lack of absolute/persistent insulin deficiency;
- absence of pancreatic autoantibodies.

Not infrequently the distinction between T1DM and T2DM at initial presentation may be difficult.

Management

All patients with T2DM require the same type and degree of educational support and clinical follow-up as for patients with T1DM. Long-term management goals are the same as for T1DM (see 📖 p.408).

Specific treatment goals should in addition include the following:
- aim to improve insulin sensitivity and insulin secretion;
- manage obesity and its comorbidities via lifestyle changes;
- screening and management of T2DM comorbidities such as hyperlipdaemia and hypertension.

Mild (incidental) T2DM should initially be managed with lifestyle interventions aimed at lowering caloric intake (low fat; reduced CHO diet) and increasing physical activity. Where these interventions fail, pharmacological therapy is added. In children, the oral insulin sensitizing agent metformin is added as a first step; however, if glycaemic targets remain difficult to achieve insulin therapy should be included.

Other forms of diabetes mellitus

Maturity onset diabetes of young (MODY)

A clinical heterogeneous group of disorders characterized by an autosomal dominant mode of inheritance, onset usually before the age of 25yrs, and non-ketotic diabetes at presentation. The condition is due a primary defect in β-cell function and insulin secretion. Six different types have been identified due to mutations in 6 different genes (see Box 12.3).

Neonatal diabetes mellitus

Rare (1/400 000–500 000 live births). Defined as hyperglycaemia requiring insulin therapy occurring in the first few weeks of life, transient (50–60%) and permanent forms are recognized.

- *Transient neonatal diabetes mellitus (TNDM):* disorder of developmental insulin production that resolves spontaneously in the postnatal period. IUGR is evident at birth and FTT and hyperglycaemia occur in the first few days. Most patients will achieve remission and insulin independence within 1yr. However, in many, persistent diabetes recurs in late childhood/adulthood. TNDM is usually sporadic. Chromosome 6 abnormalities are observed in many (paternal duplications; paternal isodisomy; methylation defects).
- *Permanent neonatal diabetes mellitus (PNDM):* rare, and may be associated with a number of clinical syndromes (IPEX syndrome—diffuse autoimmunity; severe pancreatic hypoplasia associated with IPF-1 mutation; Walcott–Rallison syndrome).
- *KCNJ11 related diabetes mellitus:* activating mutations of the KCNJ11 gene encoding the Kir62 subunit of pancreatic β-cell K+-AJP sensitive channels. Typically present in infancy and requires insulin initially. Later, treatment with oral sulphonylurea possible. Molecular genetic testing for this condition is recommended in all children with DM <1yr. This condition is associated with developmental delay and epilepsy in some cases (DEND syndrome).

Cystic fibrosis related diabetes (CFRD)

The prevalence of CFRD increases with age (~9% between ages 5 and 9yrs; 26% between ages 10 and 19yrs). It is primarily due to a defect in pancreatic insulin secretion, although modest insulin resistance is also recognized. Insulin is recommended for all patients with CFRD.

Severe insulin resistance syndromes

A rare, heterogeneous group of disorders. Genetic mutations resulting in insulin receptor and post-receptor signalling defects underlie the mechanism of severe insulin resistance. Hyperinsulinaemia is present. Common clinical features include acanthosis nigricans and evidence of ovarian hyperandrogenism in females. Syndromes associated with severe insulin resistance include:

- type A insulin resistance;
- Donohue's syndrome;
- Rabson–Mendenhal syndrome;
- partial-lipodystrophy.

Box 12.3 Types of MODY

MODY 1
- 5% of MODY cases
- Mutation in *HNF4α* gene (20q)
- Presents/onset at adolescence: <25yrs age
- Severe hyperglycaemia
- Oral agents/insulin therapy often required
- Microvascular complications: frequent/high risk

MODY 2
- 10–63% of MODY cases
- Heterozygous for mutation in glucokinase gene (7p)
- Altered glucose sensing by pancreatic β-cell
- Presents incidentally/onset early childhood
- Mild hyperglycaemia
- Diet therapy alone
- Complications: rare

MODY 3
- 20–70% of MODY cases
- Mutation in *HNF1α* gene (12q24)
- Presents/onset adolescence/<25yrs age
- Severe hyperglycaemia
- Oral agents/insulin therapy often required
- Microvascular complications: frequent/high risk

MODY 4
- Rare
- Heterozygous for mutation in *IPF-1* gene (13q)
- Onset post-pubertal
- Moderately severe diabetes
- Microvascular complications: rare

MODY 5
- ? Rare
- Mutation HNF-1β/TCF2 gene (17cen-q21.3)
- Onset post-pubertal
- Severe diabetes
- Associated renal insufficiency
- Microvascular complications: unknown

MODY 6
- Rare
- Mutation *NeuroD1/β2* gene (2q32)
- Onset post-pubertal
- ? Severe diabetes
- Microvascular complications: unknown

Goitre

A goitre is an enlargement of the thyroid gland. It may be congenital or acquired. Thyroid function may be normal (euthyroid), underactive (hypothyroid), or overactive (hyperthyroidism). Enlargement is usually 2° to increased pituitary secretion of TSH, but may, in certain cases, be due to an infiltrative process that may be either inflammatory or neoplastic.

Congenital goitre

The commonest causes of congenital goitre are due to the transplacental transmission of factors that interfere with foetal thyroid function from the mother to the foetus:
- maternal antithyroid drugs;
- maternal iodine exposure;
- maternal hyperthyroidism (Graves's disease).

Other rare causes include:
- thyroid teratoma;
- endemic iodine deficiency;
- thyroid hormone biosynthetic defects (e.g. Pendred syndrome).

Acquired goitre
- Simple (colloid) goitre.
- Multinodular goitre.
- Acute thyroiditis.
- Graves's disease.
- Anti-thyroid chemical exposure: iodine intoxication.
- Anti-thyroid drugs: lithium, amiodarone.

Simple (colloid) goitre

This is a euthyroid, non-toxic goitre of unknown cause. It is not associated with disturbance of thyroid function and is not associated with either inflammation or neoplasia. Thyroid function tests and radioisotope scans are normal. It is most common in girls during or around the peripubertal years. Treatment is not needed, although follow-up is recommended.

Multinodular goitre
- Rare.
- A firm goitre with single or multiple palpable nodules.
- Thyroid function studies usually normal, although TSH and anti-thyroid antibody titres may be elevated. Abnormalities on thyroid US and areas of reduced uptake on radioisotope scanning may be seen.

Solitary thyroid nodule

Solitary nodules of the thyroid are uncommon. Approximately 15% may be associated with underlying thyroid cancer. Careful evaluation is required. Potential causes of a solitary thyroid nodule include:

- benign adenoma;
- thyroglossal cyst;
- ectopic, normal thyroid tissue;
- single median thyroid gland;
- thyroid cyst or abscess;
- thyroid carcinoma.

Investigation should include radioisotope (^{99m}Tc) scan. Cold nodules or nodules that feel hard on palpation, or are rapidly growing should raise suspicion of thyroid cancer. Biopsy and surgical excision are indicated.

Thyroid carcinoma

Thyroid cancer is rare in childhood. Many carcinomas of the thyroid in the past were associated with previous direct irradiation to the head and neck tissues for other conditions. Carcinomas of the thyroid are histologically classified as being either papillary, follicular, or mixed. They are usually slow growing. Girls are affected twice as often as boys. Presentation is usually with a painless thyroid nodule. Cervical lymph node involvement is often evident at time of diagnosis. Metastases to the lung may be observed radiologically, but are usually asymptomatic. Diagnosis is established by biopsy. Radioisotope scans (^{123}I or ^{99m}Tc) demonstrate reduced uptake. Thyroid function tests are usually normal.

Treatment and prognosis

Thyroidectomy (subtotal or complete) is indicated. Radioiodine therapy after surgery is often given. Post-ablative oral thyroid hormone replacement therapy is needed. Prognosis is usually very good, even with presence of cervical node and/or metastases at diagnosis.

Medullary thyroid cancer

See 📖 pp.440, 615.

Congenital hypothyroidism

Hypothyroidism may be due to a number of conditions that result in insufficient secretion of thyroid hormones. Congenital hypothyroidism is a relatively common condition, occurring in approximately 1/4000 births. It is twice as common in girls than in boys.

Aetiology

The causes of congenital hypothyroidism include the following:
- *Thyroid dysgenesis (85%):* usually sporadic; resulting in thyroid aplasia/hypoplasia, ectopic thyroid (lingual/sublingual).
- *Thyroid hormone biosynthetic defect (15%):* hereditary, e.g. Pendred's syndrome.
- Iodine deficiency (rare UK; but common worldwide).
- *Congenital TSH deficiency (rare):* associated with other pituitary hormone deficiencies.

Clinical features

Usually non-specific; they are difficult to detect in first month of life. They include:
- umbilical hernia;
- prolonged jaundice;
- constipation;
- hypotonia;
- hoarse cry;
- poor feeding;
- excessive sleepiness;
- dry skin;
- coarse faecies;
- delayed neurodevelopment.

Diagnosis

In most developed countries there are national neonatal biochemical screening programmes.
- Test in 1st week of life.
- Blood spot—filter paper collection (e.g. 'Guthrie card').
- TSH (high) and/or fT4 (low) estimation.

Thyroid imaging is also recommended to determine whether the cause is due to thyroid dysgenesis or due to hormone biosynthetic disorder.
- Thyroid US.
- Radionucleotide scanning (^{99}Tc or ^{131}I).

Treatment

Without early hormone replacement therapy a number of adverse sequelae may occur.
• Neurodevelopmental delay and mental retardation.
• Poor motor coordination.
• Hypotonia.
• Ataxia.
• Poor growth and short stature.

The earlier the treatment with oral thyroid hormone replacement therapy is initiated the better the prognosis: levothyroxine (initial dose 10–15micrograms/kg/day).

Monitoring therapy

Monitor serum TSH and T4 levels:
• Every 1–2mths 1st year; every 2–3mths age 1–2yrs; every 4–6mths age >2yrs.
• Maintain T4 level in upper half of normal range; TSH in lower end of normal range.

Transient hyperthyrotropinaemia

This is uncommon and is usually detected at the time of neonatal thyroid screening. It is characterized by slightly elevated serum TSH level in presence of otherwise normal serum T4 levels. It is probably due the transplacental transmission of maternal thyroid antibodies to the child *in utero*. Presumed cases do not need treatment, but must be monitored. TSH levels that remain persistently elevated after a few months or low T4 levels should be treated with oral levothyroxine.

Acquired hypothyroidism

A relatively common condition with an estimated prevalence of 0.1–0.2% in the population. The incidence in girls is 5–10 times greater than boys.

Aetiology

Acquired hypothyroidism may be due to a primary thyroid problem or indirectly to a central disorder of hypothalamic–pituitary function.

Primary hypothyroidism (raised TSH; low T4/T3)
- Autoimmune (Hashimoto's or chronic lymphocytic thyroiditis).
- Iodine deficiency: most common cause worldwide.
- Subacute thyroiditis.
- Drugs (e.g. amiodarone, lithium).
- Post-irradiation thyroid (e.g. bone marrow transplant—total body irradiation).
- Post-ablative (radioiodine therapy or surgery).

Central hypothyroidism (low serum TSH and low T4)
Hypothyroidism due to either pituitary or hypothalamic dysfunction.
- Intracranial tumours/masses.
- Post-cranial radiotherapy/surgery.
- Developmental pituitary defects (genetic, e.g. *PROP-1*, *Pit-1* genes): isolated TSH deficiency; multiple pituitary hormone deficiencies.

Clinical features

The symptoms and signs of acquired hypothyroidism are usually insidious and can be extremely difficult to diagnose clinically. A high index of suspicion is needed.
- *Goitre:* primary hypothyroidism.
- Increased weight gain/obesity.
- Decreased growth velocity/delayed puberty.
- Delayed skeletal maturation (bone age).
- *Fatigue:* mental slowness; deteriorating school performance.
- *Constipation:* cold intolerance; bradycardia.
- *Dry skin:* coarse hair.
- *Pseudo-puberty:* girls—isolated breast development; boys—isolated testicular enlargement.
- *Slipped upper (capital) femoral epiphysis:* hip pain/limp.

Diagnosis

Diagnosis is dependent on biochemical confirmation of hypothyroid state.
- Thyroid function tests: high TSH/low T4/low T3.
- Thyroid antibody screen. Raised antibody titres:
  - antithyroid peroxidase;
  - anti-thyroglobulin;
  - TSH receptor (blocking type).

Treatment

- Oral Levothyroxine (25–200 micrograms/day).
- Monitor thyroid function test every 4–6mths during childhood.
- Monitor growth and neurodevelopment.

Hyperthyroidism (thyrotoxicosis)

- *Thyrotoxicosis:* refers to the clinical, physiological, and biochemical findings that result when the tissues are exposed to excess thyroid hormones.
- *Hyperthyroidism:* denotes those conditions resulting in hyperfunction of the thyroid gland leading to a state of thyrotoxicosis.

Causes of thyrotoxicosis

Due to hyperthyroidism

- *Excessive thyroid stimulation:*
  - Graves's disease (🕮 p.426)
  - Hashimoto's disease (Hasitoxicosis; 🕮 p.428)
  - neonatal (transient) thyrotoxicosis (🕮 pp.124, 427)
  - pituitary thyroid hormone resistance (excess TSH)
  - McCune–Albright syndrome (McAS; 🕮 p.441)
  - hCG-secreting tumours
- *Thyroid nodules (autonomous):*
  - toxic nodule/multinodular goitre
  - thyroid adenoma/carcinoma (🕮 p.421)

Not due to hyperthyroidism

- *Thyroiditis:*
  - subacute
  - drug-induced
- Exogenous thyroid hormones

Clinical features (all causes)

Thyrotoxicosis may be associated with the following symptoms:
- hyperactivity/irritability;
- poor concentration; altered mood; insomnia;
- heat intolerance/fatigue/muscle weakness/wasting;
- weight loss despite increased appetite;
- altered bowel habit—diarrhoea;
- menstrual irregularity;
- sinus tachycardia; increased pulse pressure;
- hyperreflexia; fine tremor;
- pruritis.

Investigations

- *Thyroid function tests (serum):* raised T4 and T3; suppressed TSH.
- *Thyroid antibodies:* antithyroid peroxidase; anti-thyroglobulin; TSH receptor antibody (stimulatory type).
- *Radionucleotide thyroid scan:* increased uptake (Graves's disease); decreased uptake (thyroiditis).

Graves's disease

Graves's disease is an autoimmune disorder with genetic and environmental factors contributing to susceptibility. Several HLA-DR gene loci (DR3; DQA1*0501) have been identified as susceptibility loci and there is often a family history of autoimmune thyroid disease (girls > boys). Graves's disease occurs due to a predominance of stimulating type autoantibodies to the TSH receptor.

Clinical features

In addition to those of hyperthyroidism (see 📖 p.424), Graves's disease is characterized by specific features:
• Diffuse goitre (majority).
• *Graves's ophthalmopathy:* exophthalmos/proptosis; eyelid lag or retraction; periorbital oedema/chemosis; ophthalmoplegia/extraocular muscle dysfunction.

Diagnosis

Clinical suspicion of Graves's disease requires confirmatory blood test:
• *Thyroid function tests:* high T4/high T3/low TSH.
• *Thyroid antibody screen:* antithyroid peroxidase; anti-thyroglobulin +ve; TSH receptor antibody (stimulatory type) +ve; radionucleotide thyroid scan—increased uptake.

Treatment

The aims of therapy are to induce remission of Graves's disease with antithyroid drugs (carbimazole or propylthiouracil) and, if necessary, to bring the symptoms of thyrotoxicosis (anxiety, tremor, tachycardia) under control using a β-blocking agent (propranolol). Two alternative regimens are practised.
• *Dose titration regimen:* antithyroid treatment titrated to achieve normal thyroid function.
• *Block and replace regimen:* antithyroid treatment maintained at the lowest dose necessary to induce complete thyroid suppression and therapeutic hypothyroidism. In this situation replacement thyroxine therapy is also necessary to achieve euthyroidism.

Antithyroid therapy is usually given for 12–24mths in children, before considering a trial off treatment. Thyroid function (serum-free T4; TSH levels) should be monitored at regular intervals (1–3mths).

Prognosis

Following completion of treatment 40–75% of children will relapse over the next 2yrs. Relapses may be treated with a further course of antithyroid drugs, although definitive therapy with radioiodine is being offered as the first-line treatment. Thyroid surgery is another approach for management of relapses. Following ablative treatment (either radioiodine or surgery), lifelong thyroxine replacement therapy will be required.

Neonatal thyrotoxicosis (see 📖 p.124)

- Rare and due to the passive transfer of maternal thyroid antibodies from a thyrotoxic mother to the foetus.
- Affected neonates are irritable, flushed, and tachycardic. Weight gain is poor and cardiac failure may be present.
- The condition is self-limiting. Supportive treatment, e.g. beta blocker therapy, is required.

Thyroiditis

Inflammation of the thyroid gland that may result in goitres. Initial thyrotoxicosis is usually followed by hypothyroidism. Recognized causes include:
- autoimmune thyroiditis (Hashimoto's);
- acute suppurative (pyogenic) thyroiditis;
- subacute (de Quervain) thyroiditis.

Autoimmune thyroiditis (Hashimoto's)

This is the most common cause of thyroid disease in childhood and adolescence and is the most common cause of hypothyroidism in developed countries.
- Characterized by lymphocytic infiltration of the thyroid gland and early thyroid follicular hyperplasia, which gives way to eventual atrophy and fibrosis.
- Associated with a positive family history of thyroid disease. There is an increased risk of other autoimmune disorders (e.g. type 1 diabetes).
- 4–7 times more common in females than in males.
- Children with Down's or Turner's syndrome are at increased risk.
- Peak incidence is in adolescence, although may occur at any age.

Presentation

Clinical presentation is usually insidious with a diffusely enlarged, nontender, firm goitre. Most children are asymptomatic and biochemically euthyroid. Some children may present with hypothyroidism. A few children may have symptoms suggestive of hyperthyroidism, i.e. 'Hashitoxicosis'.

The clinical course is variable. Goitres may become smaller and disappear or may persist. Many children who are initially euthyroid eventually develop hypothyroidism within a few months or years of presentation. Periodic follow-up is therefore necessary.

Investigations

- Diagnosis can be established by thyroid biopsy (but not indicated).
- Thyroid biochemistry may be normal or abnormal.
- Anti-microsomal thyroid antibody titres are usually raised, whereas anti-thyroglobulin titres are increased in only approximately 50%.

Treatment

Only required for the management of either hypothyroidism (see 📖 p.424) or hyperthyroidism if present (see 📖 p.426).

Acute suppurative thyroiditis

This is uncommon. Often preceded by respiratory tract infection.
  Organisms include *Staphylococcus aureus*, streptococci, and *Escherichia coli* (rarely, fungal infection). Abscess formation may occur.

- Presentation is with painful tender swelling of thyroid.
- Thyroid function is usually normal; however, hyperthyroidism may occur.
- Recurrent infection should raise suspicion of the presence of a thyroglossal tract remnant.
- Treatment requires administration of antibiotics and surgical drainage of abscess if present.

Subacute thyroiditis (de Quervain's)

- A self-limiting condition of viral origin, associated with tenderness and pain overlying the thyroid gland.
- Symptoms of thyrotoxicosis may be present initially, although hypothyroidism may develop later.
- Treatment includes non-steroidal anti-inflammatory agents and, in severe cases, corticosteroids (prednisolone). Beta-blocker therapy, e.g. propranolol, may help to control thyrotoxic symptoms.

Adrenal insufficiency

- 1° *adrenal failure:* results in both reduced glucocorticoid (cortisol) and mineralocorticoid (aldosterone) production. Adrenocorticotrophin (ACTH) levels are elevated due to reduced cortisol negative feedback drive.
- 2° *adrenal failure:* is due to either reduced corticotrophin-releasing factor (CoRF) or reduced ACTH production (or both) and results in reduced cortisol production only. Mineralocorticoid activity remains normal as this is mainly regulated by the angiotensin–renin system.

Causes of adrenal insufficiency

Primary

Acquired

- Autoimmune adrenalitis (Addison's disease).
- Adrenal infection, e.g. tuberculosis.
- Adrenal haemorrhage/infarction.
- Iatrogenic: adrenolectomy; drugs (e.g. ketoconazole).

Congenital

- Congenital adrenal hyperplasia (🕮 p.436).
- Congenital adrenal hypoplasia (🕮 p.439).
- Adrenoleucodystrophy.
- Familial glucocorticoid deficiency.

Secondary

- Defects of hypothalamus/pituitary structures:
  - congenital—pituitary hypoplasia;
  - intracranial masses: tumours (e.g. glioma, germinoma); craniopharyngioma;
  - intracranial inflammation: Langerhan's histiocytosis;
  - intracranial infections;
  - cranial radiotherapy/irradiation;
  - neurosurgery;
  - traumatic brain injury.
- Suppression of hypothalamic–pituitary–adrenal axis:
  - glucocorticoid therapy;
  - Cushing's disease (after pituitary tumour removal).

Clinical features

The age of onset and manifestations will depend on the underlying cause. Clinical features may be subtle and a high index of suspicion is often required. Typically, clinical features are gradual in onset with partial insufficiency leading to complete adrenal insufficiency with impaired cortisol responses to stress and illness (adrenal crises):

- anorexia and weight loss;
- fatigue and generalized weakness;
- dizziness (hypotension);
- salt craving (primary adrenal insufficiency);
- hyperpigmentation (primary adrenal insufficiency);
- reduced pubic/axillary hair (primary adrenal insufficiency);
- hypoglycaemia (neonates/infants).

Diagnosis

Basal serum cortisol and ACTH

Note: Random basal cortisol levels are often within the normal range and cannot be relied on. Inappropriately low basal cortisol during 'stress' suggests adrenal insufficiency. A basal cortisol level of >550nmol/L usually excludes this diagnosis. An elevated early morning (09.00 hours) ACTH level for the level of cortisol is suggestive of primary adrenal insufficiency.

Adrenal stimulation tests

Usually required to establish a diagnosis of adrenal insufficiency and are used to demonstrate inappropriately low serum cortisol responses to physiological or pharmacological stimulation of the adrenal glands.

- *Insulin tolerance test:* considered the gold standard test. Insulin-induced mild hypoglycaemia is used to assess the integrity of the entire hypothalamic–pituitary–adrenal axis. Serum cortisol response to hypoglycaemia (>550nmol/L) is normal.
- *ACTH stimulation (synacthen) test:* serum cortisol is measured at baseline and at +30 and +60min after IV/IM of synthetic ACTH (short synacthen test). Serum cortisol response >550nmol/L at 60min is considered normal. Recent onset secondary adrenal insufficiency may produce a normal response to a short synacthen test.

Other investigations

- *Serum electrolytes:* serum sodium (low); serum potassium (high).
- Adrenal antibody titres (Addison's disease).
- *Adrenal imaging:* US; CT scan.
- Adrenal androgen profile: serum/urine.
- Molecular genetic studies.
- *Pituitary imaging:* CT or MRI scan.

Adrenal insufficiency: treatment

Primary adrenal insufficiency requires both glucocorticoid and mineralo-corticoid replacement therapy. 2° adrenal insufficiency requires glucocorticoid therapy only.

- *Glucocorticoid therapy:*
  - *hydrocortisone*—oral 12–15mg/m^2/day in 2–3 divided doses per day. Usually about two-thirds of the dose is given in the morning, in an attempt to mimic normal diurnal variation in cortisol secretion.
  - During times of illness and stress (e.g. infection, trauma, surgery) patients are advised to increase their normal daily maintenance dose of hydrocortisone by 2 to 3 times.
- *Mineralocorticoid therapy:* fludrocortisone—oral 50–150micrograms/ day. Monitor BP and plasma renin levels.

Adrenal crises

An adrenal (or Addisonian) crisis is an acute exacerbation of an underlying adrenal insufficiency brought on by 'stresses' that necessitate increased production and secretion of cortisol from the adrenal gland. This is a life-threatening emergency and should be treated if there is a strong clinical suspicion rather than waiting for confirmatory test results. Typical causes include infection, trauma, and surgery. Symptoms include:

- nausea/vomiting;
- abdominal pain;
- lethargy/somnolence;
- hypotension.

Treatment

- Immediate IV bolus of hydrocortisone followed by 6-hourly repeat injections.
- IVI fluids/glucose.

Adrenal excess

A state of glucocorticoid (cortisol) excess. The commonest cause of hypercortisolaemia is iatrogenic, due to exogenous steroids. Hyperfunction of the adrenal cortex resulting in excess cortisol secretion may have 1° (adrenal or ACTH-independent) or 2° (ACTH-dependent) causes. The term Cushing's disease applies to an ACTH-secreting pituitary tumour. All other causes of glucocorticoid excess are often referred to as Cushing's syndrome.

Causes of adrenal (cortisol) excess

- Iatrogenic.
- *1° adrenal hyperfunction (ACTH-independent):*
  - adrenal tumour (carcinoma/adenoma);
  - nodular adrenal hyperplasia;
  - McAS (📖 p.441).
- *2° adrenal hyperfunction (ACTH-dependent):*
  - Cushing's disease—pituitary ademona/hyperplasia;
  - ectopic ACTH secretion (tumour).

In young children (<5yrs) adrenal disorders are the most common, non-iatrogenic, cause of hypercorticolism. In neonates and infants, McAS should be considered. In older children and adolescents Cushing's disease is most common.

Clinical features

All causes of hypercortisolaemia are characterized by the following pattern of clinical signs and symptoms.

- *Obesity:* central adiposity—face, trunk, abdomen.
- 'Moon' faecies.
- *Buffalo hump:* prominent/enlarged posterior cervical/supraclavicular fat pads.
- Muscle wasting.
- Proximal muscle weakness.
- *Skin abnormalities:* thinning (rare in children); easy bruising; striae (abdomen/thighs).
- Hypertension.
- *Growth impairment:* reduced growth velocity; short stature.
- Pubertal delay/amenorrhoea.
- Osteoporosis.

Note: Other signs may be present depending on the underlying cause. Children with adrenal tumours may have signs of abnormal virilization and masculinization (early pubic hair, hirsuitism, acne, clitoromegaly) due to excess adrenal androgen secretion.

Investigations

These are directed at establishing a diagnosis of hypercortisolism and thereafter at differentiating between ACTH-dependent and ACTH-independent causes (see Box 12.4).

Box 12.4 Investigations to determine the following

Is hypercortisolism present or not?
- *Serum cortisol circadian rhythm:*
  - midnight serum cortisol. *Note:* Patients must be asleep at time of sampling for test to be valid
  - Loss of normal diurnal variation—raised midnight value observed.
- *Urinary free cortisol excretion: 24hr collection*
- *Dexamethasone suppression test:*
  - overnight test (1mg dexamethasone at midnight)
  - low dose test (0.5mg every 6hr for 48hr)
  - failure of suppression of plasma cortisol levels is observed

Cause of hypercortisolism
- *Plasma ACTH:* high in ACTH-dependent causes
- *Dexamethasone suppression test:*
  - high dose test (2mg every 6hr for 48hr)
  - in Cushing's disease serum cortisol levels decrease by approximately 50%. Ectopic ACTH secretion: no suppression.
- CoRF test
- CT scan of adrenal glands
- MRI scan of brain
- Bilateral inferior petrosal sinus sampling

Management

Cushing's disease
- Preoperative treatment in order to normalize blood cortisol levels:
  - metyrapone;
  - ketaconazole.
- Pituitary surgery: transsphenoidal surgery.
- Pituitary radiotherapy.

Adrenal disease/tumour
- Surgery, i.e. adrenalectomy.

Congenital adrenal hyperplasia

Congenital adrenal hyperplasia (CAH) is a family of disorders character-ized by enzyme defects in the steroidogenic pathways that lead to the bio-synthesis of cortisol, aldosterone, and androgens. The relative decrease in cortisol production, acting via the classic negative feedback loop, results in increased secretion of ACTH from the anterior pituitary gland and to sub-sequent hyperplasia of the adrenals. All forms of CAH are inherited in an autosomal recessive manner, and their clinical manifestation is determined by the effects produced by the particular hormones that are deficient and by the excess production of steroids unaffected by the enzymatic block.

The causes of CAH include deficiencies in the following steroidogenic pathway enzymes:

- 21α-hydroxylase (CYP21);
- 11β-hydroxylase (CYP11);
- 3β-hydroxysteroid dehydrogenase;
- 17α-hydroxylase/17–20 lyase (CYP17);
- side-chain cleavage (SCC/StAR).

Deficiency of the 21-hydroxylase enzyme is the most common form of CAH, accounting for over 90% of cases.

21α-hydroxylase deficiency

CAH due to deficiency of the 21α-hydroxylase enzyme arises as a result of deletions or deleterious mutations in the active gene (CYP21) located on chromosome 6p. Many different mutations of the CYP21 gene have been identified, causing varying degrees of impairment of 21α-hydroxylase ac-tivity that result in a spectrum of disease expression. CAH can be classified according to symptoms and signs and to age of presentation.

- *Classic CAH:* includes a severe 'salt wasting' form that usually presents with acute adrenal crisis in early infancy (usually males at 7–10 days of life), and a 'simple virilizing' form in which patients demonstrate masculinization of the external genitalia (females at birth) or signs of virilization in early life in males.
- *Non-classic (late onset) CAH:* this presents in females with signs and symptoms of mild androgen excess at or around the time of puberty.

The incidence of CAH due to 21α-hydroxylase deficiency has been reported to be in the region of 1 in 10,000–17,000 in Western Europe and the USA, with an overall worldwide figure of approximately 1/14,000 births.

Diagnosis

'Classic' CAH is diagnosed by demonstrating characteristic biochemical abnormalities, which are present regardless of severity, age, and sex of the infant:

- elevated plasma 17-hydroxyprogesterone levels;
- elevated plasma 21-deoxycortisol levels;
- increased urinary adrenocorticosteroid metabolites.

Note: It may be difficult to distinguish elevated androgen levels from the physiological hormonal surge that occurs in the first 2 days of life. These tests should be postponed or repeated after 48hr of age.

In the 'salt-wasting' form, the aldosterone deficiency results in hyponatraemia, hyperkalaemia, and metabolic acidosis. However, these are not specific findings and can cause diagnostic confusion with children presenting with more common causes of renal tubular dysfunction, such as acute pyelonephritis.

Treatment

Glucocorticoid replacement therapy

Required in all patients. In addition to treating cortisol deficiency, this therapy also suppresses the ACTH-dependent excess adrenal androgen production. Standard therapy usually consists of: hydrocortisone: oral $15mg/m^2$/day in 3 or 4 divided doses.

As in other disorders associated with cortisol insufficiency, during periods of stress and illness increased amounts (e.g. double or triple dose) of glucocorticoid therapy are required.

Mineralocorticoid therapy

For the salt-wasting form of CAH only: fludrocortisone: oral 50–300micrograms/day.

Sodium chloride therapy

Resistance to mineralocorticoid therapy is usually seen in infancy. Sodium chloride supplements are often required during this period of life to maintain normal electrolyte balance. Once a normal solid diet is established salt supplements may be discontinued.

Sodium chloride solution: oral, added to feed, 2–10mmol/kg/day in divided doses.

Urogenital surgery

Reconstructive surgery (clitoral reduction and vaginoplasty) is usually performed in infancy in females with significant virilization of the external genitalia.

Long-term management and monitoring

Regular monitoring of patients by a specialist team is required in order to ensure the child's optimal growth and development.

Mineralocorticoid excess

The principal mineralocorticoid secreted by the adrenal gland is aldosterone. Increased production may result from a primary defect of the adrenal gland (primary hyperaldosteronism) or from factors that activate the renin–angiotensin system (secondary hyperaldosteronism). Hypokalaemia and hypertension are typical features.

Primary hyperaldosteronism

Characterized by hypokalaemia and hypertension. There is suppression of the renin–angiotensin system with low plasma renin levels. Children may have no symptoms, the diagnosis being established after the incidental finding of hypertension. Chronic hypokalaemia may result in muscle weakness, fatigue, and poor growth.

Causes of primary hyperaldosteronism

- Bilateral adrenal hyperplasia
- Adrenal tumours
- Glucocorticoid-remediable hyperaldosteronism

Secondary hyperaldosteronism

This occurs when excess aldosterone production is secondary to elevated renin levels. Hypertension may or may not be present.

Causes of secondary hyperaldosteronism

Associated with hypertension
- Renovascular malformations/stenosis
- Primary hyperreninaemia
- Juxtaglomerular tumour
- Wilm's tumour (🕮 p.668)
- Post-renal transplantation
- Urinary tract obstruction
- Phaeochromocytoma

No hypertension
- Hepatic cirrhosis (see 🕮 p.344)
- Congestive cardiac failure
- Nephrotic syndrome (see 🕮 p.378)
- Bartter's syndrome (see 🕮 p.386)
- Anorexia nervosa (see 🕮 p.594)
- Syndrome of apparent mineralocorticoid excess: type 1 and type 2 variants

Mineralocorticoid deficiency

Reduced aldosterone production or activity is rare and may be due to congenital or acquired causes.

- Aldosterone synthase deficiency:
  - type 1;
  - type 2.
- Pseudohypoaldosteronism:
  - type 1;
  - type 2.
- Hyporeninaemic hypoaldosteronism.
- Hyperreninaemic hypoaldosteronism.
- Transient hypoaldosteronism in infancy.
- Congenital adrenal hyperplasia:
  - 17α-hydroxylase (CYP17) deficiency;
  - 11β-hydroxylase (CYP11) deficiency.
- Congenital adrenal hypoplasia.
- Primary adrenocortical insufficiency.
- Iatrogenic hypoaldosteronism.

Inherited endocrine syndromes

Multiple endocrine neoplasia

This is a family of endocrine neoplasia syndromes that are inherited in an autosomal dominant manner:
- multiple endocrine neoplasia (MEN) type 1;
- MEN type 2;
- Von Hippel–Lindau (VHL) syndrome.

The molecular genetic defects for these syndromes have been identified and genetic screening is available. Patients with these conditions require close surveillance and screening (biochemistry, radiology, etc.).

Multiple endocrine neoplasia (MEN) type 1

The condition is characterized by the following clinical features.
- Hyperparathyroidism (90%). Due to parathyroid hyperplasia. Usually presents in second decade of life.
- Pancreatic endocrine tumours (75%). Typically multifocal, pancreatic islet cell tumours. Include insulinoma (60%); gastrinoma (30%); VIPoma (rare); glucagonoma (rare). Present in adulthood.
- Pituitary adenomas (10–65%). Prolactinoma (60%); GH-secreting (30%).
- Other features: thyroid adenoma; thymic/bronchial carcinoid tumours; lipomas.

Multiple endocrine neoplasia type 2

MEN type 2 belongs to a family of three syndromes (MEN type 2A; MEN type 2B; familial medullary thyroid cancer) characterized by activating mutations in the *RET* proto-oncogene. Medullary thyroid cancer is a common feature in all the syndromes.

MEN type 2A
- Medullary thyroid cancer (90%).
- Phaeochromocytoma (50%).
- Parathyroid ademona (25%).

MEN type 2B
- Medullary thyroid cancer (90%).
- Phaeochromocytoma.
- Mucosal/intestinal ganglioneuromas.
- Marfanoid body habitus.
- Hirschsprung's disease.

Familial medullary thyroid cancer
Isolated medullary thyroid cancer.

von Hippel–Lindau syndrome (VHL)

This condition is due to a mutation in the *VHL* gene. This is a tumour repressor gene that is located on chromosome 3.
   The condition is characterized by the following features:
- *Retinal haemangioblastomas (40%):*
  - Uncommon before age 10yrs.
  - Bleeding and retinal detachment.

- *CNS haemangioblastomas:* 75% occur in cerebellum.
- *Phaeochromocytomas (20%):* bilateral in 40%.
- *Renal cysts and carcinomas:*
  - Late feature: from 4th decade.
  - Occur in 70% by age 60yrs.
- *Pancreatic neuroendocrine tumours:* uncommon. 50% malignant. Most are non-functioning tumours, but may be secreting (insulin, glucagons, VIP).
- *Simple adenomas/cysts:* uncommon.
  - Pancreas; liver; epididymis; lung.
  - Meningioma.

McCune–Albright Syndrome

Characterized by the following triad of clinical features:
- *Skin:* hyperpigmented (*café au lait*) macules.
  - classically, irregular edge (so-called 'coast of Maine' appearance);
  - do not cross midline.
- *Polyostic fibrous dysplasia:*
  - slowly progressive bone lesion;
  - any bones, although facial/base of skull bones most commonly affected.
- *Autonomous endocrine gland hyperfunction:*
  - ovary most commonly affected;
  - precocious puberty (gonadotrophin-indepdent);
  - thyroid (hyperthyroidism);
  - adrenal (Cushing's syndrome);
  - pituitary (adenoma—gigantism);
  - parathyroid (hyperparathyroidism).

Neurofibromatosis

See also 📖 pp.531, 662, 946. Two types of neurofibromatosis (NF) are recognized. Type 1 (NF-1; also known as von Recklinghausen's disease) is an autosomal dominant condition due to a mutation of the *NF-1* gene (📖 Chapter 25).

NF-1 may be associated with endocrine abnormalities:
- Hypothalamic/pituitary tumours: optic glioma (15%).
- GH deficiency.
- Precocious puberty.
- Delayed puberty.

Hypocalcaemia

Most causes of low calcium (hypocalcaemia) can be explained by abnormalities of vitamin D or PTH metabolism or by disordered kidney function. The principal manifestations of hypocalcaemia are related to neuromuscular irritability and include tetany and paraesthesiae.

- Hypocalcaemic seizures (grand-mal type) or laryngeal spasm may occur acutely.
- Cardiac conduction abnormalities (prolonged QT interval, QRS and ST changes, and ventricular arrhythmias) may be seen.

Chronic hypocalcaemia may be asymptomatic. The child's age is helpful in determining the differential diagnosis of hypocalcaemia.

> ### Causes of hypocalcaemia
>
> *Early neonatal causes*
> - Prematurity
> - Maternal diabetes
> - Maternal pre-eclampsia
> - RDS
>
> *Late neonatal causes*
> - Cow's milk hyperphosphataemia
> - Maternal hypercalcaemia
> - Congenital hypoparathyroidism
>
> *Causes in infancy*
> - Nutritional rickets
> - Pseudohypoparathroidism type 1a
>
> *Childhood causes*
> - Pseudohypoparathyroidism type 1b
> - Hypoparathyroidism
>
> *Iatrogenic causes*
> - Chemotherapy agents, e.g. cisplatin
> - Anticonvulsant agents, e.g. phenytoin

Investigations

- Plasma calcium.
- Plasma phosphate.
- Serum PTH. *Note:* Low or even normal PTH concentration implies failure of PTH secretion.
- Plasma vitamin D.
- Plasma magnesium.
- X-ray of skull. Chronic hypocalcaemia: basal ganglia calcification may be seen.

Treatment

Acute treatment See 📖 p.93.

Chronic treatment
- Should be directed at the underlying cause.
- Oral calcium supplements, together with oral vitamin D therapy in the form of calcitriol (1-α calcidiol) are often required to maintain plasma calcium levels within the normal range.

Hypoparathyroidism

Low serum parathyroid hormone levels in childhood may be due to the following:
- *Failure in parathyroid development (agenesis/dysgenesis):*
  - isolated defect: X-linked recessive;
  - associated with other abnormalities, e.g. DiGeorge syndrome, Kearnes–Sayre syndrome.
- *Destruction of parathyroid glands:*
  - autoimmune—type 1 autoimmune polyendocrinopathy;
  - surgery (post-thyroidectomy);
  - radiotherapy.
- *Failure in PTH secretion: magnesium deficiency.*
- *Failure in PTH action: pseudohypoparathyrodism.*

Investigations
- *Plasma calcium:* low.
- *Plasma phosphate:* high.
- *Serum PTH:* low.

Pseudohypoparathyroidism (PHP)

Characterized by end-organ resistance to the actions of PTH. It is a genetic disorder due to a defect in the G_s α-adenylate cyclase signalling system common to the PTH receptor and other endocrine receptors belonging to the G protein-receptor family (e.g. TSH, LH, FSH). See Table 12.2.

Table 12.2 Classification of pseudohypoparathyroidism (PHP)

Classification	Pathophysiology	AHO*	Other hormone resistance	Urinary cAMP response to PTH
PHP Ia	GNAS1 mutation	Yes	Yes	Decreased
Pseudo PHP	GNAS1 mutation	Yes	No	Normal
PHP Ib	G_sα-related protein	No	No	Decreased
PHP Ic	? Receptor signal transduction	Yes	Yes	Decreased
PHP II	cAMP dependent protein	No	No	Normal

* AHO, Albright hereditary osteodystrophy (short stature and short metacarpels).

Rickets

A disorder of the growing skeleton due to inadequate mineralization of bone as it is laid down at the epiphyseal growth plates. There is a characteristic widening of the ends of long bones and characteristic radiology. *Osteomalacia* occurs when there is inadequate mineralization of mature bone. Both rickets and osteomalacia may be present at the same time.

Causes

Malnutrition and calcium deficiency are common causes worldwide. Vitamin D deficiency is rare in developed countries, although inadequate exposure to sunlight and exclusive breastfeeding of 6–12mths during infancy are well recognized causes.

Calcium deficiency Dietary; malabsorption.

Vitamin D
- *Vitamin D deficiency:* dietary; malabsorption; lack of sunlight; iatrogenic (drug-induced, e.g. phenytoin therapy).
- *Defect in vitamin D metabolism:* vitamin D-dependent rickets type I (1α-hydroxylase deficiency); liver disease; renal disease.
- *Defect in vitamin D action:* vitamin D-dependent rickets type II.

Phosphate deficiency
- *Renal tubular phosphate loss (isolated): hypophosphataemic rickets:*
  - X-linked (see 📖 p.445);
  - autosomal recessive;
  - autosomal dominant.
- *Acquired hypophosphataemic rickets:*
  - Fanconi syndrome (see 📖 pp.372, 384);
  - renal tubular acidosis;
  - nephrotoxic drugs.
- Reduced phosphate intake.

Clinical features
- Growth delay or arrest.
- Bone pain and fracture.
- Muscle weakness.
- Skeletal deformities:
  - swelling of wrists;
  - swelling of costochondral junctions ('rickety rosary');
  - bowing of the long bones;
  - frontal cranial bossing;
  - craniotabes (softening of skull).

Diagnosis
- *Laboratory (see Table 12.3):*
  - plasma calcium/phosphate/alkaline phosphatase/PTH;
  - vitamin D metabolites (25-hydroxyvitamin-D3 (25 OHD)/1,25-dihydroxyvitamin-D3 (1,25 OHD)).
- *Radiological:* X-ray of wrists (generalized osteopenia/widening, cupping and fraying of metaphyses).

There are three characteristic stages in disease progression:
- *Stage 1:* low plasma calcium/normal plasma phosphate.
- *Stage 2:* normal plasma calcium (restored due to compensatory hyperparathyroidism).
- *Stage 3:* low plasma calcium and phosphate—advanced bone disease.

Stages 1 and 2 are biochemically evident only. Stage 3 has clinical features.

Table 12.3 Laboratory findings in different types of rickets

	Plasma Ca	Plasma PO4	ALP	25, OHD	1,25 OHD	PTH
Vit. D deficiency	↓	↓	↑	↓	↓	↑
VDDR, type I	↓	↓	↑	↔	↓	↑
VDDR, type II	↓	↓	↑	↔	↑	↑
X-linked hypophos-phataemic	↔	↓	↑	↔	↔	↔ or ↑
Renal tubular acidosis	↓ or ↔	↓	↑	↔	↔ or ↑	↔

Vitamin D-dependent rickets (VDDR) type I

Autosomal recessive condition. Due to a deficiency in renal 1α-hydroxylase, the enzyme responsible for the conversion of 25-hydroxyvitamin-D3 to 1, 25 dihydroxyvitamin-D3. The condition is due to mutations in the 1α-hydroxylase gene, P450c1α.

Patients usually present with evidence of severe clinical rickets within the first 24mths of life.

Treatment Requires replacement dose of 1, 25 dihydroxyvitamin-D3 (calcitriol).

Vitamin D-dependent rickets type II

Autosomal recessive condition. This disorder is due to mutations in the vitamin D receptor gene, leading to end-organ resistance to vitamin D. The condition is also referred to as vitamin D resistant rickets.

Clinical, laboratory, and radiological features are similar to those seen in vitamin D deficiency and VDDR type I. However, a striking feature observed in the majority of patients with VDDR-type II is sparse body hair development or total alopecia. This finding is usually present at birth or develops during the 1st year of life.

Treatment with supraphysiological doses of 1, 25 dihydroxyvitamin-D3 (e.g. up to 60mcg/day of calcitriol) is often successful, although responses are highly variable.

Hypercalcaemia

There are a number of different causes of high plasma calcium levels:
- William's syndrome.
- Idiopathic infantile hypercalcaemia.
- Hyperparathyroidism.
- Hypercalcaemia of malignancy.
- Vitamin D intoxication.
- Familial hypocalciuric hypercalcaemia.

Other uncommon causes include: sarcoidois and other granulomatous disease; chronic immobilization; renal failure; hyperthyroidism; Addison's disease; iatrogenic, e.g. thiazide diuretics.

Clinical features

Symptoms and signs of hypercalcaemia are non-specific.
- *GI:* anorexia; nausea and vomiting; failure to thrive; constipation; abdominal pain.
- *Renal:* polyuria and polydipsia.
- *CNS:* apathy; drowsiness; depression.

Investigations

Laboratory
- Plasma calcium (total and corrected for albumin).
- Serum PTH.
- Vitamin D metabolites.
- U&E/LFTs.
- TFT.
- Urinary calcium excretion (UCa:UCr ratio; 24hr UCa).

Radiological Renal US scan (screen for nephrocalcinosis).

Treatment

Acute treatment See ☐ p.447.

Chronic treatment Directed at the underlying cause.

Hyperparathyroidism

Uncommon in children, excessive production of PTH may result from a primary defect of the parathyroid glands or may be secondary and compensatory to either hypocalcaemia or hyperphosphataemic states.

- 1° *hyperparathyroidism*:
  - parathyroid adenoma;
  - parathyroid hyperplasia: MEN type 1; MEN type 2; neonatal severe form.
- 2° *hyperparathyroidism*:
  - *hypocalcaemic states*—rickets;
  - *hyperphosphatemia*—chronic renal failure.
- *Transient neonatal hyperparathyroidism: m*aternal hypoparathyroidism.

Primary hyperparathyroidism

Rare in children. In the neonatal period it usually associated with generalized parathyroid hyperplasia. In older children it is usually due to a parathyroid adenoma and most often associated with MEN type 1.

Transient neonatal hyperparathyroidism

Observed in neonates born to mother with previously undetected and/ or untreated hypoparathyroidism or pseudohypoparathyroidism. Chronic intrauterine hypocalcaemia results in hyperplasia of the foetal parathyroid glands.

Neonatal severe hyperparathyroidism
See Familial hypocalciuric hypercalcaemia.

Hypercalcaemia of malignancy

Rarely, in children with endocrine tumours (e.g. phaeochromocytoma) or other tumours (e.g. lymphoma), production of humoral factors such as PTH-related peptide (PTHrP) results in hypercalcaemia.

Treatment requires resection and removal of the tumour to reverse the hypercalcaemic state. Interim control can be achieved with a single IV infusion of a bisphosphonate agent, e.g. pamidronate. The latter enhances calcium bone resorption.

Familial hypocalciuric hypercalcaemia

Autosomal dominant disorder caused by a mutation of the calcium-sensing receptor (*CaSR*) gene. This is a benign, mostly asymptomatic disorder, which is often an incidental finding during routine biochemistry analysis. Plasma calcium levels are raised (but usually <3mmol/L), and urinary calcium excretion is low. PTH levels are inappropriately normal for the degree of hypercalcaemia.

Note: Those homozygous for the mutation have severe, life-threatening primary hyperparathyroidism at birth. This form of neonatal severe hyperparathyroidism requires immediate parathyroid surgery.

Posterior pituitary: syndrome of inappropriate antidiuretic hormone secretion

Heterogeneous disorder characterized by hypotonic *hyponatraemia* and impaired urinary dilution that cannot be accounted for by a recognized stimulus to ADH secretion. Plasma ADH is elevated or inadequately suppressed. Several different types of pathogenic mechanisms are likely to be responsible for this. There are many causes of SIADH (Box 12.5).

> **Box 12.5 Causes of SIADH**
>
> - *Congenital:* agenesis of corpus callosum
> - *Acquired:*
>   - *CNS*—traumatic brain injury, cerebrovascular bleeding
>   - *Tumours*—brain, lung, thymus
>   - *Infection*—pneumonia, meningitis, encephalitis, TB
>   - *Neurological*—Guillain–Barré syndrome
>   - *Respiratory*—asthma, pneumothorax
>   - *Drugs*—vincristine, cyclophosphamide

Up to 15% of children presenting with brain trauma or infection develop SIADH. Clinical features include development of: confusion; headache; lethargy; seizures and coma.

Symptoms do not necessarily depend on the concentration of serum sodium, but on its rate of development. Slow, gradual development of hyponatraemia may be asymptomatic.

SIADH diagnostic criteria

- Hyponatraemia (serum Na^+ <135mmol/L)
- Hypotonic plasma (osmolality <270mOsm/kg)
- Excessive renal sodium loss (>20mmol/L)
- No hypovolaemia or fluid overload
- Normal renal, adrenal, and thyroid function
- Increased plasma ADH

Management

Treatment of the underlying cause is necessary. Fluid restriction is the mainstay of therapy.

- Hypertonic (3%) saline solution may be used to correct severe hyponatraemia, or hyponatraemia resistant to fluid restriction.
- Slow correction of hyponatraemia is essential to avoid rapid overcorrection with possible complication of central pontine demyelination.
- Longer-term management/treatment with demeclocycline may be effective for fluid balance by inducing nephrogenic DI.

Hypopituitarism

Hypopituitarism refers to either partial or complete deficiency of the anterior and/or posterior pituitary function. Hypopituitarism may be congenital or acquired, secondary to pituitary disease or to hypothalamic pathology that interferes with pituitary function. Clinical features depend on the type of hormone deficiency, its severity, and rate of development.

Congenital hypopituitarism

Mutations in pituitary transcription factor genes (e.g. *HESX-1*, *PIT-1*, *LHX-4*) can result in isolated or multiple anterior pituitary hormone deficiencies.

A number of specific inherited genetic defects have been characterized. Abnormalities in the hypothalamic–pituitary structures and other midline brain structures (e.g. septo-optic dysplasia; optic nerve hypoplasia; absent corpus callosum) are often detected on imaging.

Acquired hypopituitarism

Potential causes of pituitary hormone deficiency include the following:
- Intracranial (parapituitary) tumours.
- *Cranial irradiation/radiotherapy:* GH axis is the most sensitive to radiation damage, followed by gonadotrophin, and adrenal axes, and finally by thyroid axis.
- Traumatic brain injury.
- *Inflammatory/infiltrative disease:* Langerhan's cell histiocytosis; sarcoidosis.
- Pituitary infarction (apoplexy).
- Intracranial infection.

Investigations

- *Basal hormone levels:* e.g. LH/FSH; TSH, fT4; prolactin; cortisol (9 a.m.); IGF-I.
- *Dynamic endocrine testing:* specific tests to assess secretory capacity of the anterior pituitary gland.
- *MRI scan:* brain.

Treatment involves adequate and appropriate hormone replacement therapy and, where applicable, management of underlying cause.

Posterior pituitary: diabetes insipidus

The posterior pituitary gland secretes two hormones, arginine vasopressin (AVP) and oxytocin.

Diabetes insipidus (DI) is defined as the inappropriate passage of large volumes of dilute urine (<300mOsm/L). Due to either deficiency in AVP production (cranial DI) or resistance to its actions at the kidney (nephrogenic DI). The most common cause of DI is primary deficiency of AVP production (i.e. cranial DI). This may be acquired or inherited in origin.

Classification of diabetes insipidus

Cranial DI

Inherited/familial
- Autosomal dominant
- Autosomal recessive
- X-linked recessive (Xq28)
- Wolfram syndrome (4p WFS1)

Congenital
- Midline craniofacial defects
- Holoprosencephaly

Acquired
- Intracranial tumours
  - Craniopharyngioma
  - Germinoma
- Traumatic brain injury
- Infiltrative/inflammation:
  Langerhan's cell histiocytosis
- CNS infection

Primary polydipsia
- Psychogenic
- Dipsogenic (abnormal thirst)

Nephrogenic DI

Inherited/familial
- Autosomal dominant:
  Aquaporin-2 gene
- Autosomal recessive:
  Aquaporin-2 gene
- X-linked recessive:
  ADH receptor-2 gene

Acquired
- Idiopathic
- Drugs (lithium; cisplatin)
- Metabolic (hypercalcaemia)

Children present with polydipsia, polyuria, and nocturia, which must be distinguished from more common causes. Infants may exhibit failure to thrive, fever, and constipation. Other symptoms may be related to the underlying cause, e.g. headache, visual acuity/visual field impairment.

Diagnosis

When suspected, assessment of 24hr urinary volume and osmolality under conditions of *ad libitum* fluid intake should be undertaken. Serum osmolality, U&E (Na$^+$), and blood glucose should also be measured.

Blood hypertonicity (serum osmolality >300mOsm) with inappropriate urine hypotonicity (urine osmolality <300mOsm) should be demonstrated. Diabetes mellitus and renal failure should be excluded.

A water deprivation test (see Box 12.6) and assessment of responses to exogenously administered ADH is required to diagnose the type of DI. Other tests to determine the underlying cause of DI will also be needed (e.g. cranial MRI imaging).

Box 12.6 Water deprivation test

Should be carried out in conditions of strict monitoring and in centres with experience with this test:
- Allow fluids overnight. If primary polydipsia is suspected consider overnight fluid deprivation to avoid over hydration
- Commence fluid deprivation at 8 a.m.
- Serum osmolality, serum Na^+, urine osmolalitiy. Each time urine sample voided
- Duration of water deprivation is seldom longer than 8–12hr in children and 6–8hr in young infants. In any case, the water deprivation is terminated if there is either:
  - urine osmolality concentrated: ≥800mOsm/kg or
  - thirst becomes intolerable or
  - 5% dehydration (5% weight loss) or
- Serum osmolality: ≥300mOsm/L.
- In those with inadequate urinary concentration, desmopressin is administered: DDAVP 0.1mg/kg to maximum of 4mg IM
- Interpretation of results: see table that follows

| | Urine osmolality (mOsm/kg) | |
	After fluid deprivation	After DDAVP
Cranial DI (CDI)	<300	>800
Nephrogenic	<300	<300
Primary polydipsia	>800	>800
Partial CDI/polydipsia	>00–800	<800

Treatment

Cranial DI Synthetic analogue of ADH, DDAVP, which has a longer duration of action, can be given intranasal or oral. Dose required varies considerably and must be titrated for each patient. The dose and frequency of administration (1–3 times a day) is adjusted to maintain 24hr urine output volume within the normal range. Water retention should be avoided. It is essential to educate all patients and families about the hazards of excessive water intake. Patients with an intact thirst sensation mechanism should achieve this.

Nephrogenic DI Correction of underlying metabolic or iatrogenic causes, if possible. Maintenance of an adequate fluid input is essential. Thiazide diuretics (e.g. hydrochlorthiazide), amiloride, and prostaglandin synthase inhibitors (e.g. indomethacin) can be effective.

Primary polydipsia Treatment is often difficult. Behaviour modification strategies usually required.

Polycystic ovarian syndrome

Polycystic ovarian syndrome (PCOS) is a common (5 to 10%) heterogeneous condition, affecting females of reproductive age that is increasingly identified in the adolescent population. It is a life-long condition characterised by chronic anovulation, disordered gonadotrophin release, ovarian and adrenal hyperandrogenism, and insulin resistance.

The pathogenesis of PCOS is uncertain, however, both genetic and environmental factors are thought to play a role. Risk factors include low birth weight for gestational age, premature adrenarche, atypical early pubertal development and obesity. A family history of PCOS is often observed.

The current diagnostic criteria for PCOS are defined as the presence of any two of the following three features:
• Oligo-and/or anovulation.
• Clinical or biochemical evidence of hyperandrogenism, provided other aetiologies of androgen excess (e.g. congenital adrenal hyperplasia, androgen-secreting tumours, Cushing's syndrome) have been excluded.
• Polycystic ovaries on US scan (i.e. the presence of 12 or more follicles in each ovary, measuring 2–9mm in diameter, and/or increased ovarian volume (>10mL)).

The clinical and biochemical features of the syndrome are variable and the combination and degree of expression of these features vary between individuals.

Typical signs and symptoms develop during or after puberty and may include any of the following:
• oligo/amenorrhea;
• hirsuitism;
• acne;
• obesity;
• acanthosis nigricans.

Laboratory finding include:
• Elevated androgen concentrations (e.g. testosterone; dehydroepiandrosterone sulphate (DHEAS)).
• Elevated plasma LH:FSH ratio.
• Decreased sex hormone binding globulin (SHBG) concentrations.
• Hyperinsulinaemia (fasting, oral glucose tolerance test (OGTT), IVGT samples).
• Decreased IGFBP-1 concentrations.

PCOS is recognized to have important long-term health implications and is particularly associated with a range of abnormalities that are characteristic of the metabolic syndrome. These include hyperinsulinaemia, impaired pancreatic β-cell function, the development of obesity, hyperlipidaemia, and an increased risk of T2DM and cardiovascular disease in later life. In addition, chronic anovulation is thought to carry an increased risk of endometrial cancer.

Treatment of PCOS is symptomatic and is directed at the presenting clinical problems. Lifestyle modifications are an important first-line intervention particularly when obesity is evident. Other treatment approaches include the use of the following drugs:

- Metformin (insulin sensitizer).
- Combined oral contraceptive pill (suppress ovarian hyperandorgenism).
- Spironolactone (anti-androgen).
- Cyproterone acetate (synthetic progesterone—anti-androgen).
- Flutamide (anti-androgen).

Cosmetic treatments such as electrolysis, laser hair removal, waxing, and bleaching, and use of topical depilatory creams may be used when hirsutism is a predominant clinical feature.

Growth and puberty

Normal growth

Normal human growth can be divided into two distinct phases: prenatal (foetal) and postnatal.

Prenatal/foetal growth

This is the fastest period of growth, accounting for around 30% of eventual height. Factors that determine growth during this period include maternal size, maternal nutrition, and intrauterine environment. Hormonal factors such as insulin, insulin-like growth factor (IGF)–II, and human placental lactogen are important regulators of growth during this period.

Postnatal growth

This is classically divided into three overlapping periods.

Infantile period

From birth to 18–24mths of age. Rapid but decelerating growth rate (growth velocity range: 22–8cm/yr). Growth is largely under nutritional regulation during this period. Some infants (15–20%) may show significant catch-up or catch-down in length and weight. By age 2yrs, height is more predictive of final adult height than at birth.

Childhood period

From age 2yrs until onset of puberty. Characterized by a slow, steady growth velocity (range 8–5cm/yr). Growth is primarily dependent on growth hormone (GH), provided there is adequate nutrition and health.

Puberty

Growth during this period is dependent on growth hormone (GH) and the actions of sex steroid hormones (testosterone and oestrogen). This combination induces the characteristic 'growth spurt' of puberty. In both males and females, oestrogen induces the maturation of the epiphyseal growth centres of the bones, eventually resulting in fusion of the growth plates, the cessation of linear growth, and the attainment of final height.

Sex differences in growth during puberty

The onset of the pubertal growth spurt is earlier in females compared with males. Females are therefore, on average, taller than males between the ages of 10 and 13yrs. In males, the pubertal growth spurt is later in onset and greater in magnitude. As a result males are, on average, 12–13cm taller than females at final height.

Normal puberty

Puberty is a well-defined sequence of physical and physiological changes occurring during the adolescent years that culminates in attainment of full physical and sexual maturity.

- Nocturnal, pulsatile, secretion of the hormone luteinizing hormone-releasing hormone (LHRH) by the hypothalamus is the first step in the imitation of puberty. This results in the pulsatile secretion of the gonadotrophin hormones LH and FSH by the anterior pituitary gland. LH stimulates sex hormone production from the gonads.
- The age of onset of puberty is earlier in females (mean (range) 10.5 (8.5–12.5)yrs) compared to males (12.0 (10–13.5)yrs). In each sex, puberty progresses in an orderly or 'consonant' manner through distinct stages (see Table 13.1).
- In females, the first sign of puberty is breast development, followed by pubic hair growth and growth acceleration. Menarche (the onset of menstruation) occurs, on average, 2.5yrs after the start of puberty (average age 13.0yrs).
- In males, the first sign of puberty is an enlargement of testicular size to greater than 4mL in volume. Pubic hair development and growth acceleration follow.

Pubertal growth spurt

In females, peak growth (height) velocity occurs relatively earlier in girls (Tanner stage 2–3) compared with boys (Tanner stage 3–4; testicular volumes 10–12mL).

Note: The age of onset of puberty varies slightly between children of different races. In Afro-Caribbean and African-American children, average age of onset of puberty may be earlier compared with that of White children.

Table 13.1 The normal stages of puberty ('Tanner stages')

Boys

Stage	Genitalia	Pubic hair	Other events
I	Prepubertal	Vellus not thicker than on abdomen	TV* <4mL
II	Enlargement of testes and scrotum	Sparse long pigmented strands at base of penis	TV 4–8 mL Voice starts to change
III	Lengthening of penis	Darker, curlier and spreads over pubes	TV 8–10 mL Axillary hair
IV	Increase in penis length and breadth	Adult type hair but covering a smaller area	TV 10–15mL Upper lip hair Peak height velocity
V	Adult shape and size	Spread to medial thighs (Stage 6: Spread up linea alba)	TV 15–25 mL. Facial hair spreads to cheeks Adult voice

Girls

Stage	Breast	Pubic hair	Other events
I	Elevation of papilla only	Vellus not thicker than on abdomen	
II	Breast bud stage: elevation of breast and papilla	Sparse long pigmented strands along labia	Peak height velocity
III	Further elevation of breast and areola together	Darker, curlier and spreads over pubes	
IV	Areola forms a second mound on top of breast	Adult type hair but covering a smaller area	Menarche
V	Mature stage: areola recedes and only papilla projects	Spread to medial thighs (Stage 6: spread up linea alba)	

* TV, testicular volume: measured by size-comparison with a Prader orchidometer. Source: Tanner JM (1962) *Growth at adolescence*, 2nd edn. Oxford: Blackwell Scientific Publications.

Assessment of growth

Growth must be measured accurately. Equipment used to measure weight and height must be regularly maintained, checked, and calibrated. Ideally, growth measurements should be carried out by someone specifically training and experienced in measurement techniques (e.g. an auxologist). This will minimize measurement error.

Assessment of height

- From birth to age 2yrs, length is measured horizontally using a specifically designed measuring board (e.g. Harpenden Neonatometer). Two people need to ensure that child is lying straight with legs extended.
- In children, aged ≥2yrs, standing height is measured against a wall-mounted or free-standing stadiometer. A specific technique is required, with the person measuring applying moderate upward neck traction to the child's head with the child looking forward in the horizontal plane.
- Measurement of sitting height using a modified stadiometer and calculation of the leg length (standing height *minus* sitting height) allows an estimate of upper and lower body segments and body proportion.

Growth data interpretation

Weight and height measurement data should be plotted on a simple sex and age range appropriate standard growth centile chart (e.g. the UK 1990 Growth Reference charts). A UK-WHO growth chart for children from birth to 4yrs of age has been developed based on the WHO child growth standards. These describe optimal growth of healthy breast-fed children. Previous UK growth charts based on data from studies on breast- and formula-fed children, do not reflect normal weight fluctuations of breast-fed infants in first few weeks (see Fig. 13.1). Height measurements should be plotted on specific population growth charts where necessary or applicable, e.g. Turner's syndrome; Down's syndrome.

Single growth measurements should not be assessed in isolation from other previous measurements. Serial measurements are used to show a pattern of growth and to determine growth rate. To minimize error in the assessment of growth rate, calculation of height velocity (cm/year) should be taken from measurements a minimum of 6mths apart, ideally using the same equipment and by the same person.

Final height and target height

Final height is the height reached after the completion of puberty and is estimated to be achieved when growth velocity has slowed to <2.0cm/year. This can be confirmed by finding epiphyseal fusion of the small bones of the hand and wrist on assessing the bone age X-ray.

Final height is largely genetically determined. A target height range can be estimated in each individual from their parent's heights, first calculating the mid-parental height (MPH).

MPH (boys) = [(Mother's ht (cm) + Father's ht (cm))/2] + 6.5cm

MPH (girls) = [(Mother's ht (cm) + Father's ht (cm))/2] − 6.5cm

Target height range = MPH ± 10cm

Bone age

This is a measure of skeletal maturation, which can be assessed by the appearance of the epiphyseal centres of the long bones. Conventionally this is quantified from X-rays of the left hand and wrist, with either compared with standard radiograph images (e.g. Gruelich and Pyle method) or assessed using an individual bone scoring system (Tanner–Whitehouse methods).

The difference between bone age (BA) score and chronological age at the time of assessment may be used as an estimation of the tempo of growth. The BA may also be used as an indicator of the likely timing of puberty, which usually starts when BA is around 10.5yrs in females and 11.5yrs in boys. The relationship between BA and age of onset of menarche is more robust.

Girls usually reach skeletal maturity at a BA of 15.0yrs and boys when BA is 17.0yrs. The BA can therefore be used as an estimation of the remaining growth potential and can be used to predict final adult height.

Assessment of puberty

Puberty stage can be rated using the Tanner staging system. This involves identification of pubertal stage particularly by assessment of stage of breast development in girls and of testicular volume (by comparison with an orchidometer) in boys.

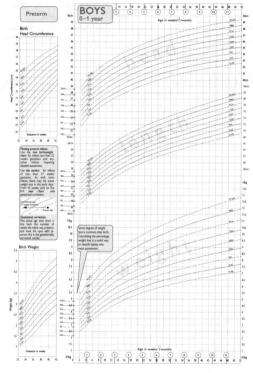

Fig. 13.1 (a) Boys child growth charts 0–1.

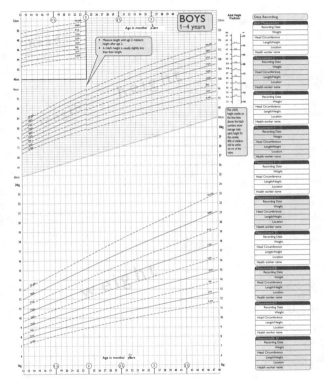

Fig. 13.1 (b) Boys child growth charts 1–4.

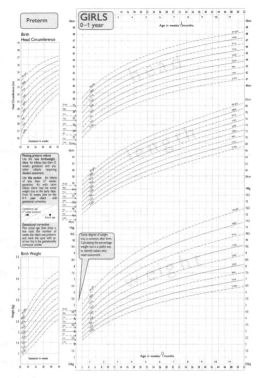

Fig. 13.1 (c) Girls child growth charts 0–1.

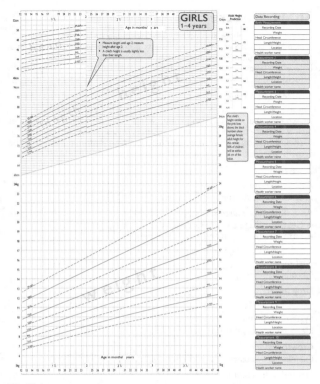

Fig. 13.1 (d) Girls child growth charts 1–4.

Short stature

Defined as a height 2 SDs or more below mean for the population. On a standard growth chart this represents a height below the 2nd centile. *Note:* abnormalities of growth may be present long before height falls below this level and can be identified much earlier by monitoring growth velocity and observing a child's height crossing centile lines plotted.

Causes of short stature

These are summarized in the Box 13.1. The most common cause is familial, where either one or both parents will also be short. Height correlates well with parental height and is probably of polygenic inheritance, but it should be noted that short parents may have a dominantly inherited growth disorder.

Assessment

Antenatal history
Pregnancy illness/drugs/complications

Perinatal/infancy history
- Gestational age and complications
- Birth weight (length and head circumference)
- Feeding and weight gain

Past medical
Chronic asthma

Drug history
Corticosteroids

Systematic enquiry
Headaches/visual disturbance

Growth history
Examine previous growth records if available

Neurodevelopmental
- Developmental delay.
- School performance.

Family history
- Short stature/pubertal delay.
- Endocrine disease.

Examination
- Measure height; weight; head circumference.
- General systems examination.
- Puberty (Tanner) staging.
- Observe for goitre; dysmorphic features; malnutrition.
- Assess growth velocity over (a minimum of) 6-monthly intervals.
- Measure parent's height and calculate MPH and family height target.

Box 13.1 Causes of short stature

- Familial (genetic) short stature
- Constitutional delay in growth & puberty (📖 p.468)
- Intrauterine growth retardation (📖 pp.111, 468)
- Growth hormone deficiency (📖 p.470)
- Other endocrine disorders, e.g. hypothyroidism (📖 p.424), Cushing's syndrome (📖 p.434)
- Dysmorphic syndromes:
  - Turner syndrome (📖 pp.469, 948)
  - Noonan syndrome (📖 p.941)
  - Down syndrome (📖 p.936)
- Coeliac disease (📖 p.336)
- Chronic renal failure (📖 pp.366–369)
- Chronic inflammatory disorders (📖 p.469): inflammatory bowel disease (📖 p.332); rheumatic disease (📖 p.772)
- Skeletal dysplasia (📖 p.766): achondroplasia/hypochrondroplasia
- Metabolic bone disease: X-linked hypophosphataemic rickets (📖 p.445)
- Malnutrition

Investigations

The following baseline screening tests should be carried out:
- U&E (renal function).
- FBC and CRP (chronic disease/inflammation).
- Calcium and phosphate (bone disorder).
- Karyotype (chromosomal abnormalities, especially Turner's syndrome).
- Thyroid function tests.
- Serum IGF-I (and IGFBP-3) (GH deficiency).
- Coeliac disease antibody screen.
- Urinalysis.

Where clinically indicated:
- Bone age X-ray.
- GH provocation test.

Management

This will depend on the underlying cause (see later sections of this chapter). The diagnosis of a child with short stature is often a shock to the family, and they should be offered detailed, reliable information about their child's condition and informed where to get additional support and advice. In the UK the Restricted Growth Foundation (www.restricted-growth.co.uk) is a good resource. Familial short stature does not require any specific treatment.

Note: Most short children are psychologically well adjusted. Where there are problems from being teased and bullied at school or poor self-esteem, psychological intervention measures may be needed.

Constitutional delay in growth and puberty

Relative short stature occurs because of a delay in the timing of onset of puberty. It is a variation in the timing of normal puberty, rather than an abnormal condition. It usually presents in early adolescence, although it may be recognized in earlier childhood. There is often a familial basis, often having occurred in one of the parents. It is much commoner in males, although this may reflect a bias in the level of concern.

Characteristic features include short stature and delayed pubertal development by greater than 2 SDs. Typically, there is a mild degree of skeletal disproportion with evidence of a shorter back (sitting height percentile) relative to leg length. There is invariably delay in BA maturation, which usually remains consistent over time. Height velocity is appropriate for BA.

Laboratory investigations are normal, including GH provocation tests.

Management

Usually no treatment is required as the onset of puberty and the accompanying growth spurt will occur spontaneously and an appropriate final adult target height is achieved.

Treatment is sometimes indicated in those adolescents who have difficulty coping with their short stature or with the delayed physical development. Administration of sex steroids for a period of 3–6mths can be used to induce pubertal changes and to accelerate growth rate (boys: testosterone 50–100mg IM every 4wks).

Intrauterine growth retardation

See also 🕮 p.111. IUGR refers to reduction and restriction in expected foetal growth pattern. IUGR affects 3–10% of pregnancies and 20% of stillborn infants are thought to have evidence of IUGR. Perinatal mortality rates are 4–8 times higher for growth-retarded infants, and morbidity is present in 50% of surviving infants.

Growth outcome

In placental causes of IUGR, 'catch-up growth' occurs after birth in the majority of infants during the first 1–2yrs of life, with infants regaining their genetically determined weight and height centiles. However, in approximately 15–20% of infants with IUGR, catch-up growth does not occur and patients are at risk of short stature. Recent studies also implicate IUGR in adult onset of hypertension and CHD, and in early onset obesity, polycystic ovarian disease, and type 2 diabetes. These studies suggest that IUGR has long-term effects on insulin sensitivity and on endocrine function.

Turner's syndrome

See also 📖 p.948. This condition must always be considered in girls presenting with short stature, or height below parental target height range. Karyotype confirms the diagnosis.

The majority of girls with Turner's syndrome will not have the classical phenotype of dysmorphic features and it may be difficult to identify, particularly where there is mosaicism in the karyotype.

- Short stature is frequent. Typically growth rate begins to falter from age 3–5yrs and is due to an underlying skeletal dysplasia.
- Ovarian dygenesis and consequent gonadal failure result in loss of the pubertal growth spurt.
- Mean final height is consistently 20cm below the norm.

Treatment with daily SC injections of high dose recombinant human growth hormone (rhGH 10mg/m^2/wk) increases final height, although individual responses are variable. Oral oestrogen (ethinylestradiol) is required to induce puberty between ages 12 and 14yrs. Combination therapy, which also includes the anabolic steroid, oxandrolone, may further improve final height.

Coeliac disease

Also see 📖 p.336. Coeliac disease may be asymptomatic or atypical in its presentation with few if any gastrointestinal symptoms or signs. Poor height velocity and evolving short stature may be a presenting feature.

Chronic inflammatory disorders

Poor growth and short stature is a common feature of long-term inflammatory conditions such as inflammatory bowel disease and rheumatic disorders. It may be a presenting feature in Crohn's disease when GI symptoms are initially minimal (see 📖 p.332).

Short stature is due to long-term use of immunosuppressive agents (e.g. corticosteroids) and to the generation of inflammatory factors (e.g. IL-6). Both lead to GH/IGF-I resistance and suppression of bone growth.

Management should be aimed at minimizing inflammation, and reducing immunosuppressive therapy. rhGH may have a role in treatment.

Skeletal dysplasias

This heterogeneous group of disorders includes achondroplasia and hypochrondroplasia. Most disorders are characterized by severe short stature and often evidence of disproportion in body segment development. Skeletal survey may allow identification of specific condition (see 📖 pp.766–767, 950).

Growth hormone deficiency

Physiology: secretion

GH is secreted from the somatomammotropic cells of the anterior pituitary gland in a pulsatile pattern. Secretion is diurnal and largely nocturnal and is controlled by a rhythmically changing equilibrium between two hormones secreted by the hypothalamus: GH releasing hormone (GHRH) and GH-inhibiting hormone (or somatostatin). GHRH induces GH synthesis and secretion whenever somatostatin is low. Different factors act at the level of the hypothalamus to regulate GH hormone secretion. GH secretion is regulated by negative feedback by circulating insulin-like growth factor-I (IGF-I) at the pituitary and hypothalamus, and by short loop-feedback by GH on the hypothalamus.

Causes of growth hormone deficiency

These may be primary (or congenital) or secondary (acquired) in origin. In clinical practice the most frequent cause of GH deficiency is 2° to cranial radiotherapy (Box 13.2).

> ### Box 13.2 Causes of GH deficiency
>
> *Primary or congenital causes*
> • Idiopathic/isolated
> • Congenital hypopituitarism (see 📖 p.449)
> • Midline brain anomalies
>
> *Secondary or acquired causes*
> • *Intracranial tumours:* craniopharyngioma
> • Cranial irradiation/radiotherapy
> • Psychosocial deprivation
> • Traumatic brain injury
> • *Inflammatory/infiltrative disease:*
>   • Langerhan's cell histiocytosis
>   • sarcoidosis
> • Intracranial infection

Clinical features

Presentation depends on the age of onset of GH deficiency.

GH deficiency in infancy

May present with hypoglycaemia. Co-existing deficiencies in the adrenal, thyroid, and gonadal axes may cause prolonged jaundice and micropenis. Size at birth and growth during the 1st year of life may be normal as growth during this period is not GH-dependent.

GH deficiency in childhood

Typically presents with slow growth rate and short stature. Other characteristics include increased subcutaneous fat, truncal obesity, and decreased muscle mass. Children with congenital GH deficiency develop relative hypoplasia of the mid-facial bones, frontal bone protrusion, and delayed dental eruption. Delayed closure of the anterior fontanelle may also be observed.

Investigations

Laboratory

- *Baseline/random serum IGF-I and IGFBP-3:* GH-dependent and may be low in GH deficiency, but normal levels do not exclude GH deficiency.
- GH provocation tests.

All tests should be performed in the morning after an overnight fast and serial blood samples are collected. The insulin tolerance test (ITT) is considered the gold-standard test. GH provocation test should only be performed in those centres with experience and with appropriate technical and laboratory support.

Assessment commonly used in children/adolescents

Pharmacological stimulation tests

- Insulin tolerance test (gold standard; children aged ≥5yrs)
- Glucagon stimulation tests
- Clonidine test
- Arginine test

Physiological tests

- Exercise
- Overnight or 24hr GH serum profiles
- Random serum IGF-1 and/or IGFBP3 level

Radiological

- Bone age
- MRI scan of brain (hypothalamic/pituitary structures)

NICE criteria for diagnosis of GH deficiency[1]

- GHD is primarily a clinical diagnosis supported by auxological, biochemical, and radiological findings. Confirmation of the diagnosis is usually by GH provocation testing
- Two such tests should be used in children with suspected isolated GH deficiency together with evaluation of other aspects of pituitary function
- Definition of a normal GH response remains arbitrary as there is a continuous spectrum of GH secretory ability in childhood—peak GH concentrations <20mIU/L (7microgram/L) have traditionally been used to support the diagnosis

Reference

1 NICE (2010). *Guidance on the use of human growth hormone (somatropin) in children with growth failure,* Technology Appraisal Guidance, No. 188. London: NICE.

Growth hormone deficiency: management

GH deficiency is treated with rhGH, which is administered as a once daily SC injection ($0.7-1.0$mg/m^2/day or $23-39$microgram/kg/day).

- Treatment should be undertaken in experienced centres.
- Responses to treatment (height velocity increase) and dose adjustments should be reviewed once every 6mths.
- Catch up growth optimal if GH therapy is started as early as possible.

Transition to GH deficiency care in adulthood

Treatment with rhGH is continued until final adult height is achieved. At this point the GH deficiency should be reconfirmed, particularly in those with isolated or so-called idiopathic GH deficiency where the cause is unclear. Up to 50% of patients with the latter may have normal GH secretion when retested in early adulthood. Those patients with persisting GH deficiency should be offered the opportunity to continue rhGH therapy ($0.2-0.5$mg/day). Studies have demonstrated that rhGH replacement in adulthood may maintain lean body mass, muscle strength, and bone mineral density. In addition, improved quality of life has been reported with treatment.

Cranial irradiation and GH deficiency

Cranial radiotherapy used in the treatment of tumours (intracranial, face, and nasopharynx) may cause GH deficiency. The GH axis is the most sensitive to radiotherapy, followed by the gonadal and adrenal axes, and finally the thyroid axis, which is least sensitive. There is a good correlation between radiotherapy dose and the occurrence of hypothalamic–pituitary dysfunction (Table 13.2). Risk of dysfunction is also related to dose fractionation (single is more toxic than divided), and age (younger more sensitive).

Table 13.2 Correlation between radiotherapy dose and GH deficiency

Radiotherapy dose (Gy)	% GH-deficient*
18	
24	55
25–45	68–76
>45	100%

* Assessed 4yrs after radiotherapy.

Pyschosocial deprivation

Children subjected to physical or emotional abuse may exhibit growth failure. This may be due to a reversible inhibition of GH secretion that improves within 3–4wks of being removed from the adverse environment. Catch-up growth is usually dramatic.

GH insensitivity syndrome

Moderate to severe short stature may be due to GH resistance. This may be due to a defect in the GH receptor or to a defect in post-receptor GH signalling.

Complete GH insensitivity syndrome (GHIS) results in severe short stature. It may be inherited as an autosomal recessive trait (Laron syndrome). Affected individuals have high GH levels and low circulating IGF-I levels. Exogenous rhGH administration fails to increase IGF-I levels further (IGF-I generation test).

Tall stature

Referral for tall stature is much less common than that for short stature. Socially, it is more acceptable to be tall, particularly for boys. Nevertheless, tall stature, particularly when it is associated with inappropriately increased growth rates, may indicate an underlying growth disorder.

Causes of tall stature

In the majority tall stature is genetic in origin and inherited from tall parents. Other causes, although rare, need to be considered:
- Familial.
- Early (normal) puberty.
- Obesity.
- *Endocrine disorders:*
  - precocious puberty (see 📖 p.480);
  - GH excess;
  - pituitary adenoma;
  - androgen excess;
  - congenital adrenal hyperplasia (📖 p.436);
  - hyperthyroidism (📖 p.425);
  - aromatase enzyme deficiency (very rare);
  - oestrogen receptor defects (very rare).
- Chromosomal abnormalities: Klinefelter's syndrome (XXY); XYY; XYYY (📖 p.938).
- *Other syndromes:* Marfan (📖 p.940), homocystinuria, Soto, Beckwith–Wiedemann (📖 p.949).

History

A detailed history should be obtained.

Perinatal/infancy history
- Size at birth.
- Birth weight (head circumference).
- Feeding and weight gain.

Systematic enquiry E.g. headaches/visual disturbance.

Growth history
- Examine previous growth records if available.
- Recent growth acceleration.
- Signs of puberty.

Neurodevelopmental
- Developmental delay.
- School performance.

Family history
- Tall stature.
- Early puberty.
- Endocrine disease.

Examination

- *Measure:*
  - height;
  - weight;
  - head circumference.
- Puberty staging (Tanner).
- Observe dysmorphic features; goitre.
- Assess growth velocity over a minimum 6-monthly interval.
- *Measure parents' heights and calculate:*
  - MPH;
  - family height target.

Investigations

The following baseline screening tests should be carried out:

- Karyotype (chromosomal abnormalities—Klinefelter's syndrome).
- Thyroid function tests/serum IGF-I (and IGFBP-3).
- Sex hormone/LH and FSH levels.
- Androgen levels (DHEAS; 17-OH progesterone).
- BA X-ray.

Where clinically indicated GH suppression test (i.e. modified oral glucose tolerance test; GH levels normally suppressed to low levels).

Management

In familial tall stature, reassurance and information about predicted final height are usually sufficient. Early induction of puberty using low dose sex-steroid to advance the pubertal growth spurt and to cause earlier epiphyseal closure is occasionally considered. However, this produces variable results and there is a theoretical risk of complications (including thromboembolic disease and oncogenic risk).

Delayed puberty: assessment

This is defined as the lack of initiation and progress of pubertal development > +2 SD later than the average age of onset of puberty for the population. In the UK, this is to >14yrs for females and >16yrs for males.

The causes of delayed puberty are shown in Box 13.3.

History

A detailed history should screen for the many possible physical and functional causes of delayed puberty. Make careful enquiry about age at puberty onset (including menarche in females) in other family members.

Examination

- Measure height, weight, head circumference.
- Puberty (Tanner) staging.
- Review previous growth records if available.
- Measure parents' heights and calculate MPH and family height target.

Investigations

The following baseline screening tests should be carried out.

Blood

- LH and FSH levels.
- *Sex hormone*: oestrogen/testosterone.
- Karyotype (chromosomal abnormalities).
- Thyroid function tests.
- Routine biochemistry and inflammatory markers (e.g. CRP).

Radiological

- BA X-ray.
- Pelvic US (ovarian morphology).
- Abdominal US (e.g. intra-abdominal testes).
- MRI scan brain.

Tests

- *hCG stimulation test (3- or 21-day test):* measurement of testosterone pre- and post-hCG (as indicator of functional testicular tissue).
- *GnRH (LHRH) test:* measurement of basal and post-GnRH LH and FSH levels (an indicator of hypothalamic–pituitary function).

Note: It is difficult to distinguish constitutional delay in growth and puberty (CDGP) from other causes of hypogonadotrophic hypogonadism (HH) using current tests. In both conditions basal and stimulated gonadotrophin (LH/FSH) levels are low. Differentiation may only be possible after induction of puberty with sex steroid therapy and attainment of final height, when reassessment of the hypothalamic–pituitary gonadal axis should be repeated after withdrawal of treatment.

Box 13.3 Causes of pubertal delay

Constitutional delay of growth and puberty

Hypogonadotrophic hypogonadism
Low/undetectable basal and stimulated gonadotrophin levels:
- *Congenital:*
  - Kallman's syndrome
  - congenital hypopituitarism (e.g. LHX-3; PROP-1; see 📖 p.449)
  - isolated LH deficiency
  - isolated FSH deficiency
  - other causes of gonadotrophin deficiency, e.g. congenital adrenal hypoplasia (DAX-1 gene)
  - syndromic associations, e.g. Prader–Willi syndrome
- *Acquired:*
  - intracranial tumours (e.g. craniopharyngioma)
  - cranial irradiation
  - traumatic brain injury
  - Langerhan's cell histiocytosis
  - anorexia nervosa
  - excess physical training
  - chronic childhood disease, e.g. inflammatory bowel disease

Primary gonadal failure (hypergonadotrophic hypogonadism)
High basal and stimulated gonadotrophin levels
- *Congenital:*
  - chromosomal disorders, Turner's syndrome, Klinefelter's syndrome
  - gonadal dysgenesis
  - LH resistance
  - disorders of steroid biosynthesis (e.g. congenital adrenal hyperplasia: StAR; CYP17; 3βHSD (see 📖 p.436))
- *Acquired:*
  - chemotherapy
  - gonadal irradiation (local radiotherapy)
  - gonadal infection (e.g. mumps orchitis)
  - gonadal trauma/gonadal torsion
  - cranial irradiation
  - autoimmune (ovarian)

Delayed puberty: management

- Children with CDGP may be treated with a short course of sex steroid therapy to promote physical development and growth (see Constitutional delay of growth and puberty).
- Children with permanent gonadotrophin deficiency or gonadal failure requiring complete induction of puberty and thus long-term treatment can have puberty induced with gradually increasing doses of sex steroids over a period of 2–3yrs.
  - *Boys:* testosterone esters by IM injection. Incremental increases in dose, starting from 50mg every 4–6wks to 250mg every 3–4wks.
  - *Girls:* ethinylestradiol, oral. Increasing doses every 6mths, starting from 2micrograms/day increasing to 5–20micrograms/day. A progesterone (e.g. norethisterone or levonorgestrel given on days 14 to 21 of the cycle only) should be added when the dose of ethinylestradiol is 10–15micrograms/day or when vaginal bleeding or spotting is first observed.
- The aim of long-term sex steroid therapy is the maintenance of secondary sexual features, libido, and menstruation in females. There are also positive benefits in terms of bone mineralization and cardiovascular health.

Note. In males, testosterone therapy does not promote testicular growth and testicular size remains prepubertal unless spontaneous puberty occurs.

Constitutional delay of growth and puberty

This is the most common cause of delayed puberty. Usually observed in boys, this condition reflects a delay in the timing mechanisms that regulate the onset of puberty. There is often a family history of delayed puberty in parents or siblings.

- Children presenting with CDGP are invariably healthy.
- Onset and progress through puberty will occur normally with time.
- Children achieve a final adult height in keeping with their predicted familial target range.

It is likely that most children with CDGP are not referred for medical attention, as they and their parents will not perceive that there is a problem. However, for many others, concerns about the lack of physical development and the lack of anticipated adolescent growth spurt would be a source of much anxiety and psychological stress.

There is often evidence of delayed or slow growth in childhood, which is most pronounced in the peripubertal years due to lack of anticipated growth spurt. Children will also have evidence of delayed skeletal maturation on bone age assessment.

No specific therapy is required. For many children and families, explanation of the benign nature of the condition and reassurance that puberty will occur normally is sufficient. However, children who are experiencing significant social or psychological difficulties may request treatment. In this situation, low dose sex steroids may be used (e.g. boys: testosterone, 50mg IM monthly for 4–6mths). This approach will:

• induce sexual development;
• promote an increase in growth rate;
• stimulate activation of the hypothalamic–pituitary–gonadal axis.

Thus puberty may continue once the administration of sex steroids has been stopped.

Any decision regarding whether therapy is required or not must include the views of the child and their parents, who should be part of the decision process.

Hypogonadotrophic hypogonadism

This indicates impaired gonadotrophin release from the pituitary gland. Congenital and acquired causes are recognized (see Box 13.3, 🕮 p.477). The condition is characterized by low or undetectable gonadotrophin levels either under basal or stimulated (GnRH test) conditions.

Congenital causes of HH may be characterized by micropenis and undescended testis at birth in boys, whereas in girls physical signs are absent.

Kallmann syndrome (KS)

A genetic disorder characterized by the association of HH and anosmia (absent sense of smell). This arises due to a defect in the co-migration of GnRH releasing neurons and olfactory neurons that occurs during early foetal development. X-linked, autosomal dominant, and autosomal recessive modes of inheritance are recognized. The X-linked form of KS results from a mutation in the *KAL* gene (encoding the glycoprotein, anosmin-1). It is also characterized by a range of clinical features including synkinesia (mirror-image movements), renal agenesis, and visual problems as well as craniofacial anomalies, although their expression is highly variable.

Precocious puberty

This is defined as the early onset and rapid progression of puberty. Age criteria vary. In White European children, precocious puberty (PP) is defined as <8yrs in females and <9yrs in males.

Classification and causes

PP is either central or peripheral in origin. The various causes of PP are as follows.

Central (true) PP (gonadotrophin-dependent)

- Idiopathic (familial/non-familial).
- *Intracranial tumours:* e.g. hypothalamic hamartoma, craniopharyngioma, astrocytoma, optic glioma.
- *Other CNS lesions:* hydrocephalus, arachnoid cysts, traumatic brain injury, cranial irradiation.
- *Secondary central PP:* early maturation of the hypothalamic–pituitary–gonadal axis due to long-term sex steroid exposure, e.g. congenital adrenal hyperplasia (CAH), McCune–Albright syndrome.

Puberty occurs as a consequence of early physiological (true) activation of the hypothalamic–pituitary–gonadal axis (central). A normal sequence of pubertal development is observed.

Central PP may also be idiopathic and familial. Girls with central PP are more likely to have idiopathic central PP, whereas in boys there is a much greater risk of intracranial tumours.

Peripheral PP (gonadotrophin-independent)

- *Gonadal:* McCune–Albright syndrome; ovarian tumours (e.g. benign cyst; granulosa cell tumour); testicular tumour; familial testitoxicosis (LH receptor-activating mutation).
- *Adrenal:* CAH; adrenal tumour (carcinoma; adenoma).
- *Human chorionic gonadotrophin (HCG)-secreting tumours:* e.g. CNS (chorioepithelioma; dysgerminoma).
- Iatrogenic (exogenous sex-steroid administration).

Puberty is due to mechanisms that do not involve physiological gonadotrophin secretion from the pituitary. The source of sex steroid may be endogenous (gonadal or extragonadal) or exogenous. Endogenous hormone production is independent of hypothalamic–pituitary–gonadal activity. An abnormal sequence of pubertal development is usually observed.

Assessment

History

A detailed history should be obtained:
- Age when first signs of pubertal development observed.
- Which features of puberty are present and in what order did they appear?
- Evidence of growth acceleration.
- Family history: careful enquiry about the age of onset of puberty (including age of menarche in females) within other family members.

Examination

- Puberty (Tanner) staging.
- Measure height; weight; head circumference.
- Review previous growth records if available.
- Measure parents' heights and calculate MPH/family height target.
- *Skin lesions:* e.g. *café-au-lait* marks (McCune–Albright; NF-1).
- Abdominal/testicular masses.
- *Neurological examination:* visual fields; fundoscopy.

Investigations

Baseline screening tests should be considered.
- Plasma LH and FSH levels.
- *Plasma sex hormone:* oestrogen/testosterone.
- *Other serum androgen levels:* e.g. 17-OH progesterone, DHEAS, androstendione.

In addition, undertake the following:
- *Urine:* steroid profile (sex/adrenal steroids).
- BA X-ray.
- Pelvic US (ovarian morphology; testicular masses).
- Abdominal US, e.g. adrenal glands.
- MRI scan brain.
- *GnRH (LHRH) test:* measurement of basal and post-GnRH LH, and FSH levels as indicator of hypothalamic–pituitary function.

Precocious puberty: management

Diagnosis

The diagnosis is based on demonstrating progressive pubertal development and increased growth rate, together with laboratory evidence of increased sex steroid production. Distinguishing central and peripheral PP and PP from other normal variants of pubertal development may be difficult (see Table 13.3). In CPP there is evidence of consonance in sequence of pubertal development in keeping with the normal physiological activation of puberty.

Table 13.3 Characteristic findings of disorders of pubertal development

	Sequence of pubertal changes	Height velocity	Sex steroids	LH/FSH (basal/ stimulated)	BA
Central PP	Consonant	++	++	++, LH predominant	++
Peripheral PP	Usually non-consonant	++	++	Pre-pubertal; suppressed	++
Premature thelarche	Breast tissue only	N	N	Pre-pubertal/ FSH +	N
Thelarche 'variant'	Breast tissue only	+	N	Pre-pubertal/ FSH +	N/+
Premature adrenarche	Pubic hair; skin changes only	N	N/DHEAS +	Pre-pubertal; suppressed	N

BA, Bone age; +, slightly raised or advanced; ++, raised or advanced; N, normal.

Management

The management of precocious puberty is aimed at the following:

- *Detection and treatment of underlying pathological causes of PP:* this is especially important in males in whom early puberty is invariably due to organic disease.
- *Reducing the rate of skeletal maturation, if necessary:* accelerated skeletal maturation and growth rate occur and will result in the affected child being tall during childhood relative to peers. However, skeletal maturation exceeds concomitant growth and thus growth potential is reduced, growth is complete prematurely, and final adult height is reduced and potentially below the predicted expected familial target height range.
- *Reducing and halting, if necessary, the rate of physical pubertal development.*
- *Addressing potential behavioural and psychological difficulties:* sexual and reproductive characteristics advance inappropriately for age, leading to mature appearance. Early menstruation occurs in girls, and spermatogenesis and ejaculation in boys. Sexualized behaviour may occur and interactions with age-peers and adults may be based on assumed, but age-inappropriate, mental and social expectations.

Before therapy is considered, it is essential that an explanation of the physiology and physical consequences of precocious puberty should be discussed with the parents and the child. The decision on therapy should be made jointly with the parents.

Treatment of precocious puberty

Central PP

- Suppression of the hypothalamic–pituitary–gonadal axis with a long-acting GnRH analogue is the only currently effective treatment for central PP. These agents work by providing continuous stimulation of the GnRH receptor on the pituitary gonadotrophes, resulting in down-regulation of the receptor and thus decreased LH and FSH secretion.
- GnRH analogues are administered by either SC or IM injection, monthly (or 3-monthly in depot preparations).
- Treatment efficacy should be assessed by monitoring growth rate and pubertal stage. In addition, serum LH and FSH levels (basal and stimulated) should be measured to ensure hypothalamic–pituitary–gonadal axis suppression.

Variants of normal puberty

These include premature thelarche and premature adrenarche. Neither condition is associated with pubertal activation of the hypothalamic–pituitary–gonadal axis.

Premature thelarche

- Isolated premature breast development occurring in the absence of any other signs of puberty.
- Typically, females present in infancy and usually by 2yrs of age.
- Breast development is due to the action of physiological or mild increases in the amounts of circulating oestrogen.

The clinical course is characterized by a waxing and waning of breast size, normal growth (height) rate, and the absence of any further sexual development. Breast development may be asymmetrical, and there is usually a resolution of any breast enlargement by age 4–5yrs.

The cause is unknown, but small increases in basal and stimulated serum FSH levels are usually observed. In contrast LH levels remain suppressed in the prepubertal range. Ovarian follicle development is often observed, but no changes in ovarian or uterine size are seen. Serum oestradiol levels are increased when measured by sensitive assays, but typically within normal range by standard radioimmunoassay.

The condition is benign. Bone maturation, age of onset of menarche, and final adult height are not affected. Management is conservative with re-evaluation of growth and puberty stage at 3–6-monthly intervals.

Thelarche variant

- An intermediate condition between premature thelarche and central precocious puberty.
- It represents a non-progressive form of early pubertal development.

Patients have evidence of breast development, increased growth rate, and advanced skeletal maturation on bone age assessment. There may also be evidence of ovarian enlargement and raised serum oestradiol levels. For most patients the tempo of progression of pubertal development will be slow and they will have laboratory findings within normal range for age. Management is usually conservative with regular re-evaluation of growth and pubertal status at 3–6 monthly intervals. Decisions to treat (as for central PP) are based on height velocity and final height predictions.

Premature adrenarche

Early onset of pubertal adrenal androgen secretion is a common variation of normal pubertal development. Premature adenarche is the result of premature secretion of androgens from the zona reticualris of the adrenal gland.

- Children typically present with premature appearance of androgen-dependent 2° sexual hair development (axillary hair, pubic hair, or both), acne, and axillary (body) odour.
- Patients may have mild acceleration in height velocity and slight increase in BA.
- Laboratory investigations reveal an increase in serum DHEAS levels that are appropriate for pubic hair stage rather for than age.
- Serum concentrations of testosterone and 17-OH progesterone are normal.

When evaluating patients for premature adrenarche it is important to assess for clinical signs and symptoms that might indicate another cause of excess androgen production (e.g. adrenal tumour; congenital adrenal hyperplasia). The later are characterized with signs of virilization, rapid growth rate, and significantly advanced bone age.

Premature adrenarche is a benign condition. The timing of onset of true puberty is normal and final adult height is unaffected. Management is conservative with reassurance after exclusion of other causes of adrenal androgen excess. Symptomatic treatment may be required if adrenarche is pronounced, particularly in females who may go on to develop features of ovarian hyperandrogenism and the polycystic ovarian syndrome.

Disorders of sex development

Terminology

- *Sexual determination* refers to the process that occurs from the time of conception until the foetal bipotential gonad has been fully determined as either an ovary or testis.
- *Sexual differentiation* refers to the process that occurs from the time gonadal sex is determined until 2° sexual characteristics are fully expressed and fertility achieved.

Disorders of sexual development

The complex process of sexual determination and differentiation may be interrupted. Numerous disorders that can result in genital ambiguity and uncertainty about an infant's sex are recognized. Disorders of sexual differentiation may be classified as genetic defects of gonadal determination (Box 13.4) or defects in androgen biosynthesis, metabolism, and action (excess or deficiency).

Box 13.4 **Genetic disorders of gonadal determination**

- *Gonadal dysgenesis:*
  - 45 XO (gonadal dysgenesis)
  - 46 XY (gonadal dysgenesis)
  - 46 XX (gonadal dysgenesis)
  - 45 XO/46 XY (mixed gonadal dysgenesis)
- True hermaphroditism
- 46 XX or 46 XY sex reversal
- Camptomelic dysplasia (SOX-9 mutation)
- DAX-1 mutation
- Denys–Drash syndrome (WT-1 mutation)

Virilization of 46 XX infants (female pseudohermaphrodite)
- *Excessive androgen production:* congenital adrenal hyperplasia—21α-hydroxylase deficiency; 11β-hydroxylase deficiency; 3βHSD
- *Defect in androgen exposure:* placental–foetal aromatase deficiency
- Maternal steroid exposure

Under-virilization of 46 XY male (male pseudohermaphrodite)
- *Defect in testosterone production:*
  - Leydig cell hypoplasia/agenesis
  - *defects of testicular and adrenal steroidogenesis*—StAR; 3βHSD; 17α-hydroxylase/17,20 lyase deficiency
- *Defect in testosterone metabolism:* 5α-reductase deficiency
- *Defects in testosterone action:* androgen insensitivity syndrome: complete or partial

---

Assessment

History

A detailed history should be obtained and should include:

- *Family history:* ambiguous genitalia; disorders/problems of puberty; inguinal hernia.
- *Prenatal history:* maternal health; drugs taken during pregnancy; maternal virilization during pregnancy.
- History of previous stillbirths or neonatal death?

Examination

- *General examination:* dysmorphic features or midline defects; state of hydration; BP.
- *Are the gonads palpable?* If 'yes' they are likely to be testes or ovotestes.
- *Assess the degree of virilization:*
  - Prader stage (Fig 13.2).
  - External masculinization score.
- *Measure the length of the phallus:*
  - Normal term penis is about 3cm (stretched length from pubic tubercle to tip of penis).
  - Micropenis is a length <2.0–2.5cm.
- *Penis:* presence of chordee.
- *Vagina:* locate opening?
- Appearance of labioscrotal folds.
- Position of urethral opening.
- *Skin—pigmentation of genital skin:* hyperpigmentation with excessive adrenocorticotrophin (ACTH) and opiomelanocortin in CAH.

In preterm girls clitoris and labia minora are relatively prominent. In preterm boys, testes remain undescended until 34wks gestation.

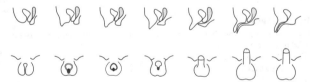

Fig. 13.2 Prader staging: virilization. Reproduced from Prader A. (1058). Die Haufigkeit der kongenitalen adrenigenitalen syndrome. *Helv Paediatr Acta* **13**: 5–14 and 426–31. With kind permission of Springer Science and Business Media.

Disorders of sex development: management

Investigations

Laboratory

- *Genetic sex determination:* FISH for Y and X chromosomes; karyotype (takes 3–5 days).
- Serum electrolytes.
- Blood sugar (hypoglycaemia).
- *Adrenal androgens:* plasma testosterone; 17-OH progesterone; urine steroid profile; LH and FSH.
- Molecular genetic studies; blood (DNA).

If a male/mosaic karyotype is confirmed, further investigations are directed at establishing whether testicular tissue is capable of producing androgens:
- hCG stimulation test;
- testosterone: DHT ratio;
- androgen receptor binding studies;
- genital skin biopsy (fibroblast).

Imaging studies

- *US scan pelvis:* anatomy of urogenital sinus/vagina/uterus.
- *US scan abdomen:* renal anomalies.
- Urogenital sonogram.
- MRI.

Internal examination

- Examination under anaesthesia (+/– cystography).
- Laparoscopy.
- Gonadal biopsy.

Management

This is professionally challenging and requires a multidisciplinary team including the following:
- Paediatric endocrinologist.
- Neonatologist.
- Paediatric urologist.
- Gynaecologist.
- Geneticist.
- Radiologist.
- Psychologist.
- Clinical biochemist.

Most infants presenting with a disorder of sexual differentiation will present with ambiguous genitalia at birth.
- Parents and their relatives will be anxious to know the sex of their newborn baby.
- Decisions about an infant's sex (sex assignment) must be delayed until the multidisciplinary team has carried out a thorough assessment.
- Birth registration must be delayed until this has been completed and an agreement on sex assignment has been made with the parents (see Box 13.5).

Box 13.5 General principles of sex assignment

Virilized females
- Should be brought up as female
- *Clitoromegaly:* clitoral reduction (clitoroplasty) in infancy/childhood
- Vaginoplasty is deferred until late childhood/early adolescence

Under-virilized male
Decision regarding sex assignment is more complex. Depends on the following:
- Degree of sexual ambiguity
- Underlying cause if known
- Potential for normal sexual function and fertility
- *Phallic size:*
  - if >2.5cm, reconstructive surgery more likely to be successful
  - a trial of IM testosterone or topical dihydrotestosterone cream may improve phallic size

Gonadectomy is required:
- If dysgenetic testis
- If complete androgen insensitivity syndrome (AIS)
- If decision to raise as female

Hormone replacement therapy
- Testosterone therapy if decision to raise as male
- Oestrogen therapy if decision to raise as female

Psychological support
- Experienced counselling is essential
- Patient support groups are available

Issues regarding assignment of gender, timing of reconstructive surgery, and hormone replacement therapy are complex. Current consensus on management is largely based on expert opinion.[1]

Reference
1 Hughes IA, Houk C, Ahmed SF, et al. (2006). Consensus statement on the management of intersex disorders. *Arch Dis Child* **91**(7): 554–63.

Androgen insensitivity syndrome

This condition is due to defects in the androgen receptor and results in a spectrum of under-virilized phenotypes in the 46XY patient.

Complete AIS

Deletions of the gene and certain mutations can result in a completely female phenotype.

- External genitalia are unambiguously female, with normal clitoris, hypoplastic labia majora, and blind-ending vaginal pouch. Müllerian structures are absent.
- Testes may be located in the abdomen, inguinal canal, or labia.
- AIS should be strongly suspected and excluded in any female presenting with inguinal hernia.
- Patients with complete AIS often present in adolescence with primary amenorrhoea.
- At puberty, serum levels of testosterone and LH are elevated. Conversion of testosterone to oestradiol in the testis and in peripheral tissues results in normal breast development.
- Pubic and axillary hair development is absent or sparse.
- Diagnosis is confirmed by demonstrating 46XY karyotype.

In view of the potential risk of malignant transformation if retained, removal of the testis either soon after diagnosis or after the completion of puberty is carried out. After gonadal removal, oestrogen replacement therapy is given.

Partial AIS

Certain mutations of the androgen receptor gene result in a partial form of AIS. There is a wide spectrum of phenotypic expression ranging from ambiguous genitalia to a normal male phenotype presenting with fertility difficulties. There is, however, poor genotype–phenotype correlation and patients with the same mutation present with different phenotypes.

Management is much more challenging. Sex assignment depends on the degree of genital ambiguity.

True hermaphroditism

Individuals have both ovarian tissue with follicles and testicular tissue with seminiferous tubules either in the same gonad (ovotestis) or with an ovary on one side and a testis on the other. The aetiology of this condition is unclear. In 70% of cases the underlying karyotype is 46XX; 20% 46XX/46XY; 10% 46XY.

Ovotestes may be present bilaterally and may be located in the inguinal canal. The external genitalia are most often ambiguous, although in 10% phenotype may be female. The degree of feminization and virilization that occurs varies widely. Management is dictated by sex assignment. Dysgenetic testicular tissue should be removed because of the risk of malignant transformation.

Micropenis

Micropenis is often an incidental finding on newborn examination.

An intact hypothalamic–pituitary–gonadal axis is required for the formation of a normal-sized phallus and for descent of the testis. Both GH and the gonadotrophins are required for phallic growth.

The finding of micropenis warrants assessment of hypothalamic–pituitary function and exclusion of both GH deficiency and HH. Micropenis may also be part of a syndrome causing ambiguous genitalia.

Evaluation

Penile size

- Measured from pubic tubercle to tip of stretched penis in a term baby.
- Normal size at birth is usually >3cm.
- Micropenis <2.2–2.5cm (varies with ethnicity).

General examination

- Dysmorphism.
- Midline craniofacial defects.

Ophthalmic examination

Optic nerve hypoplasia/septo-optic dysplasia.

Investigations

- US of head for midline defects.
- MRI head.
- *Anterior pituitary hormone levels (basal and stimulated):* ACTH and cortisol; GH (IGF-I, IGFBP3); LH and FSH; TSH and fT4.
- Karyotype.

Management

Referral to a paediatric urologist is often required. If severe micropenis is present a decision regarding sex assignment will be needed.

Treatment with a short course of IM testosterone or topical application of dihydrotestosterone cream may stimulate penile growth and improve appearances.

Gynaecomastia

This is a condition affecting boys in which there is hyperplasia of the glandular tissue of the breast resulting in enlargement of one or both breasts. It is a common condition with 3 well-defined time periods of occurrence:
- neonatal;
- puberty;
- during older adult life.

It is due to either an imbalance in the normal systemic or local oestrogen/androgen ratio. An absolute or relative increase in oestrogen levels, local breast tissue hypersentivity to oestrogens, or a decrease in the production, or action of free androgen levels may induce gynaecomastia.

Aetiology
A number of diverse causes are recognized (Box 13.6). Gynaecomastia must be differentiated from pseudogynaecomastia, which is breast enlargement due to fat accumulation.

Box 13.6 Classification and causes of gynaecomastia

- Pubertal gynaecomastia
- Neonatal gynaecomastia
- *Impaired gonadal function:*
  - hypogonadotrophic hypogonadism
  - hypergonadotrophic hypogonadism
- Androgen insensitivity syndrome
- Adrenal tumours
- *Testicular tumours:*
  - Leydig cell tumour
  - Sertoli cell tumour
  - germ cell tumour
- *Iatrogenic:*
  - exogenous hormones, e.g. oestrogen, anabolic steroids
  - ketoconazole
  - psychoactive drugs, e.g. diazepam, phenothiazines
- Alcohol excess
- Cannabis

Pubertal gynaecomastia

This is most common cause of gynaecomastia in children and adolescents. The exact cause remains unclear. Proposed mechanisms include alterations in the rate of change in oestrogen and androgen production during puberty and/or hypersensitivity of breast tissue to oestrogen.

May affect 40–50% of children to some degree. It also depends on ethnicity and nutritional status. Usual age of onset of development is just before puberty (ages 10–12yrs), peaking during puberty (age 13–14yrs). In the majority of children the gynaecomastia usually involutes after 1–2yrs and is generally resolved by end of puberty (age 16–17yrs).

The diagnosis is established by excluding other possible causes of gynaecomastia by taking a detailed clinical and family history, and examination.

Investigations should include:
- serum oestrogen, testosterone, LH, FSH;
- serum prolactin;
- LFT; thyroid function tests;
- karyotype.

Where testicular/adrenal/hepatic tumour is suspected the following investigations should be considered:
- US abdomen/testis;
- MRI abdomen/testis;
- serum βhCG levels.

Management

Reassurance and explanation are usually sufficient for pubertal gynaecomastia. In severe cases where pubertal gynaecomastia is causing significant pyschological distress or where gynaecomastia persists beyond puberty, surgical resection of excess glandular breast tissue is warranted. The role of medical therapy with aromatase inhibitors or with selective oestrogen receptor blocking agents (e.g. tamoxifen) is currently unclear.

Neurology

Examination

This is the most useful tool in assessing children with neurological disorders. Nevertheless, it is neglected and often thought difficult. With a few simple tricks it is both easy and enjoyable for doctor, child and parent.

Children with mental age >4 years who can walk

Older children can undergo the full 'adult' neurological examination by making it a game. Pay particular attention to their:
• affect;
• gait and spine;
• head size;
• *skin*: neurocutaneous stigmata.

Children able to walk with a mental age <5 years

Such children can be examined by stealth, then moving onto a game. Observe the play and note:
• Gait, watch how they walk, narrow/normal/wide based, heel/toe strike, walk in a straight line 'on a tight rope', turn quickly around (cerebellar function); symmetric or asymmetric, do they perform the Gower's manoeuvre (assessing proximal muscle strength).
• Visual acuity, hearing, speech.
• Behaviour,
• Movements.

Examine:
• Skin, spine, and head circumference.
• Co-ordination (taxis) and formation of movement (praxis) by simple games. 'Take this bread from my hand', 'Pretend to open a door'.

Cranial nerves (II, III, IV, VI)

• Look at the child's eyes. Do they fix and follow?
• Move an interesting toy and watch child's eye movements. Get the child to look at you. Will they look left or right when the toy comes in from each side of their visual field? Is there a squint, is it the common type—non-paralytic—where they can move the eyes fully, but with asymmetry?
• Get a carer to stand behind you and wiggle their nose. Ask the child to 'see if you can count how many times daddy wiggles his nose', then look at their fundi by asking them to look at daddies nose and ask him to keep the child gaze on her.

Other cranial nerves

• Watch the facial movements (VII).
• Say something with your hand covering your mouth and see if the child responds appropriately (VIII).
• Does the child dribble excessively? Ask a carer or watch them swallow and listen to their articulation of speech (IX, X).
• Children love to stick out their tongues and shrug their shoulders (XI, XII).

Neuromuscular and peripheral examination

Children who can walk, run, jump, hop, and spring up form the ground well are very unlikely to have an abnormality of the peripheral neurological system that will be identified on further examination. However, if there is an abnormality do the following.

- Remove clothes as far as underwear if the child is happy.
- Look at the gait. Where does the foot strike? Heel or toe? Is it waddling, asymmetrical, is there abnormality of posture?
- Observe the muscle bulk and joint positions with particular reference to scoliosis, lordosis, hip flexion, ankle inversion, or eversion.
- Assess the upper limbs for joint ranges, tone, and power, by having a game with the child. Laugh and keep praising them. Use an adult tendon hammer and elicit the reflexes, but place your thumb over the biceps and brachioradialis.
- Have another game as you assess the same in the lower limbs.
- Try to categorize the pattern into increased or decreased tone. Is it mainly unilateral; or bilateral, but mainly in the legs, or in all four limbs, and possibly the bulbar muscles?

Sensation

If indicated assess sensation by asking them to close their eyes and say 'Luton' every time they feel your touch. Note that children do not like closing their eyes with a stranger, so reassure them by doing it first on daddy, then with eyes open (briefly), finally with their eyes closed. Move around dermatome by dermatome, but move irregularly when you will touch them, otherwise they may say they can feel it by guessing when the next touch is likely to come.

Examination: children aged <5 years who can't walk

Observe and note the following:
- Developmental stage. Can they see, hear, or move?
- Do they vocalize?
- Are they dysmorphic? Are their orthoses, e.g. wheelchair, visible?

Examination

Don't rush to get the child's clothes off as you will frighten them. Examine the following:
- Skin for neurocutaneous stigmata;
- Spine;
- Fundi;
- Head circumference (when they like you, or at the end of the examination if you haven't managed to break the ice).
- Check for dysmorphic features.

Cranial nerves (II, III, IV, VI)

- Check visual acuity. Will they fix on a small toy or large object, e.g. toy, face, bright light? If they do not fix are they pupil responses, i.e. is the child blind? Will they follow it?
- Are their eyes symmetrical with a full range of movement, when following small and large toys?
- Other cranial nerves.
- Will they respond to a quiet, moderate, or loud sound (VIII)?
- Elicit a smile, or wait to see if there is a grimace (VII).
- Ask about or watch their swallow (IX, X).

Neuromuscular and peripheral examination

- *Observe their best motor function:* antigravity movement; rolling over; lifting head up; sitting up; or pulling to stand.
- Place your little fingers in their hands while lying supine. Do they have a primitive grasp reflex? Then pull them up off their bed, watching for head lag, which would imply low tone, reduced power, or both.
- If child has head control, see if they can sit with or without support.
- Pick them up under their armpits. Do they slip through your hands (a sign of hypotonia)?
- Then assess their parachute and moro reflexes (see 🕮 pp.145, 558).
- *Power:* observe the movements and pattern of any paucity.
- *Tone:* gently manipulate joints, but take care to avoid trauma.
- *Reflexes:* use an adult tendon hammer and elicit the reflexes, but place your thumb over the tendons.
- *Co-ordination:* if age-appropriate, assess fine motor ability by presenting an attractive target for them to take or grasp with either a primitive or pincer grasp.
- Sensation is difficult to access in children with mental age <2. A clue to an abnormality may be inferred from other signs (e.g. skin, peripheral motor system).

Congenital abnormalities

There are many disorders that can affect the brain. The majority are classed as disorders of neuronal migration or cortical dysplasia and are thought to either be genetically programmed, due to gene mutation, or a disruption of foetal development due to a deleterious process between the 6th and 16th week of pregnancy, e.g. vascular or viral. They are normally associated with developmental delay, may have a cerebral palsy, and can have very troublesome epilepsies.

Investigation

This is normally initiated after an abnormality is licked up on standard MRI scan of the head. Unless the disorder is likely to have been caused by a single process, e.g. mutation in the *Lis1* gene causing the majority of children with isolated lissencephaly, then it is important to perform a full examination and look for other stigmata of a genetic or acquired disorder. For example, dysmorphic features, for the former, and stigmata of infection for the latter.

Most children will benefit from exact radiological classification of the abnormality, and associated changes on examination/history, then targeted genetic investigation. If this fails, then karyotype and micro array analyses should be undertaken.

Lissencephaly 'smooth brain'

There is absence of normal gyri on the cerebral cortex (Fig. 14.1). The children may have unusual facial appearance, difficulty swallowing, failure to thrive, seizures, and severe learning disability. Hands, fingers, or toes may be deformed. It may be associated with other diseases including, Miller-Dieker and Walker-Warburg syndromes. Where multiple genes are deleted, e.g. Miller-Dieker, then wider malformations are seen. In isolated lissencephaly, the majority will either have a change within the Lis1 gene, or it is completely lost (Miller-Dieker).

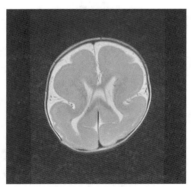

Fig. 14.1 T2-weighted axial MRI images of a lissencephalic brain.

Pachygyria
Here, there is a paucity of gyri vs the absence in lissencephaly. Although milder, it is associated with a very similar range of complications and management is similar.

Heterotopia
In these disorders there is abnormal positioning of the white/grey matter (Fig. 14.2). It is more commonly used to describe abnormal migration of grey matter. It can be a single area, multiple, nodular or a band. Milder than either of the above, many children will be normal, or present later in life with events such as new onset seizures.

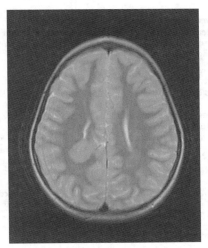

Fig. 14.2 T2-weighted axial MRI scan, showing a isolated area of heterotopia in the right hemisphere.

Cortical dysplasias
These can occur as either a very small or large lesion. Either can be associated with learning difficulties, and especially seizures. One in particular is very well recognized—*perisylvian polymicrogyria*—which is associated with very troublesome seizures and bulbar difficulties. There is a particular type of cerebral palsy which primarily affects the bulbar muscles (unlike diplegias, hemiplegias and quadripleagias, where bulbar signs are normally much milder than those in the limbs. It is known as *Worster-Drought syndrome*.

Agenesis of the corpus callosum
Can occur as an isolated finding, or in more widespread disorders, e.g. Aicardi Syndrome. It is isolated, children may be almost normal, but as in other disorders there is a significant chance of learning difficulties, and especially seizures.

Paroxysmal episodes: not epilepsy

Up to one-third of children diagnosed with 'epilepsy' actually have non-epileptic events. In adolescents presenting to emergency teams in 'status epilepticus', over half turn out to have non-epileptic psychologically induced episodes. Think carefully about other paroxysmal episodes (such as those described below) before diagnosing a form of epilepsy and treating the child with anticonvulsants.

Aetiology

It is best to consider the cause of paroxysmal episodes according to the age of the child.

Neonates and infants

- *Benign neonatal sleep myoclonus:* these are single or repetitive episodes of jerking of arms and legs (typically while falling asleep after a feed) and sparing the face.
- Shuddering attacks.

Older infants and toddlers

- *'Breath-holding attacks' and RAS:* history of suddenly going limp (or syncope), which may be followed by clonic jerking (e.g. RAS). On closer questioning at least 1 episode has been triggered by a noxious stimulus (e.g. banging head). Typically, there is a short cry and then the child goes limp, collapses to floor, and may have brief jerking movements. Other episodes are characterized by 'blue' breath-holding where the child starts to cry for any reason, the crying builds up, and then the child collapses to the floor at the end of expiration.
- *Masturbation and other gratification phenomena:* when the child is bored they indulge in self-stimulation. In girls, the legs are held outstretched, and the eyes are glazed. Sweatiness almost invariably raises the possibility of a tonic seizure and these episodes are commonly mistreated as epilepsy.
- *Febrile myoclonus:* short jerks associated with high fever.
- *Benign paroxysmal vertigo of childhood:* acute onset of fear, nausea, vertigo, and unsteadiness if forced to walk. Rarely, the child vomits and they may have nystagmus.
- *Benign paroxysmal torticollis:* acute episodes of head tilt, similar to the nystagmus seen in benign paroxysmal vertigo.
- *Night terrors:* while in deep sleep, about 1–2hr after bed, the child suddenly wakes up and is inconsolable. This lasts some 10–20min and then child 'wakes', looks confused, rolls over, and sleeps again.

Childhood

Daydreaming

This episode can appear very similar to an absence seizure. However, the latter will occur at home during activity as well as at school. Classical absences, as part of an idiopathic generalized epilepsy (see 🕮 p.512), can be elicited on an EEG (taken during normal and sleep deprived state) in over 95% of cases. They are short, associated with abrupt psychomotor arrest and immediate resumption of activity, speech, and thought.

Absences as part of a focal seizure disorder will only very rarely occur without some other suggestive feature such as an automatism, abnormal movement, or postictal state.

Syncope
- Also known as fainting.
- Occurs from age 7mths onwards. There may well be a history of precipitating events (e.g. fright, head bang, sudden standing, hair-brushing).
- Often the child has an aura of loss of vision, tingling, and auditory phenomen, this is followed by loss of consciousness and posture change: falls over if standing. Not all syncopal events result in a loss of tone. In some, the fall is accompanied by increased tone.
- Myoclonic jerks may follow for a few seconds. Useful tools in diagnosis include: a history of a precipitant; jerking lasting less than 20secs; and the movements may not be rhythmic.
- If in doubt assume that it is syncope until there is evidence otherwise (see Psychologically determined paroxysmal events (PDPE)).

⚠ **Caution** If there is a history of sudden death in the family, or of syncope induced by sudden physical stress such as exercise or sleep, long QT syndrome should be investigated.

Psychologically determined paroxysmal events (PDPE)
This is a less pejorative term to describe episodes of psychological origin that used to be described as hysteria, and more recently as pseudoseizures, malingering, factitious or conversion disorders. The episodes are a psychological phenomenon, although identifying or looking for the psychological causes at time of diagnosis can be misleading or even counterproductive. There is no single event that will separate them from epilepsy. Some children rarely may even have both.

Features suggestive of, but not diagnostic of PDPE

- Events triggered by specific situations
- Events with convulsive movements that are not explained anatomically, e.g. left arm jerking, then lull followed by right leg
- Thrashing movements that wax and wane, +/– pelvic thrusting
- Eyes open during the episode
- Slumping to the floor in a dramatic manner. Falls without injury
- Violence, rather than violent movements
- Gain from the situation
- Generalized movements with rapid return to normal

These features are not diagnostic. There is no *never* or *always*. In particular, young people can injure themselves and pass urine in PDPE, which are often misreported as a diagnostic feature of genuine seizures (see 📖 p.505).

Paroxysmal episodes: general management

Assessment

History
The majority of paroxysmal episodes can be classified with a careful history. No episode can be safely classified, even after EEG and MRI, if an adequate history has not been taken. Take details of the following:
- *First episode:* when, where, what happened, and the child's responsiveness; how long, recovery, and talk to the witness.
- *Subsequent episodes:* situation, precipitants, duration, frequency.
- Full medical history, family history, developmental and psychosocial history.

Video
If you are unsure about the diagnosis, then request the carers to take a video recording of the event. Do not investigate or treat until the diagnosis is confirmed. Children are safer off treatment, when the clinician is unsure, if the caution below is followed. Even when you are sure of the diagnosis, it is good clinical practice to request video recording of all different paroxysmal events, since the episodes or events may evolve.

> ⚠ **Caution** Even when the diagnosis could be a non-epileptic disorder, until this is confirmed, the carers should be advised how to manage a genuine seizure. The child should avoid specific dangers:
> - injury from fall
> - proximity to swimming water without an identified lifeguard
> - unprotected heat
> - moving objects and machinery

Management

Infantile non-epileptic disorders, syncopal episodes and jerks
Allay the carers' concerns over the diagnosis.

Psychologically determined paroxysmal events
See 📖 p.503. PDPE can be difficult to treat, but these patients do respond to well organized management. The principal areas include the following:
- Unambivalent diagnosis explained to both the parent and the child/young person.
- Acknowledgement/acceptance by the young person, carers and all health professionals that these are non-epileptic.
- Stabilization phase where the family is developing understanding.
- Strengthen coping abilities and remove gain from the behaviour.
- Psychological support is essential. Some families will feel very threatened when the possibility is raised of looking at psychological issues that may have triggered these events in the child.

Seizures and childhood epilepsies

One per cent of children will have had one seizure, not associated with fever, by the age of 14yrs. The majority of these seizures will be generalized tonic–clonic episodes.

Forms of epilepsy

The two main forms of epilepsies can be categorized as having generalized or focal seizures.

Generalized seizures

These can be described as follows:

- *Myoclonic:* with shock-like movement of one/several parts or the whole body.
- *Tonic:* with sustained contraction and stiffness.
- *Clonic:* with rhythmic jerking of one limb, one side, or all of the body. (See how this contrasts with the description of psychologically determined clinical events, 📖 p.503).
- *Tonic–clonic:* a combination of the above forms.
- *Absence:* these are episodes of abrupt psychomotor arrest lasting 5–15s in younger children, but can be longer in the older child. They can be associated with retropulsion of the head, upward deviation of eyes and eyelid, or perioral myoclonia. (You should note that facial myoclonia can be asymmetrical and give the impression of a 'focal' seizure).

Focal seizures

These seizures start in one area of the brain and then may spread, and ultimately generalize. If the latter part of the event is witnessed it may be described incorrectly as being primarily generalized. The semiology depends on the locality of the initial electrical activity. 'Typical' seizure semiology includes the following:

- *Occipital:* multicoloured bright lights spreading from one area of homonymous visual fields.
- *Centroparietal:* sensorimotor phenomena spreading from one limb and marching up one side of the body.
- *Temporal:* feelings of gastric discomfort, strangeness, anxiety, memory disturbances (e.g. familiarity, 'déjà vu'), autonomia (e.g. automatisms such as nose rubbing), and contralateral clonic or dystonic movements.
- *Frontal:* dystonic posturing and strange guttural noises.

Status epilepticus (StE)

StE can be convulsive with tonic/clonic movements. Alternatively, it can be non-convulsive with impairment of consciousness and often subtle twitching. Technically, StE is a seizure lasting for more than 30min, or repeated seizures lasting more than 30min without recovery of consciousness in between. Practically, though, the treatment algorithm for StE can be used once a convulsive seizure has lasted longer than 5min (see 📖 pp.80–81).

Seizures: management

First unprovoked seizure

- *History:* a full account of personal, social, and family history should be obtained.
- *Examination:* perform a thorough examination looking for markers of neurological diseases, particularly skin and dysmorphism.
- *Electroencephalography (EEG):* there is debate as to whether an EEG should be obtained. The current opinion is that, in most children, it is unlikely to influence management. Few specialists would start therapy at this point whatever the EEG showed. With expert neurophysiology a more accurate prognosis may be given, which in turn may influence therapy.
- *Imaging:* MRI is not indicated after a single seizure alone. However, if abnormality is found on physical examination then MRI is very important to exclude a space-occupying lesion.

Febrile seizures

These can occur in infants or small children. Most last a minute or two, but it can be just a few seconds. Others last for more than 15min.

- Typically, these children have no prior neurological disease or focal deficits on examination. Here are some key facts about febrile seizures.
- They occur in up to 4% of all children, generally between the ages of 6mths and 6yrs (although it is unusual to have one's first episode when aged >4yrs).
- These children may have a temperature ≥39°C, however the temperature may have become normal by the time it is measured.
- The seizure tends to occur during the first day of fever.
- Children prone to febrile seizures are not considered to have epilepsy.
- Recurrence risk of seizures is 35% over lifetime; 25% during the next 12mths.
- The vast majority of febrile seizures are harmless.
- 95–98% of children who have experienced febrile seizures do not go on to develop epilepsy.
- Children who have febrile seizures that are lengthy, affect only part of the body, recur within 24hr, or who have neurological abnormalities have a higher incidence of subsequent epilepsy.

Categorization

- *Simple febrile seizures (typical):* generalized tonic–clonic activity lasting <15min with associated fever.
- *Complex febrile seizures (atypical):* these occur in up to 15% of cases and are characterized by focal seizure activity, or prolonged seizure longer than 15min, or multiple seizures within a day.
- Convulsive seizures that occur in a child with no neurological problems, in the context of an intercurrent infection, even without a recorded fever, are normally classified as febrile.

Management of febrile seizure

Safety
- Move any danger away from the child and consider their privacy
- Place the child on a protected surface on their side
- It is good practice to note the time

Assistance
- The family should call for help if unfamiliar with febrile seizures
- Then call ambulance

Treatment
- If the seizure lasts >10min, the child should be treated for status epilepticus
- Once the seizure has ended, the child should be assessed for the source of the fever, investigated, and treated appropriately
- Consider admission and observation, especially if this is the first episode

Meningitis?
- Consider meningitis if the child shows symptoms of stiff neck, extreme lethargy more than 4hr post-seizure, abundant vomiting, or is <12mths old
- If there is concern perform a lumbar puncture as long as the child is not encephalopathic

Seizure prevention and home care
- There is poor evidence to support interventions to prevent febrile seizures
- Parents should give standard antipyretics early in any febrile illness
- Parents should get expert advice if a previous seizure lasted >10min

Epilepsies: neonatal

See also 📖 p.134. Neonatal seizures are rarely part of a benign epilepsy syndrome, expert advice should be sought.

- They are more commonly a symptom of underlying, severe cerebral dysfunction.
- Seizures are never generalized tonic–clonic seizures because the brain has not matured enough to produce synchronous epileptic activity.

Management

- *History:* is there a family history of similar convulsions with benign prognosis? Take a history for cerebral insults such as hypoxia-ischaemia. Is there a relevant family history, including consanguinity?
- *Examination:* look for neurocutaneous stigmata and dysmorphic features.
- *Blood investigations:* FBC; CRP; blood glucose; serum electrolytes (calcium and phosphate).
- *Lumbar puncture:* CSF glucose, red blood cell count (RCC), and white cell count (WCC); CSF microscopy and growth culture; CSF lactate and glycine; CSF latex agglutin (group B streptococci).

Epileptic encephalopathy If no cause is evident consider the investigations for epileptic encephalopathy (see Box 14.1). Follow advice of the biochemist for further investigation or management of relevant results

Drug treatment

- *Phenobarbital:* treat by loading with 20mg/kg IV. Continue on 5mg/kg once daily for at least 2wks.
- *Pyridoxal phosphate 10mg/kg/qds PO:* if the infant is unresponsive to Phenobarbital, treat with pyridoxal phosphate. If possible wait for 48hr to assess effect.
- *Clonazepam:* if the pyridoxal phosphate has proved ineffective or the seizures continue to give the child significant cardiorespiratory compromise, commence infusion of IV clonazepam at 5micrograms/kg/min increasing as seizures continue up to a maximum of 20micrograms/kg/min.

Box 14.1 Investigations for epileptic encephalopathy

Examinations

- *Wood's light:* tuberous sclerosis
- *Ophthalmology:* retinitis pigmentosa, phakomata, and other ophthalmological markers of neurological disorders
- *MRI:* neuronal migration defects, structural abnormalities

Blood: routine

- *U&E, urate:* renal and purine disorders
- *Liver function tests:* liver dysfunction
- *Ammonia:* urea cycle defects and liver failure
- *Lactate:* mitochondrial disease
- *Thyroid function tests:* thyroid disease
- *Chromosomes:* major structural chromosomal abnormalities

Blood: special biochemistry

- *Plasma amino acid (including glycine and serine) and total homocysteine:* aminoacidaemias and defects in homocysteine remethylation
- *Transferrin isoelectric focusing:* congenital defects of glycosylation
- *Biotinidase:* biotinidase deficiency
- *Carnitine profile:* mitochondrial fatty acid β-oxidation defects

Blood and CSF

- *Plasma glucose matched with CSF glucose:* glucose carrier transport deficiency
- *CSF lactate:* mitochondrial cytopathies
- *CSF glycine and serine:* non-ketotic hyperglycinaemia and 3-phosphoglycerate dehydrogenase deficiency

Urine

- *Amino and organic acids:* amino and organic acidurias, sulphite oxidase deficiency, and molybdenum cofactor deficiency
- *Purine and pyrimidine:* disorders of purine and pyrimidine metabolism
- *Creatine to guanidinoacetate ratio-* disorders of creatine metabolism

Epilepsies: infantile

Infantile epilepsies are challenging and expert advice should be sought.

Benign myoclonic epilepsy of infancy

This form of epilepsy requires no further investigation or therapy providing that what is observed meets the following criteria.

- Myoclonic seizures only.
- No other seizure type.
- Normal interictal EEG.
- Normal development.

West's syndrome

The diagnosis of this condition is based on a classic triad.

- *Infantile spasms:* short tonic contraction of trunk with upward elevation of arms; may be confused with gastro-oesophageal reflux or colic.
- *Developmental:* delay or regression.
- *Hypsarrhythmia:* on the EEG.

Often children have only some of these or the EEG is reported as being chaotic, with high voltage sharp and slow waves, but not 'classical hypsarrhythmia'.

Investigations

Take a thorough history and examination and make sure that you have excluded tuberous sclerosis (see 📖 pp.530, 947). Then, use the series of investigations on the previous page for epileptic encephalopathy.

Treatment

Children with West's Syndrome are best cared for at home.

Prednisolone therapy

- *Step 1:* 15mg* oral/tds for the first week
- *Step 2:* Continuing seizures. Increase oral dose to 20mg*, qds
- *Step 3:* at 14 days. Withdraw—in four steps over 15 days

* This is the complete dose, NOT per kg

Note: The child will be immunosuppressed whilst and for 2wks after therapy. Many will develop hypertension, it is useful to let the GP know the dose of nifedipine should the child become hypertensive. Some authors prefer ACTH IM injections, but evidence of its superiority is poor, and administration is more difficult

Second line therapy is with oral vigabatrin First 24hr: 25mg/kg bd, Next 2 days: 50mg/kg bd, Day 4—if there are continuing seizures—75mg/kg, twice daily for no more than 20wks, due to the risk of visual field damage.

Severe myoclonic epilepsy of infancy

Seizures occur from the first year onwards, and include:
- prolonged (>1hr) febrile and shorter afebrile seizures;
- focal seizures;
- atypical absences;
- segmental myoclonia.

Investigations
- *EEG:* may be normal initially, but may develop photosensitivity (i.e. within 12mths in 50%) and generalized discharges once the seizures are frequent.
- *Genetics:* over 70% have a mutation in the SCN1a gene. However, if negative and the clinical picture is atypical, then use the screening investigations for epileptic encephalopathy (📖 p.509).

Treatment
The treatment should follow a sequence, adding anticonvulsants if there is no response. Lamotrigine should be avoided. The sequence is as follows:
- Start with sodium valproate.
- Add clobazam.
- Consider stiripentol if resistant to therapy (needs expert supervision).

Myoclonic astatic epilepsy

A condition with:
- myoclonic astatic seizures;
- myoclonic jerks;
- generalized tonic–clonic seizures.

The EEG demonstrates predominantly generalized discharges once seizures are established. Seek advice about further investigation and treat as for idiopathic generalized epilepsy (📖 p.513). Seizures in this condition are likely to be unresponsive, so consider using the ketogenic diet early in refractory cases.

Lennox–Gastaut syndrome

A condition with:
- Tonic seizures with trunk flexion (often evolving out of infantile spasms).
- Atonic seizures, myoclonic jerks, atypical absences.

Invariably there is developmental delay once the seizures are established. This condition rarely responds to drugs. Seek advice about further investigation and treat as for an idiopathic generalized epilepsy (📖 p.513), initially, then getting expert help.

Epilepsies: mid to late childhood (1)

Idiopathic generalized epilepsies

These epilepsies are better described as genetic epilepsies. The diagnosis of epilepsy rests on the history. The EEG helps with classification. It should be remembered that generalized discharges on EEG (particular with photic stimulation) may occur in children without seizures. There is no need for MRI or blood tests after the first episode. Seizures include combinations of:

- typical absences;
- myoclonia;
- tonic seizures and generalized tonic–clonic seizures;
- myoclonic jerks.

In these patients more than 80% of standard, and 95% of standard + sleep-deprived EEG recordings will show generalized discharges.

Myoclonic absence epilepsy

- Typical absences with short symmetrical jerks of mainly the upper limbs with abduction and elevation.
- Early onset <5yrs of age.
- EEG demonstrates generalized discharges of 3cycles/s spike and wave, that are not well formed and, in addition, may have short bursts of polyspikes.
- Poor prognosis and can deteriorate into an epileptic encephalopathy, may require treatment with the ketogenic diet.

Childhood absence epilepsy

- Previously known as '*petit mal*'.
- Typical absences only, but very frequent.
- Present during the first decade.
- Rarely develop generalized tonic–clonic seizures.
- Absences can be associated with mild myoclonia, asymmetry, or automatisms.
- EEG demonstrates regular bursts of 3cycles/s spike and wave.

Juvenile absence epilepsy

- Onset towards the end of the first and during the second decade.
- All have absences.
- Up to 30% have myoclonic jerks.
- Majority develop generalized tonic–clonic seizures during second decade if untreated.
- EEG discharges more fragmented and irregular than in childhood absence epilepsy, with more bursts of polyspike.
- Prognosis is guarded even after many years of being seizure-free as an adult, relapse is common.

Juvenile myoclonic epilepsy
- Onset in the second decade.
- Invariable myoclonic jerks classically within the first hour of awakening.
- High risk of generalized tonic–clonic seizures, up to 80% of adolescent girls will have further generalized tonic–clonic seizures if they withdraw medication completely.
- EEG may have absences and photosensitivity; discharges are more fragmented and irregular than in juvenile absence epilepsy with bursts of polyspike.

Treatment of idiopathic generalized epilepsies
- *First-line:* sodium valproate is normally used as first-line therapy, except in childhood absence epilepsy, where ethosuximide can be considered. In girls aged >9yrs, families should be counselled that it is up to twice as likely to produce seizure freedom as other drugs. Some experts (but not others) consider it may stimulate appetite and increase the incidence of polycystic ovary syndrome. Both of which reverse on drug withdrawal. All experts agree that it is significantly more teratogenic than other anti-epileptic drugs if taken during pregnancy at a dose of more than 1000mg per day.
- *Second-line:* lamotrigine is the next choice, but take note that it needs to be introduced more slowly when sodium valproate is being used concurrently.
- *Third-line:* there is no consensus. Some clinicians advocate using a benzodiazepine and suggest clonazepam as the most effective. However, it is extremely difficult to withdraw if it is used in moderate to high dosage. Therefore, others advise using clobazam, topiramate, or levetiracetam.

Epilepsies: mid to late childhood (2)

Idiopathic focal epilepsies

The term idiopathic focal epilepsy, or benign focal epilepsy, is used less frequently due to the severity of the seizures in some children.

Benign childhood epilepsy with centrotemporal spikes—Rolandic Epilepsy'

The classic presentation of this condition is:

- Predominantly nocturnal sensorimotor seizures.
- Onset in one side of face or a hand, then spreading down one side and may generalize.
- EEG may be relatively normal whilst awake.
- EEG in slow wave sleep or drowsiness will develop frequent centrotemporal spike and wave discharges with an easily recognizable shape and distribution.

The majority of children with this condition have infrequent, short seizures and the decision whether to treat or not is taken after discussion with the parents and child. Some clinicians feel strongly that therapy should be the same as in idiopathic generalized epilepsy, but others will consider using carbamazepine.

Benign childhood occipital seizure syndrome (Panayiotopoulos syndrome)

- Young children (aged 1–7yrs).
- *Bizarre seizures:* prolonged (<30min), stereotyped episodes of encephalopathy often associated with ictal vomiting, headache, and eye deviation.
- Often misdiagnosed.
- Heterogeneous EEG abnormalities.
- Good prognosis.
- Treatment is rarely indicated.

Landau–Kleffner syndrome (LKS) and electrical status in slow wave sleep

These conditions are considered to be an extreme variant, marked by the following:

- Intellectual regression with relatively few seizures.
- Striking language impairment—an epileptic aphasia in LKS.
- EEG may show non-specific abnormalities in the waking state, but once drowsy or in slow wave sleep the EEG develops electrical status.

They are difficult to treat and normally refractory to first-line drugs. Steroids are advocated and have been shown to be of temporary benefit. They may even improve long-term outcome.

Focal epilepsies

These epilepsies are symptomatic of a focal area of dysfunction, but the electrical discharges may generalize (i.e. secondary generalization).

- While the electrical discharges are focal, consciousness may be maintained (previously known as simple partial seizures).
- When the discharges become more widespread consciousness will be impaired or lost (previously known as complex partial seizures).
- They all may develop into a secondarily generalized seizure. At that point it is not possible to classify them if the onset has not been witnessed.
- Their expression will depend on the principally affected area of the brain.

Frontal lobe epilepsies

These children tend to have short, but frequent seizures—particularly arising out of sleep. They are often associated with asymmetric dystonic posturing and brought on by loud noises. Recovery can be quick and they may be difficult to assess on the EEG.

Temporal lobe epilepsies

The seizures affect memory and emotion with disturbances such as '*déjà vu*', fear, abdominal discomfort, and automatisms.

Occipital lobe epilepsies

These episodes are associated with simple multicoloured blobs of light in one side of a visual field. They often produce headache and vomiting.

Management of focal epilepsies

Investigation

MRI is always indicated. Children rarely have malignant brain tumours. However, they can have dysplasias, gliosis, and benign tumours. The temporal lobe may show hippocampal sclerosis.

Treatment

- *First-line:* carbamazepine is generally recommended.
- *Second-line:* therapy is widely debated. There are few good studies comparing anti-epileptic drugs against each other. However, sodium valproate is a logical choice amongst the older anticonvulsants (but not in girls >9yrs of age). Of the newer anticonvulsants, lamotrigine, topiramate, and levetiracetam could be used, but licensing conditions should be noted.

Headache

Children with headache are commonly referred to general paediatricians.
- Over 90% will have chronic childhood headache, with no identifiable physical cause.
- Some have migraine.
- Malignant brain tumours obstructing CSF flow, causing hydrocephalus and consequent headaches, are less common. These are almost always associated with focal signs on examination or a suggestive history (see 📖 pp.653, 662), if present for more than 6wks.

Chronic, tension type headache

This form of headache is:
- regular;
- often frontal;
- not associated with vomiting, paraesthesia, visual disturbance, or abnormality on examination (including BP).

History

The headache may be reported to be severe enough to take time off school, but with few objective signs of pain. A full history is important, not only to exclude migraine and symptoms of raised ICP, but also to elucidate stresses that may be causing the headache or gains the child may have from the behaviour. It should be assumed to be chronic if present for more than 6wks.

Treatment

- Reassure the family that, with the thorough history and examination, migraine and tumours can be excluded.
- It is inappropriate to perform either a CT or an MRI scan.

Sympathize with the family over the problem and suggest analgesia, but at best it is likely to make no difference. Therefore dosage and number of drugs should be reduced to the minimum acceptable. Encourage the child or young person to continue doing all the normal activities for somebody of their age. 'I can't take away the headache, but the more normal things you do and the fewer drugs you take, the less you will notice the pain'.

Raised ICP

This is a potent cause of headache and will be associated with either or both of the following:
- *Abnormal examination:* in particular, heel–toe walking, finger–nose co-ordination, eye movements, and fundi (i.e. papilloedema).
- *Severe short history:* vomiting, morning headache, visual disturbance.

Clinically, the main concern is a *mass obstructing CSF flow*, particularly a malignant posterior fossa tumour. Therefore the children need expert opinion on neuroimaging as soon as possible. MRI superior, but CT head is performed if MRI not immediately available.

However, the ICP can be raised without abnormality evident on CT scan. In some of these children there may be thrombosis of a cerebral sinus. Therefore, MRI and MRV are recommended.

A subgroup has raised pressure of unknown cause—idiopathic intracranial hypertension, where the only sign on examination will be papilloedema +/– reduced visual acuity, with normal cranial imaging, except for the lateral venous sinuses, which can look compressed.

Idiopathic intracranial hypertension (IIH)

IIH or benign IH or pseudotumour cerebri typically is associated with obesity, female sex, and adolescence. It is important to exclude secondary cases caused by:

- *Drugs:* steroid withdrawal; vitamin A; thyroid replacement; oral contraceptive pills; phenothiazines.
- *Systemic disease:* iron deficiency; Guillain–Barré syndrome; systemic lupus erythematosus.
- *Endocrine changes:* adrenal failure; hyperthyroidism; hypoparathyroidism; menarche; pregnancy; obesity.
- *Head injury.*

History

Early morning headache blurred or double vision, vomiting.

Examination and investigation

- *General:* check BP.
- *Neurology:* there may be ataxia.
- *Eyes:* papilloedema; scotoma on visual field testing.
- *Imaging:* normal.
- *Lumbar puncture:* raised ICP (>20cm CSF); normal CSF cell count, protein, and glucose.

Management

- Weight loss in the obese.
- Try and remove the causal medication.
- *Diuretics:* to reduce CSF formation (e.g. acetazolamide, furosemide).
- *Steroids:* may be effective, but can cause rebound problems when withdrawn.
- Serial lumbar punctures or surgical intervention.
- *Monitoring of eyes and visual fields:* most patients without visual deficit do well, but some patients with eye problems may deteriorate.

Headache: migraine

Up to 10% of children may have migraine. These are debilitating episodes and the criteria are listed below. If they occur frequently (more than 4 times per month for more than 3mths), the diagnosis is unlikely. If the headache occurs daily then the term chronic headache should be used and managed as described on ☐ p.516.

Treatment

- *Exclude triggers:* such as diet, dehydration, overtiredness, and stress.
- *Paracetamol and domperidone:* these can be tried initially, at the onset of symptoms, as they will treat the headache and nausea.
- *Prophylaxis:* if the migraine is frequent enough to disrupt schooling or social activity, then consider prophylaxis. The evidence-base for different therapies is poor. Initially try a 3mths trial of pizotifen. If this is not effective, then try propranolol. Antidepressants such as amitriptyline have also been used. Sumatriptan may be used in children older than 12yrs at the onset of symptoms, if other treatments are ineffective.

Diagnostic criteria for paediatric migraine

Migraine without aura

A At least 5 attacks fulfilling B–D
B Headache attack *lasting 1–48hr*
C Headache has at least *two of the following:*
- Bilateral (temporal or frontal) or unilateral location
- Pulsating quality
- Moderate to severe intensity
- Aggravation by routine physical activity
D During headache, at least *one of the following:*
- Nausea and/or vomiting
- Photophobia and/or phonophobia

Migraine with aura

A *Idiopathic recurring disorder:* headache that usually *lasts 1–48hr*
B At least *two attacks fulfilling C*
C At least *three of the following:*
- One or more fully reversible aura symptoms indicating focal cortical and/or brainstem dysfunction
- At least one aura developing gradually over >4min, or two or more symptoms occurring in succession
- No aura lasting >60min
- Headache follows in <60min

Bell's palsy

- Acute paralysis of the muscles of facial expression may be unable to close the eye on the affected side.
- Normally unilateral, but may be bilateral lower motor neuron lesion.
- 2° to oedema of the facial nerve as it passes through the temporal bone.

Aetiology

- Idiopathic.
- Varicella and other viruses.
- *Borrelia burgdorferi* (Lyme disease), particularly if bilateral.

Examination

- *Check:* whether other branches of the facial nerve are affected, e.g. hyperacusis.
- *Full systemic examination:* in particular, look for signs of leukaemia and vasculitides.
- *Full neurological examination:* look for other signs, the presence of which would exclude an idiopathic Bell's palsy.

Investigation

- FBC and film (leukaemia).
- Varicella titres.
- Borrelia investigation, in suspicious cases, only after discussion with microbiology as this is a difficult infection to either refute or confirm.

Treatment

- *Steroids:* evidence for the use of steroids is limited, but the general opinion is to use 2mg/kg (maximum 60mg) prednisolone, once daily for 5 days if the symptoms are less than 7 days old.
- *Aciclovir:* recent evidence indicates that oral aciclovir (40mg/kg/day) for 10 days, irrespective of varicella status, may be useful.

Prognosis Most children will either recover fully or recover to a good degree. When this does not occur after 6mths, referral for facial nerve grafting is appropriate.

Acute disseminated encephalomyelitis

ADEM is an immune mediated disease. It usually occurs following a viral infection, but may follow other infections or vaccination. It involves auto-immune demyelination, it is similar to multiple sclerosis- although mono-phasic. ADEM produces multiple inflammatory lesions in the brain and spinal cord, particularly in the white matter. Usually these are found in the subcortical/central white matter and cortical gray-white junction of both cerebral hemispheres, cerebellum, brainstem, and spinal cord, but other areas including the basal ganglia may also be involved.

Presentation
- The average age around 5–8yrs old.
- Abrupt onset and a monophasic course.
- Symptoms usually begin 1–3wks after infection or vaccination and include fever, headache, drowsiness, coma, and seizures.
- Average time to maximum severity about four and a half days.
- Additional symptoms include hemiparesis, paraparesis, and cranial nerve palsies.

Diagnosis

This is based on finding typical changes on MRI- as above in the subcor-tical/central white matter, cortical gray-white junction, cerebellum, brain-stem, and spinal cord. The basal ganglia may also be involved (Fig. 14.3). CSF may show a mild lymphocytosis, with normal glucose, but there may be a mild rise in protein.

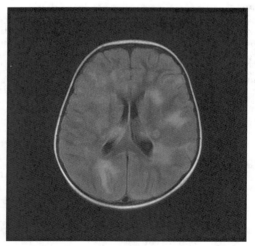

Fig. 14.3 MRI head scan of child with ADEM on FLAIR sequence, which shows the subcortical/central white matter, cortical gray-white junction lesions well.

Treatment

It is important to exclude other causes of encephalopathy (📖 pp.72–79, 552). Then supportive measures such as hydration/feeding, bulbar function and respiration should be instituted. Pulsed intravenous methylprednisolone is widely recommended as definitive treatment, and is normally associated with improvement within days.

ADEM may relapse once or twice, it is then called M(ultiple)DEM.

Multiple Sclerosis rarely occurs in childhood, but becomes more common as children approach adulthood. It presents with demyelinating plaques, which differ from ADEM in their distribution- more periventricular white matter, and with much less encephalopathy, seizures, and coma, but more focal neurological signs.

Stroke in childhood

Cerebrovascular stroke—although commonly presenting with congenital hemiplegia—is rare in childhood, but it does cause significant morbidity. The cause can be arterial-ischaemic, haemorrhagic, or venous in origin. The majority of cases will have a likely cause identified on history and/or examination. The main causes are:

- sickle cell disease;
- congenital cardiac defects;
- cerebral infection;
- trauma (arterial dissection).

Management

Children with stroke will need initial attention to ABC (see 📖 p.46) and treatment of acute conditions such as mastioditis/meningitis before early transfer to a specialist unit.

Investigation

Once stable all children will require brain imaging—preferably magnetic resonance imaging and angiography of both cerebral and neck vessels, rather than CT scan (although CT will show the distribution of injury and exclude haemorrhage). Even with a known cause such as trauma, all children require screening for underlying thrombophilia as these conditions may co-exist. If there is no obvious cause then the investigations in the box should be considered.

Treatment

After stabilization, acute treatment should be undertaken in a specialist centre. Subsequent management, although acute, would be undertaken with the same team and aims as that outlined for cerebral palsy.

Investigation for stroke

Blood: haematology
- *FBC, ESR:* polycythaemia
- *Thrombophilia screen, fibrinogen:* thrombophilia

Blood: biochemistry
- Electrolytes, magnesium
- Liver function tests
- *CRP:* inflammation
- *Plasma lactate and CSF lactate:* mitochondrial disorders
- *Fasting glucose:* diabetes
- *Fasting lipid screen:* hyperlipidaemias
- *Thyroid function tests:* Hashimoto thyroiditis/encephalopathy
- *Ammonia:* urea cycle disorders
- *Homocysteine (free and total):* methyltetrahydrofolate reductase (MTHFR) deficiency can also be picked up by common mutation analysis on the thrombophilia screen, and if symptomatic has a raised plasma homocysteine
- Serum iron, total iron binding capacity, ferritin, red cell folate, and vitamin B_{12}: iron deficiency and other nutritional disorders
- *Plasma amino acids:* aminoacidurias
- *Carnitine (acyl, free, and total):* β-oxidation defects

Urine: biochemistry
Urine organic and amino acids: homocystinuria, MTHFR deficiency

Blood immunology and infection screen
- *IgG, IgM, IgA:* immunodeficiency
- *Titres for infection screen of: Mycoplasma, Chlamydia, Helicobacter, Borrelia, Brucella;* viruses (echo, Coxsackie, Epstein–Barr, *Varicella,* hepatitis B)
- *ASOT, Anti DNAase B:* streptococcal disease
- *ANA, ANCA, anticardiolipin and antiphospholipid antibody:* SLE and autoimmune disease

Imaging studies
- *Magnetic resonance imaging and angiography of head/neck:* vascular disease, particularly dissection and thromboembolism
- *Echocardiogram:* endocarditis and other cardiac disease

Acute abnormal movements

Ataxia

An abnormality in gait that is wide-based, staggering, and unsteady may have a number of causes including:

- Posterior fossa tumours.
- Inborn errors of metabolism.
- Poisoning.
- Brainstem encephalitis.
- *Post-infectious or autoimmune:* acute cerebellar ataxia.
- Trauma.
- Vascular disorders.
- *Congenital malformations:* Dandy–Walker.
- *Neurological:* olivopontocerebellar degeneration, ataxia–telangiectasia (at), adrenoleucodystrophy, Friedreich's ataxia (FrA).
- Conversion disorders.

Clinical review

- *Speech:* increased separation of syllables and varied volume—scanning speech.
- *Neurology:* sensory disturbance in proprioception, positive Romberg, nystagmus with eye movement.
- *Systemic:* immunodeficiency in AT; hypertrophic cardiomyopathy and diabetes in Fanconi's anaemia (FA).

Investigation

Cerebral imaging, if cause not found plasma and CSF analysis for the above, with particular reference to assessing for varicella, streptococcal and other infections, and for inborn errors of metabolism, e.g. urea cycle disorders.

Chorea

Jerk-like movements may involve the face, arms, or legs. In childhood the causes include:

- *Drugs:* anticonvulsants, psychotropics, benzodiazepine withdrawal after intensive care.
- *Systemic illness:* Sydenham's chorea, SLE, hyperthyroidism.
- *Genetic:* Huntington's chorea, glutaric aciduria and other inborn errors of metabolism, benign familial chorea.
- *Other:* pregnancy.

Streptococcal infection

Sydenham's chorea is often associated with streptococcal infection. It occurs in older children particularly girls. It is frequently misdiagnosed as being psychogenic, particularly as it may be associated with emotional liability. It is characterized by the onset of a mild to moderate chorea (may be unilateral) that is more distal, in a well child (possibly with recent infection).

- About 20% of rheumatic fever cases include chorea.
- *Treatment:* high-dose penicillin V 500mg, oral, bd., for 10 days; then daily prophylaxis.

- Sodium valproate is the first line treatment, if inborn errors of metabolism are unlikely, as it can cause metabolic decompensation.
- Benzodiazepines, phenothiazine, haloperidol may control the movement.
- Improvement may occur over weeks to months.

Paediatric autoimmune neuropsychiatric disorder associated with streptococcus (PANDAS)

PANDAS has specific diagnostic criteria and is accompanied by behavioural problems, e.g. obsessive–compulsive disease and tics. There is some debate as to whether it represents a separate entity.

Conversion or 'psychologically mediated' disorders

A high percentage of children older than 7yrs who present with rapidly progressing and bizarre neurological symptoms, with no sign of systemic illness, and retained consciousness have a conversion disorder. These children are more likely to be teenage girls. However, it is important that this fact should not prejudice your clinical assessment—major oversights and mistakes can be made. These children tend to be well and have signs that cannot be explained anatomically, e.g. paralysis of one leg and the contralateral arm, sensory disturbances that do not fit a typical neuropathy, and visual phenomena.

The initial diagnosis should be that of a genuine physical disorder until **all** assessments (medical, psychological, and social) are complete.

⚠ *Examination must be thorough.* You may reveal inconsistent signs such as an inability to lift the leg off bed, but the child is able to walk across the room. Video can be very helpful, especially if a second opinion is needed/the signs intermittent.

Investigation

These should only be undertaken if clinically indicated, as there is a risk of a false positive

Imaging Sophisticated imaging is at the physician's discretion, but the family is likely to become very distressed if a psychological diagnosis is given while there are outstanding investigations. Therefore correlate all the relevant information, decide if it is either psychological or a physical disorder. If unsure refer for expert opinion.

Treatment If confident it is psychological follow the strategy for PDPE (📖 pp.503–504).

Subdural haemorrhage in a child under 2 years

Children under 2yrs presenting with subdural haemorrhage (SDH) are an important cause of morbidity and mortality. A significant number will have been caused by purposeful, inflicted, trauma, as part of an acceleration/deceleration injury. In the investigation of non-accidental head injury (NAHI) it is important to differentiate inflicted injury and other causes of SDH. This section aims to help doctors and other staff thoroughly investigate the child presenting with SDH.

- This section assumes that the child is stable clinically (airway, breathing, circulation) and relevant teams are being contacted for further opinions.
- The investigations will take at least a week to perform, therefore there is no 'hurry' to produce definitive report/guidance for other professionals until results are available.
- Do not use the term 'shaken baby syndrome'. Shaking is a possible mechanism of injury, and not a syndrome, and should be considered in the context of other mechanisms of non-accidental head injury.
- NAHI is a leading cause of death and disability in children, particularly if cerebral injury is part of the spectrum of damage. Bleeding from torn bridging veins into the subdural space is the hallmark of non-accidental head injury. When infants who developed a SDH after infection or neurosurgical intervention are excluded, in retrospective studies, 24–82% of cases with SDH were highly suggestive of abuse in different series.

Differential diagnosis of SDH

- Trauma, traumatic labour.
- Neurosurgical complications, cranial malformation (aneurysm, arachnoid cyst).
- Cerebral infections.
- Coagulation and haematological disorders.
- Metabolic (glutaric aciduria, galactosaemia).
- Biochemical disorders (hypernatraemia).

Symptoms/signs of acute SDH

- Encephalopathy (irritability, crying, inconsolability, unsettled behaviour, lethargy, meningism, decreased or increased tone, seizures, impaired consciousness).
- Vomiting, poor feeding.
- Breathing abnormalities, apnoea.
- Pallor, shock.
- Tense fontanelle.
- Early post-traumatic seizures occur more frequently in inflicted than in non-inflicted head injury.

Symptoms/signs of subacute or chronic SDH

- Expanding head circumference.
- Vomiting, failure to thrive.
- Neurological deficit/s.

Retinal haemorrhages ('haemorrhagic retinopathy')

- Although strongly associated with NAHI, retinal haemorrhages are not specific for the diagnosis, nor can they be dated with precision. In NAHI haemorrhagic retinopathy can typically affect all retinal layers. It shows different ages and stages of resorption. It can be found throughout the retina to the ora serrata.
- Vitreous haemorrhage is frequent.
- Retinal haemorrhage may be unilateral or asymmetric in terms of number and distribution, however, some victims have none at all (15–25%). In severe life threatening trauma (motor cycle, great height) retinal haemorrhage is found in less then 3%. Retinal haemorrhages in newborns are seen in vacuum-assisted deliveries in up to 75% and in spontaneous vaginal deliveries in up to 33%. They resolve by 2wks after birth, at the latest by 6wks, in the great majority. A consultant ophthalmologist with expertise in the assessment of the eyes in children suspected to have NAHI should examine the child.

Fractures

- Since skull fractures may be missed by bony windows on CT, a plain skull film should be obtained.
- Skull fractures do not heal by callus formation and so dating of an injury is especially difficult. If the edges are round and smooth it is likely to be more than 2wks old.
- If the skull fracture is depressed or has branching, crossing, or stellate fracture lines, it is highly suggestive for NAI, whereas accidental fractures typically are linear, parietal, and over the vertex.
- The typical non-skull fracture of child abuse is the metaphyseal fracture caused by twisting the limb. It can also occur from birth injury (e.g. breech extraction). The 'bucket handle' and 'corner' type metaphyseal fractures are very suggestive for NAI. It is very important to target X-ray imaging on the metaphyses, as wider imaging can miss fractures (see 📖 pp.758, 923, 1000).

Brain imaging

- The initial investigation is likely to be CT, but MRI will also be necessary in most cases (Fig. 14.4).
- MRI is more sensitive in identifying SDH's of different signal characteristics, posterior and middle cranial fossa bleeds, and parenchymal changes in the brain.
- CT scans may miss small subdural bleeds. Blood along the tentorium, interhemispheric haemorrhages, and SDHs in multiple sites or of different densities were almost exclusively seen in NAI. While acute haemorrhage may be isointense with brain on T1-weighted images, acute or subacute blood is more likely to be moderately hyperintense on these sequences.

- T2-weighted sequences may also show high intensity, although this may be difficult to separate from the adjacent signal in CSF. The FLAIR sequence suppresses the signal from normal CSF, allowing the high signal haemorrhage to be visualized.
- In the early acute stage when the blood clot is solid it may not be impressive. However, as it breaks down by fibrinolysis and water is drawn into the haematoma a marked effusion may become visible. Due to the dynamic changes of pathology sequential brain imaging is recommended in order to capture the evolution of different lesions. Within 2–4wks contusions and tears are at their most prominent.
- Encephalomalacia may be apparent and even early atrophy. By 2–3mths atrophy is well established. Areas of contusion and hypoxia-ischaemia have evolved into cysts, and SDH should be clearing.
- A neuroradiologist with experience in NAHI should report/review all scans.

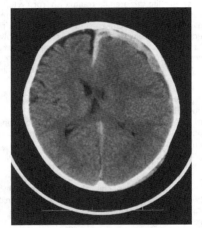

Fig. 14.4 CT head scan of subdural haemorrhage, overlying right frontal lobe, but extending posteriorly and along the falx. Highly suggestive of NAHI. This child also had extensive retinal haemorrhages and was found to have fractures consistent with inflicted injury on skeletal survey.

Coagulation and haematological disorders

- For the exclusion of thrombocytopenia, anaemia and malignancy: do platelet count, FBC and blood film. Renal and liver function tests rule out these acquired coagulation defects.
- The 'coagulation screen' comprises of PT, APPT, Thrombin time, Fibrinogen and 'Mixing studies' (50:50 mix) to exclude inhibitor.
- Factor assays are available for factor II, V, VII, VIII, IX, XI, and 'von Willebrand's disease'. An α 2 antiplasmin deficiency is diagnosed by a thromboelastogram (TEG). Platelet function disorders, vitamin C

deficiency, Factor XIII, and collagen disorders are extremely difficult to diagnose in a child under 2yrs and are very rare conditions.
- Therefore, investigations for these disorders should only be done after discussion with Paediatric haematologist, and on good clinical grounds.

Glutaric aciduria type 1 (GA1)

The exclusion of GA1 is fraught with difficulty. The best approach is to obtain the urine and blood, however, to delay further investigation until other investigations are back. As an example, if the child has multiple fractures, or malicious injuries these would not have been caused by GA1. In such an instance the investigations for organic acids, acylcarnitines, or even a skin biopsy are inappropriate.

Management

- Take full social, medical, family history, including report from social services and police on all adults in household/caring for child.
- CT head and MRI head/spine when possible.
- Skeletal survey.
- Clotting assessment (see Coagulation and haematological disorders, 📖 p.528).
- Take urine to store in case of need to check organic acids.
- Arrange ophthalmology assessment.

Unless sure that there has been accidental trauma, arrange a full conference around the child with relevant professionals, including social services, who may invite police attendance (their responsibility). Remind them: the investigations will take at least a week to perform, therefore there is no 'hurry' to produce definitive report/guidance for other professionals until results are available.

Neurocutaneous disorders

Tuberous sclerosis complex (TSC)

See also 📖 pp.372, 947 and Fig. 14.5.
- TSC is an autosomal dominant inherited disorder affecting brain, skin, heart, kidney, eye, and lung.
- The disorder is caused by haematomata affecting the above organs, although other neoplasms also occur.
- Two genes have been identified: TSC 1 and 2. About 1/3 of cases are inherited, the others de novo mutations.

Diagnosis of TSC

The diagnosis is made when a child has either 2 major, or 1 major and 2 minor criteria.

Major criteria	Minor criteria
• Facial angiofibromas	• Pits in dental enamel
• Ungual fibroma	• Rectal polyps
• Hypomelanotic macules (>3)	• Bone cysts
• Shagreen patch	• Cerebral white matter 'migration tracts'
• Subependymal (subE) nodules	• Gingival fibromas
• subE giant cell astrocytoma	• Non-renal haematoma
• Retinal nodular haematoma	• Retinal achromic patch
• Cardiac rhabdomyohomata	• Confetti skin lesions
	• Multipale renal cysts

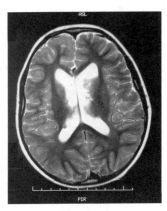

Fig. 14.5 T2-weighted MRI scan of the head showing multiple sub-ependymal nodules, lining the walls of the ventricles.

Management

Treatment is symptomatic depending on the organ-specific effects of the haematoma and neoplasms. All cases require expert assessment:

- Recurrence risk in family members.
- Symptomatic epilepsies, particularly if West syndrome occurs.
- Cardiac rhabdomyomata need to be referred to cardiology support, but if echo/ECG is normal, then they can be discharged as these do not develop postnatally.
- Renal complications are very rare * under 9yrs, but after this bi-annual renal ultrasound with regular enquiry for renal function/loin pain is needed. Polycystic kidney disease can occur if there is contiguous deletion of the neighbouring gene.
- Pulmonary lymphangiomatosis occurs very rarely in childhood, and only in girls. Regular screening is not indicated, unless a history given of respiratory symptoms.
- Ophthalmological haematomata need to be referred to ophthalmology. If fundi are normal, patients can be discharged as these lesions do not develop post-natally.

Neurofibromatosis

See also ⬚ pp.441, 662, 836, 946. There are 2 distinct AD disorders, characterized by multiple benign tumours of the peripheral nerve sheath.

NF1: chromosome 17

The diagnosis is based on having at least 2 of the following:

- >6 *café au lait* macules: >5mm diameter before puberty; >15mm diameter after puberty.
- Skin fold or axillary freckling.
- 1 Neurofibroma or a plexiform neurofibroma.
- 1 Lisch nodule in iris.
- Optic glioma.
- Skeletal dysplasia.
- Affected first-degree relative.

The management of this condition is symptomatic and depends on the local effects of the neurofibroma. However, all cases require expert assessment of:

- recurrence risk in family members (they need assessment annually);
- neoplasia and optic gliomata;
- renal artery stenosis;
- skeletal dysplasia;
- cognitive performance.

NF2: chromosome 22

The diagnosis is based on having 1 major or 2 minor criteria.

- *Major criteria:*
  - unilateral vestibular Schwannoma and first-degree relative with NF2;
  - bilateral vestibular Schwannomas.
- *Minor criteria:*
  - meningioma;
  - Schwannoma;
  - ependymoma;
  - glioma;
  - cataract.

The management of NF2 is complex as the tumours themselves do not need to be removed when identified in many cases, although they may be symptomatic.

Sturge–Weber syndrome

- *Leptomeningeal angiomatosis:* associated with a port wine naevus in the distribution of the first branch of the trigeminal nerve.
- Children may be very well, but can have severe focal epilepsies, learning disability, hemiplegia, glaucoma, and transient stroke-like episodes, and severe headaches.
- *Diagnosis:* on facial appearance and CT ± MRI scan.

Macrocephaly and microcephaly

Macrocephaly

Macrocephaly is defined as a head circumference above the 99.6th centile. The majority of such children will have a benign and familial cause for this condition. However, hydrocephalus and degenerative disorders need to be considered.

History
- Take a full history including developmental progression.
- Are there any features of autism or degenerative disorders?
- Are there signs of raised intracranial pressure?

Examination
- Perform a thorough examination.
- Plot OFC on a growth chart along with previous measurements.
- Look at the skin for signs of neurofibromatosis (see 📖 p.836).

Findings and investigation
- *Abnormal:* if there are any abnormalities these will need further investigation.
- *Normal:* if the examination is normal, try and compare the child's head circumference with parental head circumferences. If they are all large, then the likely diagnosis is familial macrocephaly. If the parents' head circumferences are normal, then the child's condition is probably benign, but it would be appropriate to follow measurements for the next 12mths. If there is crossing of centiles then perform a CT scan, looking for hydrocephalus.

Some children, boys more than girls, present with macrocephaly, mild developmental delay/hypotonia. If there is nothing else in the history and examination then manage as above. They will, however, need to be investigated for the developmental delay (📖 pp.564–565, 942–943).

Microcephaly

See also 📖 p.171. Microcephaly is defined as a head circumference below the 0.4th centile. It is associated with a small brain. The majority of these children will have developmental and neurological abnormalities.

History
- Take a full history including developmental progression and infection during pregnancy.
- Was Guthrie screening done (phenylketonuria)?

Examination
- Perform a thorough examination.
- Plot OFC on a growth chart along with previous measurements.
- Look for features of craniosynostosis—spiral CT head if likely.

Investigation
- Repeat PKU screening.
- Obtain a karyotype, plasma lactate, maternal and child's TORCH infection screen, plasma and urine for amino and organic acidaemias.
- MRI scan.

Management
Obtain genetic advice. There may be a recurrence risk of up to 25% (autosomal recessive microcephaly) if no cause is found.

Hydrocephalus
See also 📖 p.170. Hydrocephalus may be present irrespective of whether there is obstruction to cerebrospinal fluid flow. The causes are:
- *Obstructive (non-communicating):* aqueduct stenosis, posterior fossa and other tumours.
- *Communicating:* meningitis, subarachnoid haemorrhage, IVH.

Clinical features
- *History:* older children may present with a history of headache and vomiting; babies usually present because there is concern about head growth (i.e. crossing centiles) and delay in development.
- *Examination:* plot OFC on a growth chart along with previous measurements; macrocephaly or bulging fontanelle in those with open sutures; 'sunsetting' of the eyes; papilloedema; hyperreflexia; spasticity; poor head control.
- *Diagnosis:* cranial imaging looking for enlarged ventricles. Imaging may also reveal associated congenital abnormalities such as Arnold–Chiari malformation.

Treatment
- *Neurosurgical referral* for placement of ventricular shunt system or other surgery *urgently*.
- Children with shunt systems in place are at risk of shunt blockage, infection (e.g. ventriculitis), and subdural haematoma. Acute changes in behaviour, new onset headache, or persistent fever will need to be assessed with these problems in mind. Again, referral to the neurosurgical team for imaging and CSF sampling will need to be carried out.

Degenerative disorders

There are many disorders that can present with *developmental regression*, that is, 'loss of skills' and/or neurological deterioration, i.e. developing new neurological signs, or progressive intellectual deterioration. These signs always require intensive investigation.

History

- *Full developmental history:* try and exclude autism.
- *Family and social history:* with particular emphasis on consanguinity.
- *Medical history:* check for other organ involvement—eyes, hearing, cardiac, endocrine, respiratory, viscerae.

Examination

- *All systems:* storage disorders often involve other systems besides the brain, particularly face and viscera.
- *Neurological examination:* this must be thorough. Look particularly for evidence of ataxia, myoclonus, dementia, dystonia, and pyramidal signs.

Investigations

See also 📖 pp.537, 942, 956, 960. History should guide a rational approach to investigation, e.g. a family history of a similar disorder in a girl would make x linked disorders much less likely.

- *MRI:* this form of imaging will give the largest yield. Look particularly at the white matter for leucodystrophies and see if there are any structural abnormalities (Fig. 14.6).
- *Other laboratory investigations:* these are outlined in the Box 14.2.

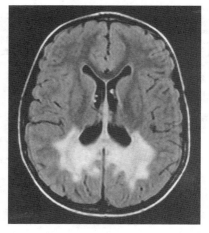

Fig. 14.6 Axial FLAIR sequence MRI head of a boy with adrenoleukodystyrophy showing dramatic signal in the posterior white matter bilaterally, during the acute deterioration seen in this condition.

Box 14.2 Investigations for developmental regression

Blood biochemistry
- *U&E:* renal failure
- *Liver function tests:* liver disease
- *Plasma glucose and matching CSF glucose:* glucose carrier transport (GLUT1) deficiency
- *Plasma lactate and matching CSF lactate:* mitochondrial cytopathy
- *Ammonia:* urea cycle defects
- *Thyroid function tests:* thyroid disease
- *Urate:* Lesch–Nyhan disease and purine disorders
- *Plasma amino acids:* aminoacidopathies
- *Very long chain fatty acids:* peroxisomal disorders
- *Copper level:* Menkes disease
- *Caeruloplasmin:* Wilson disease

Special blood investigations
- *Vacuolated lymphocytes:* Batten's disease and other storage disorders
- *WBC enzymes including Batten's enzymes:* lysosomal storage disorders and Batten's disease

Urine
- *Amino and organic acids:* organic acidurias, MTHFR deficiency, sulphite oxidase deficiency
- *Urate, creatinine, purine, and pyrimidine over 24hr:* Lesch–Nyhan, purine/nucleotide phosphorylase deficiency
- *Hydroxybutyric acid:* succinate semialdehyde dehydrogenase deficiency
- *Mucopolysaccharides:* mucopolysaccharidoses

Tissue biopsies
- *Liver:* Alper's disease
- *Skin (choelesterol esterification):* Niemann–Pick type C
- *Muscle:* mitochondrial disease
- *Rectal:* Batten's disease

Eyes
Ophthalmology review: retinitis pigmentosa and other ophthalmological markers of neurological disorders e.g. cherry red spots

Electrophysiology
- *Visual evoked responses:* Batten's disease
- *EEG:* status epilepticus and regular spike wave discharges (e.g. progressive myoclonic epilepsies, such as lafora body, gangliosidoses)

Neuromuscular disorders

See also the floppy infant (📖 p.136). In children with neuromuscular problems, first think about the anatomical site that is affected (Fig. 14.7).
- Brain (see Cerebral insult 📖 p.539).
- Spine (see Spinal cord lesions 📖 p.539).
- Anterior horn cell (see 📖 p.540).
- Peripheral nerve (📖 p.541).
- Neuromuscular junction (📖 p.544).
- Muscle (📖 p.546).

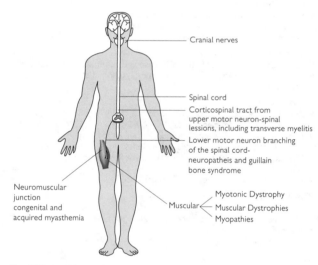

Cranial nerves

Spinal cord

Corticospinal tract from upper motor neuron-spinal lesions, including transverse myelitis

Lower motor neuron branching of the spinal cord-neuropatheis and guillain bone syndrome

Neuromuscular junction congenital and acquired myasthemia

Muscular
- Myotonic Dystrophy
- Muscular Dystrophies
- Myopathies

Fig. 14.7 An example of a motor neuron.

Cerebral insult

Any brain insult may make a child unreactive and move less. In these children there may be obvious signs of cerebral dysfunction such as encephalopathy. Facial movement and peripheral power are good if the child is able to follow commands. However, they may have low tone in the trunk, with relatively better tone at limb extremities. Good examples are Down or Prader-Willi syndromes. Reflexes should be present. If there is damage to the upper motor neuron then there will be spasticity with increased tone and brisk reflexes, e.g. cerebral palsy.

Spinal cord lesions

Spinal tumours and transverse myelitis should produce a rough level, beneath which there will be upper motor neuron signs or a sensory level or both. Spinal cord tumours are normally associated with a number of signs including constipation and urinary symptoms. There are particular signs which should always be investigated.

When to worry about a spinal cord lesion

- Neurological signs, particularly when objective, e.g. hyperreflexia and paresis, at a level beneath C1
- Back pain with no other signs in children under 11yrs
- Change in urinary function or bowel habit with back pain in older children

---

Transverse myelitis

Quick onset (i.e. in days and sometimes hours) of weakness, and/or anaesthesia, and/or urinary dysfunction, and/or bowel disturbance, often within a week of a minor viral infection. It may be associated with back pain. Although later on there will be upper motor neuron signs, where there is an acute presentation, there may be reduced reflexes and power for the first days. However, where the weakness continues there will be a gradual increase in the reflexes and tone. Urgent imaging of the cord by spinal MRI with gadolinium required to exclude cord compression, and in many cases will confirm appearances of myelitis.

Management

- *Immediate admission for monitoring* of respiratory status (use FVC; see 📖 p.49). Review for urinary and GI disturbance. Feeding/swallowing assessment.
- Early introduction of physiotherapy and occupational therapy to avoid joint contracture.
- Control of pain.
- *Methylprednisolone:* IV treatment (30mg/kg, given over a period of at least 30min for 3 days) normally used initially, if no response consider other immune-modulatory therapy.

Anterior horn cell disorders
Disorder here produces flaccid, areflexic limb, normally sparing the face.

Polio
- Now rare. May still be seen following vaccination, or in immigrants.
- Long-term, the limb becomes flaccid and wasted.

Spinal muscular atrophies
See also 📖 p.945. Confirmation of these conditions includes fibrillation on EMG and homozygous deletion of survival motor neuron (SMN) gene.
- *Type 0 (neonatal form):* very severe, often with arthrogryposis.
- *Type 1 (Werdnig–Hoffman):* severe with onset in the first months of life. Typically, there are 'bright eyes', severe hypotonia, 'frog-like posture', areflexia, and weakness that is present more in the legs than arms. Normally fatal by 2yrs of age.
- *Type 2:* onset in the first years of life with low tone, peripheral weakness, absent reflexes, and scoliosis.
- *Type 3:* adolescent onset with progressive weakness and gait disturbance, loss of reflexes, and low tone.

These disorders will have similar DNA results, so do not make a prognosis on the basis of the DNA result. They are very complicated, and will need to be reviewed by specialists, with reference to:
- An accurate prognosis based on clinical assessment.
- Advice on appropriate therapies e.g. invasive ventilation for type 1.
- Multidisciplinary support for occupational, physio and speech therapies, as well as dietary, respiratory, neurological, psychological and social support.

Peripheral neuropathies

Charcot–Marie–Tooth disease (hereditary motor and sensory neuropathies)

This refers to a group of disorders with mainly autosomal dominant inheritance:

- The *hallmark is progressive distal weakness*, initially presenting in the lower limbs with peroneal muscle weakness and atrophy.
- Also there is *clumsiness and loss of fine motor control.*
- Later, these patients *develop sensory disturbances* with pins and needles in a glove and stocking distribution.

The most common types are:

- *Type 1:* demonstrates reduced conduction velocities on nerve conduction studies due to demyelination.
- *Type 2:* near normal nerve conduction and symptoms due to axonal degeneration.
- *Type 3:* has an onset much earlier and is sometimes called Dejerine–Sottas syndrome. Characterized by very slowed motor nerve conduction velocities.

The diagnosis of these conditions is based on the clinical picture, nerve conduction studies, and genetic analysis of the P0, PMP 22, (AD) and, less commonly, the *Connexin 32* gene (X chromosome). There are now other genetic tests available including mitofusin 2 and ganglioside-induced differentiation-associated protein (GDAP).

Treatment is symptomatic with physiotherapy and orthoses in order to encourage joint mobility and maintain range of movement. Particular emphasis is put on the avoidance of contractures in the hands—'clawing', as well as peroneal muscle weakness, with foot drop and shortening of the Achilles tendons.

Other neuropathies

Neuropathy may also occur in many systemic disorders, including the following conditions:

- Leucodystrophies.
- Porphyria.
- Diabetes.
- Uraemia.
- Hypothyroidism.
- Vitamin deficiencies (B_1, B_6, B_{12}, and E).
- Autoimmune disorders such as SLE.
- Acutely as part of the Guillain–Barré syndrome (G-BS).

Guillain–Barré syndrome

G-BS is an acute, potentially fatal, demyelinating polyneuropathy. It often follows an intercurrent infection, classically *campylobacter enteritis*. Initially, there are motor signs that progress up the body. That is, first there is gait disturbance, which then progresses to involvement of the arms, and then respiratory and bulbar involvement in severe cases. Children may complain of muscle pain, which can mask the weakness. Sensory involvement also occurs, but this feature may be overlooked.

Aetiology
- EBV, cytomegalovirus.
- Measles, mumps.
- Enteroviruses.
- *Mycoplasma pneumoniae*.
- *Borrelia burgdorferi*.
- *Campylobacter*.

Diagnosis
The differential diagnosis includes myasthenia gravis, polio, spinal cord compression/myelitis, and botulism. The main diagnostic features of G-BS are as follows.
- *Clinical picture:* muscle weakness, with loss of reflexes in an ascending fashion.
- *Nerve conduction studies:* demonstrate characteristic features.
- *Cerebrospinal fluid:* elevated protein, but this does not occur at onset.
- *Variants:* Miller–Fisher variant includes bulbar cranial nerve involvement, ophthalmoplegia, ataxia, and areflexia.
- The bladder should be spared.

Course
- *Onset:* starts 1–2wks after an antecedent illness.
- *Ascending weakness:* the initial deterioration, normally lasts <2wks.
- *Plateau phase:* symptoms are static, normally lasts for 1–2wks.
- *Recovery:* should begin within 2–4wks, in a descending manner, though full recovery sometimes takes a number of months. The reflexes are the last to recover.

Management
- *Immediate admission for monitoring:* of respiratory status (use forced vital capacity (FVC); see 📖 p.49) and autonomic involvement. Dysautonomia leads to tachycardia, fluctuating BP, and GI disturbance. Pain control. Feeding/swallowing assessment.
- Early introduction of physiotherapy and occupational therapy to avoid joint contracture.
- Control of pain.
- *Immunoglobulin:* IV treatment (400mg/kg/day for 5 days) is normally used initially, with plasmapheresis reserved for refractory cases. Note risk of transmissible infection and allergic reactions to IVIG.

Neuromuscular junction

Autoimmune myasthenia gravis

The hallmark of this condition is fluctuating, fatiguable weakness. At onset 50% of patients have ptosis with, eventually, more than 80% developing it. The condition is caused by autoantibodies against the nicotinic acetylcholine (ACh) receptor, which blocks transmission at the neuromuscular junction. Normally, the condition is insidious, but sometimes an acute onset of fluctuating weakness of the extra-ocular, facial, oropharyngeal, respiratory, and limb muscles may present.

Diagnosis

- *Clinical picture:* fatiguability of power/reflexes, particularly upward gaze with eyelids/elevation, fluctuating weakness of the extra-ocular, facial, oropharyngeal, respiratory, and limb muscles.
- Electrophysiological assessment of the neuromuscular junction (NMJ) in affected muscles.
- *Response to a trial of edrophonium:* video recording is essential as response may be brief.
- ACh-receptor antibodies are present in more than 50% of cases.

Management

- Immediate assessment of respiratory status using bedside measurement of FVC.
- Immediate assessment of bulbar function looking at swallowing.
- *First-line:* cholinesterase inhibitors such as pyridostigmine with steroids.
- *Refractory cases:* acute, severe cases may respond to plasmapheresis. Subsequent immunosuppression, azathioprine, ciclosporin, methotrexate, and thymectomy. Needs to be monitored by an expert.
- Outpatient management of NMJ and muscular disorders (📖 p.548).

Congenital myasthenia gravis (CMG)

These are mainly a group of autosomal recessive disorders. However, can rarely be caused by passive transfer of maternal antibodies, which quite often have a predeliction for the foetal NMJ. Unlike the better known acquired version, they are caused by congenital abnormalities in the release, receptors for or recycling of acetylcholine at the NMJ. Despite 'less publicity', they contribute a much greater part of neuromuscular practice as they are lifelong and cannot be cured completely, so require expert management.

Presentation

In some cases as neonates, with arthrogryposis +/– bulbar/respiratory insufficiency +/– facial weakness +/– limb girdle weakness. One symptom is particularly noteworthy—laryngeal palsy, as this is a rare condition, and very likely to be caused by a CMG if there are no other ENT problems.

Diagnosis

- Clinical picture, including examination of mother (passive transfer of maternal antibodies).
- Electrophysiological assessment of the NMJ in affected muscles.
- *Response to a trial of edrophonium:* video recording is essential as response may be brief.
- ACh-receptor antibodies are not normally present if the mother is unaffected.

Management

Outpatient management of NMJ and muscular disorders (📖 p.548).

Muscular disorders

Muscular dystrophies

Are a group of congenital disorders that are characterized by dystrophic change on muscle biopsy. They can affect muscles in different patterns and are characteristically associated with a raised creatine kinase enzyme.

Duchenne muscular dystrophy (DMD)

See also 📖 p.944. This condition classically presents within the first 4yrs with delayed motor milestones and mild speech delay. DMD is an X-linked recessive condition that lies at the severe end of the spectrum of disorders and is due to a molecular abnormality of dystrophin.

Examination
- Waddling lordotic gait.
- Calf hypertrophy.
- *Weakness in limb girdles (lower more than upper):* Gower's sign.
- Sparing of the facial, extra-ocular, and bulbar muscles.

Investigation
- Markedly raised creatine kinase.
- *Genetic analysis:* this does not differentiate between the milder Becker muscular dystrophy (BMD) and more severe DMD, therefore expert interpretation is required.
- Outpatient management of NMJ and muscular disorders (📖 p.548).

Myotonic dystrophy

See also 📖 pp.136–137, 944. Autosomal dominant disorder with expanded CTG trinucleotide repeats on chromosome 19 (and anticipation when transmitted from mother).
- *Congenital form:* severe cases may present in the neonatal period and are almost always of maternal inheritance. Infants present with hypotonia, feeding difficulty, tent-shaped mouth, and respiratory impairment. Treatment is supportive, but, notably, the symptoms become less disruptive as the child grows.
- *Later onset form:* children present with hypotonia, myopathic face, and global developmental delay. Later complications include diabetes mellitus, cataracts, and cardiac involvement. The diagnosis will initially be made by the characteristic clinical picture.

Diagnosis
Confirmation can be made on examination of both parents and DNA analysis. EMG demonstrates the characteristic myotonic discharges, but is not needed for diagnosis.

Management
See Management of neuromuscular junction and muscular disorders, 📖 p.548.

⚠ **Caution** There is a particular risk of malignant hyperthermia during general anaesthesia.

Congenital myopathies

See also 📖 pp.136–137. These are a group of mainly autosomal recessive disorders characterized by:
• muscle weakness;
• hypotonia;
• variable involvement of the facial, bulbar, and extra-ocular muscles.

The congenital myopathies can be associated with arthrogryposis and if present in the neonate, may improve with good management for the first years.

Diagnosis
• Clinical picture.
• EMG and nerve conduction studies.
• DNA analysis.
• Muscle biopsy is used when the commoner disorders (myotonic dystrophy, DMD, and spinal muscular atrophy) have been excluded.

Management (see 📖 p.548)

Management of neuromuscular junction and muscular disorders

These disorders are rare, severe and complicated. They need to be managed by a good local service with on going advice from a specialist centre. Key components of care include:

- Assessment for power, joint ranges, and contractures. With appropriate advice from physio- and occupational therapists.
- Access to speech therapy and dietary assessment.
- Consideration on appropriate management of respiratory, cardiac and other systems' complications.
- Liaison with allied services, particularly education/social services.
- Genetic counseling for the child and other family members.
- Psychological support for the child and family.

It should be noted that, although a specialist centre will need to be involved, they will fail, if they do not liaise and empower a good local service, and the child/family, with the above key parts. Their advice on the projected trajectory and likely complications for the specific disorder should inform the exact local management plan.

⚠ **Caution** There is a particular risk of malignant hyperthermia during general anaesthesia for most neuromuscular disorders, so make sure child, parents and all relevant professionals are alerted, particularly family practitioners.

Cerebral palsy

- *Definition:* a chronic disorder of movement and/or posture that presents early (i.e. before the age of 2yrs) and continues throughout life.
- *Causation:* CP is caused by static injury to the developing brain.
- *Associations:* children with CP are at increased risk of impairments including vision, hearing, speech, learning, epilepsy, nutrition, and psychiatric.
- *Clinical forms:* most children will have a mixed disorder, but some can have pure components of spasticitiy, choreoathatosis, or very rarely ataxia.

Spastic CP

This is the commonest label and children can be hemiplegic, diplegic, or quadriplegic. Monoplegic cerebral palsy is extremely rare, and normally a misdiagnosis as the clinician has not examined the arm effectively. Spasticity is a stretch-related response characterized by a velocity-dependent, increased resistance to passive stretch. It is caused by disruption to the spinal reflex arc by the upper motor neuron. It will affect all the skeletal muscles and causes the following:

- Increased tone and reflexes.
- Clasp knife phenomenon on rapidly stretching tendons often described as a 'catch'.
- *Leg:* ankle plantar flexion, and either valgus or varus deformity of foot.
- *Hip:* flexion, limited adduction, and often internal rotation.
- *Wrist:* flexed and pronated.
- *Elbow:* flexed.
- *Shoulder:* adducted.
- Bulbar muscles may be spastic giving dysphagia and dribbling.

Choreoathetosis

Condition presents as a 4-limb disorder with greatly increased tone while awake and less so during the early stages of sleep. These patients do not have the stretch-related response and increased reflexes of pure spastic CP. However, there may be combinations of these features in mixed CP. As the child matures they will often develop fixed reduction in joint range of movement and then the signs will be more difficult to distinguish from those of spastic CP. They almost always have bulbar problems.

Ataxic cerebral palsy

This form of CP is extremely rare and poorly understood. It is also known as the disequilibrium syndrome. Children have a congenital ataxia giving them a striking loss of balance in the early years (i.e. disequilibrium). They often have a mild diplegia and are thought to be aetiologically distinct from the other types of CP, where hypoxia and ischaemia are thought to be causal factors. It may be that congenital ataxia is a better than applying cerebral palsy—see Investigation of CP.

Investigation of CP

- CP is a descriptive term of disability and not the cause.
- The key factor is a static neurological insult.

- May well be given in the history. Beware associations being used to explain CP; factors such as prematurity may lead to complications, but the child needs a comprehensive assessment to exclude other disorders—esp. progressive ones. All children need investigation.
- *History:* the cause may be evident from a good history, in particular for prematurity and periods of hypoxic ischaemia.
- *Imaging:* MRI scan of the brain, with particular reference to the pyramidal tracts in children with spasticity and the basal ganglia in others (Fig. 14.8). If there is a problem in the history, e.g. hypoxic ischaemic encephalopathy, then there should be signs of this on the imaging. Where imaging does not confirm a static insult, seek expert opinion.

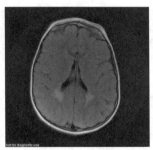

Fig. 14.8 T2-weighted axial images of bilateral periventricular leucomalacia.

Management of CP

- *Complex multidisciplinary input.:* the primary therapists are the child's carers as they will provide at least 90% of the therapy to the child. In the early years, experts in speech, physiotherapy, and occupational therapy will support this treatment.
- *Posture and movement:* optimize function by improving symmetry, joint ranges, muscle length and power. Treatments and support include stretching exercises, orthoses (e.g. ankle foot orthosis), wheelchair for mobility, sleeping and standing systems, and botulinum toxin (Botox) to the gastrocnemius. Surgery is used as a last resort.
- *Communication:* with speech therapy and aids.
- Independence with a tailored educational program, aids under supervision from occupational therapy.
- *Cognition and learning support:* with a tailored educational programme.
- *General medical:* watch for seizures, constipation, malnutrition, and behavioural or psychiatric disturbance.

Note: Dopamine-responsive dystonia will very rarely present with an unexplained diplegia and normal MRI. All these children will need a trial of co-careldopa with a gradually increasing dose of up to 10mg/kg/day of the dopa component over 3mths. If there is not a significant improvement then the child is unlikely to be dopa-sensitive.

Acute encephalopathy (See also 📖 pp.72–79.)

Encephalopathy is defined as a degeneration of brain function, due to different causes. However, in practical terms it is thought to denote a process with impaired cognition, ± focal neurological signs. It normally is matched by a typical EEG trace: with an abundance of slow waves. There is reduced consciousness as assessed by the GCS—📖 p.76.

Note: The difference between encephalopathy and encephalitis—the latter being encephalopathy 2° to an infective process—mainly viral. It is thought that CSF with normal WCC excludes encephalitis.

Assessment

The cause will be apparent within the history in the majority of cases, e.g. meningitis, trauma, or HIE. Consider/ask about potential causes:

- *Infections:* viruses as well as bacterial, e.g. meningitis.
- *Metabolic:* including mitochondrial dysfunction, check for consanguinity.
- *Autoimmune:* e.g. ADEM, thyroiditis.
- *Increased ICP:* e.g. tumours obstructing CSF.
- *Lack of oxygen or blood flow:* hypoxia-ischaemia.
- Trauma.
- Toxins (inc. solvents, drugs, alcohol, and metals).
- Radiation.
- Nutrition.

If not, or to confirm then perform a full neurological examination—with particular reference to assessment of the conscious state and place on the GCS, eye movement, fundi, bulbar control (can the child manage secretions?), upper motor neuron signs in limbs. Also check for other system involvement—skin, immune, and viscerae.

Management

These children are very sick, and at risk of cardiorespiratory compromise, until a diagnosis has been made, and they have a secure plan to manage the encephalopathy. Management should be performed simultaneously to investigation.

Is the GCS<8? If so proceed to intubation/ventilation, keep the CO_2 between 4 and 5kpa.

- Treat shock if present. If not, then IV fluids at 60% of normal daily volume requirements. Early consideration for NG feeding, if too unwell too feed orally.
- Unless there is a conformed non-infective diagnosis, treat as if meningitis (🕮 pp.78–79, 720–721). Also treat with acyclovir (🕮 p.79) for Herpes, and oral clarithromycin for mycoplasma pneumoniae.
- Check, full blood count, CRP, ESR, glucose and renal/liver function. If cause unclear, check serum ammonia, lactate, acylcarnitine profile, urine organic acid profile and store for further assessment as needed, e.g. toxicology.
- *Only when stable*, perform LP make sure there is a full WCC, glucose, protein, lactate and stored sample for subsequent viral analysis/immunology as needed.
- Neuroimaging is essential, but should only be performed once the child is stable. Always give enhancement, if possible scan the spine as well, and get MRI rather than CT, although the latter is better than nothing.

Further therapy will depend on the case, and should only happen within a centre with a paediatric neurology service and the intensive care unit.

Child development

Managing and living with disability

A diagnosis of a child with disability is invariably devastating for the family concerned. Parents will react in different ways and their needs and support will vary. Health professionals should provide clear, practical information and should be open, realistic, and honest in their approach. It is vital not to withhold information.

A multidisciplinary team that comprises specialist paediatricians, physiotherapists, occupational therapists, language therapists, and specialist nurses (e.g. community paediatric, epilepsy, learning disability) should be involved in the co-ordination and provision of care for the child with disability and their family. There should also be close liaison with social care and education. A key worker should take responsibility for co-ordinating appointments and information.

Many aspects of a child's disability will change with time and their ongoing and long-term needs will require regular reevaluation.

- Mobility problems.
- Hearing and vision difficulties.
- Communication difficulties
- Self-care and continence issues.
- *Educational provision:* special schooling; statements of special educational needs.
- Feeding difficulties.
- Sleeping difficulties.
- Behaviour problems.

Social considerations

These are just as important as the medical needs and social care.is often able to provide support and advice for the family.

A child with a disability is a 'child in need' according to the Children Act and therefore is entitled to an assessment, which can include

- Provision of temporary respite care for parents.
- Provision of suitable accommodation, e.g. wheel chair access; bathroom access.
- Financial support, e.g. disability living allowances.

Transition of care to adult services must be carefully planned and co-ordinated.

Normal development

Early child development is best divided into four functional areas:
- gross motor (📖 p.558);
- fine motor (📖 p.559);
- speech (language and hearing) (📖 p.560);
- social (emotional and behavioural) (📖 p.561).

Cognitive development refers to higher intellectual function and develops as the child gets older. Development is the result of a combination of hereditary and environmental factors. The environment must meet the child's physical and psychological needs. Developmental progress is about the acquisition of functional skills. There is remarkable consistency in the pattern of skills acquisition, although there is a wide normal range.

Gross motor development

Key motor developmental milestones

Head control
- *Newborn:* head lag on pulling to sit; head extension in ventral suspension.
- *6wks:* lifts head on lying prone and moves it from side to side.
- *3mths:* infant holds head upright when held sitting.

Primitive reflexes 'Primitive' reflexes are found in normally developing infants that *disappear by 4–6mths* (Box 15.1).

Box 15.1 Primitive reflexes

- *Moro reflex:* sudden head extension causes symmetrical extension of limbs followed by flexion
- *Grasp reflex:* fingers/toes grasp an object placed on the palm/sole
- *Rooting reflex:* head turns to tactile stimulus placed near the mouth
- *Stepping reflex:* infant held vertically, will step on a surface when foot is placed on it, followed by an up step by the other foot
- *Asymmetric neck reflex:* lying supine, if head turned, a 'fencing posture' is adopted: outstretched arm on the side the head is turned

Sitting
By *6–8mths* an infant usually can sit without support. To achieve this, the baby must have developed two reflexes:
- Propping or parachute reflex in response to falling.
- Righting reflex to position head and body back to the vertical on tilting.

Children not sitting by 9mths should be referred for evaluation

Locomotor skills
An infant initially becomes mobile, usually by crawling, but some will bottom shuffle and others will commando crawl (creep).
- *By 10mths* infants are usually cruising round the edge of furniture.
- *By 12mths* 50% of infants are walking independently; however, the age range for this is broad.

Children not walking by 18mths must be referred for evaluation

Further development of motor skills
Children learn to run and jump and *by 24mths* they start to kick a ball
- *Age 3yrs:* can jump from a bottom step, stand on one leg briefly, and pedal a tricycle.
- *Age 4yrs:* can balance on one leg for a few seconds, go up and down stairs one leg at a time, and pedal a bicycle with stabilizers.
- *Age 5yrs:* can skip on both feet.

Fine motor development

Fine motor development and vision

Fine motor skills are dependent on good vision. Therefore fine motor skills are usually assessed alongside visual development.

Early visual alertness

- *A newborn infant* will fix and follow a near face or light moving across the field of view.
- *By 6wks* infant is more alert and will turn the head through 90° to follow an object.
- *By 3–4mths* a baby will spend a lot of time watching their hands (i.e. hand regard).

Note: Some infants may demonstrate an intermittent squint. Fixed squints and all those persisting beyond the 8-week check must be referred to an ophthalmologist (see 📖 Chapter 24 pp.908–910).

Early fine motor skills

As the primitive grasp reflex starts to decrease infants will start to reach for objects.

- *At 6mths:*
  - grip is usually with the whole palm (palmar grasp);
  - holds objects with both hands and will bang them together;
  - transfers objects between hands.
- *By 10mths* infant is developing a pincer grip using thumb and first finger.
- *By 12mths* infant will use index finger to point to objects.

Preschool fine motor development

Fine motor skills can be assessed with pencil control and with building bricks (Table 15.1).

Table 15.1 Fine motor skill developmental milestones

Age	Pencil skills	Brick building
18mths	Scribbles	
2yrs		Builds 6-brick tower
2.5yrs	Copies a circle	Builds 8-brick tower *or* train with 4 carriages
3yrs	Draws a circle	Copies/makes bridge
4yrs	Draws a cross	Copies/makes steps
4.5yrs	Draws a square	
5yrs	Draws a triangle	

Speech and language development

Speech is assessed in conjunction with hearing (📖 p.896). Impaired hearing will affect language development. Age of acquisition of language is very varied.

Early signs of normal hearing and vocalization

- *Newborn* will quieten to voices and startle to loud noises.
- *By 6wks:* responds to mother's voice.
- *By 12wks:*
  - will vocalize alone or when spoken to;
  - begins to coo and laugh.

Early language development

- *At 6mths* will use consonant monosyllables, e.g. 'ba' or 'da'.
- *By 8mths* will use non-specific two-syllable babble, e.g. 'mama' or 'dada'.
- *By 13mths* two-syllable words become appropriate and develops understanding of other single words (e.g. 'drink' or 'no').
- *By 18mths:*
  - vocabulary of 10 words;
  - demonstrate 6 parts of the body.

Phrase and conversation development

Conversation becomes increasingly complex with sentence development in the 2nd year.

- *By24mths* begin to combine 2 words together progressing to 3-words phrases by the age of 2yrs (e.g. 'Give me toy' or 'get me drink').
- *By 3yrs* knows age, name and several colours.

Social, emotional, and behavioural development

Early social development
- *At 6wks:*
  - starts smiling;
  - becomes increasingly responsive socially.
- *At 10mths* shows separation anxiety when separated from parent and an increased wariness of strangers.
- *By 10mths* begins to wave 'good-bye'.

Social and self-help skills development
- *At 8mths* begins to start to feed self using fingers.
- *At 12mths* will drink from a cup.
- *At 18mths* uses spoon to feed self.
- *By 2yrs* removes some clothes and will soon start to try to dress self.

Bladder and bowel training

Very variable. Some children are potty trained by 2yrs, but others can be much older when they develop this behaviour. Night-time dryness always takes longer. 10% of 5-year-olds still wet the bed at night.

Symbolic play
- *By 24mths* children start to copy actions and activities that they see around them (e.g. feeding a doll, making tea, dusting, and cleaning).
- They progress in the 2nd year to play on their own or alongside peers in parallel play.
- *From 3yrs* they start to have interactive play, taking turns and following simple rules.

Cognitive function
Cognition refers to higher mental function.
- *Pre-school children:*
  - thought processes are called pre-operational; children are at the centre of their world;
  - 'magical' thinking and play with toys as if they were alive.
- *Junior school age:* thoughts become operational and thought processes are more practical and orderly.
- *Teenage years:* formal operational thought has developed including abstract thought and complex reasoning.

Developmental assessment

The Denver Developmental Screening test (Box 15.2) is used as a relatively quick test of children's abilities and as an assessment of whether they have achieved their age-appropriate developmental milestones (Fig. 15.1).

Box 15.2 How to use the Denver Developmental Screening test

- A vertical line is drawn at the child's chronological age
- If premature, subtract the months of prematurity from the chronological age (up until the age of 2yrs)

Developmental assessment should always consider developmental progress over time within each area of skill. The pattern and rate of attainment of developmental milestones may also vary.

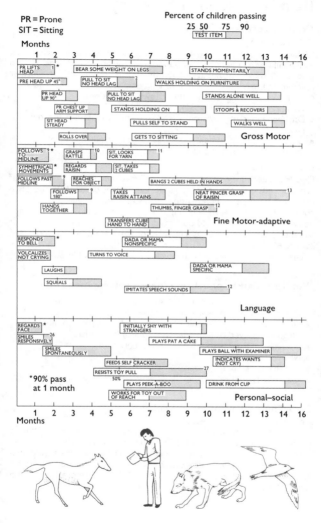

Fig. 15.1 Denver developmental screening.

Neurodevelopmental delay

Common presentations

Delayed walking

Children may show early delay in the acquisition of motor milestones, with a failure to crawl or sit unsupported at the appropriate age. A child who is not walking at the age of 18mths should be referred for a further opinion, and may need to see a physiotherapist or a specialist paediatrician. It is important to exclude the following conditions:

- Cerebral palsy (see 📖 p.550).
- Duchenne muscular dystrophy (DMD) or other muscular disorders (📖 p.546).
- Global neurodevelopmental delay as part of a syndrome or other unidentified cause (📖 pp.537, 564–565, 942, 956, 960).

Delayed speech

Delayed speech may be an isolated finding, either in the production of actual sounds or in the use of language. Language is divided into receptive language (language comprehension) and expressive language (speech to communicate). A speech and language therapist should assess language delay. A hearing test should be considered especially if the child has not had their hearing screened as a neonate or there are other concerns (see 📖 pp.560, 896).

The causes of delayed speech development are shown in Box 15.3.

Box 15.3 Causes of delayed speech development

- *Familial:* a family history of language delay where parents have been late in developing language skills or have had speech therapy
- *Hearing impairment:* chronic otitis media (glue ear) is a common cause for delayed or poor clarity of speech in the pre-school age
- *Environmental:* poor social interaction/deprivation
- *Neuropsychological:*
  - global developmental delay
  - autistic spectrum disorder

Global neurodevelopmental delay

See also 📖 pp.537, 565, 942, 956, 960.

Global developmental delay indicates a delay in all skill areas. Often it is more pronounced in fine motor, speech, and social skills. The degree of gross motor deficit is variable. There are many causes of developmental delay (see Box 15.4), although in some cases the cause will remain unknown. If the delay is severe or profound then it is more likely that a cause will be found.

Box 15.4 Causes of global neurodevelopmental delay

Genetic
- Chromosomal disorders, e.g. Down syndrome, fragile X
- Duchenne muscular dystrophy
- Metabolic syndromes, e.g. phenylketonuria

Congenital brain anomalies e.g. hydrocephalus or microcephaly

Prenatal insult
- Teratogens, e.g. alcohol and drugs
- Congenital infections, e.g. rubella, CMV, or toxoplasmosis
- Hypothyroidism

Perinatal insult
- Complication of extreme prematurity, e.g. intraventricular haemorrhage; periventricular leucomalacia
- Birth asphyxia
- Metabolic disorder, e.g. hypoglycaemia or hyperbilirubinaemia

Postnatal events
- *Brain injury:* trauma; anoxia, e.g. suffocation or drowning
- *CNS infection:* e.g. encephalitis/meningitis
- *Metabolic:* e.g. hypoglycaemia

Learning difficulties/disabilities

- Learning difficulty categorized as mild, moderate, severe, or profound.
- Cognitive function can be assessed by an IQ (intelligence quotient) test (Table 15.2), but it may be difficult to assess all skill areas, especially in preschool age group—assessment can be significantly affected by language problems and motor skills.

Table 15.2 Cognitive function assessment using an IQ test

Assessment	IQ
Normal	70
Mild learning difficulty	50–69
Moderate learning difficulty	35–49
Severe learning difficulty	20–34
Profound learning difficulty	<20

Mild learning disability may only be detected once a child is in school. A child with moderate learning difficulty will need significant support in their education. One with severe difficulties will learn basic personal care and develop simple speech, but will always need supervision. A child with profound difficulty is unlikely to develop speech and will always be dependent.

Developmental co-ordination disorder

See also 📖 p.988. Previously known as dyspraxia

Developmental co-ordination disorder (DCD) is where there are difficulties in learning specific motor and fine motor skills There are often associated problems with motor planning, proprioception and sensation(maybe hypo/hypersensitive to touch, taste, smell) Children tend to be clumsy and poorly co-ordinated, but may also have specific difficulties in writing, learning to dress, and remembering daily routine. DCD may also affect reading.

Physiotherapists and occupational therapists will assess the child and the nature of their difficulties and provide appropriate supportive strategies and training programs to help the child manage in school.

Communication difficulties

Children may have an isolated language disorder and difficulty with social skills. However, when these two development problems are present on a background of other difficulties (limited play, obsessions and lack of social awareness), autism must be considered (see 📖 p.602).

Child and family psychiatry

Prevalence

- The prevalence of child and adolescent mental health problems is similar across many Western countries (~14–20%).
- ~50% of those meeting symptom requirements for a diagnosis are also experiencing significant functional impairment.
- As a consequence at any one time around 10% of children and adolescents are suffering from a clinically significant diagnosable mental health disorder (based on ICD-10 diagnostic criteria).[1]
- Mental disorders are more common in boys than girls (11% compared with 8%), and in teens compared with preteens 5–10yr olds—10% boys, 6% girls; 11–15yr olds—13% boys, 10% girls).[1]
- <20% children with mental health difficulties actually receive specialist care and most remain undiagnosed.
- Applying the disability-adjusted life year (DALY) methodology, the burden of neuropsychiatric conditions affecting children is predicted to double by the year 2020.[2] The then US Surgeon General, David Satcher, summarized in 2001, 'the burden of suffering experienced by children with mental health needs and their families has created a health crisis in this country'.[3]
- Anybody can suffer from a mental health problem. However, adverse mental health is more commonly experienced by individuals from deprived or abusive backgrounds, from families that are financially disadvantaged or emotionally troubled. Single parent families and members of ethnic minority groups are over represented. These groups may also experience specific barriers to accessing child and adolescent mental health services that are predominantly clinic- or hospital-based.

References

1 Department of Health (2000) *The Mental Health of Children and Adolescents in Great Britain.* London: Stationery Office.
2 World Health Organization (1999). *Making a difference.* Geneva: WHO.
3 Report of the US Surgeon General's Conference on Children's Mental Health (2001). *A national action agenda.* Washington DC: Department of Health and Human Services.

Classification, categories, and dimensions

As is the case in general medicine and paediatrics diagnosis is used in child and adolescent psychiatry to;
• Collect and organize information collected at assessment.
• To guide treatment planning.
• To inform about prognosis.

Classification systems assist with the standardization of the diagnostic process and the use of a reliable and effective classificatory system can serve several important functions;
• Their use results in a greater precision in planning treatment at both the individual and population levels.
• They are a prerequisite for the conduct of many types of clinical research and facilitate the communication of research findings.
• They allow for the collection of epidemiological data a process which is central to health-care planning at international, national, and local levels.

The two most influential diagnostic systems are the World Health Organization's International Classification of Diseases (ICD) and the American Psychiatric Association's *Diagnostic and statistical manual* (DSM) system. Current versions are ICD-10 and DSM-V, although revisions are underway for both. Both are categorical systems. They both include sections describing disorders first diagnosed in childhood and adolescence, but also allow children and adolescents to meet criteria for most 'adult' mental health disorders. A key requirement of both systems is that they insist that both symptoms and associated impairments be present in order for a diagnosis to be made.

Notwithstanding these clear benefits there has been some resistance to the introduction of standardized diagnostic systems into routine clinical practice in child and adolescent mental health. Some clinicians believe this categorical approach is overly restrictive and propose that a dimensional approach whereby 'cases' represent the extreme end of a continuum is more appropriate. Supporters of the dimensional view suggest it is less stigmatizing for children, evoke a more holistic management strategy than a limited medical model, and, for some presentations, has more predictive validity than the categorical/diagnostic model. Drawbacks of the dimensional approach include difficulties deciding when to treat and an over reliance on symptoms at the expense of impairment. Unfortunately debates over 'categorical' versus 'dimensional' often become unnecessarily polarized and it is important to remember that they are not mutually exclusive from each other.

Comorbidity and causation

The aetiology of most common mental health problems is poorly understood. In most cases there appears to be interplay between genes and environment with polygenic pathways, multiple potential environmental risk factors and complex gene × environment interactions and associations (Fig. 16.1). As a consequence the simple relationship depicted by example 1 is rare. Example 1 does, however, remind us that one condition may develop into another, e.g. the progression of oppositional defiant disorder to conduct disorder. Reverse causality is also possible e.g. head injury caused by impulsive risk taking behaviours 2° to ADHD. It is also the case that the presenting condition, for instance depression, may be 2° to earlier struggles with an eating disorder (example 2). The co-occurrence of disorders is common in child and adolescent mental health. Disorders A and B in examples 3 and 4 above are comorbid. An example of 3 is sexual abuse acting as a non-specific risk factor for later drug and alcohol use and deliberate self-harm. In example 4, the two conditions may co-occur, but are aetiologically unrelated. Other potential relationships between A and B are possible and indeed most cases will be much more complex than depicted here.

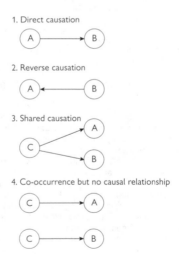

Fig. 16.1 Comorbidity and causation.

Developmental perspective

A cross-sectional understanding, effectively a snap-shot in time, is not usually informative about the child's pre-presentation strengths and vulnerabilities, and has been shown to have little predictive validity about future development. A developmental model acknowledges that the individual's needs, demands, skills and contributions change over time. Infant, child, and adolescent stages of development are described, as being embedded within the, also changing, emotional and material resources of the primary caregivers, which in turn exist within evolving social and community resources and cultural factors such as a given group's typical way of expressing emotion, reaction to adversity, and morals about acceptable behaviour.

- Some factors, such as a genetic vulnerability, act continuously, but variably across time.
- Some care giving influences, such as coercive parenting styles, are often seen as developmental continuities, unless an active process of change is undertaken.
- Children can be described as being on a normal, or abnormal, trajectory, either globally or for a range of constructs such as regulation of mood, impulsivity, emotional reciprocity, etc.

The usefulness of this perspective lies in understanding whether a recent presentation is a continuation of a long-standing behavioural or emotional state or a recent discontinuity from a normal trajectory. The former usually involves continuity of causative factors. Such presentations require more complex interventions, over longer periods and generally have a more guarded prognosis.

The heuristic bio-psychosocial is another framework that helps the clinician avoid reductionist and simple formulations for complex presentations.

Systemic thinking

No child is an island. No family should be one. Children and families present within the context of systems; nuclear and extended families as well as the local and school communities. They are also affected by regional and national phenomena such as employment and poverty gradients and access to services.

Systemic thinking involves viewing the child within the context of the family and these broader systems. Such understanding is especially important when treatment systems intersect around complex psychosocial presentations. The difficulties some physicians caring for adolescents with anorexia nervosa experience in balancing the various inputs from mental health therapists, dieticians, school teachers and heads, the child, and parents is a good example.

Understanding the family system is essential: whether the parents work together or undermine the other one's parenting; the function of sibling subsystems; whether there are typical alliances (i.e. father and son going to the football) or unhealthy alliances (i.e. cross-generation grouping to remove someone from family activities). Other types of questions that could be asked include;

- Has a child been elevated into a decision-making role?
- Has one parent been demoted?
- Is a child an 'identified' rather than actual patient, e.g. the child is presented with withdrawn behaviour when the real problem is an imminent parental separation?
- Have healthcare staff been unwittingly triangulated by some family members to exclude others from carer roles?

There are a number of schools of systemic thinking, but all tend to focus on understanding a number of key issues about the family and their relationship with the environment;

- Family functioning, roles, and relationships.
- Attitudes and beliefs within the family.
- Patterns of communication and interaction.
- Problem solving abilities.
- Strengths within the family.
- Social and cultural backgrounds.

Assessment

A thorough assessment and understanding of the presenting difficulties forms the basis for any treatment interventions offered for children, young people, and their families or carers. As mental health problems rarely occur in isolation, with comorbidity the norm, it is essential that any assessment is sufficiently comprehensive to ensure that a clear and complete formulation of the presenting problems has been made.

An assessment will usually have 4 major components:
- Identification of problems, history, signs and symptoms.
- The information gathering stages.
- Evaluation/synthesis.
- Care/treatment planning.

The psychiatric history and examination of child and adolescent mental health problems bears many similarities to that of adults. However, there are several differences in detail and emphasis. The assessment will usually be conducted as part of a joint interview with parents and the child/young person and will often require more than one visit. The general processes include;
- Clinical interview with the parent(s)/carers.
- Clarify presenting complaints with systematic evaluation of psychopathological symptoms and description of how problems developed over time.
- Developmental history.
- Pre and post-natal factors.
- Early developmental history (e.g. milestones, language, attachment, sleep, feeding problems, early temperament).
- Medical history (esp. tics and epilepsy, and psychosis for adolescents).
- Medication (esp. anticonvulsants, antihistamines, sympathomimetics, steroids).
- Family history, functioning, problems coping styles, warmth and hostility, social networks and other resources.
- Interview with the child/young person.
- Functioning in the family, the school and the peer group.
- Emotional problems and self-esteem.
- Self report rating scales may be useful as supplement especially for emotional symptoms in those 9yrs and older.
- Behavioural observation during clinical examination can be very useful when problems are seen, but an absence of observed problems during assessment does not mean they are not there. Also look for social disinhibition and evidence of language disorder during observation.
- Systematic screening for psychiatric symptoms/disorders.
- Physical examination.

Preschool or school information is invaluable—if parents' consent. Whilst classroom observation may be helpful a narrative report of behaviour and behaviour problems seen within school setting is often adequate.

History taking

Why have multiple informants?

Neither parents nor their children and adolescents may, be aware of or see the whole picture. They may also withhold information from you. Which of us does not on occasion operate a need to know policy? As an example, the teenage girl with anorexia nervosa who wants to avoid admission may exaggerate the amount she is eating and minimize her level of exercise.

Whom to get information from?

This is a balance between 'the more sources the better' and the demands of confidentiality and time.
- A good starting point is the referral details and information from both the young person and members of the family.
- Information from the school should also be sought though this may not be practicable in an emergency situation.
- Where relevant, others should be approached, e.g. social services, child and adolescent mental health services, youth offending teams.

Example The child is brought to Accident and Emergency with an unexplained and suspicious injury. Collaboration with other agencies is essential if child protection concerns exist. Local information-sharing protocols protect practitioners and expedite this work (see 🕮 pp.1005–1009, 1038).

Interviewing the family

To an extent the family interview is an efficient way of gathering information and hearing the views of the patient, siblings, and parents all at one go. However, to see it this way is missing the point. It is an opportunity to learn so much more.
- Are there obvious tensions or conflicts?
- Is tension between the parents diffused by the child's behaviour?
- Are the children allowed appropriate autonomy, or do they rule the roost?
- Is one parent a 'switchboard' through which all communication is routed?
- Are family members able to listen to each others' views?
- Is disagreement tolerated?
- Is there a family 'story' that informs how they interact around the presenting problem? Examples include, 'no-one listens to us', 'we have tried our best and can't do any more', 'it is all this child's fault', and 'he/she cannot be helped, but at the same time someone has to do something about her/him'. This sort of mixed message around a scapegoated child can often be very difficult to work with.

Family structures are variable. Often times the interview is with one parent. Sometimes it can be illuminating if grandparents are also present. Are there coalitions across generations (e.g. grandparent and child), in effect combining forces to undermine one of the parents?

A further area to note is how the family responds to you. Are you treated as a threat, a messiah, a parent/grandparent, or just a doctor? Do you feel pulled to take sides in a dispute?

Communicating

See also 📖 pp.20, 794, 1034–1035.

Tips for communicating with children

- Children's anxiety is often decreased if first interviewed with an adult they trust.
- Assume children do not fully understand why they are being seen.
- Often children assume they are 'in trouble'.
- Often children equate doctors with physical illness, often with painful procedures such as injections. Rarely have they met a 'talking doctor'.
- Be prepared to see a child several times to gain trust and rapport.
- Learn and/or practise child-appropriate communication, i.e. drawing, colouring, storytelling, pretending, building, making, exploring, appreciating tall tales, talking about current TV, technology, books. Do not take over play; follow the child's lead and still behave like a sensible adult.
- Practise age-appropriate language.
- Do not undermine the parents' efforts by appearing too competent.

Tips for communicating with adolescents

- Don't assume they have chosen to be there.
- Understand they may be ambivalent about recognizing they have a problem, dealing with, or denying it. They may see you as a source of help or as a threat—or both.
- Discuss the context of your conversation—why are you meeting?
- Discuss what you will do with what she/he tells you (confidentiality and its limits may be crucial).
- It may be helpful to ask about neutral areas first.
- Be prepared to ask closed questions accepting a yes or no answer.
- Speak plainly. Avoid talking like an adult pretending to be a teenager.
- Convey your desire to understand by checking whether you are getting it right. 'I am hearing that unless something changes pretty quick you are not going to be able to go to school any more. Have I got it right?'
- Do ask the adolescent what she/he would like to happen, but as above accept they may have mixed feelings.
- Be patient. Unless it is an acute situation consider continuing your assessment over more than one session.
- Do see the adolescent alone as well as with his/her parents.

Asking the difficult questions

About sexual abuse

See also 📖 pp.801, 1002. Sexual and other forms of abuse are common specific and non-specific vulnerability factors fors poor mental health and must be excluded as aetiological factors. The clinician's task is to find an approach to asking about abuse that they are comfortable with and appear to the child to be comfortable with. One approach is a hierarchical set of questions.

- *Introductory comment:* 'I ask these questions to all children I see.'
- *Ask child to respond to a broad, non-leading statement:* 'Some children tell me something has happened to them that they wish had never happened.' Child's response may be verbal or non-verbal affirmation, denial, or looking perplexed; they may not understand the question at all.
- *Ask more specific questions:* 'Some things are done by other people…' or '… are touched in places they wished they had not been touched.'
- *Ask very specific questions:* 'Some people are touched in places like their private parts/vagina/penis (language depends on age, may also point or draw picture), has this happened to you?'

Partial affirmation or non-verbal cues that suggest possible abuse should be followed up during later appointments. One caveat is there are differences between a purely forensic and a clinical interview. In both settings open, non-leading questions are preferable. Local protocols will also guide assessments.

About suicidal ideation and intent

Clinicians must ask about suicidal thinking, especially in adolescents with any depressive features. Asking does not create or promote suicidal thinking. Again, a hierarchical approach is used effectively by many clinicians.

- *Introductory comment:* 'I ask these questions to everyone I see.'
- *Ask adolescent to respond to a broad statement:* 'Some young people tell me that they feel life is not worth living anymore.' Again look for responses that may be verbal or non-verbal affirmation or denial.
- *Ask more specific questions:* 'Have you considered what it would be like to not be alive' or 'Some people think it would be better to be dead.'
- *Ask very specifically to clarify risk and extent of planning:* 'Have you thought of killing yourself?'; 'Have you ever made a plan to kill yourself? 'Have you ever lost control and started your plan?'

As above, partial affirmation or non-verbal cues that suggest possible abuse should be followed up during later appointments.

Depression

Loose usage of the words 'depression' and 'depressed' causes much confusion. They can refer to a mood, which may be appropriate, a symptom, or a mental disorder.

Prevalence

Approximately 10% of 10-yr-olds are reported by parents and teachers, and 20% of 14-yr-olds report themselves to be often miserable. However, the rate of diagnosable depressive disorder in a community sample of 11–16-yr-olds is closer to 3%. The discrepancy is due to those who suffer low moods, but do not meet full diagnostic criteria.

Aetiology

Genes increase both the risk of developing depression and of experiencing negative life events. Post-pubertally females are twice as likely as males to become depressed and possible links to oestrogen levels, either *in utero* or post-puberty, have been suggested. Females may also be more influenced by lack of positive relationships, close friendships, or a supportive peer network. Environmental factors include; early adversity and attachment difficulties, negative or traumatic life events or abuse, death of a parent, drug and alcohol abuse, and bullying. Psychosocial factors include; social isolation and negative interpersonal relationships, poor academic achievement, unstable family environment, parental drug and alcohol abuse.

Clinical features

Diagnosis of depressive disorder requires that mood is persistently lowered and accompanied by a loss of interest and enjoyment and/or increased fatigability for more than 2wks with a significant effect on functioning. There should also be at least two of the following symptoms;

- Reduced concentration and attention.
- Reduced self-esteem and self-confidence.
- Ideas of guilt and unworthiness.
- Bleak and pessimistic views of the future.
- Ideas or acts of self-harm.
- Diminished appetite.
- Disturbed sleep.

Depressive disorders are frequently recurrent so it is always important to ask about past episodes.

Dysthymia is a chronic enduring depressed state lasting for over a year, but without the intensity of a depressive episode.

Amongst those referred to child psychiatric clinics, comorbidity is common, e.g. conduct disorder, obsessive compulsive disorder.

Management[1]

Initial assessment should identify:

- Significant risk of self-harm or suicide.
- Significant lack of self-care or neglect.
- Symptoms of manic episode or psychotic disorder.

- Comorbid psychiatric disorder.
- Previous history of moderate or severe depressive episodes.

When these are present, referral to a specialist child and adolescent mental health service is appropriate

First line treatment for mild depressive disorder with symptom duration less than 4wks

Supportive therapy and psychoeducation about depressive disorders are effective first line interventions in 30% of children and adolescents with recent onset of mild to moderate depressive symptoms. Advice should be given on sleep hygiene, nutrition, activity, and exercise. If there is no response to supportive management after 2–3mths, young people should be referred to Tier 2/3 CAMHS services for more intensive psychological therapy.

Treatment for moderate to severe depressive disorders

Psychological therapies are recommended as first line treatments for treating child and adolescent depressive disorders. Recommended practice is that a block of psychological therapy should be undertaken prior to consideration of antidepressant medication. Supported approaches are cognitive behavioural therapy (CBT) and interpersonal therapy. Brief family therapy may be effective in some cases.

Response to treatment should be reviewed after 12wks

If there is a good response to treatment the course of therapy should be completed and follow up should be provided for 12mths after remission of symptoms (or 2yrs if the patient has had one or more previous episode of depression).

Where there is a poor response to treatment after 12wks the assessment, formulation, and treatment plan should be reviewed and comorbid diagnoses considered and any significant environmental factors investigated. If a diagnosis of depression remains, consider alternative psychological therapy and/or antidepressant medication. The most commonly used medications are the selective serotonin re-uptake inhibitor antidepressants. Recently there has been concern about side-effects (including increased suicide) as well as efficacy. In the UK fluoxetine is the only medication that is currently recommended for use as an antidepressant in children. Tricyclics appear ineffective and should not be used.

Prognosis

Whilst recovery from a depressive disorder is likely, this may take months or in some cases years. Prognosis is worsened by increasing severity of disorder and by the presence of comorbid oppositional defiant disorder. Even in those who have made a good recovery, further depressive episodes are not uncommon. Prolonged follow-up is, therefore, wise.

Reference

1 National Collaborating Centre for Mental Health (2005) *Depression in children and young people.* British Psychological Society. London: BPS. ℘ http://guidance.nice.org.uk/CG28/Guidance/pdf/English.

Suicide and non-fatal deliberate self-harm

Suicidal thoughts are common; they become abnormal when there is intent and/or plan when suicide is considered the only option.

- *Suicide* is very rare in pre-pubertal children, but incidence rises through the teenage years. It is the fourth commonest cause of death in the 15–19-yr age group (UK, 4–8 per 100,000) with a male:female ratio of 4:1.
- *Non-fatal deliberate self-harm* is far more common, with some 7% of those aged 15–16yrs having engaged in an act of deliberate self-harm in the previous year, and 10% in an act of deliberate self-harm in their lifetime. Actual self-harm is more common in females, with a female:male ratio of reported self-harm in the previous year of 4:1. Thoughts of self-harm are also more common in females, with a rate of 22.4% girls and 8.5% boys.

Predisposing characteristics to completed suicide include:
- Psychiatric disorder (such as conduct disorder, depression, substance misuse, ADHD and psychosis).
- Social isolation.
- Physical illness.
- Low self-esteem.

Relevant family factors include a family history of abuse and neglect or of psychiatric illness and suicide, and family dysfunction.

Methods of self-harm

Those who kill themselves use a range of methods, most commonly:
- drug overdose;
- inhaling car exhaust fumes;
- hanging;
- suffocating;
- shooting (in countries where guns are easily accessible).

The majority of non-fatal deliberate self-harm is through overdosing, generally with analgesics or prescribed drugs.

Cutting is very common, particularly amongst adolescent girls. Unless the cutting is deep and over the site of major blood vessels, it should not be seen as necessarily linked to suicide or attempted suicide. Those who cut describe it as easing a build-up of bad feelings, resolving emotional numbness, or sometimes as a form of self-punishment.

Assessment

Careful assessment should happen soon after the self-harm. It should include the young person, the family, and information from other sources such as the family doctor or social services. Initial assessment should identify:
- Injuries from self-harm.
- Likely/potential effects of ingestion of substance.
- The child/young person's capacity to consent to or refuse treatment.

- Presence or absence of mental illness.
- Risk of further episode of self-harm.

Appropriate medical treatment should be provided. A further separate interview should be conducted with the child once the acute situation is stable. Take a general history and address:
- History of act of self-harm.
- Circumstances leading up to self-harming behaviour.
- Degree of suicidal intent at time of deliberate self-harm.
- Intensity, frequency and duration of self-harm thoughts.
- Behaviour at time of overdose/self-harm.
- Impulsivity or planned nature of the self-harm episode.
- Help seeking or help avoiding behaviour.
- Ongoing plans for further self-harm or suicide.
- Previous history of self-harming behaviours.
- A full mental state assessment.

A clinical interview with the parents should include:
- A corroborative history of events surrounding self-harm episode.
- An exploration of parental response to the episode of self-harm.
- An assessment of family functioning and support for the child.
- Identification of symptoms suggesting a psychiatric disorder.

Management

First treat the physical effects of the self-harm episode and arrange a mental health assessment. Following risk assessment, make sure that appropriate levels of supervision are in place. Consider access to medication and other means of self-harm. If there are significant concerns about ongoing suicide risk, consider admission to an inpatient unit. If there are concerns about child protection, a referral should be made to social work. Treat any comorbid psychiatric disorder.

Management options for deliberate self-harm.

Aims of intervention
- Address self-esteem issues.
- Improve interpersonal skills and address relationship difficulties.
- Improve communication skills.
- Learn more helpful ways to communicate emotions.

Family work
Family support and counselling with more structured and intensive family therapy may be appropriate.

School based interventions
- Entire school programmes focusing on self-esteem peer relationships.
- Peer support programmes.
- Development and implementation of anti-bullying policies in school.

Prognosis 10% of those who self-harm will repeat within a year. A significant proportion will kill themselves within 5yrs—4% of girls and 11% of boys.

Bipolar disorder

The diagnosis of bipolar disorder (BiPD) in children and adolescents remains controversial due to concern about how best to operationalize and apply the diagnostic criteria to children and young people in general and pre-pubertal children in particular.

Prevalence

There have been few epidemiological studies addressing this issue. All epidemiological studies have reported mania as being very rare or non-existent in prepubertal children. A number of epidemiological surveys of 9–18-yr-olds estimated the prevalence of mania to be between 0–0.6%. Large retrospective surveys of adults with bipolar disorder have noted that onset before age 10 occurs in 0.3–0.5% of patients, although many more described mood symptoms (commonly depression) beginning in childhood. Over recent years several groups in the US have proposed that early onset bipolar disorder is much more common than previously reported. A closer inspection of these cases (most of whom have ADHD and/or oppositional defiant disorder) suggests that they do not in fact meet the full diagnostic criteria and that they are probably better charac-terised as having severe mood dysregulation.

Clinical features

Because of the controversy surrounding the recent increases in the diag-nosis of early onset bipolar disorder, and the symptom overlap with other disorders, clinicians are recommended to reserve this diagnosis for those who have clearly met the diagnostic criteria for a manic episode. The symptoms with the best specificity are;

- elevated mood;
- grandiosity/inflated self-esteem;
- pressured speech;
- racing thoughts;
- decreased need for sleep;
- hypersexuality.

Differential diagnosis

Differential diagnoses include, schizophrenia, schizoaffective disorder, ADHD, conduct disorder, substance abuse, autism spectrum disorders, organic causes, e.g. acute confusional states, epilepsy (pre or post ictal confusional states) and medication side effects, e.g. akathisia due to neuro-leptics. Sexual, emotional, and physical abuse may present with hypervigi-lance, disinhibition, and hypersexuality.

Management

The current evidence for both drug and psychological treatments of bipo-lar disorder in children and adolescents is extremely limited and treatment should be carried out by specialist child and adolescent mental health services. The goals of therapy will include reduction in core symptoms, psycho-education, relapse prevention, and facilitating normal growth and development.

Pharmacotherapy

Most of the recommendations for the pharmacotherapy of BiPD in children and adolescents are based on findings in adults. Neither the effectiveness nor the safety of anti-manic (this term is used as there is no agreed definition of mood stabilizer), antipsychotic and anticonvulsant medications in early and adolescent onset bipolar disorder is not yet established. To date only lithium in licensed in the UK for treatment of bipolar disorder in those 12yrs and older.

Prognosis

Longitudinal studies show:
- Children with ADHD do not have an increased risk of BiPD in later life.
- No studies have demonstrated that pre-pubertal mania progresses to the classic adult disorder.
- Very low rates of conversion of depression to mania among pre-pubertal children.
- Adolescent onset BiPD tends to have a relapsing and remitting course similar to adult presentations.
- Around 20% of adolescents who have an episode of major depression experience a subsequent manic episode by adulthood. This is predicted by:
  - depressive episode of rapid onset with psychomotor retardation and psychotic features;
  - family history of affective disorder especially mania;
  - history of mania or hypomania following antidepressant treatment.
- Adolescents presenting with an initial manic episode show higher relapse rates (approximately 50% during 5yr follow-up).
- The presence of psychosis is associated with chronicity.

Anxiety disorders

Diagnostic criteria

One disorder is specific to children and adolescence: separation anxiety disorder (SAD). Other anxiety disorders that may occur in children and adolescents include: generalized anxiety disorder (GAD), panic disorder (with and without agoraphobia), simple and social phobias, and post-traumatic stress disorder (PTSD). Specific physical and cognitive symptoms are described for each disorder. Developmental principles apply.

- Very young children experience 'stranger danger', later simple phobias, and SAD with the beginning of the school years.
- Middle childhood presentations include fears of animals, the dark, burglars, and anxiety-related abdominal pain.
- A recrudescence or first presentation of SAD may occur at the onset of secondary schooling.
- Adolescents may experience social phobia, and panic with or without agoraphobia.

Prevalence

Rates vary by disorder. SAD and GAD are not uncommon presentations to tertiary clinics. Panic disorders are less common.

Differential diagnosis

Child abuse may present as an anxiety disorder. Anxiety and depression often co-occur and mood should always be assessed. Acting out behaviour may be due to anxiety. Truancy must be differentiated from school refusal 2° to separation anxiety. Prominent physical symptoms, esp. without typical anxiety-related onset (e.g. Monday morning stomach pains), should be investigated. Occasionally, you must decide 'who has the anxiety', the child not wanting to go to school or the parent.

Treatment

CBT is the treatment of choice for anxiety disorders, general principles include the following:

- Clarity of diagnosis and psycho-education of child and parents (over-investigation often causes more anxiety).
- Helping child to face their fears, usually by hierarchical desensitization. Rapid exposure techniques (flooding or implosion) are rarely used.
- Identification of unhelpful, distorted, or maintaining cognitions, challenging these cognitions, and practising more functioning thinking.
- Skills acquisition, e.g. progressive muscle relaxation, guided imagery.
- Parents as motivators and behavioural coaches.
- Early relapse identification.

Medication is usually reserved for when there is either no response or only an incomplete response to psychological therapy. The selective serotonin reuptake inhibitors (SSRIs) have been shown to have short term benefit in the treatment of anxiety disorders, in children and adolescents.

Prognosis

Untreated anxiety disorders predict later internalizing conditions in girls and externalizing disorders in boys. Short-term outcome of treatment is positive, especially in conjunction with parental support.

Post-traumatic stress disorder

Prevalence

No unitary prevalence—all traumatic events vary in threat exposure and individual responses vary by developmental stage, past experiences, and competencies. Prevalence varies from 100% of children taken hostage to 10% after natural disasters. Girls may report more PTSD symptoms.

Diagnostic criteria

A range of psychopathology may be experienced following an emotionally traumatic event, dependent on pre-existing vulnerabilities, event exposure, and related loss and grief. PTSD occurs as a response to an exceptionally threatening or catastrophic event. This leads to:

- *Re-experiencing phenomena:* e.g. nightmares, flashbacks, and intrusive memories.
- Persistent avoidance of reminders of the trauma.

And either:

- Inability to recall, either partially or completely, some important aspects of the period of exposure to the stressor, or;
- Persistent symptoms of increased psychological sensitivity and arousal: e.g. difficulty falling or staying asleep, irritability or outbursts of anger, difficulty concentrating, hyper-vigilance, exaggerated startle response.

Emotional numbing and detachment is also often reported.

Age-specific symptoms

Younger children often present as regressed with altered sleep and feeding routines; exhibiting clingy, anxious, or aggressive behaviour; or engaging in post-traumatic play. Young children cannot report emotional numbing or detachment; parents report these symptoms as a 'personality change'.

Differential diagnosis

Other anxiety disorders including event-related phobias, GAD, OCD, or, if of lesser severity, an adjustment disorder. Comorbidity with depression is common. If trauma is repetitive expect disruptive behaviours in boys and early evidence of personality dysfunction in teenagers.

Treatment

If severe, treatment can be complex and take time. Interventions include cognitive strategies such as identifying and modifying dysfunctional schema, behavioural strategies including prolonged re-exposure, skills acquisition such as relaxation techniques, supportive therapy, and family interventions to monitor for secondary impairment and altered family functioning. Eye movement desensitization and reprocessing (EMDR) has a role. Psychopharmacology may provide some symptomatic relief.

Prognosis

Many children seem to be resilient to traumatic events, but long-term problems including symptom chronicity, generalization of fears, and generalized impairment have been reported—especially if parents have been unable to help the child manage their trauma. A history of chronic, repetitive trauma, such as sexual abuse, is overrepresented in other mental health presentations including drug and alcohol abuse, bulimia.

Obsessive compulsive disorder

Diagnostic criteria

- *Obsessions:* recurrent persistent thoughts, images or impulses that are distressing, time-consuming and functionally impairing. Young people recognize these thoughts as their own, and perceive them as unhelpful and at times senseless.
- *Compulsions:* mental or physical behaviours, completed in an attempt to neutralize anxiety caused by the obsessional thoughts or images.
- *Rituals and habits:* present in 2/3 pre-school children. They are similar in form and content to compulsions in OCD, but:
  - are less frequent and intense;
  - do not impact on functioning;
  - do not cause distress.

A diagnosis of OCD requires symptoms to be present on most days for at least 2 successive weeks and be a source of distress or interference with activities. Children are not required to have insight into the nature of their thoughts to meet the criteria for a diagnosis of OCD.

Prevalence

Prevalence of OCD in children and adolescents is estimated as 0.5%. This is lower than in the general population where estimates of prevalence vary between 1 and 3%. 30–50% of adults who have been diagnosed with OCD will have had symptoms before age 18yrs. Onset is more common in boys pre-puberty and girls post-puberty.

Treatment

Age and developmentally appropriate psycho-education and guided self-help regarding both the psychological and biological perspectives of OCD are essential components of treatment for all children and young people. CBT (usually conducted in a 12-wk block of weekly therapy) and pharmacotherapy are effective and often required for more severe cases. Fluvoxamine and sertraline are licensed for the treatment of OCD in children and adolescents.

Prognosis

The course of OCD may be acute or chronic. Longitudinal studies of adults who with a diagnosis of OCD suggest that prognosis is variable, but that most people fall into one of three patterns. 40% will recover and experience only mild symptoms, 40% will experience a fluctuating illness course with symptoms remitting and relapsing. 20% will develop chronic illness pattern.

Attachment disorder

Definition and diagnostic criteria

The key feature of attachment disorders is a pattern of abnormal social functioning that is apparent during first 5yrs of life, and is associated with a significant disturbance in emotional functioning. These patterns persist into later childhood and adolescence in spite of changes in the child or young person's environment. Two patterns of attachment disorders are described;

Disinhibited attachment disorder

Associated with an 'institutional' style of care in early life, with care being provided by a number carers and the absence of a specific primary care giver. The child is unduly friendly with strangers, does not seem to mind who looks after her/him, and forms superficial relationships easily. Such children may be overactive, aggressive, show emotional liability, or poorly tolerate frustration. The incidence of disinhibited attachment disorder is not well characterized, but is relatively low in the general population. Significant rates of disinhibited attachment disorder are however, reported in children raised in institutional care from birth.

Reactive attachment disorder

These children fail to respond appropriately to social interactions and display a fearfulness and hypervigilance which is not responsive to reassurance. Contradictory or ambivalent social responses may also be present. Parental abuse, neglect, and severe maltreatment are highly significant aetiological factors. The severity and duration of abuse or neglect influences the severity of the disorder. The prevalence of inhibited attachment disorder is low and not all children who experience significant abuse and neglect will develop an inhibited attachment disorder.

Differential diagnosis Includes autism spectrum disorder, PTSD, ADHD, anxiety disorders, and selective mutism.

Treatment

The focus of interventions is to ensure a secure nurturing care setting which provides consistent behavioural management and emotional responses. Infants and young children often have the capacity to alter their behaviour in response to sensitive and emotionally responsive parenting. There is less evidence for significant change in older children.

Children with severe attachment disorders may require placement in a therapeutic residential unit.

Prognosis

Children with attachment disorders have significant difficulties with interpersonal relationships and are at greater risk of developing mental health problems in adolescence and adulthood. Duration of inadequate care is linked to outcome. Children who are placed with appropriate carers before age two have a better outcome.

Schizophrenia

Schizophrenia is characterized by disorders of thought, perception, mood, and sometimes posture. Peak onset is in young adult life. Prevalence in mid teens is ~0.25% with equal numbers of males and females. Schizophrenia is very uncommon in the pre-pubertal child, when it does occur in this age group it is more common in boys.

Causes

There is a significant genetic contribution with heritability estimates as high as 82 and first-degree relatives having a 12-fold increase in risk of developing the illness. Several pre- and perinatal factors also appear to be important. These include maternal infections, stressful events during pregnancy and obstetric complications.

Clinical features

The features of schizophrenia are complex. Refer to a standard adult psychiatric text for a more complete description of terms and their meaning. Onset may be insidious or acute. Core features of schizophrenia include the following:

- *Thought disorder:* thoughts inserted or removed from one's head or broadcast to others or disorganized with abnormal speech patterns.
- *Auditory hallucinations:* external voices discussing the patient or commenting on his/her behaviour.
- *Delusions:* fixed beliefs that are false not open to reason, and not in keeping with the patient's developmental or cultural context.
- *Disorders of posture:* holding abnormal postures.

Differential diagnosis

Important differential diagnoses include affective psychosis (bipolar disorder/psychotic depression), drug-induced psychoses, and psychoses secondary to other organic conditions (see also 📖 pp.956, 976), temporal lobe epilepsy, autism spectrum disorder.

Assessment

As a schizophrenia-type psychosis can be caused by organic conditions, it is essential that signs of these be sought. Include full neurological examination, and check for thyroid, adrenal, or pituitary dysfunction, and drug screen.

Management

Schizophrenia is often complex and difficult to treat. Children and adolescents will require both:

- Specific therapies, aimed at reducing the core symptoms.
- General therapies, relating to the psychological, social, and educational needs of the child/young person and their family.

The aim is usually to deliver treatment on an out-patient basis, but it may occasionally be necessary to consider day or in-patient treatment.

Traditional psychotherapies have little effect, but learning based therapies and those that increase family support and reduce intrusive and critical interactions can improve functioning and decrease relapse rates.

Antipsychotic medication, most commonly the newer atypical antipsychotics with preferable side-effect profiles, is often effective. Relapses are fewer when families are supportive, but not intrusive or critical.

The acute phase can progress to a chronic state with poor motivation and inactivity. Clozapine (an atypical antipsychotic drug) may ameliorate this, but can cause agranulocytosis so ongoing blood monitoring is essential.

Prognosis

Prognosis is relatively good for a single acute episode in a previously well functioning teenager. However, it is worse for insidiously developing illness particularly in a child with pre-existing developmental difficulties. The differentiation between schizophrenia and affective psychosis may be particularly difficult and it is not uncommon for patients' diagnoses to switch between the two.

Somatoform disorders and typical consultation–liaison presentations

This is a poorly defined area with a whole host of overlapping terms, and confusions between descriptive terms and implied aetiology. Some of the terms in common usage are:

- *Psychosomatic:* a very general and rather unhelpful term that can include both illnesses brought on by stress, e.g. tension headache and physical symptoms secondary to psychiatric illness, e.g. hypothermia secondary to malnutrition in anorexia nervosa.
- *Somatoform disorders:* physical symptoms with no organic basis. These are subdivided into:
  - conversion disorders;
  - chronic fatigue syndrome;
  - pain syndromes, hypochondriasis;
  - somatization disorder.

Whilst many of these terms are entrenched, and so unlikely to disappear, the concept of somatoform disorders has been much criticized on the following grounds:

- It implies a cause that is not demonstrable and often intuitively does not appear to be correct.
- It is often unacceptable to patients and parents and is therefore an obstacle to forming a collaborative relationship.
- Its use may result in missing psychiatric or physical diagnoses.
- There seems little relationship between this term and other diagnoses commonly applied to the same patients in non-mental health settings, e.g. irritable bowel, chronic fatigue.

Conversion disorder

See also 📖 p.525. Conversion disorder is characterized by the presence of physical symptoms (e.g. paralysis, seizures, and sensory deficits) or mental symptoms (e.g. amnesia), but without any evidence of physical cause. Previously called hysteria. Proposed underlying mechanism is transformation of emotional conflict into mental or physical symptoms. The postulated splitting off of mental processes from each other is referred to as dissociation. There may be secondary gain, e.g. when the child who is being bullied at school develops paralysis, which keeps him at home. Conversion disorders are rare in childhood, particularly before the age of 8yrs.

Treatment

Principles of treatment include attempts to resolve any apparent emotional difficulties, avoidance of unnecessary physical investigation, removal of secondary gain, and help in returning to normal life.

Prognosis Generally favourable.

Chronic fatigue syndrome See 📖 pp.990–991

Recurrent non-organic abdominal pain

See also 📖 pp.310, 991. The child's complaints of recurrent abdominal pain are not found to have a physical basis.

- Common, affecting ~10–15% of children at some point, usually between 5 and 12yrs (no apparent gender or social class bias).
- There may be associated symptoms of other pains, nausea, or even vomiting.
- Pains are usually episodic and relapsing though may be more persistent.
- An uncommon variant is the periodic syndrome where episodes of pain are associated with vomiting, headache, and low grade pyrexia. This is thought by some to be a form of migraine.

Differentiation from organic pathology may be difficult. Features that may help include the diffuseness of the pain, the tendency not to be woken by it, pains elsewhere in the body, anxiety, and depression in child and parent, and the lack of positive findings on physical examination.

Treatment
Generally a combination of reassurance, education about the links between stress and the body, psychological treatment where appropriate and avoidance of unnecessary physical investigation and treatment.

Prognosis
Short-term outcome is usually favourable though it is not known whether this is due to or in spite of treatment. In the longer term further episodes of non-organic pain are found in a large minority of cases.

Selective eating

This is a condition of younger children that in most, though not all, resolves in the teenage years. These children eat only a limited range of foods. In severe cases the restriction may be to only 3 or 4 foods. It is surprising that most children seem to ingest all the required nutrients in their very limited diet. To treat, a mixture of reassurance and encouragement seems to be the best approach. More active intervention is indicated when the child is malnourished and usually entails a gradual hierarchical desensitization programme.

Anorexia nervosa

Epidemiology

Anorexia nervosa is the third commonest chronic illness in teenage girls. Prevalence in the Western world is ~0.5%. Whilst varying with age, a sex ratio of 9:1 (girls:boys) is fairly typical. Pre-pubertal cases are rare, but do occur. Bulimia nervosa is generally of youth onset.

Causes

Often unclear in individual cases; however, genetic pre-disposition, a perfectionist personality, and low self-esteem seem to be implicated. Dissatisfaction with weight and shape is relatively common in children as young as 8yrs and is presumably a vulnerability factor. The pathway into anorexia nervosa is through weight loss, either due to a desire to lose weight or for some other reason such as depression/anxiety or, sometimes, viral illness.

Diagnostic criteria

- Dietary restriction (may be accompanied by vomiting, exercise, laxative abuse, or other weight control methods) leading to significant and unhealthy self-induced weight loss (e.g. to less than 85% of expected body weight for height or age or a BMI < 17.5) or to stunting of expected growth.
- Intense fear of gaining weight even when severely underweight.
- Body image distortion with dread of fatness.
- Amenorrhoea (may be 1° or 2°).

In younger teenagers anorexic thoughts may often be either absent or hidden, e.g. fear of becoming fat may be absent because they 'know' they can control their weight. Individuals who exhibit significant weight-losing behaviours, not explained by depression, a specific phobia, or physical illness, may be referred to as having an atypical eating disorder.

Treatment

The evidence-base for treatment is small. Management of anorexia nervosa in children and young people requires a team effort and virtually all cases will require intensive treatment with more than one therapeutic modality. The key to success in individual treatment is the engagement with the therapist rather than the type of therapy provided. Involvement of the family through family therapy seems to be important.

Treatment is likely to be lengthy and to involve attention to anorexic behaviours, to recognizing and not acting on anorexic thoughts and feelings, and to returning to aspects of normal function such as school and home life. It is far preferable to work collaboratively with the young person. At times compulsory treatment (requires use of the Mental Health Act) may be needed.

Clearly, correction of dangerous weight loss or its secondary complications may be urgent. Patients who are unable or unwilling to manage adequate oral nutrition may need nasogastric feeding. In any rapid refeeding plan the risks of refeeding syndrome (📖 p.322) should be remembered.

Prognosis

Anorexia nervosa is a serious psychiatric disorder that carries a significant risk of mortality as well as considerable morbidity. Although some cases of anorexia in children and young people are mild and resolve without intensive treatment programmes, many will go on into adult services with chronic eating problems. Whilst the quoted long term outcomes for anorexia generally accept that a third will recover full, a third will make a partial recovery and a third with have chronic symptoms, this is taking into account the lifetime course of the illness. The prognosis for teenagers is generally better than for adults with most making a full recovery. This can, however, take years, and an interim step may be to learn how to live with the illness rather than be controlled by it.

The risks to physical long term health are greater without early attention to malnutrition and long term problems include:

- growth retardation;
- delayed or arrested puberty;
- reduced bone density;
- higher likelihood of low birth weight baby.

Risk factors for poorer outcome

- late onset;
- excessive weight loss;
- vomiting and purging as part of the clinical picture;
- poor social adjustment;
- poor parental relationships;
- being male;
- chronic course of illness.

Bulimia nervosa

Epidemiology

Bulimia nervosa is rare before the age of 13yrs. Although onset of the disorder is generally in mid- to late teens, it is unusual to present for help before early twenties. In teenagers, bulimia may occur alongside other externalizing teenage behaviours such as sexual promiscuity, drug taking drinking, and self-harming. 90% + of cases are female and is distributed right across the social classes. In adult women, the incidence is 1–1.5% and it is 2–3 times more common than anorexia nervosa in adolescents. Bulimia is associated with westernized lifestyle with a lower prevalence in developing countries and rural areas. There may, or may not be, a preceding history of anorexia nervosa.

Causes

Similar factors contribute to the aetiology of bulimia nervosa as are found for anorexia nervosa. Additional risk factors include:
- adverse family life events;
- family history of obesity;
- parental substance misuse;
- family history of affective disorder;
- poor social network;
- critical parents.

In contrast to anorexia nervosa, bulimia is associated with high expression of emotions, impulsivity, and a chaotic lifestyle.

Diagnostic features
- Persistent preoccupation with eating. Craving for food with recurrent episodes of binge eating, associated with feeling out of control.
- Regular use of mechanisms to reduce weight gain from binging (e.g. vomit-induction, laxatives, diuretics, appetite suppressants, excessive exercise).
- Morbid fear of fatness.
- Body weight higher than required for the diagnosis of anorexia.

Repeated vomiting and/or laxative abuse may result in serious electrolyte disturbance, seizures, tetany, haematemesis, or stomach rupture.

Management

Usually best managed by a multidisciplinary team and including the family from the start. Cognitive behavioural therapy including educational input about healthy eating, starvation, and binging. Motivational interviewing and family therapy can also be helpful. Pharmacotherapy, e.g. fluoxetine, rarely used, but may reduce food craving.

Prognosis

Full recovery occurs in up to 50% of cases. Between 66–75% show at least partial recovery at 10-yr follow up. Bone density follow up shows no osteopenia or osteoporosis in recovered bulimic patients.

Oppositional defiant and conduct disorders

Oppositional defiant disorder (ODD) and conduct disorder (CDD) are related disruptive behaviour disorders, typified by defiance, disobedience, and violation of social rules and the rights of others.

Epidemiology

- Prevalence varies greatly depending on the age of the sample and the diagnostic criteria used.
- Both CDD and ODD are more common in males.
- ODD is more common in younger children (<10yrs).
- ODD prevalence in 5–10yr olds is around 4.8% boys and 2.1% girls.
- CDD prevalence increases with age: ~1% in children and 4% in adolescents.

Causes

Longitudinal studies of delinquency suggest the causes are complex. Many are likely to have an underlying genetic vulnerability and an association with various pre- and perinatal risk factors. Subsequent exposure to coercive parenting (intrusive parenting and subsequent reinforcement of child counterattack and parent withdrawal) early in life has also been implicated. Later involvement of vulnerable individuals with a deviant peer group predicts a CDD pathway as does a variety of psychosocial risk factors, e.g. low socioeconomic status, peer relationship difficulties, parental mental illness, and child maltreatment, neglect, and abuse.

Clinical features

The name ODD is highly descriptive, i.e. hostile, negativistic, and defiant, particularly to the parents. The defiant behaviour pattern must last at least 6mths and cause impairment across a variety of domains. CDD is defined by more serious aggressive behaviour and rule violations, property damage, theft, arson, truancy, and running away, which again must have been present for at least 6mths and result in functional difficulties.

Differential diagnosis

Comorbidity with other disruptive behaviour disorders is common, e.g. ADHD (📖 p.600). Speech and language deficits may be comorbid or on a causal pathway.

Management

Prevention is the best approach. Early intervention with ODD in very young children using universal parenting programmes targeting coercive parenting and parental abuse is indicated. If ODD and CDD are established, programmes that employ intensive interventions that involve children, parents, and other participants in the child's social ecology have proved effective.[1] Multisystemic therapy is an example of such an intervention. Remedial education is likely to be needed and can also be helpful as self-esteem rises.

Psychopharmacology research on disruptive behaviour disorders, other than ADHD, presently provides no definitive guidelines.
- ADHD comorbidity should be treated.
- Planned, premeditated aggression is not an indication for drug therapy.
- Impulsive aggression or aggression in an individual with prominent affective symptoms may prove responsive to a 5-HT blocking agent or an atypical antipsychotic (e.g. risperidone). Further research is required before these pharmacological strategies can be demonstrated to be both safe and effective enough to be used in routine clinical practice.

Prognosis

Management of established disruptive behaviour disorders is difficult. Children often fail at school. Poor prognosis with ODD is associated with;
- early onset of symptoms;
- longer duration of symptoms;
- comorbid mood, anxiety, ADHD, impulse control and substance use disorders;
- development of conduct disorder.

Two patterns of CDD are described. Early onset- (onset before the age of 11yrs) and adolescent onset-CDD. Whilst adolescent onset CDD is most often self-limiting and does not typically persist into adulthood, early onset CDD is associated with a particularly poor prognosis. This is also the case for conduct disorder which is comorbid with ADHD. Almost 50% of all youths that initiated serious violent acts before the age of 11 continued this type of offending beyond the age of 20 twice the rate of those who started in adolescence. Approximately 40% of prepubertal children with conduct disorder may develop antisocial personality disorder and most antisocial adult report a history consistent with conduct disorders as a child.[2]

References

1 National Institute for Health and Clinical Excellence (2006). *Parent-training/education programmes in the management of children with conduct disorders*. London: NICE. http://guidance. nice.org.uk/TA102/Guidance/pdf/English

2 Farrington DP. (1998). Predictors, causes and correlates of youth violence. In: *Youth violence* Tonry M, Moore MH (eds). Chicago: University of Chicago Press.

Attention deficit hyperactivity disorder

ADHD is a complex neurodevelopmental disorder.

Prevalence

Rates of diagnosis vary greatly both between and within different countries. In the US, Netherlands, and Germany, rates are much higher than in the UK, which is much higher than those in France, Italy, and Spain. A recent systematic review identified 102 studies, across all world regions. Overall prevalence of ADHD was 5.3 %. Prevalence for children 6.5% and for adolescents 2.7%. ADHD is 2–3 times more common in boys. Prevalence decreases with increasing age. Differences between studies mainly accounted for by the use of differing diagnostic criteria, the source of information used to elicit symptoms and whether impairment was required to be present in order for the diagnosis to be made. After adjustments were made to account for these methodological issues, the prevalence in North America and Europe were similar.

Causes

ADHD displays considerable heterogeneity at the genetic, pathophysiological, cognitive, and behavioural levels of analysis. Whilst the exact aetiology of ADHD is unknown considerable research supports a strong genetic component (heritability of 0.7) with non-shared environmental factors contributing most of the residual variance. Environmental factors are likely to include prenatal exposure to nicotine, pre and perinatal obstetric complications and low birth weight, exposure to lead and other environmental toxins. Gene-environment interactions seem likely to be particularly important, but have not yet been studied extensively.

Diagnostic criteria

- *Inattention:* e.g.
  - fails to attend to detail;
  - difficulty sustaining attention;
  - does not follow through;
  - difficulty organizing tasks, easily distracted;
  - reluctant to engage in tasks that require sustained mental effort.
- *Hyperactivity:* e.g.
  - often fidgets;
  - leaves seat in classroom;
  - runs and climbs excessively;
  - often on the go;
  - acts as if driven by a motor.
- *Impulsivity:* e.g.
  - often blurts out answer before the question has finished;
  - has difficulty waiting turn;
  - interrupts and butts in.

Symptoms must be present for at least 6mths, be present before age 7yrs, and result in impairment in 2 or more functional domains or settings. In DSM-IV inattentive, hyperactive–impulsive, and combined subtypes are described. The ICD-10 criteria are more restrictive and only include those with severe, pervasive and impairing combined ADHD in the diagnostic category *hyperkinetic disorder*. This results in a lower prevalence for hyperkinetic disorder of around 1.5%.

Differential diagnosis In young children it may be difficult to differentiate age-appropriate boisterousness and activity from ADHD symptoms. Inattention may be due to under-stimulation of above-average children or seen in children in classroom settings too advanced for their mental age. ADHD symptoms common in PTSD (📖 p.586) and autism spectrum disorders (📖 p.602).

Common comorbidities

- Disruptive behaviour disorders (ODD and CDD) (see 📖 p.598; 42–68%).
- Anxiety (22–37%).
- Depression (12–17%).
- Learning, speech, and language disorders are also overrepresented.

Treatment

- *Psychopharmacology:* drug therapies include psychostimulants (methylphenidate, dexamfetamine) and the non-stimulant atomoxetine.
- *Behavioural interventions:* integrated home–school behaviour management, token economies, and parent effectiveness training. The effectiveness of family interventions is inconclusive.

A multisite randomized controlled trial (NIMH-MTS study) of combined subtype ADHD found that, over 14mths, carefully organized medication was superior to either behavioural treatment or community care (which usually included less well organized medication treatment) for core symptoms and that a combination of behavioural and medication therapies were equally better for related symptoms compared with usual care.[1]

Current UK[2] and European practice suggests that for those, over 6yrs of age, where ADHD is severe, pervasive, and impairing ADHD (ICD-10 hyperkinetic disorder) medication will usually be the first choice treatment. For those with less severe ADHD behavioural interventions are suggested as the first choice treatment with medication reserved for those who either fail to respond to the behavioural treatments or for whom behavioural treatment is not possible.

Prognosis

- 70–80% continue to display symptoms and impairments as adolescents.
- 50–65% as adults.
- Only 10–20% reach adulthood without any psychiatric diagnosis, functioning well, and without symptoms of their disorder.
- Pharmacological treatments may be continued into adulthood

Reference

1 See reference list at: 🔗 http://www.rcpsych.ac.uk/mentalhealthinfo/mentalhealthand growingup/adhdhyperkineticdisorder.aspx
2 National Collaborating Centre for Mental Health (2008) *The NICE guideline on diagnosis and management of ADHD in children, young people and adults.* London: British Psychological Society and Royal College of Psychiatrists. 🔗 http://guidance.nice.org.uk/CG72/Guidance/pdf/English

Autism spectrum disorders

Disorders in this cluster, also called pervasive developmental disorders (PDD), have common clinical features in the areas of communication, social relatedness, movement, and intrapersonal relations. Nosological issues include the diagnostic distinctiveness of syndromes and whether presentations can change over time. Autism spectrum disorders include:
- Autism (prevalence ~1/1000).
- Rett's syndrome (prevalence 1/15 000).
- Asperger's disorder (prevalence 3–4/1000).

Aetiology

It is likely that the autism spectrum disorders are heterogeneous in aetiology. Most believe there are underlying complex genetic vulnerabilities with subsequent environmental influences and factors that trigger gene expression. Recent functional neuroimaging studies have led to a wide variety of neurobiological hypotheses. It is likely numerous neural systems are involved with a focus on areas typically implicated in emotional regulation such as the limbic lobe. (See references for Cochrane reviews discussing benefit of diet, vitamins, and auditory integration training.[1-3])

Clinical features

- Usually identified in the pre-school years, but may be found later in individuals with above average IQ.
- Problems with social interactions include appearing aloof, impaired non-verbal behaviours, difficulty establishing friendships, and poor or absent emotional reciprocity.
- Language problems include marked delay of or lack of speech, inability to converse, and abnormal speech including stereotypical speech.
- Behaviour problems include preoccupied, stereotypical behaviours (e.g. hand flapping). In adolescence aggressiveness, mood variability, and sexually inappropriate behaviour can be problematic.
- Mental retardation, language delay, ADHD, and medical complications such as epilepsy often coexist with an autism spectrum diagnosis.

Management

No single intervention appears superior. Psychosocial interventions, often with an emphasis on behaviour management and parent involvement, can often lead to increased child skills and have high parent satisfaction. However, such improvement does not usually lead to significant changes either on standardized measures or improve the overall developmental trajectory. Recent studies with atypical neuroleptics (e.g. risperidone) hold much promise for improvement of global functioning. For an in-depth discussion of recent assessment, aetiological, and treatment research.[4]

Prognosis

- 70% remain severely handicapped.
- 50% develop useful speech.
- 5% will lead independent adult lives.

References

1 Millward C, Ferriter M, Calver S, *et al.* (2004). Gluten and casein-free diets for autistic spectrum disorder. *Cochrane Database Syst Rev* 2004;(2):CD003498.
2 Nye C, Brice A. (2002). Combined vitamin B6–magnesium treatment in autism spectrum disorder. *Cochrane Database Syst Rev* 2002;(4):CD003497.
3 Sinha Y, Silove N, Wheeler D, *et al.* (2004). Auditory integration training and other sound therapies for autism spectrum disorders. *Cochrane Database Syst Rev* 2004;(1):CD003681, publ. 2.
4 Volkmar FR, Lord C, Bailey A, *et al.* (2004). Autism and pervasive developmental disorders. *J Child Psychol Psychiat* **45**(1): 135–70.

Individual psychotherapy

All health professionals working with children talk to the children by themselves sometimes. All try to be helpful, and probably most of us are helpful at least some of the time. So in what way is psychotherapy different from an informal helpful chat? Perhaps the key elements are that the treatment is delivered by a trained therapist who carries out therapy within a theoretical framework. There are a wide range of individual therapies including the following.

Behaviour therapy

This is brief and is directed at encouraging desired behaviours and the eliminating problem behaviours. Problems are dealt within a behavioural framework rather than through focus on underlying thoughts, feelings, or past causes.

Cognitive behaviour therapy

As above, but with a wider focus on thoughts and attribution of meaning, as well as behaviour. This is one of the better researched therapies, though there remains a shortage of trained therapists. CBT involves the keeping of diaries and homework carried out between sessions.

Psychodynamic psychotherapy

Longer-term treatment directed at underlying problems and the presenting symptom. Central to treatment are theories of the unconscious mind. The patient is encouraged to use their relationship with the therapist to explore dysfunctional patterns of behaviour. The therapist is able to comment on these and help the patient to understand new ways of relating. Therapy in the younger age group may be based more around play materials such as animals, crayons, and paper. Just to complicate matters there are also play therapists who are not necessarily psychodynamic in their orientation.

Which therapy is best?

The inevitable question arises as to which therapy is better. It is difficult to answer as short therapies directed to diagnostic related groups are easier to evaluate. In particular there is a growing body of evidence to support the use of CBT in a range of conditions. That being said it is also probably true those well motivated, intelligent, articulate patients without previous problems and from well functioning families are likely to do better with whichever therapy. Non-specific factors about therapists (e.g. empathy, good listening, and warmth) may be pre-requisites to effective treatment whatever the model.

Family therapy

This term covers a wide range of treatments with a similar diversity of theoretical underpinnings. They share the idea that problems are affected by the communication between family members and such communication can serve to maintain or to ameliorate their difficulties.

One of the points of difference concerns understanding of the problem. Family therapy based on systems theory might identify recurring dysfunctional patterns of interaction and typically might hypothesize that the presenting problem in one family member is a manifestation of this. Such a view, of pathology being located between, rather than within people, may be at odds with the Western focus on the individual. An example of such an approach is the school-refusing child who is being kept home to act as a buffer between parents who are in conflict. The child's presence may prevent dangerous escalation, but may also interfere with the parents' ability to resolve their differences. Therapy in this case might focus on helping the parents to address their difficulties without involvement of the child, and for the child to trust his/her parents to do this and to get on with being a child, e.g. going to school.

An alternative is to help the family members to be aware that they are feeling overwhelmed by the problem, have lost confidence, and are not seeing that they do have the resources to deal with it. They might be helped to think of occasions when they have overcome difficulties without the help of their child; or to see how they do this and more often. The child may be helped to see that he/she does, at times, overcome his/her fear and gets on with being a child, and can do more of this.

Finally, we can consider family therapy for multifactorial illnesses, such as autism. This is not a product of any particular family pattern or dysfunction. However, this does not mean that the family cannot be helped to manage this better. Such an approach is likely to focus on support, on psycho-education, and on helping the family to address the developmental (independence) issues, which are there for any family, but so much more difficult when there is a child with chronic illness or disability.

Outcome

The heterogeneity of family therapy, the wide variety of problems it is used to address, and sometimes an overemphasis on complex theory that can seem a long way from clinical practice have contributed to a dearth of outcome research. There is evidence though for effectiveness in a range of conditions including anorexia nervosa (AN) (see 📖 p.594).

Contraindications

Non-clinicians often see family therapy as a potential panacea for all family based problems. Unfortunately this is not the case and family therapy is not always the correct way to address such difficulties. Family therapy is not possible if the family cannot, or will not, attend. It is contraindicated in families where one member is being severely scapegoated. Unless there is reason to believe that such a family is open to the idea of doing things differently once this pattern is identified, family therapy should be discontinued.

Psychopharmacotherapy

Societal views exist about medication for mental health in general and specifically for children. Not all mental health professionals hold positive views about psychoactive medications or believe them to be safe and effective treatments for mental health disorders. Some non-professional groups are openly antagonistic. Whilst there is some clear evidence to support the use of medications for some children and adolescents with some disorders in some situations, it is also true that more research and stronger evidence is urgently required.

Until recently prescribing for children and adolescents with mental health problems has not benefited from age-specific pharmacokinetic studies, nor had there been extensive work establishing the pharmaco-dynamics of psychoactive medications. As a consequence for almost all psychopharmacological situations, other than ADHD, one usually assumes that the pharmacodynamic effect in children is the same as that in adults. Similarly, there has been relatively little attention paid to pharmacovigilance and many questions about drug safety remain unanswered.

Data supporting efficacy and effectiveness also remain relatively sparse and the current evidence-based medicine summaries do not comprise a comprehensive review of child and adolescent mental health prescribing (see Cochrane Library). Many protocols are listed; over time it is hoped there will be more consistent coverage from completed reviews. Despite this lack of evidence, psychotropic medication prescribing has increased exponentially over the past 15yrs. Fortunately, recent changes in legislation in the US and Europe have meant that far more psychiatric drugs are being trialled and licensed for use in children.

For specific prescribing information, indications, contraindications, precautions, side-effects, and dosage regimes the reader should consult an up-to-date formulary and the primary literature. One reference text offers the following useful headings in a section on general principles.[1]

• First do no harm.
• Know the disorder and use drugs when indicated.
• Choose the best drug.
• Understand the drug and its properties.
• Minimize drug use and dosage.
• Keep things simple.
• Avoid polypharmacy.
• Don't be a fiddler or follow fads.
• Take particular care with children.
• Establish a therapeutic relationship.
• Compliance (adherence) with treatment.

Whilst some mild mental health presentations may respond to medication alone, in individuals with multiple comorbidities, impairment across domains, or distressed parents, medication is almost invariably adjunctive to or part of a more comprehensive and sophisticated management plan.

Reference
1 Werry JS, Aman MC. (1999). *Practitioner's guide to psychoactive drug for children and adolescents*, 2nd edn. New York: Plenum Medical Book Co.

Haematology

Peripheral blood film

Table 17.1 FBC and blood film abnormalities and their causes

Abnormality	Cause(s)
Acanthocytes	Abetalipoproteinaemia, severe liver disease, Vitamin E deficiency in premature neonates, hereditary acanthocytosis
Basophilia	Myeloproliferative disorders, chronic myeloid leukaemia (CML), basophilic leukaemia, reactive disorders, e.g. ulcerative colitis, infection
Basophilic stippling	Ineffective erythropoiesis; haemoglobinopathies, recovering bone marrow, lead poisoning
Echinocytes (Burr cells)	Renal failure, pyruvate kinase deficiency, liver disease, HUS, burns
Elliptocytes	Hereditary elliptocytosis (□ p.616)
Eosinophilia	Parasitic infections, allergic states, e.g. asthma, eczema, drugs, polyarteritis
Fragmented red blood cells (RBC)	Microangiopathic and mechanical haemolytic anaemias, DIC (□ p.625), HUS (□ p.376), renal failure
Heinz bodies (intracellular Hb precipitate)	G6PD deficiency (□ p.618), haemoglobinopathies, post-splenectomy, hyposplenism, Heinz body haemolysis
Howell–Jolly bodies (intracellular DNA fragments)	Normal neonatal blood picture, hyposplenia, post-splenectomy, megaloblastic anaemia
Leucocytosis	Leukaemia (□ p.656)
Lymphocytopenia (lymphopenia)	Infection, mainly viral, malignancy, stress, vomiting, burns, anorexia, drugs, SLE, Crohn's disease, immunodeficiency states (SCID, diGeorge syndrome, acquired, e.g. HIV), marrow failure, aplastic anaemia, leukaemia
Lymphocytosis	Viral and non-viral (pertussis, mycoplasma, malaria) infection, leukaemia, atypical lymphocytosis (EBV, CMV, adenovirus), stress, exercise, status epilepticus
Macrocytic RBCs	Vitamin B$_{12}$ or folate deficiency (□ p.615), aplastic anaemia (□ p.626), normal neonatal blood picture (□ p.192)
Microcytic RBCs	Iron deficiency (□ p.614), thalassaemia (□ p.622), anaemia of chronic disease
Monocytopenia	Autoimmune disorders, e.g. SLE, drugs, e.g. corticosteroids, chemotherapy
Monocytosis	Chronic bacterial infection, malaria, typhoid, TB, infective endocarditis, post-chemotherapy
Neutropenia	See □ pp.627, 724

Neutrophilia	Infection, inflammation, chronic bleeding, post-splenectomy, drugs, e.g. corticosteroids
Reticulocytosis/polychromatic RBCs	Haemolysis, bleeding, response to haemotinics (e.g. iron), marrow infiltration
Sickle cells	Sickle cell anaemia (📖 p.620)
Spherocytes	Normal neonatal blood picture, hereditary spherocytosis (p.616), immune mediated haemolytic disease, post-splenectomy
Target cells	Severe iron deficiency (📖 p.614), sickle cell disease, thalassaemia, liver disease, post-splenectomy, asplenia
Thrombocytopenia	See 📖 pp.642–643
Thrombocytosis	See 📖 p.641

Anaemia

Red cell indices vary considerably with age. Haemoglobin (Hb) at birth may be as high as 22g/dL, but then falls rapidly to about 11g/dL by 3mths. A mild hypochromic microcytic picture normally seen between 6mths and 6yrs. Sex differences in red cell indices do not appear until puberty.

Symptoms and signs of anaemia
- Fatigue, lethargy.
- Pallor.
- Poor feeding, anorexia.
- Poor growth.
- Dyspnoea on exertion.
- Rarely stomatitis or koilonychia.

Diagnostic approach to anaemia

History
- Familial/ethnic causes (sickle cell, thalassaemia).
- Diet (cow's milk, vegan).
- Overt blood loss.
- Duration of symptoms.
- Drug history, e.g. NSAIDs.

Examination
- Height and weight (FTT, malabsorption).
- Dysmorphic features, e.g. micrognathia, cleft palate, abnormal/absent thumbs (Fanconi's anaemia, Diamond–Blackfan anaemia).
- Jaundice (haemolysis).
- Adenopathy/organomegaly (underlying malignancy).

FBC and film (See Table 17.2)
- *Red cell indices:* mean cell volume (MCV), mean cell haemoglobin (MCH), mean corpuscular haemoglobin concentration (MCHC) (anaemia may be microcytic, macrocytic, normocytic, and/or hypochromic).
- *RBC:* spherocytes, sickle cells, Howell Jolly bodies.
- Other cytopenias.

Table 17.2 Investigations for different anaemia types

Anaemia type	Investigate for
Microcytic anaemia	Iron deficiency, thalassaemias, sideroblastic anaemias, anaemia of chronic disease
Macrocytic anaemia	Bone marrow failure syndromes (reticulocytopenic anaemias; pure red cell aplasia, aplastic anaemia, Diamond–Blackfan anaemia), myelodysplastic syndromes, megaloblastic anaemia (B_{12}/folate deficiency), dyserythropoeisis, drugs
Normocytic anaemia	Haemolysis, sequestration, anaemia of chronic disease, recent significant bleeding, combined iron and B_{12}/folate deficiency, i.e. severe malnutrition
Haemolytic anaemia	Investigate as described on p.612

Haemolytic anaemias

Haemolysis causes reduction in the normal mean RBC survival of 120 days. Causes can be intrinsic (RBC membrane defects, enzyme defects, or haemoglobinopathies) or extrinsic (immune mediated or mechanical RBC fragmentation).

Diagnosis

History

- *Symptoms:* e.g. headache, dizziness, fever, chills, dark urine, back or abdominal pain (intravascular haemolysis).
- *Possible precipitating factors:* e.g. infection, medications, foods such as fava beans in G6PD deficiency.
- *Ancestry:* e.g. African, Mediterranean, or Arabic ancestry is suggestive of G6PD deficiency in boys.
- *Family history:* e.g. gallstones in spherocytosis.

Examination Specific examination should include temperature, pallor, jaundice, splenomegaly. Look for leg ulcers.

Investigations

FBC and blood film

- Increased reticulocyte count suggests increased RBC production in response to haemolysis or blood loss.
- *Platelet count:* thrombocytopenia with normal clotting suggests HUS, thrombotic thrombocytopenic purpura (TTP); with abnormal clotting suggests DIC.
- *Pancytopenia:* consider viral infection, malignancy, hypersplenism.
- *Abnormal blood film:* e.g. spherocytes or other RBC abnormalities, malaria parasites, features of RBC fragmentation (schistocytes, burr cells).

Specific tests include the following:

- *Unconjugated bilirubin:* raised level = increased RBC destruction.
- *Lactate dehydrogenase:* raised activity = increased RBC production.
- Free plasma Hb, haemoglobinuria, haemosiderin in urine (all increased in intravascular haemolysis).
- Coombs antiglobulin test to establish if there is immune or non-immune haemolysis. Positive direct Coombs test (DCT) = antibodies on RBC surface. Positive indirect Coombs test = antibodies in serum.
- If DCT +ve, screen serum for red cell isoimmune antibodies, e.g. neonatal rhesus or ABO haemolytic disease (see b Chapter 6, p.xxx,).
- If DCT +ve, IgG- and C3- specific reagents suggest warm and cold antibody autoimmune haemolysis respectively.
- IgM for mycoplasma; CMV; EBV; rubella; for cold antibody autoimmune haemolysis.
- Hb electrophoresis for sickle cell anaemia, thalassaemias, unstable Hbs, e.g. Hb Koln.
- Flow cytometry for hereditary spherocytosis.
- RBC enzyme assays for RBC enzyme defects, e.g G6PD.
- If history suggestive, immunophenotyping (CD55 + CD59) for paroxysmal nocturnal haemoglobinuria (PNH).

Deficiency anaemias

Iron deficiency
Commonest nutritional deficiency. Occurs in 10–30% of those at high risk:
- Preterm, LBW infants, multiple births;
- After exclusive breastfeeding >6mths, delayed introduction of iron-containing solids, excessive cow's milk (protein enteropathy);
- Adolescent females (growth spurt and menstruation);
- Low iron-containing diet due to poverty, fad diets, or strict vegans.

Causes
- *Dietary:* commonest cause, e.g. prolonged and exclusive consumption of cow's or breast milk with late introduction of iron containing solids.
- *Infancy and early childhood:* low level of dietary iron, e.g. high milk intake (low iron), GI blood loss, e.g. cow's milk protein enteropathy.
- ↑ *Demand due to rapid growth:* e.g. following prematurity or puberty.
- *Malabsorption:* e.g. coeliac disease, IBD.
- *Rarely blood loss:* e.g. Meckel's diverticulum, oesophagitis. Bleeding may be occult into cysts, tumours or 2° to drugs, e.g. NSAIDs.
- *Intestinal parasites:* e.g. hookworm (in less developed world).

Presentation
- Most cases are subclinical. Onset of symptoms of anaemia is usually insidious. Profoundly iron deficient toddlers usually adapt to their anaemia and tolerate surprisingly low Hbs.
- Pallor, lethargy, poor feeding, breathlessness (only in severe anaemia).
- May also develop symptoms associated with iron deficiency, including neurological effects of listlessness and irritability (infants), mood changes, reduced cognitive and psychomotor performance (can occur at levels of mild/moderate deficiency before anaemia develops), and rarely, pica (eating unusual items, e.g. soil, chewing on pencils).

Diagnosis Iron deficiency anaemia is a sign not a diagnosis—always look for underlying cause (usually dietary or GI disease).
- *FBC:* Hb ↓, MCV & MCH & MCHC ↓ (below normal range for age), platelets often raised.
- *Blood film:* microcytic, hypochromic anaemia.
- *Serum ferritin ↓ (indicative of iron stores):* it may be low before anaemia. Check C-reactive protein, as ferritin may be falsely raised due to acute phase reaction (↓ serum iron and ↑ total iron binding capacity (TIBC) confirms iron deficiency).

Treatment Give 5mg/kg elemental iron/day (as oral ferrous salt) given in 2–3 divided doses (max dose of 200mg/day). Response in reticulocyte count is usually within 5–10 days. Continue for 3mths after Hb normalizes to replenish body stores. If indices don't improve once Hb normalized, screen for thalassaemia trait.

Prevention in high risk groups
- Iron supplementation in preterm infants.

- Encourage iron-containing diet, e.g. iron fortified formulas and breakfast cereals, meat, green vegetables, beans, egg yolk, foods rich in vitamin C ($\uparrow$ iron absorption).
- Avoid prolonged cow's milk consumption to detriment of solids intake.

Macrocytic anaemia

Vitamin B$_{12}$ deficiency Vitamin B$_{12}$ (cobalamin) usually sourced from animal products. Vegan or other diets lacking meat most at risk. Alternatively, can have defective absorption due to intrinsic factor deficiency (congenital autosomal recessive (AR) or juvenile autoimmune pernicious anaemia), defective B$_{12}$ transport (transcobalamin II deficiency), intestinal disease causing malabsorption (ileal resection, IBD, coeliac disease), or bacterial over-growth in small bowel.

Folate deficiency

A common nutritional deficiency worldwide. *Causes* include:
- Malnutrition (marasmus, kwashiorkor), goat's milk feeding.
- Malabsorption, e.g. coeliac disease, IBD, other small intestinal disease;
- Increased requirements, e.g. rapid growth, chronic haemolytic anaemias (give daily folic acid prophylactically), hypermetabolic states (infection, hyperthyroidism), severe skin disease.
- Drugs, e.g. phenytoin, valproate, trimethoprim, nitrofurantoin.
- *Disorders of folate metabolism:* Lesch–Nyhan syndrome; orotic aciduria.

Presentation for folate or vitamin B$_{12}$ deficiency

- Insidious onset of pallor, fatigue, anorexia, glossitis, developmental delay, and hypotonia.
- In severe cases, subacute combined degeneration of cord (rare in children): paraesthesia of hands/feet, ataxic gait, loss of vibration sense.

Diagnosis of macrocytic anaemias

- *Macrocytic anaemia:* Hb $\downarrow$, MCV $\uparrow$ (above the normal range for age, i.e. >82 aged 1yr, >90 aged 6–12yrs or >125fL as a newborn).
- WBC $\downarrow$, hypersegmented neutrophils, platelets $\downarrow$, bilirubin $\uparrow$.
- $\downarrow$ Serum B$_{12}$ or $\downarrow$ folate level (red cell folate level is more reliable than serum folate, which reflects recent intake).
- Bone marrow, if indicated, shows megaloblastic appearance.
- Rarely, intrinsic factor autoantibodies or test of B$_{12}$ absorption, e.g. Schilling test.

Treatment

Improve diet. Depending on whether vitamin B$_{12}$ or folic acid is deficient:
- *B$_{12}$ deficiency:* IM hydroxocobalamin (1mg)—usually response is within 1wk. Watch K$^+$ level as it may drop. Treat 3 times/wk until Hb normal; then give 2–3-monthly if the underlying problem persists (important to identify cause).
- *Folate deficiency:* daily oral folic acid (500micrograms/kg). Response is prompt (within few days).
  - look for underlying cause (usually GI).
  - ⚠ *never treat with folic acid alone unless serum B12 level is known to be normal,* as subacute combined degeneration of the cord can be precipitated.

Red blood count membrane defect anaemias

Hereditary spherocytosis (HS)

- Autosomal dominant (AD) in 75% cases. Incidence ~1/5000 (northern European).
- Various RBC membrane skeletal defects occur; commonest involves ankyrin (~50–60%).
- Mild to moderate anaemia in compensated cases. Anaemia can be severe with transfusion requirement.
- Splenomegaly is usually present.
- Infection exacerbates haemolysis with worsening jaundice.
- Aplastic (red cell) crisis can occur with parvovirus B19 infection. The severity of anaemia depends on degree of baseline haemolysis (worst in those with high reticulocyte counts due to sudden decompensation).
- Folate deficiency can occur with massively increased RBC turnover so oral supplementation with 5mg/day folic acid should be given routinely.
- Laboratory investigation includes: ↑ reticulocytes, ↑↑ spherocytes on blood film; red cell indices may be slightly low, but clue is in the MCHC, which is raised, i.e. hyperchromic due to the spherical shape of the RBCs. Direct Coombs test −ve (excludes autoimmune causes).
- In the past the osmotic fragility was performed, but now diagnosis can be made on clinical and basic haematological features of indices, reticulocytes and blood film. Diagnosis in difficult cases can be made by flow cytometry, but is expensive and usually not clinically warranted.
- Provide supportive treatment, e.g. folic acid supplementation, blood transfusion if anaemia severe during aplastic crises.
- Ideally, if splenectomy is indicated it is best performed after 5yrs of age but before puberty. Consider if:
  - anaemia is not compensated and child is not thriving physically, socially, or educationally;
  - chronic haemolysis resulting in gallstone formation;
  - persistent jaundice is a rare indication for cosmetic reasons.
- Splenectomy requires pre-operative vaccination against *pneumococcus*, *Haemophilus influenza* type B (HiB) and *meningococcus* C, as well as post-operative 5-yearly boosters, annual influenza vaccination, lifelong penicillin V prophylaxis (250mg bd from 5yrs until adolescence, then 500mg bd).

Hereditary elliptocytosis (HE)

Heterogeneous group of disorders with mainly AD inheritance. Incidence 1:25,000. Severity varies from asymptomatic chronic compensated haemolysis (majority) to transfusion dependence. Presentation and management similar to HS. Blood film shows elliptical RBCs.

Hereditary pyropoikilocytosis

In this disorder RBCs are extremely sensitive to raised temperature. Hb usually 77–9g/dL. Jaundice and splenomegaly present. Good response to splenectomy in those severely affected.

Hereditary stomatocytosis

This condition has AD inheritance and is of variable severity.

Red blood count enzyme defect anaemias

Glucose-6-phosphate-dehydrogenase deficiency (G6PD)

- *X-linked recessive:* disease occurs in heterozygous males and homozygous females, with variable expression in heterozygous females (depending on Lyonization).
- Endemic in Mediterranean, South-East Asia, West Africa, and Middle East.
- There are over 400 enzyme variants. African (A–) (10–60% enzyme activity) and Mediterranean (3% activity) are most clinically relevant.
- RBC G6PD levels fall rapidly as cells age, with impaired elimination of oxidants and reduced cell integrity.
- Intermittent acute haemolytic episodes (intravascular haemolysis) are associated with febrile infections (most common), oxidant drugs (antimalarials, sulphonamides, dapsone, aspirin, phenacetin, ciprofloxacin), foods (fava beans), chemicals (naphthalene - common in moth balls, henna).
- May present as neonatal jaundice or chronic haemolytic anaemia.

Laboratory investigation
- Normal during non-haemolytic state.
- During haemolysis, findings of RBC destruction (bite cells and Hb puddling (ghost cells)), increased RBC production (raised reticulocyte count), spherocytes and Heinz bodies on blood film, DCT –ve.
- Definitive diagnosis is by measuring reduced G6PD enzyme activity (may be falsely normal during acute haemolysis; repeat 6wks later).

Management
Avoid oxidant drugs and foods, maintain good urine output with fluids, transfuse if required, give folate supplements in chronic haemolysis or in patients recovering from acute episodes, treat hyperbilirubinaemia in newborns.

Pyruvate kinase (PK) deficiency

A rare congenital autosomal recessive (AR) condition. Chronic haemolytic anaemia results from deficiency of pyruvate kinase. Enzyme deficiency leads to ↓ RBC ATP generation and ↑ 2,3- diphosphoglycerate (DPG) production (shifts O_2 dissociation curve to right). Severity is variable. Neonatal jaundice is common. Patients can have persistent, severe hyperbilirubinaemia. Parvovirus B19 infection can cause (red cell) aplastic crisis. Laboratory findings are of ↑ RBC destruction and production, ↓ PK enzyme level. Blood film pre-splenectomy not very informative.

Management
- Oral folate supplements.
- Blood transfusion if symptomatic anaemia.
- Support of aplastic crisis, e.g. blood transfusion.
- Splenectomy in severe cases.

Sickle cell disease

- SCD is autosomal recessive. The most severe form is homozygous sickle haemoglobin HbSS, with less severe disease in compound heterozygotes, e.g. HbSC, HbSD, HbSβ^0, or HbSβ$^+$ thalassaemia. A mutation in codon 6 of β-globin gene (chromosome 11) with single amino acid substitution (glutamine for valine).
- Found in Caribbean, Africa, Middle East, Mediterranean, and India. In Jamaica, carrier rate is 10%, with disease (HbSS) in 1 in 300 births. HbC carriers represent 3.5% of Jamaicans. Heterozygous carriers of HbS have increased resistance to malaria, accounting for the high gene prevalence in malarial regions. In England SCD now occurs in more than 1 in 2000 live births.

The disease is due to vaso-occlusion and haemolysis. RBCs show ↑ blood viscosity, reducing flow through small vessels causing tissue infarction. Sickle RBCs are prematurely destroyed resulting in a haemolytic anaemia.

Clinical features

A spectrum of disease, ranging from asymptomatic to severe, frequent crises and organ damage. Usually presents between 3mths and 6yrs.
- *Infancy:* high HbF is protective (reduces tactoid formation) in the first months of life. Common problems are dactylitis, splenic sequestration and pneumococcal sepsis (if not vaccinated and on penicillin V prophylaxis).
- *Young children:* infection from encapsulated organisms (if not vaccinated and on penicillin V prophylaxis) and parvovirus, vaso-occlusive crises in long bones, upper airway obstruction, stroke.
- *Older children:* vaso-occlusive crises, avascular necrosis and stroke.
- Risk of pneumococcal sepsis greatest in the first 3yrs of life.

Sickle crises and problems

- *Vaso-occlusive (VOD)crises:* presents as excruciating pain in bones and joints, commonly involving hands and feet, becoming more central with increasing age. Dactylitis is an early manifestation of disease. It is precipitated by cold weather, dehydration, infections and hypoxia.
- *Acute chest syndrome:* can be precipitated by chest infection with shortness of breath, cough, chest pain, falling SpO$_2$. CXR changes may be late, and progress within hours. Prompt treatment essential.
- *Sequestration:* body organs trap sickled RBCs. Splenic sequestration is more common in first year; later liver and lung sequestration occurs. Rapid fall in Hb may be fatal. Recurrent episodes warrant splenectomy.
- *Stroke:* most common in 5–10-yr-olds, and by 20yrs up to 20% will have had silent stroke. Untreated, mortality is 20%; recurrence rate is 70% within 3yrs. Requires prompt treatment with exchange transfusion to reduce HbS <20%. All UK children over the age of 2yrs require an annual transcranial Doppler: those with high velocity flow should start serial exchange transfusion to prevent stroke.
- *Infections:* patients are functionally hyposplenic by 1yr, resulting in high risk of infection from *Pneumococcus*, *Meningococcus*, *Haemophilus* Inf. B. Ensure vaccination is up to date and give penicillin V prophylaxis.

- *Aplastic crises:* typically after infection with parvovirus B19. Reticulocytes and consequently Hb falls. Spontaneous recovery usually occurs in 10 days. The patient may require transfusion.
- *Priapism:* affects 3–5% of pre- and 30–40% of post-pubertal boys. May be acute fulminant (painful, lasting >3hr) or minor 'stuttering' priapism (shorter <3hr, self-limiting episodes). May result in erectile dysfunction. Major episodes require urgent urology. Recurrent stuttering priapism is managed with exercise, warm baths or oral etilefrine.
- *Avascular necrosis:* hip joint, humerus or any bone.
- *Renal impairment:* hyposthenuria (urine concentration defect) with high urine output and susceptibility to dehydration. Enuresis is common. Papillary necrosis causes haematuria. Chronic renal failure can occur later.
- *Retinopathy:* small vessel occlusion → neovascularization → vitreous haemorrhage → resorption → fibrous strands → retinal detachment. More common in HbSC disease. Surveillance needed. Treat with photocoagulation (see ▢ p.920).
- *ENT problems:* adenotonsillar hypertrophy is common and may lead to nocturnal hypoxia precipitating crises. Ask about 'snoring'.
- *Leg ulcers:* uncommon in childhood.
- *Growth and development:* generally delayed although final height is usually normal. Specific SCD growth charts exist.

Diagnosis

- In the UK all newborns are screened
- *Clinical suspicion:* required in unscreened population
- *Haematology:* Hb 5–9g/dL, reticulocytes ↑, sickle cells on blood film. Hb electrophoresis (HPLC) is definitive test.
- *Routine screening* of Afro-Caribbean children prior to anaesthesia.
- *Prenatal diagnosis:* may be performed on fetal red cells or fibroblasts.

Management of acute crises

- *Investigations:* Hb ↓, reticulocytes ↑, blood culture, U&E, creatinine, LFT, CRP (↑ with sickling/infection), group and save, CXR.
- *Hydration:* aim for 150% normal maintenance (oral or IV).
- *Analgesia:* titrate to severity of pain. Initially treat at home with simple analgesia, e.g. paracetamol, NSAIDs; give opiates if required.
- *Antibiotics:* broad spectrum cephalosporin, after blood culture if fever >38°C. Add a macrolide if atypical pneumonia.
- *Oxygen:* to maintain arterial oxygen saturation (SaO$_2$) >95%. Keep warm.
- *Blood:* transfusion for aplastic crisis, sequestration, or anaemia; exchange transfusion for sequestration, chest syndrome, or stroke.

Maintenance treatment

- *Avoid precipitating factors:* e.g. hypoxia (air travel), cold, dehydration.
- *Vaccination:* see ▢ p.728.
- *Lifetime oral penicillin V prophylaxis.*
- *Daily oral folic acid.*
- *Hydroxycarbamide (hydroxyurea):* may reduce crises and need for blood. A rise in MCV shows compliance and myelosuppression is most common adverse effect. Use in patients with moderate to severe disease.
- *Bone marrow transplantation:* if successful is curative.

Thalassaemia

A inherited defect in synthesis of one or more globin chains (globin chain linked to haem group = Hb) resulting in imbalanced globin chain production → ineffective erythropoiesis → precipitation of excess chains → haemolysis → variable severity anaemia.

- At birth the major Hb is HbF ($\alpha_2\gamma_2$). By the end of the first year of life and into adulthood the major Hb is HbA ($\alpha_2\beta_2$), ~2. 5% is HbA$_2$ ($\alpha_2\delta_2$), and only 1–2% is HbF.
- HbA ($\alpha_2\beta_2$) is comprised of two α globin chains that are encoded by *two* α-globin genes on each chromosome 16 (i.e. each cell has 4 α-globin genes), designated as ($\alpha\alpha/\alpha\alpha$).
- The two β globin chains are encoded by only *one* β-globin gene on each chromosome 11, designated (β/β).
- HbF has 2 α globin chains combined with 2 γ ($\alpha\alpha/\gamma\gamma$). HbA$_2$ has 2 α chains combined with 2 δ chains ($\alpha\alpha\delta$).
- There are various forms of thalassaemia, e.g. β thalassaemia (β chains are not produced), α thalassaemia, δ-β thalassaemia.
- Thalassaemia genes can be null mutants, which make no globin chains, e.g. β° or α°, or can make minimal amounts of globin chains, e.g. β^+, or α^+.
- Thalassaemia major describes the homozygous disease state, e.g. (β°/β°)
- Thalassaemia minor (also called thalassaemia trait) describes carriers (heterozygotes) of either β° or β^+ genes or α° or α^+ genes.
- Thalassaemia intermedia describes the spectrum of phenotypes between major and minor (i.e. 3 α gene deletion causes HbH disease, or a β^+ mutation with another β^+ mutation).

The severity of anaemia and clinical picture are related to the number and nature of gene mutation and deletions and consequent imbalanced globin chain production. Thalassaemia is common in malaria-affected regions of the world (the trait is probably protective), i.e. parts of Africa, Mediterranean, Middle East, India, and Asia.

α-thalassaemia

- Silent α-thalassaemia ($\alpha\alpha/\alpha-$): one α gene deletion. Asymptomatic.
- α-thalassaemia trait ($\alpha\alpha/--$) or ($\alpha-/\alpha-$): Two α gene deletion. Asymptomatic with hypochromic microcytic picture (Hb may be ↓, MCV ↓, MCH ↓). May mimic iron deficiency, if RBC >5.0 × 10^{12}/L with microcytic, hypochromic film, then thalassaemia trait more likely.
- Hb H disease ($\alpha-/--$): Three α gene deletion or equivalent. Variable chronic anaemia with mild hepatosplenomegaly and jaundice. Hypochromic anaemia with target cells and reticulocytes ↑. HbH inclusions (tetramers of β globin) are seen on special staining. Folic acid supplements required, and occasionally transfusions. Splenectomy may be beneficial.
- Hb Bart's hydrops fetalis ($--/--$). Four α gene deletion. Causes hydrops fetalis leading to stillbirth or early neonatal death. Hb analysis shows mainly Hb Bart's (γ4). Most often seen in South-East Asia where frequency of ($\alpha\alpha\ --$) carriers is high.

β-thalassaemia

This disorder is not obvious until γ chain production falls off at around 6mths of age and HbF ($\alpha\alpha/\gamma\gamma$) levels fall.

β thalassaemia trait

- (β°/β) or (β^+/β).
- Asymptomatic with mild Hb ↓, MCV ↓, MCH ↓.
- HbA_2 characteristically ↑ on Hb electrophoresis to > 3.5%.
- No treatment required, but important to detect for genetic counselling purposes, especially if partner also has haemoglobinopathy.

β thalassaemia major

Presentation

- Presents in first year to 18mths as HbF drops, but no Hb A is made leading to anaemia.
- Severe anaemia (3–9g/dL); markedly ↓ MCV and MCH, ↑ reticulocytes, target cells, and nucleated RBCs.
- Secondary growth and development failure.
- Extramedullary haematopoiesis causes skeletal deformity (frontal bossing of skull, maxillary swelling) and hepatosplenomegaly in older children who are not adequately transfused.
- Hb electrophoresis shows mainly HbF, but no HbA.

Management

- Regular transfusions (every 3–4wks) to maintain Hb level that suppresses extramedullary haematopoiesis and sustains growth and development.
- Iron overload is major problem, with haemosiderosis affecting the heart, liver, endocrine organs, and pancreas.
- Chelation of iron starts when ferritin level >1000micrograms/L (usually following 10–20 transfusions). Desferrioxamine by SC infusion 5–7 nights per week. Side-effects include: cataracts, hearing loss, *Yersinia* gut infections. Alternatively, in children over 6yrs give desferiserox (a new oral iron chelator). Start at dose of 20mg/kg/day and monitor renal function.
- Splenectomy may help if massive splenomegaly or increased transfusion requirements.
- Bone marrow transplantation is the only cure and is usually successful when carried out as a planned procedure in a unit that specializes in the procedure, and in well chelated patients with no end organ damage. The procedure well carries significant risks.

Thalassaemia intermedia

Has a variable phenotype depending on the genotype from asymptomatic to a moderately severe anaemia, similar to thalassaemia major, that may require intermittent transfusions. This disorder is usually due to co-inheritance of an ameliorating condition, e.g. triplicated α globin chains, and HbF (hereditary persistence of fetal Hb), α thalassaemia trait.

Immune haemolytic anaemia

In this group of disorders, RBCs react with autoantibody +/− complement, which leads to their destruction by the reticuloendothelial system. Many drugs can induce antibody-mediated haemolysis, e.g. penicillins, cephalosporins, ibuprofen, anti-malarials, rifampicin, antihistamines. Mechanisms are variable. Immune haemolytic anaemia can be divided into isoimmune and autoimmune forms.

Isoimmune

See 🕮 p.194. Sensitization induces maternal red cell antibodies that cross placenta and haemolyse foetal and neonatal red cells. Usually, direct Coombs test +ve.
- Rhesus haemolytic disease.
- ABO incompatability.
- Other blood group incompatibilities, e.g. Kell, Duffy, blood groups.

Autoimmune

Warm antibody type—mostly IgG
- Rare.
- Majority are idiopathic.
- *Other causes:* drugs (e.g. penicillin), lymphoid malignancies, autoimmune diseases (e.g. SLE, IBD).
- Variable haemolytic anaemia, mild jaundice, splenomegaly, DCT +ve.
- Warm autoantibodies—often non-specific.

Treatment Give oral prednisone. If no response give rituximab (anti-CD 20 antibody). Consider splenectomy if severe or poorly responsive to immunosuppression.

Cold antibody type—mostly IgM
- Very rare in children except PCH (see Paroxysmal cold haemoglobinuria).
- RBC antibody reacts most actively <32°C to cause intravascular RBC haemolysis.
- Idiopathic or secondary to EBV or *Mycoplasma* infection.
- Acrocyanosis in cold, splenomegaly.
- Chronic haemolytic anaemia, DCT −ve for IgG, +ve for C3.
- IgM autoantibodies react best at 4°C.

Treatment Treatment rarely needed. Warmth, immunosuppression, plasma exchange, and splenectomy may help. Usually, the condition is self-limiting if there is an infectious cause.

Paroxysmal cold haemoglobinuria (PCH)
- 2° to infections (varicella, measles, syphilis) and vaccinations.
- Acute onset of intravascular haemolysis, after fever and chills.
- Due to a biphasic antibody, called Donath Landsteiner antibody.
- Antibody fixes on the cells in the cold peripheries and lyses in the central warmth of the body—protect from cold.
- Transfuse as required. Condition is self limiting.

Red blood cell fragmentation

Causes
- *Microangiopathic haemolytic anaemias (MAHA):* includes—HUS, TTP, giant capillary haemangioma (Kasabach Merritt syndrome), and DIC.
- *Infection:* e.g. meningococcal, pneumococcal, malaria (black water fever- intravascular haemolysis), viral haemorrhagic fevers, *Clostridium perfringens*.
- Burns.
- *Mechanical:* e.g. prosthetic heart valves, March haemoglobinuria.
- *Hereditary acanthocytosis:* rare genetic condition of abetalipoproteinaemia with mental retardation, ataxia, retinitis pigmentosa, and steatorrhoea.
- Envenomation from several of the worlds venomous snakes, spiders, etc.

Clinical features
Depend on underlying cause and severity of anaemia.

Laboratory investigations
- Hb ↓.
- *Blood film:* reticulocytes, nucleated RBC ⬆, RBC fragmentation, shistocytes, irregularly contracted cells, microspherocytes, acanthocytes.
- Possible platelets ↓ or clotting prolongation with consumption.
- In malaria, visible parasites on thick/thin blood film.

Treatment
- Treat underlying disease.
- Correct haematological abnormalities, e.g. blood +/− platelet transfusion, fresh frozen plasma to correct clotting abnormalities.
- Give iron or folate supplements if required.

Aplastic anaemia

Due to severe bone marrow suppression of RBC, WBC and platelet precursors (pancytopaenia). Rare. May be acquired or congenital.

Acquired aplastic anaemia

Causes Idiopathic is most common. Rarely, 2° to radiotherapy, chemotherapy, idiosyncratic reaction to drugs or chemicals (chloramphenicol, carbamazepine, phenytoin, NSAIDs, mesalazine, several solvents), viral (hepatitis A, B, C; CMV; EBV; parvovirus—more common in adults). *Note:* Bone marrow invasion, e.g. malignant cells, osteopetrosis, displaces normal marrow; causes pancytopenia, not aplastic anaemia.

Presentation
Features of pancytopenia
- *Anaemia:* due to ⇊ RBC production.
- *Infection:* particularly bacterial and fungal. Due to WCC ⇊, particularly if neutrophils <0.5 × 10⁹/L (severe aplastic anaemia, SAA), <0.2 × 10⁹/L (very severe aplastic anaemia, VSAA).
- Mucosal bleeding, purpura, and bruising. Due to platelet count ⇊.

Investigations
- *FBC:* WBC↓, platelets < 20 × 10⁹/L, reticulocytes < 20 × 10⁹/L.
- *Bone marrow aspirate and trephine:* aplasia (marrow cellularity <25%).
- CD55/CD59 immunophenotyping to exclude PNH (see Paroxysmal nocturnal haemoglobinuria (PNH)).
- Cytogenetics and chromosomal breakage studies to detect myelodysplastic syndrome (MDS), Fanconi's anaemia or dyskeratosis congenita.

Treatment
- Remove or treat underlying cause, e.g. drugs.
- Depending on severity: RBC +/– platelet transfusion.
- Bone marrow transplant (BMT) may be curative.
- Immunosuppression, e.g. rabbit anti-thymocyte globulin followed by ciclosporin is best second line therapy for those with no BMT donor.

Prognosis Depends on underlying cause. Some patients recover spontaneously. Most will progress to more severe disease, PNH or leukaemia. Long-term survival is unlikely in severe disease without good response to immunosuppressive therapy or BMT.

Paroxysmal nocturnal haemoglobinuria (PNH)
- Rare, acquired clonal disorder of marrow cells deficient in glycosylphosphatidylinositol (GPI) anchors that protect against complement lysis.
- Usually associated with background aplasia, allowing PNH clone a positive selective advantage.
- Complement lysis leads to chronic haemolytic anaemia, with intermittent haemoglobinuria but persistent haemosiduria. Urine is Hb +ve.
- High risk of recurrent and fatal venous thrombosis e.g. Budd Chiari, venous thrombosis, cerebral sagittal sinus.
- FBC: ↑ reticulocytes, ↓ WBC, and ↓ platelets
- Bone marrow is hypoplastic with erythropoietic islands.
- Flow cytometry detects CD55 and CD59 deficient cells.

Treatment Blood transfusion, iron replacement (rarely) or iron chelation, warfarin (anticoagulant therapy), immunosuppression (e.g. with steroids). Ecluzimab (anti-complement antibody) may reduce severity. BMT can be curative of both PNH and aplasia. Otherwise, median survival is 8–10yrs. Death is due to thrombosis or complications of pancytopenia.

Inherited and congenital bone marrow failure syndromes

Fanconi's anaemia (FA) This rare, autosomal recessive condition leads to progressive bone marrow failure affecting all three haemopoietic cell precursors. Associated with chromosomal fragility and defective DNA repair.

Presentation
- May present at any age, but typically at 4–10yrs.
- Usually presents with bruising and purpura or insidious onset anaemia.
- *Associations:* short stature (80%); skin hyperpigmentation (*café au lait* spots, 75%); skeletal abnormalities, particularly upper limb and thumb (66%); renal malformations (30%); microcephaly (40%); cryptorchism (20%); mental retardation (17%); deafness (7%); abnormal facies.

Investigations
- *FBC:* pancytopenia, or just thrombocytopenia initially.
- *Bone marrow:* hypoplastic, dyserythropoietic, or megaloblastic changes.
- Chemically-induced cell culture lymphocyte chromosomal breakages.
- Investigate to detect renal abnormalities or hearing loss.
- Most of the 12 FA genes have been cloned and can be screened for in families where the mutation is known. Diagnosis is essential as standard BMT conditioning is fatal and appropriate modifications are essential.

Treatment
- Supportive, e.g. RBC transfusion, hearing aids, orthopaedic.
- Immunosuppression with corticosteroids and androgens (oxymetholone).
- Successful BMT curative for haematological defects but problems post BMT as FA is a constitutional and multi-organ disorder.

Prognosis Most respond to steroids/androgens but treatment is long term. Patients not responding to immunosuppression usually die within a few years due to complications of pancytopenia or acute leukaemia.

Shwachman–Diamond syndrome
A rare autosomal recessive disorder. Most patients have mutations in the *SBDS* gene on 7q11. The condition typically affects bone marrow, pancreas and skeleton. Neutropenia occurs more than thrombocytopenia and anaemia, leading to infections due to immunocompromise. Exocrine pancreatic enzyme insufficiency causes diarrhea and FTT. Skeletal effects include metaphyseal dysostosis and dental problems. Bone marrow examination is diagnostic +/– pancreatic function testing. *SBDS* genotyping can be helpful. Treatment is supportive, e.g. pancreatic enzyme supplements. BMT is an option but survival is relatively poor (i.e. order of 50%).

Dyskeratosis congenita
This is a very rare condition with dystrophic nails, skin pigmentation, and mucous membrane (oral) leucoplakia. Bone marrow shows hypo/aplastic changes. Treatment is BMT.

Failure of red cell production (pure red cell aplasia)

Causes
- Transient erythroblastopenia of childhood (TEC).
- Diamond–Blackfan syndrome.
- Drugs.
- Viral, e.g. parvovirus B19.
- Isoimmune haemolytic disease in newborn, e.g. anti-Kell.
- Congenital dyserthropoietic anaemia (CDSs).
- Megaloblastic anaemia (aplastic phase).

Diamond–Blackfan syndrome (congenital red cell aplasia)

This is a hereditary condition of variable genetic inheritance that, by an unknown defect, leads to a specific reduction in bone marrow RBC production. The genetic basis remains unclear, however, mutations in the gene which codes for RPS19, a small ribosomal protein on chromosome 19q13.2, are found in approximately 25% of patients. The familial form (autosomal recessive) accounts for 10–20% of cases. The rest are sporadic.

Presentation
Presents in the first year of life in 95% (25% with severe anaemia in the first 6mths). Occasional late presentations with variable phenotypes can occur and 15–25% of cases undergo remission. The syndrome is associated with:
- Dysmorphic features; cleft palate, hypertelorism (Cathie's facies).
- Thumb abnormalities in 10–20%; triphalangeal thumbs; absent radii.
- Deafness.
- Renal defects (>50%).
- CHD.
- Musculoskeletal defects.
- Short stature and growth retardation.

Investigations
FBC shows normochromic anaemia with reticulocytes ↓ (<0.2%). WCC and platelet count are usually normal. Bone marrow aspirate and trephine shows absent red cell precursors, but is otherwise normal.

Treatment
Trial of oral prednisolone 2mg/kg/day (preferably once they are immune to varicella zoster). Wean over several weeks. Some 70% of patients have an initial response, but most will need, but often cannot tolerate, a maintenance dose. Give regular monthly RBC transfusion with iron chelation if unresponsive to steroids. BMT can be curative.

Prognosis
Although 20% spontaneously resolve, there is significant mortality and morbidity in the rest from steroid treatment and blood transfusion related complications (e.g. iron overload).

Transient erythroblastopenia of childhood

An acquired, self-limiting red cell aplasia. This condition is idiopathic or secondary to bacterial or viral infection (e.g. parvovirus B19, EBV), drugs, malnutrition, or congenital haemolytic anaemia (e.g. hereditary spherocytosis). Incidence is equal in boys and girls.

Typically presents at <5yrs of age with insidious onset of anaemic symptoms in the previously well child. Examination is usually normal except for signs of anaemia. The patient may have a preceding viral or bacterial infection. FBC shows normocytic, normochromic anaemia, absent reticulocytes, and normal WCC and platelet count. Bone marrow is normal except for markedly reduced erythroid precursors.

Treatment

- Remove any underlying cause, e.g. drugs.
- Monitor FBC to ensure this is not a leukaemic prodrome.
- Blood transfusion if required.

The condition spontaneously resolves (signaled by a rise in reticulocyte count), usually within weeks, but occasionally may take up to 6mths.

Polycythaemia

- Traditionally, defined as an increase in the total red blood cell mass (RCM) above age-specific normal. As normal ranges of RCM are lacking in children, a raised haematocrit/packed cell volume (Hct/PCV) above age-specific normal is used instead.
- Commonest in the newborn: exists when venous or arterial Hct >65%.
- Polycythaemia-hyperviscosity syndrome is diagnosed in infants when Hct > 65–75% and usually requires partial exchange to reduce to ~55%.
- Very rare in childhood, but seen in teenagers with early onset myeloproliferative disorders, which should be suspected if Hct is raised > 3–4 SD above age specific mean.

Causes of polycythaemia

Neonatal causes (see also ⌨ p.192)
- *Hypertransfusion:* delayed cord clamping, twin to twin transfusion syndrome, maternal–foetal transfusion
- *Endocrine:* infant of a diabetic mother, CAH, neonatal thyrotoxicosis.
- *Chronic hypoxia:* intrauterine growth retardation, placental insufficiency, high altitude
- *Maternal disease:* pregnancy-induced hypertension, cyanotic heart disease
- *Syndromic:* Down syndrome, Beckwith–Wiedemann syndrome
- *Relative polycythaemia:* due to reduced plasma volume due to dehydration, diuretic therapy

Causes in older children
- *Primary:* polycythaemia rubra vera (very rare)
- High O_2 affinity polycythaemic Hb variant (familial polycythaemia)
- *Secondary to increased erythropoietin production:*
  - Compensatory increase occurs in cyanotic CHD, severe chronic respiratory disease, chronic obstructive sleep apnoea, chronic alveolar hypoventilation, e.g. gross obesity, high altitude, abnormal Hb with high O_2 affinity
  - Inappropriately increased production with cerebellar haemangioblastoma, renal disease (renal cysts and carcinoma), hepatocellular carcinoma
- *Relative:* dehydration or diuretic therapy

Presentation
- Asymptomatic plethora occurs in most patients, particularly newborns.
- *Jaundice (newborn):* due to increased red cell turnover.
- *Hypoglycaemia (newborn):* due to increased red cell glucose consumption.
- *Hyperviscosity syndrome in newborns:* hypotonia, congestive cardiac failure, tachypnoea, seizures, abnormal renal function and NEC.
- *CNS:* cerebral irritability, seizures, strokes, cerebral haemorrhage.
- Respiratory distress, pulmonary hypertension, e.g. PPHN.
- Congestive cardiac failure.

- *Thrombosis:* e.g. renal venous thrombosis.
- *Miscellaneous:* cyanosis (PaO_2 usually normal), hepatomegaly.

Management

- Diagnosis is often obvious, e.g. cyanotic CHD.
- *FBC:* ↑ HCT, ↑ RCC, blood film.
- Exclude ↓ serum glucose or calcium, or ↑ bilirubin (newborn).
- Investigate for cause if not obvious.
- In neonates; if symptomatic or PCV >70% perform partial (dilutional) exchange transfusion over 30min with normal saline (rather than donor derived plasma products) to reduce PCV to <60%.

    Dilutional exchange volume (mL) =

    blood volume × [(observed −desired Hct)/observed Hct]

Prognosis

Prognosis is generally good unless severe hypoglycaemia or thrombotic complications occur.

Abnormal bleeding or bruising

Causes
- *Coagulation factor deficiencies:* likely if there is excessive blood loss following surgery or dentistry, recurrent bruises >1cm, muscle haematomas, or joint haemarthroses.
- *Platelet deficiency or dysfunction:* presents as purpura, petechia, mucosal bleeding e.g. recurrent epistaxis, menorrhagia, or GI or GU tract haemorrhage.
- *Microvascular abnormalities:* palpable purpura suggestive of vasculitis, i.e. not a haematological cause.

Detailed history
- Nature of bleeding.
- History of recent trauma.
- Concurrent disease.
- Age, e.g. haemorrhagic disease of the newborn several days after birth.
- Any maternal disease (if newborn), including maternal ITP.
- Diet.
- Drug history.
- Family history.

Examination
- Is the child well or unwell?
- Hepatosplenomegaly, suggests haemolysis or hypersplenism.
- *Dysmorphic signs:* e.g. absent radius in thrombocytopenia-absent radius (TAR) syndrome.
- *Signs of anaemia:* e.g. prolonged blood loss, bone marrow failure syndrome.
- *Pattern of purpura or bruising:* e.g. extensor and lower limb pattern of HSP.
- *Palpable purpura in vasculitis:* e.g. HSP.
- *Associated features:* e.g. arthritis (HSP), albinism (Hermansky-Pudlack syndrome), haemangioma (Kasabach–Merritt syndrome), eczema (Wiskott–Aldrich syndrome).

Investigations
- Initially perform coagulation screen (PT [INR], activated partial thromboplastin time (APTT)), FBC and film, U&E, LFTs, and CRP/ESR.
- Depending on presentation also consider: fibrinogen, TT (presence of heparin).
- If clotting screen abnormal, i.e. prolonged, perform a 50:50 mix to exclude an inhibitor, and if suggestive request lupus anticoagulant screen and anti-cardiolipin antibody screen. If 50:50 mix suggests a coagulation factor deficiency, then request factor assays according to whether PT, APTT or both prolonged.
- If clotting screen is normal perform:
  - platelet function assay (PFA);
  - if indicated, formal platelet function studies (need fresh blood so test is best done near to a laboratory that can perform these assays;

- von Willebrand's screen should be performed if history suggestive (mucosal bleeding), even if APTT normal (although usually slightly prolonged);
- *autoantibody screen*—anti-platelet antibodies (rarely useful!);
- bone marrow aspirate and trephine is rarely required for diagnosis of ITP, but if TAR or bone marrow failure syndrome is suspected then it is indicated.

Treatment

- *Supportive:* e.g. colloid/blood transfusion if significantly hypovolaemic or anaemic. *Note:* Send off all blood tests *before* any transfusion, including blood for viral serology and sufficient samples for coagulation factor assays.
- Correct known coagulation or platelet abnormalities if required.
- If there is catastrophic bleeding without diagnosis, treat with blood, FFP (20mL/kg) ± platelets (10–20mL/kg) as indicated until the precise defect is known.
- Avoid IM injections, arterial puncture, and NSAIDs.
- If the patient is a young male bleeding post circumcision then usually diagnosis is haemophilia, or, rarely, some other clotting factor deficiency.
- Important to involve haematologist and blood bank early in presentation to get appropriate expert help.

Outcome

The outcome depends on the cause and severity of bleed, but generally, bleeding from whatever cause can be controlled by platelet or coagulation factor transfusion, resulting in a low risk of death or permanent morbidity.

Coagulation studies

See Table 17.3

- *APTT:* principally assesses the 'intrinsic' path of the coagulation cascade.
- *PT or INR (monitoring warfarin therapy):* assesses 'extrinsic' pathway.
- *Thrombin time (TT):* only used to differentiate between heparin contamination, dysfibrinogenaemia and DIC. This test is not used routinely and needs to be requested specifically.
- *Serum fibrinogen:* useful if DIC or haemophagocytic lymphohistiocytosis (HLH) is suspected.
- *PFA: In vitro* test of platelet function. This test is easy to perform provided the platelet count >100 × 10⁹/L. Ranges in children have been produced.
- *Bleeding time:* tests platelet function. Now virtually obsolete.
- *Fibrin degradation products (FDPs):* Components released into the blood following clot degradation. Levels rise after any thrombotic event. Can be used to test for DIC. The most notable subtype of FDPs is D-dimer.
- *D-dimer:* principally used to screen adults for thrombotic disorders, e.g. deep vein thrombosis (DVT). Rarely used in children except possibly to help monitor management of DIC (possibly along with FDPs). *Note:* DIC is a clinical diagnosis and is not made my measuring D-dimers or FDPs.
- Other specific tests include screening tests of coagulation inhibitor, e.g. lupus anticoagulant, or individual clotting factor level.

Table 17.3 Common causes of deranged coagulation tests

Test	Cause(s)
PT and APTT ↔	Normal child, platelet abnormality, vasculitis, e.g. HSP, heparin
PT ↑, APTT ↔	Deficiency of coagulation factor VII: vitamin K deficiency (common in toddlers due to poor diet), warfarin therapy, liver disease
PT ↔, APTT ↑	Deficiency of factors VIII, IX, XI, XII (haemophilia A or B, von Willebrand disease, heparin therapy)
PT and APTT ↑	Deficiency of common pathway factors II, V, X, fibrinogen (rare factor deficiencies, DIC, toxic doses of warfarin and heparin, profound vitamin K deficiency)
TT ↑	Fibrinogen defect, heparin, DIC
Fibrinogen ↓	DIC, hypo/dys-fibrinogenanaemia, HLH
FDPs or D-dimers ↑	DIC
PFA ↑	von Willebrand disease, platelet dysfunction, drug effect

Note: Most clotting times are longer in healthy neonates, particularly in preterm infants. Always refer to appropriate age specific ranges.

Disseminated intravascular coagulation

DIC is the pathological activation of blood coagulation pathways that occurs in response to a variety of severe diseases. All, or some, of the following may simultaneously occur:
- Consumption of platelets and clotting factors → abnormal bleeding.
- Activation of intravascular thrombosis with both macro- and microthrombi formation leading to end-organ damage.
- Widespread activation of fibrinolysis leading to further bleeding.
- Microangiopatic haemolytic anaemia ('RBCs destroyed in fibrin mesh').

Causes in neonatal period
- *Common:* severe asphyxia, sepsis.
- *Less common:* severe IUGR, RDS, aspiration pneumonitis, NEC, rhesus isoimmunization, dead twin, severe haemorrhage, purpura fulminans, profound hypothermia.

Causes in older children
- *Common:* septicaemia (60%), severe trauma, and burns.
- *Less common:* profound shock, hepatic failure, anaphylaxis, severe blood transfusion reactions.

Presentation
- DIC usually occurs in the setting of a profoundly sick child.
- Oozing and bleeding from venepuncture sites, wounds, mucosal membranes, GI, pulmonary, and GU tracts.
- Microthrombi causing renal impairment, cerebral dysfunction, localized skin necrosis.
- Acute RDS (ARDS).
- Microangiopathic haemolytic anaemia.

Investigations Platelets ↓, PT ↑, APTT ↑, TT ↑, fibrinogen ↓ (<1g/L), FDPs ↑ (>80mg/mL) or D-dimers (non-specific, but useful in monitoring progress).

Management
- Immediately identify and vigorously treat underlying cause.
- *Supportive care:* O_2, volume replacement for shock, blood transfusion.
- *Platelet transfusion:* if uncontrolled bleeding, or pre-procedure, but not for oozing. Indiscriminant use of platelets can 'fuel the fire' and cause more thrombosis.
- Coagulation factor replacement as required to control bleeding, e.g. fresh frozen plasma (FFP), cryoprecipitate if fibrinogen <500mg/L.
- ◆ Exchange transfusion may be beneficial, e.g. sepsis, rhesus isoimmunization, or polycythaemia (removes causative toxins or antibodies, and replaces clotting factors).
- Use of heparin is controversial, but may be needed if there is large thrombi or significant organ damage from microthrombi. Seek expert advice from a paediatric haematologist.

Prognosis There is a high mortality, due to either the underlying disease or DIC-related haemorrhage or thrombosis.

Haemophilia A

Haemophilia A is a congenital bleeding disorder due to defective production of factor VIII (FVIII), with X-linked recessive inheritance. Incidence is 1:10,000–14,000 males. One-third have no family history. Carrier females are rarely symptomatic, but may have a low FVIII level. Genetic testing may be necessary to confirm carrier status. Severity depends on degree of FVIII deficiency:

- <1% activity = severe disease, with 'spontaneous' haemathroses, significant bleeding if cut, mucosal bleeds, and lumpy (pea-sized) bruises as infants. Most require prophylaxis with FVIII concentrate (see Management, p.636).
- 2–5% = moderate disease. Bleeding rarely occurs, and tends to involve muscles and soft tissues, secondary to trauma. Requires FVIII concentrate when bleeding occurs but no prophylaxis.
- 5–20% = mild disease. Rarely bleed. May present after surgery or trauma. Prophylaxis with DDAVP or FVIII concentrates for surgery.

Presentation

- *Rare in the neonate:* severe forms present in infancy with intracranial *bleeds or after circumcision:* most present as they start to mobilize.
- Easy bruising. In younger children often get pea-sized lumpy bruises.
- *Bleeding into joints (haemarthroses):* knees > ankles > elbows > hips > wrists. The joint is painful, swollen, tender, warm, with severe limitation of movement, +/– unable to weight bear. Uncontrolled recurrent bleeding can lead to degenerative joint disease.
- *IM bleeds:* can be difficult to differentiate between muscle strain and bleed. May lead to compartment syndrome, nerve compression, or ischaemic contracture.
- *Intracranial bleeds:* may be extradural, subdural, or intracerebral. Usually follows minor head trauma. All patients should seek medical attention, and those with severe disease need immediate FVIII.

Investigations

- APTT ↑ and FVIII ↓ (PT, von Willebrand factor and PFA all ↔).
- Perform cranial CT scan if any suspicion of intracranial bleed.
- US scans are useful for possible joint bleeds and muscle haematomas.

Management

- *Prophylaxis:* in severe disease, most require prophylaxis with alternate day IV FVIII concentrates to prevent spontaneous bleeds. Children with moderate or mild disease do not require regular prophylaxis.
- *Major bleeds:* treat with recombinant FVIII product except in those with FVIII inhibitors. The dose depends on bleeding site, child's weight and serum half life of FVIII (usually ~10hr). In those with severe disease on prophylactic therapy, regular screens are made to assess exactly how much FVIII is required to treat a joint or a major bleed. The dose for joint bleed aims to get FVIII to 40–50%, whilst for head injury to 100%, i.e. treat intracranial bleeds with twice the dose used for a joint bleed.

- *Major surgery:* preparation with a haematologist to plan timing and dose of factor. Give analgesia as required, but not NSAIDs (↓ platelet function).
- *Minor surgery or persistent bleeds:* IV, SC, or intranasal DDAVP in those with moderate/mild haemophilia may suffice.
- *Mouth bleeding:* tranexamic acid suspension/tablets (20–25mg/kg tds).
- *Avoid IM injections:* including vitamin K at birth, if disease suspected (give IV). All vaccinations should be given subcutaneously.
- *Educate family:* about PRICE guidelines for supportive care of a bleed: Pressure dressing, Ice (bag of frozen peas), Rest (non-weight bearing), Compress (cold if possible), Elevation of limb.
- *Daily physiotherapy:* following a bleed is important to avoid muscle weakness or contractures once joint bleeding has resolved.
- *Home FVIII treatment:* parents, and in due course the boys themselves, should be trained to give IV FVIII concentrates. Central venous 'ports' are only used when peripheral access is deemed impossible.

Complications

- *Chronic arthropathy:* 2° to recurrent joint bleeds.
- *Transmission of hepatitis B, hepatitis C, HIV:* now rare since virally inactivated plasma concentrates and recombinant FVIII concentrate is given. All children should be vaccinated against hepatitis B.
- *FVIII inhibitor development:* is suggested by bleeds not responding to treatment. Measure FVIII inhibitor titre. Difficult to treat but most are started on immune tolerance induction with high dose FVIII. Acute bleeds are treated with increased FVIII dose or other products, e.g. rFVIIa or FEIBA.

Prognosis

Excellent. Life expectancy is now normal with current recombinant therapy (prophylaxis and treatment).

Haemophilia B

Previously known as Christmas disease. X-linked recessive disease caused by defective production of factor IX (FIX). Indistinguishable from haemophilia A, although patients may be slower to bleed. It is five times less common than haemophilia A.

Investigations are the same as for haemophilia A except FIX activity is deficient, rather than FVIII.

Management principles are the same as for haemophilia A except that DDAVP is of no use. Prophylaxis in patients with severe disease is with recombinant FIX therapy, usually twice a week, (FIX plasma half-life is 25hr). Generally, 1μ/kg FIX raises the plasma level by 0.7–1%. Complications and prognosis are similar to haemophilia A.

von Willebrand disease

von Willebrand factor (vWF) functions as the carrier protein for factor VIIIC, protecting it from degradation, which facilitates platelet adhesion to damaged endothelium. Deficiency in vWF leads to reduced factor VIII activity and impaired platelet function.

- Von Wi;;ebrand disease (vWD) is an inherited bleeding disorder due to deficiency or abnormal function of vWF.
- Incidence ~1:5000.
- M = F.

There are three main subtypes:

- *Type I*: autosomal dominant. 70% of cases. Mild–moderate severity.
- *Type II*: autosomal dominant or recessive. 25% of cases. Mild–moderate severity. In Type IIb there is usually thrombocytopenia.
- *Type III*: autosomal recessive. Almost complete absence of vWF. <5% cases. Severe.

Presentation
Presentation is very variable. Type III usually has severe mucosal bleeding, but when FVIII level is very low picture is similar to haemophilia A. Other types may vary from virtually asymptomatic to easy bruising with associated excessive bleeding from dental surgery, trauma, surgery, and menorrhagia (always screen for vWD in any female with menorrhagia or iron deficiency 2° to menorrhagia).

Investigations
APTT is usually ↑ (if factor VIII activity is low); PT ↔; platelet count usually normal except in Type IIb; PFA ↑; factor VIIIC ↓; vWF antigen levels reduced and function ↓.

Note: vWF is an acute phase protein, as is FVIII, and may be raised to normal immediately after birth and following trauma, illness, or traumatic venepuncture (hence difficult to make a diagnosis of mild vWD in a child!).

Management
- Avoid NSAIDs and IM injections.
- Minor bleeding may respond to local pressure or tranexamic acid (locally with mouthwash or systemically 20–25mg/kg tds for ~4–5 days).
- More significant bleeds or minor surgery may respond to DDAVP (avoid if type IIB as further reduces platelet count).
- Severe bleeding or severe disease requires virally-inactivated plasma-derived factor VIII concentrate combined with vWD factor (no recombinant product currently available). Manage as for severe haemophilia A.

Complications
Mainly occur in undiagnosed cases. May be profoundly anaemic 2° to chronic blood loss and iron deficiency. If receiving plasma derived products there is the risk of viral infection or exposure to new variant Creutzfeldt–Jakob disease (nvCJD). Acute joint involvement is rare except in type III. In severe disease, complications are otherwise similar to haemophilia A.

Prognosis

Patients with type I and II disease rarely have severe bleeds and generally have normal life expectancy and quality of life, especially in men (no periods). Severity seems to improve with age, but also knowledge about how to manage bleeds improves with age. Even those with type III, if properly managed, should normal have life expectancy.

Other congenital clotting factor deficiencies

- Deficiency of every coagulation factor exists, but most are very rare.
- All have autosomal recessive inheritance.
- The most common defects are those of fibrinogen (e.g. dysfibrinogenaemia or hypofibrinogenaemia) and specific deficiency of factors VII, II prothrombin, V, XI, XIII, and X. Factor XII deficiency results in prolonged APTT, but no bleeding tendency.

In general, the severity of bleeding tendency varies from that of mild haemophilia to a familial bruising tendency. Most patients present with bleeding after surgery (circumcision, trauma, or dental extraction) rather than spontaneous bleeding or haemarthrosis. Can rarely present as cord haemorrhage in the neonatal period—usually caused by FXIII deficiency. Congenital afibrinogenaemia is clinically the most severe, and haemorrhagic manifestations usually appear within the first 2yrs of life. Patients with this condition require weekly IV infusions of fibrinogen.

Depending on specific deficient factor, PT and/or APTT will be increased (XIII deficiency excepted). Generally, any boy with unexplained bleeding in infancy or as a toddler with isolated raised APTT must be considered to have haemophilia until proven otherwise. Unless bleeding is catastrophic, send blood for urgent factor assays and treat with appropriate factor rather than FFP, unless in extremis.

Acquired haemorrhagic disorders

- Haemorrhagic disease of the newborn. Due to vitamin K deficiency.
  - rare early presentation occurs within 24hr of life with serious bleeding, including intracranial haemorrhage (mothers may be completely vitamin K deficient);
  - more classical presentation occurs in first week of life in breast-fed infants with GI bleeding, widespread bruising, occasionally intracranial haemorrhage;
  - late presentation occurs after the first week of life, again in breast-fed infants, and usually associated with a variety of diseases that compromise or reduce the availability of vitamin K, e.g. cystic fibrosis with diarrhoea, alpha1 antitrypsin deficiency, liver diseases.
- Coagulation factor deficiencies secondary to liver disease.
- DIC (see 📖 p.635).

Platelet function disorders

Congenital causes

All are rare and autosomal recessive. They are due to the following:
- Defective platelet membrane specific glycoproteins, which cause defective adhesion to fibrinogen, e.g. Glanzmann disease (thromboasthenia), Bernard-Soulier syndrome (BSS), vWD (usually AD) (see 📖 p.638).
- Defective or deficient platelet granules (normal release induces coagulation cascade, vasoconstriction, platelet aggregation), e.g. TAR syndrome, Chediak–Higashi syndrome.

Acquired causes

May be 2° to drugs, e.g. NSAIDs, corticosteroids, antihistamines, renal disease, liver disease, and diets rich in garlic, ginger, and Indian spices.

Presentation
- Easy bruising and purpura.
- Mucocutaneous bleeding.
- Menorrhagia.
- Positive family history is common (although in most AR syndromes both parents are unaffected).

Investigations
- Usually normal platelet count (except in BSS which usually has mild thrombocytopenia).
- ↑ Platelet size, e.g. giant platelets in BSS.
- Prolonged PFA.
- If congenital platelet functional disorder suspected, perform PFA followed by formal platelet aggregation studies using ristocetin, collagen, adenosine 5-diphosphate (ADP), arachidonic acid, and adrenaline; and platelet nucleotide ratios. Interpretation is complex, so seek haematologist help.

Treatment
- Control bleeding, e.g. apply pressure in mild cases.
- Correct underlying abnormality or stop responsible drug.
- Give tranexamic acid for minor bleeding, e.g. mouth washes or systemically 20–25mg/kg tds for < 5 days.
- Give platelet transfusion if bleeding severe or to cover for surgery. Note: Need to give HLA matched platelets to avoid HLA specific anti-platelet antibody formation, if child likely to need frequent transfusions.
- Avoid drugs that inhibit platelet function, e.g. NSAIDs and IM injections.
- Consider oral contraceptives in teenage girls to control menorrhagia.

Prognosis
Prognosis is generally good with normal life expectancy. Serious bleeding is rare, but can be difficult to manage, particularly in children with multiple anti-platelet or anti-HLA antibodies.

Thrombocytosis

Normal platelet count <450 × 10^9/L; platelet counts >1000 × 10^9/L may cause thrombosis or bleeding when platelets are dysfunctional.

Causes

Almost always, thrombocytosis in infants and children is reactive.

Increased production occurs with

- Acute or chronic infection.
- Acute or chronic haemorrhage.
- Trauma or surgery.
- Kawasaki's disease.
- Iron deficiency anaemia.
- Certain malignancies, e.g. Wilm's tumour.
- Any inflammatory disease, e.g. ulcerative colitis.
- Primary myeloproliferative disorder, e.g. essential thrombocytheaemia (ET) or in association with chronic myeloid leukaemia (CML).

Decreased destruction

Post-splenectomy. On examination look for signs of iron deficiency anaemia, bruising or bleeding, splenomegaly, signs of Kawasaki's disease (see p.716) and general ill health. The most common scenario is for the child to be totally well having recovered from an acute infection and a follow-up FBC shows a raised platelet count.

Investigations

- *FBC:* e.g. WCC ↑ in infection or signs of iron deficiency anaemia.
- *CRP/ESR:* ↑ in inflammatory/malignant conditions.
- Bone marrow aspirate only ever indicated if primary myeloproliferative disorder (MPD) such as essential thrombocytheaemia is suspected (which is very rare).

Management

- Treat underlying cause.
- Watch and wait in reactive cases, as requires no treatment.
- Give aspirin in Kawasaki's disease (one of the few indications for aspirin in children).

Prognosis

Reactive thrombocytosis generally has an excellent prognosis. Primary causes are very rare and have a variable prognosis. They are best managed by a paediatric haematologist.

Thrombocytopenia

See also 📖 p.193. Defined as <150 × 10⁹/L: as platelet count decreases
risk of bleeding and bruising increases. Risk of bleeding is moderately high
<20 × 10⁹/L and likely if <10 × 10⁹/L.

Causes

Decreased platelet production

- *Selective megakaryocyte depression:* viral (HIV, parvovirus, EBV) or
  more substantial bacterial infection, drugs, and poisons.
- *Marrow failure:* aplastic anaemia, Fanconi's syndrome, severe IUGR,
  severe maternal pre-eclampsia, neonatal sepsis.
- *Marrow infiltration:* leukaemia, neuroblastoma, osteopetrosis.
- *Marrow depression:* radiotherapy, cytotoxic drugs, drug reaction.
- *Hereditary:* Wiskott–Aldrich syndrome (X-linked recessive:
  boys present with early thrombocytopenia, eczema, and
  immunocompromise due to immunoglobulin abnormalities), BSS, TAR
  syndrome.
- *Nutritional deficiency:* vitamin B₁₂ or folate deficiency.

Increased destruction

- *Immune:* ITP (most commonly in child, rarely in mother), neonatal
  alloimmune thrombocytopenia (NAIT), SLE, drug-induced (penicillin
  or heparin-induced thrombocytopenia (HIT)), infection (e.g. malaria
  or HIV).
- *Non-immune:* DIC, giant haemangioma (Kasabach–Merritt syndrome),
  HUS, cardiac disease (prosthetic valves or cardiopulmonary bypass).
- *Hypersplenism:* platelets pool in enlarged spleen from whatever
  cause—effect is dilutional, rather than destructive.

Investigations

- *History:* drug history, family history, preceding viral illness.
- *Examination:* signs of bleeding, lymphadenopathy, hepatosplenomegaly,
  concurrent infection.
- *FBC and blood film.*
- *Serology:* anti-platelet antibodies (e.g. anti-HPA1) if NAIT suspected,
  autoimmune antibodies in those with chronic ITP, viral serology (CMV,
  EBV along with monospot if infectious mononucelosis suspected, or
  HIV if unusual unexplained thrombocytopenia).
- *Bone marrow aspirate and trephine:* very rarely required in cases of
  unexplained thrombocytopenia.
- *Cranial CT scan:* if any evidence of possible intracerebral haemorrhage.

Treatment

- Treat underlying cause if possible.
- Platelet transfusion if very low platelet count (prophylactically, and
  guided by haematologists, except for ITP) or life-threatening bleeding.
- Splenectomy, e.g chronic ITP, hypersplenism.
- Bone marrow transplant may be helpful in some inherited bone
  marrow failure syndromes.

Acute immune thrombocytopenia

ITP is caused by IgG autoimmune antibody to platelet cell membrane antigens leading to platelet destruction in the spleen and liver.

Presentation
- Most present between ages of 2 and 5yrs, but can occur at any age.
- 60% have preceding viral infection, e.g. upper respiratory tract infection (URTI).
- Bruising, purpura, petechiae, mucosal bleeding, menorrhagia.
- Intracranial bleeds very rare (< 0.5%); often associated with trauma.
- Physical examination otherwise usually normal, e.g. no splenomegaly.

Investigation
- *FBC:* platelet count ⇊, commonly platelet size ↑ due to compensatory megakaryocytosis. Otherwise FBC is usually normal.
- Testing for platelet antibodies is not clinically useful.
- Bone marrow in ITP normal, but striking increase in megakaryocytes.

Generally, bone marrow aspirate not indicated if the child is otherwise well, unless concurrent pancytopenia, hepatosplenomegaly, lymphadenopathy, or abnormally-increased blasts on FBC suggesting alternative diagnosis, e.g. aplastic anaemia, acute leukaemia, SLE (adolescent girls) or bone marrow failure syndrome.

Management
- Do not treat the platelet count, treat the patient! The aim of treatment is to stop the bleeding not 'cure' the disorder, which resolves in its own time. Increases in platelet count will usually be transient, but are usually sufficient to control current bleeding.
- Moderate bleeding can be controlled with tranexamic acid 20–25mg/kg tds for <5 days, provided haematuria is not present.
- Active treatment is required if patient experiencing *significant* bleeding, mucosal haemorrhage, or haematuria, as all are associated with increased risk of internal bleeding.
- *First line therapy:* 4mg/kg prednisolone for 4 days and then stop.
- Second line therapy: IV IgG 1g/kg over 2 days if steroids not effective, alternatively can use anti-D antibody (if patient Rh+).
- If bleeding life-threatening or intracranial, give 15–20mL/kg of platelets, start prednisolone and IV IgG and consider emergency splenectomy.
- Splenectomy for chronic ITP is indicated if disease is not steroid responsive and child over 5yrs.
- For chronic severe ITP, rituximab has been used successfully in young children. Exclude other underlying immunedysregulatory or lymphoproliferative disorders such as X-linked lymphoproliferative (XLP).
- Educate parents regarding ITP, including signs and symptoms that should prompt immediate return to hospital.
- Child can carry on with normal activities, but should avoid contact sports and NSAIDs when platelet count is low.

Prognosis: acute ITP in childhood is a self-limiting disorder and >80% spontaneously remit within 6–8wks. Presentation after 10yrs of age or female sex increases chance of chronic disease.

Thrombophilia

These haemostatic disorders predispose to venous or arterial thrombosis.

- May be inherited or acquired.
- Most inherited thrombophilias are asymptomatic or present in adult life. In children, most present in the newborn period or following thrombogenic events (trauma, surgery or pregnancy).
- Newborns requiring intensive support often have multiple thrombotic risk factors including sepsis, dehydration, polycythaemia, and central vascular lines.
- Inherited thrombophilia should be considered when there is an unexplained arterial or venous thrombosis, neonatal venous thrombosis, or positive family history.

Inherited causes

Activated protein C resistance or factor V Leiden deficiency

Commonest inherited form of venous thrombophilia. Activated protein C (APC) is an anticoagulant formed in the vascular epithelium and limits haemostasis with cofactor protein S. Over 90% of APC resistance is due to factor V Leiden (FVL) deficiency (a polymorphism present in 2–5% of population). Adults heterozygotes for FVL deficiency have 5–10 × increased risk of venous thrombosis, and homozygotes ×30. Whilst homozygous FVL deficiency will often present in children, heterozygous children are unlikely to experience a significant risk unless an additional prothrombotic risk factor is also present.

Prothrombin G20210A mutation
Similar incidence to FVL deficiency. It results in a higher average prothrombin level. Heterozygotes have a two-fold risk of thrombosis in adults.

Protein C deficiency
Thromboembolism is rare in childhood, but severe deficiency can cause life-threatening massive thrombosis in newborns, resulting in skin bruises that may become necrotic (purpura fulminans).

Protein S deficiency
Autosomal dominant. This condition is clinically similar to protein C deficiency; less likely to cause thromboembolism in children.

Antithrombin (III) deficiency
Very rare. Autosomal dominant. Associated with high thrombotic risk, generally venous.

Hyperhomocysteinanemia
May be 2° to a genetic defect or vitamin B_{12} or folate deficiency. Congenital homocystinuria is associated with thromboembolism, e.g. stroke, mental retardation, and, in later life, arteriosclerosis.

Hyperlipidaemia
Familial homozygous hypercholestrolemia can result in myocardial infarction in childhood, causing adult like atherosclerosis.

Acquired causes

Acquired thrombophilia is most commonly associated with:
- Septicaemia;
- Use of central lines;
- Takayasu's arteritis;
- Kawasaki disease;
- PNH;
- Polycythaemia;
- SLE, anti-phopholipid antibody;
- 2° to development of anti-protein S antibodies post-Varicella zoster virus (VZV) infection; can cause (as with congential deficiency) necrotic skin bruises.

Newborns, especially if preterm, are most at risk. In the newborn arterial or aortic thrombosis 2° to a UAC may lead to bowel infarction, NEC, buttock or leg infarction, renal arterial thrombosis. Most common venous thrombosis involves the renal vein.

Investigation of thrombophilia
- FBC (polycythaemia or infection).
- ESR/CRP (infection or inflammation).
- LFTs (protein C and S, and prothrombin are vitamin K-dependent factors).
- Standard coagulation screen.
- Thrombophilia 'screen'. Under guidance by your local laboratory, this usually includes APC resistance, with FVL, prothrombin G20210A variant testing, as well as protein C, protein S, antithrombin III, and homocystine levels.

Treatment
- *Acute venousthrombosis:* anticoagulate with SC low molecular weight (LMW) heparin (or sometimes IV unfractionated heparin) and then warfarin, if prolonged anticoagulation required. In neonatal purpura fulminans secondary to homozygous protein C or S deficiency, treat with FFP or protein C concentrate for 6–8wks until skin lesions have healed.
- *Recurrent thrombosis:* treatment depends on severity, presentation, coagulation defect, and risk factors. Long-term anticoagulation with warfarin may be appropriate (aim for INR of 3–4).
- *Major vessel or catheter-related thrombosis:* can be treated with fibrinolytic agents, e.g. tissue plasminogen activator (TPA), urokinase.
- *Prophylaxis:* give SC heparin during surgery or trauma in patients with established prothrombotic defects and a positive personal history. Alternatively, antithrombin III or protein C concentrate may be given if relevant.

Blood transfusion

Red blood cell transfusion

Whole blood is not usually available, but is useful when severe hypovolaemia 2° to acute blood loss occurs. Otherwise, packed RBC are preferred. Small volume QUAD or Octapus packs are preferred for newborns as multiple aliquots can be dispensed as required from a single unit to reduce donor exposure (within a 28-day period).

Formula for calculation of transfusion volume:

Packed cells volume (mL) = desired rise in Hb (g/dL) × weight (kg) × 4

Platelet transfusion

- Indicated for bleeding due to significant thrombocytopenia or as prophylaxis in patients receiving myelosuppressive chemotherapy or with bone marrow failure when platelet count <10 × 10^9/L.
- *Platelet concentrate volume:* if child's weight <15kg give 10–20mL/kg; if ≥15kg, single apheresis unit/standard 'pool' of 4U.

Albumin

- Rarely used in modern paediatrics; 0.9% saline is usually now preferred.
- 20% albumin is indicated to correct significant hypoproteinaemia.

Fresh frozen plasma

Indications
- DIC or acute blood loss.
- Emergency therapy of non-specific coagulation failure.
- To correct coagulation deficiencies where no specific concentrate available.

Volume = 10–20mL/kg (as guided by coagulation results)

Cryoprecipitate

- Rich in clotting factors VIII, XIII, fibrinogen, and vWF. The main indication is to correct clotting defects induced by massive transfusion or DIC, especially if fibrinogen <1.0g/L.
- Volume is: 1U/10kg (= 5mL/kg), or if child weighs 15–30kg give 5U (1U = 1 bag), over 30kg give 10U.

Intravenous immunoglobulin

Normal immunoglobulin is predominantly IgG and is obtained from the pooled serum of >1000 blood donations. Indications include:
- Hypogammaglobinaemia, e.g. X-linked hypogammaglobinaemia;
- Rarely, prophylaxis following infectious contact in immunocompromised, e.g. CMV, hepatitis A, measles, chicken pox;
- Immunomodulation, e.g. ITP, neonatal alloimmune thrombocytopenia;
- Specific IgGs also available, e.g. ZIG for prevention of potentially life-threatening chickenpox in immunocompromised children with no immunity.

Special requirements
CMV negative blood components
These are required for:
- Intrauterine transfusion.
- Neonates and infants up to 1yr.
- CMV seronegative recipients of allogeneic BMT (● since the introduction of universal leucocyte depletion of red cell products this is probably now unnecessary!).

Irradiated blood products (inactivates T lymphocytes)
These are required in:
- Intrauterine and neonatal exchange transfusions.
- Patients undergoing stem cell harvest for autografts (a week before until 3–6mths afterwards).
- Patients undergoing allogenic haemopoietic stem cell transplant (a week before and indefinitely thereafter).
- Patients with suspected and confirmed Hodgkin lymphoma.
- Patients receiving purine analogues such as fludarabine, clofaribine, etc., indefinitely.
- DiGeorge syndrome and other congenital T cell immunodeficiencies. Granulocyte transfusion.
- New indications are for patients being treated for aplastic anaemia with ALG and cyclosporine.

Blood transfusion reactions

Major blood incompatibability

An example is group A blood being transfused to a child with blood group O. Signs and symptoms of intravascular haemolysis may appear after only 5–10mL blood infusion with:

- Pain at venepuncture site.
- Agitation, flushing, chest/abdominal/flank pain.
- Fever, hypotension, haemoglobinaemia, haemoglobinuria, renal failure.

Treatment

- Stop transfusion immediately.
- Keep IV line open with saline.
- Monitor vital signs and urine output.
- Recheck patient and blood unit ID number.
- Give supportive care. Watch for hypotension, respiratory and renal failure.
- Inform the blood bank.

Minor incompatibilities (i.e. group O·⁺ blood given to an O- child) will not cause intravascular haemolysis but will cause sensitization and problems for future transfusions, in particular in females during later pregnancies.

Bacterial infected blood products

Most serious reactions are seen with platelets (kept at room temperature where bacteria can multiply and produce toxins). At its most severe there is sudden hypotension, fever, rigors, systemic collapse, and DIC.

Treatment

Give IV broad-spectrum antibiotics (unlikely to help as the reaction is toxin mediated but will stop the development of further sepsis), inotropic support, and intensive care support as required. Delayed reaction after a platelet transfusion, i.e. not immediate, but within a few hours, must raise the suspicion of an infected product, requiring immediate blood cultures, broad spectrum antibiotics. Alert the blood bank immediately.

Transfusion-related acute lung injury (TRALI)

Rapid onset cough and shortness of breath occur (may mimic fluid overload). TRALI is caused by donor antibodies to recipient leucocytes. There is an ARDS-like picture, with bilateral infiltrates on CXR. Respiratory support is required.

Febrile, non-haemolytic reactions

These are due to recipient anti-HLA or granulocyte antibodies, or cytokines in infused blood product. Reactions are secondary to red cell alloimmunization. Less frequent since the universal leucodepletion of blood products started in the UK in 1999. Fever and rigors occur within few hours of starting or completing the transfusion. To treat, slow transfusion rate and give paracetamol and antihistamines.

Circulatory overload

Results in pulmonary oedema, dyspnoea, headache, venous distension, signs of cardiac failure. To treat slow transfusion rate and give IV frusemide.

Transfusion-associated graft vs host disease (TaGVHD)

This occurs in patients with impaired cellular immunity. Lymphocytes in donor unit 'engraft' leading to rash, diarrhoea, liver impairment, and bone marrow failure. There is no effective treatment. Prevention is by prior irradiation of blood products (see 📖 p.647 for patients requiring irradiated blood products). Mortality is >90%.

Transfusion safety

UK rates of infection from blood products per transfused component:
- *Hepatitis B:* 1 in 1.5 million.
- *Hepatitis C:* 1 in 100 million.
- *HIV:* 1 in 5 million.
- *Malaria:* 0.5 in 1 million (US data only).
- *Bacterial infection:* 2 in 1 million for RBC, higher for platelet transfusion (up to 1 in 2000).
- *Variant Creutzfeldt-Jakob disease (CJD):* unknown (4 cases reported in UK up to 2010 in patients receiving non-leucocyte-depleted blood between 1996–1999).

Oncology

Epidemiology of childhood cancer

- Childhood cancer (age <16yrs) accounts for around 0.5% of all cancer.
- Approximately 1400 new cases of childhood cancer occur in the UK every year.
- Childhood cancer is the commonest cause of death in children aged 5–9yrs and 2nd only to accidents in teenagers aged 10–19yrs.
- The annual incidence in children under 15yrs of age is 1 in 10,000.
- One in 600 children will have cancer at some time during childhood.

Causes of cancer in childhood

Environmental factors do not appear to be clearly linked with childhood cancer. An inherited predisposition applies to a minority of tumours.

The proportion of cases by diagnostic group (ages 0–14, UK, 1989–98)

- Leukaemias, 32%.
- Lymphoma, 10%.
- CNS tumours, 24%.
- Neuroblastoma, 7%.
- Wilms' tumour, 6%.
- Bone tumours, 4%.
- Soft tissue sarcoma, 7%.
- Germ bell tumours, 3%.
- Retinoblastoma, 3%.
- Liver tumours, 1%.
- Others, 3%.

Clinical assessment: history

Include specific questions about:
- Fevers, night sweats, anorexia, weight-loss, pallor, bruising and abnormal bleeding.
- Family history, including malignancy and inherited conditions.

Also be aware that childhood malignancy may present with a variety of clinical features and so special attention should be paid to the following.

Respiratory symptoms

New episode of wheeze (usually monophonic and fixed) may be caused by intrathoracic mass. Treatment with oral steroids, based on a presumptive diagnosis of asthma, may lead to partial response in symptoms and therefore delay the diagnosis of leukaemia or lymphoma involving mediastinal lymphadenopathy compressing the airways.

Bone and joint pain/swelling

Persistent back pain should not be dismissed as innocent in children. It may reflect bone pain of bone marrow expansion (leukaemia or bone marrow metastases) or a spinal tumour.

Abdominal mass

May be:
- Painless and isolated (e.g. Wilms' tumour, ovarian teratoma).
- Associated with general malaise (e.g. B-cell lymphoma, neuroblastoma).
- Pelvic (e.g. rhabdomyosarcoma).

Raised intracranial pressure

The most common presenting features of brain tumours are:
- Headache (typically on waking).
- Vomiting.
- Ataxia.
- Papilloedema.
- Deteriorating conscious level.

Growth and endocrine disturbances

Midline CNS tumours may result in disturbance in the hypothalamic–pituitary hormone axes and present with:
- Poor feeding or failure to thrive (diencephalic syndrome).
- Polyuria and polydipsia (diabetes insipidus).
- Poor growth and short stature (growth hormone deficiency).
- Hypoglycaemia (ACTH deficiency).

Clinical examination

Thorough general examination including:
- All lymph node stations: neck, axillae, inguinal regions.
- *Skin:* assess pallor, petechiae, bruising, mucosal bleeding, signs of infection.
- *Masses:* measure dimensions of any mass and organomegaly.
- If leukaemia/lymphoma suspected, assess testes for swelling and optic fundi.

Specific diagnoses or concerns may be indicated by the following findings.

Lymphadenopathy

Malignancy accounts for a small proportion of cases of persistent lymphadenopathy in children. Possible diagnoses include acute leukaemia, non-Hodgkin's lymphoma, Hodgkin's disease, metastases from neuroblastoma or sarcoma.

Features of enlarged lymph node that should raise concern

- Diameter >2cm
- Persistent or progressive enlargement
- Non-tender, rubbery, hard, or fixed
- Supraclavicular or axillary position
- Associated with other features, e.g. pallor, lethargy
- Hepatosplenomegaly

Unexplained mass—at any site

The following features should raise suspicion of malignancy:
- Non-tender.
- Progressive enlargement.
- Diameter >2cm.
- Associated lymphadenopathy.

Neurological signs

The following should raise suspicion of a brain tumour:
- Cranial nerve deficits from direct tumour involvement.
- *False localizing signs:* III and VI nerve palsies (mass effect from raised ICP).
- Cerebellar signs (e.g. ataxia).
- *Visual disturbances or abnormal eye movements:* field and/or acuity defects (optic tract and suprasellar tumours); Parinaud's syndrome (paralysis of upward gaze) suggests pineal tumour.
- Abnormalities of gait.
- Motor or sensory signs.
- Behavioural disturbances.
- Deteriorating school performance or neurodevelopmental milestones.
- Unexplained focal seizures.
- Increasing head size (infants).

Key investigations

The most common reason for referral to a specialist is the identification of an abnormality on blood film.

Pancytopenia

Not all cell lines are equally affected, but the following problems occur as leukaemia or disseminated malignancy displaces normal bone marrow.
- Pallor, lethargy (low Hb).
- Bruising and/or petechiae (low platelets).
- *Unexplained fever,* recurrent or persistent infection (low WBC).

The following tests are used in diagnosis, staging, and assessment for prognosis, and as a baseline before starting treatment.

Laboratory tests
- FBC and film.
- Coagulation studies.
- Group and cross-match blood.
- Electrolytes; renal, bone, and liver profile; urate; lactate dehydrogenase (LDH).
- CRP, ESR.
- Ferritin and neuron-specific enolase (if neuroblastoma likely).
- Blood cultures.
- Thiopurine methyl transferase assay (in case of suspected acute lymphoblastic leukaemia (ALL)).
- Urine catecholamines (neuroblastoma, phaeochromocytoma).
- Lumbar puncture for cytospin, cell count, cytology.

Imaging
Sedation or general anaesthetic may be needed in young children when performing these procedures. The choice of imaging depends on the likely diagnosis, and may include:
- CXR.
- CT scan chest and/or abdomen.
- MRI scan (better than CT for soft tissue swellings and brain).
- Bone marrow aspirate and/or trephine.
- Technetium (^{99}Tc) bone scan.
- Meta-iodo-benzylguanidine (MIBG) scan (neuroblastoma, phaeochromocytoma).

Other investigations
These depend on the treatment being planned and may include:
- *EDTA:* glomerular filtration rate (nephrotoxic chemotherapy, nephrectomy).
- Audiology assessment (platinum chemotherapy, radiotherapy).
- Echocardiogram (anthracycline, pulmonary radiotherapy).
- Lung function (bleomycin, pulmonary radiotherapy).
- Pituitary function (suprasellar tumours, CNS surgery or radiotherapy).

Acute lymphoblastic leukaemia

This is the most common malignancy in childhood. It arises from malignant proliferation of 'pre-B' (common ALL) or T-cell lymphoid precursors. The cause is unknown, but in a minority it is associated with chromosomal aberrations. Possible links to patterns of childhood infection acting as a trigger have been hypothesized.

- ALL accounts for 25% of all childhood malignancies.
- Commonly presents in young children aged 2–6yrs.

Presentation

Typically with a short history (days or weeks), and with symptoms and signs reflecting pancytopenia, bone marrow expansion, and lymphadenopathy. Includes petechiae, bruising, pallor, tiredness, bone/joint pain/swelling, limp, lymphadenopathy, airway obstruction, and pleural effusion.

Specific diagnostic tests

- *Bone marrow:* morphology; immunophenotype; cytogenetics.
- *CSF for cytospin* (CNS rarely involved at first diagnosis).
- *Clinical examination* of testes in boys for inappropriate swelling.
- *CXR* for mediastinal mass.

Outline of 'standard' treatment

Induction (4wks)

- Steroids (dexamethasone or prednisolone) throughout induction
- Weekly IV vincristine
- IM L-asparaginase (e.g. 9 doses in 3wks or 2 doses of pegylated asparaginase)
- IV daunorubicin (2–4 doses, in intermediate and high risk cases)
- Intrathecal (IT) methotrexate (day 18)

Note Tumour lysis syndrome (📖 p.684) is a significant risk

Consolidation CNS-directed therapy

- *Low risk cases:* 4-weekly doses of IT methotrexate and continuous oral mercaptopurine.
- *Higher risk cases:* add IV cyclophosphamide, cytarabine.
- CNS-radiotherapy only for CNS +ve cases

Maintenance

Continuation treatment for at least 2yrs (3yrs for boys)

- Daily 6-mercaptopurine (6MP), weekly oral methotrexate (doses titrated according to blood count)
- 4-weekly vincristine IV bolus and 5-day pulses of oral dexamethasone
- 12-weekly IT methotrexate

Intensive blocks of chemotherapy

One or two blocks of 8wks duration, interrupting 1st year of maintenance. Combinations of oral steroid, vincristine, doxorubicin, cyclophosphamide, cytarabine, and L-asparaginase

Prognosis

Overall survival is approximately 80% with current treatment. Adverse prognostic factors include:
- Male gender.
- Age <2yrs or >10yrs.
- High WCC at diagnosis.
- *Unfavourable cytogenetics:* Philadelphia chromosome—t(9;22); MLL gene rearrangements (e.g. t(4;11) in infants); AML1 amplification;
- Poor response to induction and failure to remit by day 28.
- High level of minimal residual disease (MRD) at 28 days.

Mature B-cell ALL (Burkitt's type, L3 morphology)

Once considered a high-risk group, outlook is similar to that in standard risk ALL now that patients are treated with intensive chemotherapy according to strategy for B-cell non-Hodgkins lymphoma (see 📖 p.660).

Relapsed ALL

Extramedullary relapse (mainly CNS, testes) may present without bone marrow disease. Treatment is stratified according to risk factors, which include:
- Time from first diagnosis (risk reduces with time).
- Extramedullary relapse (lower risk, particularly if isolated).
- Minimal residual disease (MRD) status after re-induction (−ve status reduces risk).

Treatment
- Intensive re-induction and consolidation for all risk groups.
- *Low risk:* 2yrs of continuing conventional chemotherapy.
- *High risk:* BMT allograft.
- *Intermediate risk:* the role of BMT in this group is unclear; it may be based on minimal residual disease and/or availability of matched donor.
- *Radiotherapy for extramedullary disease:* given as a boost for those receiving total body irradiation (TBI) for BMT.

Prognosis
Long-term survival varies: 10–90% depending on risk (e.g. 90% in those with isolated extramedullary relapse more than 2yrs off treatment).

Acute myeloid leukaemia

Acute myeloid leukaemia (AML) accounts for ~5% of all childhood malignancies and <20% of all acute leukaemias. It is also known as acute non-lymphoblastic leukaemia (ANLL). AML results from malignant proliferation of myeloid cell precursors. AML can be subdivided morphologically using the French–American–British (FAB) classification system:

• *M1:* AML without maturation.
• *M2:* AML with maturation.
• *M3:* acute promyelocytic leukaemia (PML).
• *M4:* acute myelomonocytic leukaemia with eosinophilia (M4Eo).
• *M5:* acute monocytic/monoblastic leukaemia.
• *M6:* acute erythroleukaemia.
• *M7:* acute megakaryocytic leukaemia.

Presentation

• Symptoms and signs of bone marrow replacement (see 📖 p.656).
• Lymphadenopathy less prominent than in ALL.
• Intrathoracic extramedullary disease less common than in ALL.
• M3 may present with coagulopathy from proteolytic enzyme activity.
• Solid deposits (chloroma) occasionally seen in M2, M4, or M5.

Cytogenetics

Cytogenetic analysis shows characteristic abnormalities:
• *M1 and M2 AML:* t(8;21) translocation observed in 15% of all cases.
• *M3 AML:* t(15;17) translocation observed in 100% of cases;
• *M4Eo:* inv(16) frequently observed.

These translocations are regarded as good prognostic indicators. Other complex karyotypes are associated with poor risk.

Treatment

In AML prolonged continuation therapy is not used:
• 4 courses intensive myeloablative chemotherapy. The role of the gemtuzumab or Myelotarg (a monoclonal antibody directed against CD33) given alongside chemotherapy is being explored in the context of clinical trials.
• *PML:* all-trans retinoic acid given in induction, before chemotherapy, improves survival.
• High risk cases, including those who fail to achieve complete remission after 2 courses, are usually offered BMT in first remission.

Prognosis Overall survival is >60%.

Relapsed AML

All cases require BMT after intensive re-induction, usually in conjunction with 'FLAG' or 'FLAG-Ida' regimen (i.e. fludarabine, ara-C, and G-CSF support +- idarubicin).

Leukaemia and Down syndrome

The risk of developing acute leukaemia is increased 20–30 times, commonly either a pre-B (common) ALL or AML (especially M7). Response to chemotherapy is good and better relapse-free survival is found in those with AML. Children with Down syndrome-associated leukemia experience more complications of treatment.

Other genetic conditions predisposing to AML

- Fanconi syndrome.
- Bloom syndrome.
- Ataxia telangiectasia.
- Kostmann's syndrome.
- Diamond–Blackfan syndrome.
- Klinefelter's.
- Turner's syndrome.
- Neurofibromatosis.
- Incontinentia pigmenti.

Chronic myeloid leukaemia (adult type)

Classically associated with Philadelphia chromosome +ve disease (t(9;22) translocation). It is rare. It has a chronic phase with non-specific symptoms (fever, night sweats, and hepatosplenomegaly). During this phase the only cure is BMT. Some benefit from α-interferon therapy. The chronic phase progresses to a blast phase that is similar to acute leukaemia. BMT is required. Prognosis is worse if BMT delayed until blast crisis.

Juvenile myelomonocytic leukaemia

Classified with the myelodysplasias, it is also known as juvenile CML.

- It is rare (<1% of childhood malignancy).
- Age of onset mostly <2yrs.
- Associated with monosomy 7, NF1, and Noonan's syndrome.
- Response to chemotherapy is poor and only BMT offers a cure.

Lymphoma

There are two distinct disease entities that differ in regard to natural history, presentation, and management. Both are more common in boys than girls.

Non-Hodgkin's lymphoma (NHL)

The annual incidence of NHL is 10 per million. The majority are high-grade tumours that are divided into categories, using histology, immunophenotype, and cytogenetics (see Box 18.1).

Box 18.1 Classification of NHL

- *Lymphoblastic (90% T-cell, 10% pre-B):* 30% of all NHL. Most present with an anterior mediastinal mass. Disease may be present in bone, bone marrow, skin, CNS, liver, kidneys, and spleen. Cases with >25% blasts in bone marrow are regarded as leukaemia (ALL). Terminal deoxynucleotidyl transferase (TdT) positivity is usually observed. Translocations t(1;14) or t(11;14) may be observed
- *Mature B cell (Burkitt or Burkitt-like):* 30% childhood NHL. Occur in the abdomen, head and neck, bone marrow, and CNS. May grow rapidly. Endemic or African Burkitt's associated with early EBV infection and frequently affects the jaw. Expresses surface immunoglobulin and characteristic translocations t(8;14), t(8;22), or t(2;8)
- *Large cell lymphoma:* 15–20% childhood NHL. Subtypes—diffuse large B cell (BLCL) presents like Burkitt's; anaplastic large cell lymphoma (ALCL) involves extranodal sites (skin and bone). Lymphadenopathy often peripheral and painful. CNS or bone marrow disease is rare. ALCL is characterized by CD30 expression and t(2;5)

NHL staging (St Jude system)
- *Stage I:* single site or nodal area (not abdomen or mediastinum).
- *Stage II:* regional nodes, abdominal disease.
- *Stage III:* disease on both sides of the diaphragm.
- *Stage IV:* bone marrow or CNS disease.

Investigations
- *Tissue:* bone marrow aspirate; lumbar puncture; pleural and abdominal (peritoneal) fluid aspirate; exclusional biopsy.
- *Imaging:* CT and positron emission tomography (PET) scans.

Treatment
Lymphoblastic (T cell, pre-B cell) lymphoma is treated like ALL. Mature B cell disease is treated with short series of dose-intensive courses of chemotherapy. Risk of tumour lysis (p.684) is high.

Prognosis Survival is >70% (>90% in those with localized disease).

Hodgkin's Lymphoma

The incidence of Hodgkin's Lymphoma (HL), or Hodgkin's Disease, is very low before age 5yrs and rises with age. It is more common in patients with previous EBV infection. The histology shows Reed–Sternberg cells in an apparently reactive lymph node infiltrate.

Presentation

Progressive, painless lymph node enlargement, the most common sites being cervical (80%) and mediastinal (60%). Dissemination to extranodal sites is less common, lungs and bone marrow being most frequently involved. Fever, night sweats, weight loss (>10%) constitute 'B' symptoms and are common in advanced stages.

Subtypes

HL is divided into two subtypes, which are then further subdivided by histology. Classical HL includes nodular sclerosing (most common), mixed cellularity, and lymphocyte-depleted histology. Nodular lymphocyte–predominant HL is the other subtype, characterized by its distinctive histology and favorable prognosis.

Staging (Ann Arbor system)

- *Stage I:* single site.
- *Stage II:* more than one site and on one side.
- *Stage III:* on both sides of the diaphragm.
- *Stage IV:* disseminated disease.

Investigations

- CT of neck, chest, abdomen, and pelvis.
- FDG PET scan.
- Bone marrow aspiration and trephine (if radiological evidence of at least stage III disease).
- EBV serology and ESR.
- Isotope bone scan (generally done with stage IV disease, evidence of bone pain, or B symptoms).

Treatment

National practices differ, influenced by the balance between cure and adverse long-term effects. Low stage disease may be cured with involved field radiotherapy alone, but chemotherapy with low dose involved field radiotherapy for selected cases is now more commonly employed. Chemotherapy usually includes alkylating agents, vinca alkaloids, anthracyclines and steroids, and the addition of radiotherapy is considered essential at least for bulky mediastinal or stage IV disease. Reductions and augmentations of these therapies is being explored in the context of clinical trials and the role of PET scanning is likely to play an increasing role in monitoring of disease and determination of therapy.

Prognosis 5-yr survival >90% (stage IV, 70%; stage I, 97%).

Relapse Cure is still possible with second line therapy, including autologous stem cell transplant.

Central nervous system tumours (1)

Brain tumours are the most common solid tumours, accounting for 25% of all childhood malignancies (see Box 18.2 for classification).

> **Box 18.2 Classification of CNS tumours**
>
> - *Infratentorial tumours (>50%):* present with raised ICP, headaches and vomiting, and cerebellar ataxia
> - *Supratentorial tumours:* present with raised ICP, focal neurology, hypothalamic/pituitary dysfunction, and visual impairment
> - *Primary spinal tumours (rare):* differential diagnosis includes astrocytomas and ependymomas. They may present with cord compression
> - *CNS metastases:* of extracranial tumours (rare)

- Involvement of the multidisciplinary team is central to management of CNS tumours.
- The presenting features vary and may delay the diagnosis. For every childhood brain tumour, there are ~5000 children with migraine!

Initial management

Diagnostic imaging
- CT is quick and available. It provides essential information for emergency management of hydrocephalus.
- MRI gives better tumour definition. Combine with spinal imaging for staging of disease.

Raised intracranial pressure
This requires prompt treatment:
- Referral and transfer to a paediatric neurosurgical unit.
- Control tumour swelling with high dose steroids (usually dexamethasone).
- *CSF drainage:* initial surgery may involve CSF diversion only, biopsy, or complete resection, depending on location and likely diagnosis.

Low grade glioma (grade I, 45% CNS tumours)
- Most are pilocytic astrocytoma.
- Cerebellum and optic pathway are most common sites.
- Outcome depends on site. Posterior fossa lesions can be cured with surgery alone, whereas optic pathway tumours are relatively inaccessible and morbidity is high.

Neurofibromatosis type 1 (NF1)
See 📖 pp.531, 946.
- 50% of optic pathway low grade gliomas.
- Visual outcome better.
- Radiotherapy contraindicated - increased risk of second tumours.

High grade glioma (grade III/IV, 10% CNS tumours)

- Predominantly occur in older children and teenagers.
- Supratentorial sites predominate.
- Difficult to manage since complete resection, essential for good outcome, is difficult to achieve.
- Rarely cured. Treatment usually includes radiotherapy, with the addition of temozolamide or other agents in the context of clinical trials

Diffuse brainstem glioma

- Glioma in the region of the pons, usually high-grade and inoperable.
- Radiotherapy is the mainstay of treatment.
- Median survival <1yr.

Primitive neuroectodermal tumours (PNETs, 25% CNS tumours)

- Most common malignant brain tumours of childhood.
- Majority occur in the cerebellum (medulloblastoma).
- Peak incidence is <5yrs.
- Tumour metastases (mainly via the CSF) in 10–15%.
- 70% of localized cases can be cured, but expect significant long-term morbidity from radiotherapy.

Treatment

Treatment includes excision and craniospinal radiotherapy. Additional chemotherapy carries a survival advantage, allowing reduction in drug dose and/or field of radiotherapy, particularly in younger patients. Chemotherapy regimens include alkylating agents (e.g., Lomustine (CCNU), cyclophosphamide), platinum drugs (cisplatin, carboplatin), and vincristine. These are usually given after radiotherapy.

Central nervous system tumours (2)

Ependymoma (10% of CNS tumours)

- Periventricular sites.
- Usually present with obstructive hydrocephalus.
- 10% metastasize to the spine.
- Treated by surgical excision and involved field radiotherapy.
- Chemotherapy used in younger patients to delay radiotherapy.
- >70% survival if complete excision.

CNS germ cell tumours (5% of CNS tumours)

- Rare and more commonly seen in teenage males.
- *Midline (suprasellar or pineal):* 60% of malignant cases are germinoma, 40% non-germinomatous (secreting) malignant GCTs (GCTs; e.g. embryonal carcinoma, yolk sac tumour, mixed malignant tumours). Mature teratomas seen more in younger patients.
- *Secreting tumours:* characterized by raised markers (AFP or hCG) in either serum or CSF. (Biopsy in marker –ve cases).
- *Primary surgery for teratoma:* chemotherapy and radiotherapy for other tumour types.
- Cure in 70% secreting tumours and >90% for germinoma/teratoma.

Craniopharyingioma (10% of CNS tumours)

- Slow-growing midline epithelial tumours in the suprasellar area from 'Rathke's pouch'.
- *Treatment:* complete resection in 80%, partial resection with focal radiotherapy in the remainder. Complications include damage to the hypothalamic–pituitary structures, vision, and behaviour.

Retinoblastoma (3% of all tumours)

- Sporadic or familial (40%) forms that are unilateral or bilateral (30%) on presentation.
- *Peak incidence:* unilateral disease, 2–3yrs; bilateral disease, 0–12mths.
- *Presentation:* absent or abnormal light reflex (leucocoria), squint, or visual deterioration.
- *Treatment:* surgery, chemotherapy, and focal therapy.
- *90% 5-year survival:* inherited form at risk of second 1° malignancy, with OS being the most common.

Neuroblastoma

A malignant embryonal tumour derived from neural crest tissue with a wide spectrum of behaviour. It represents 7% of all childhood malignancies. Median age of presentation at 2yrs. Sites of involvement include:
- the adrenal glands (32%);
- the sympathetic chain:
  - abdomen (28%);
  - thorax (15%);
  - pelvis (6%);
  - neck (2%).

May be locally invasive; surrounds, rather than displaces vessels and other structures. Distant metastases to bone, bone marrow, liver, CNS, lungs, and skin (especially infants).

Presentation

Non-specific and variable. Depends on site, spread, and metabolic effects:
- Palpable mass (may be painless).
- Compression of nerves (e.g. Horner's, spinal cord), airway, veins, bowel.
- *Bone:* pain and/or limp.
- Lymphadenopathy and signs of pancytopenia.
- Sweating, pallor, watery diarrhoea, and hypertension.

Specific diagnostic tests

- Urine catecholamine (VMA or homovanillic acid (HVA)) to creatinine ratio, which is raised in >80% cases.
- ^{131}I-MIBG uptake scan: usually +ve.

Treatment

- Biological factors, such as MYCN amplification and 17q gain, strongly influence prognosis and treatment.
- Completely resected localized neuroblastoma may need no further treatment.
- Incompletely resected, stage 3 tumours require chemotherapy and possibly adjuvant radiotherapy.
- Stage 4 (disseminated) and *MYCN* +ve stage 3 tumours require induction chemotherapy, surgery, high dose chemotherapy with autologous stem cell rescue, radiotherapy and differentiation therapy with cis-retinoic acid. Targeted antibody treatment is increasingly employed as part of the approach to treatment in the context of clinical trials.
- *Exception:* young (<18 mths old) stage 4 patients with favorable biological features receive moderately intensive chemotherapy and surgery only.

Prognosis

Disseminated neuroblastoma only cured in 20–30%, despite intensive treatment. Survival in low risk cases (low stage, infants) is >90%.

Poor prognostic factors in neuroblastoma

- Age >18mths.
- Stage 3 and 4 disease.
- Raised serum ferritin.
- Raised LDH.
- Raised neuron-specific enolase (NSE).
- Unfavourable histology.
- *MYCN* oncogene amplification.
- 17q gain/1p loss.

Relapse treatment

Options include further surgery, chemotherapy, and/or radiotherapy, depending on 1° treatment. After previous high dose chemotherapy and stem cell transplant, cure is unrealistic. Treatment aimed at palliation.

Infant neuroblastoma (stage IVs)

Disseminated disease restricted to bone marrow, liver, and skin. Characteristically resolves spontaneously. Chemotherapy is only for life-threatening symptoms. Resection (complete or partial) is usually sufficient for localized disease.

Wilms' tumour (nephroblastoma)

This is an embryonal tumour of the kidney representing 6–7% of all childhood malignancies. Up to 75% present at <4yrs of age (90% <7yrs). Most causes are sporadic, but 1% have an affected family member. Wilms' tumour may be associated with the following conditions.
- Genitourinary abnormalities, e.g. horseshoe kidney, hypospadias.
- Hemihypertrophy syndrome.
- Aniridia.
- BWS (📖 p.949).
- Wilms', aniridia gonadal dyslasia, retardation (WAGR) complex.
- Denys Drash syndrome (nephropathy and genital abnormalities).
- Perlman syndrome.

Mutations of the WT1 tumour suppressor gene on chromosome 11p13 detected in Wilms' tumours; abnormalities of 11p15 are also implicated, associated with BWS.

Presentation Mostly as a visible or palpable abdominal mass. Usually painless. Haematuria and hypertension may also be seen.

Site

Bilateral cases are unusual and more often associated with genetic predisposition. Extrarenal Wilms' tumours are very rare. Metastases occur in 10% of cases, most commonly to the lung.

Investigations
- Abdominal US.
- CT scan of abdomen ('claw' sign in involved kidney).
- CXR or CT.
- Urine catecholamines to exclude neuroblastoma (prior to anaesthetic).
- Blood count and coagulation studies (a transient acquired von Willebrand-like syndrome is recognized and resolves with treatment).

Treatment
- *Surgical* excision required.
- *Chemotherapy* is used for all tumours. In stage I disease (complete resection of tumour without breach of renal capsule) is curable with vincristine, sometimes including dactinomycin which is also used for stage II disease. In higher-stage disease, doxorubicin is added. In bilateral (stage V) disease, the aim is to maximize response to chemotherapy prior to performing bilateral nephron-sparing surgery.
- *Local or abdominal radiotherapy* required for incomplete resection (stage III disease). In the presence of metastases (stage IV), surgery to primary tumour is delayed until resolution of metastases with chemotherapy and radiotherapy is also added. Carboplatin, cyclophosphamide, and etoposide are usually reserved for unresponsive or recurrent disease.

Prognosis Overall survival ranges from 770% for stage IV disease to >95% for stage I.

Relapse

- Follow-up should include regular CXR as well as abdominal ultrasound as pulmonary relapse is twice as common as local recurrence.
- Surgery, second-line chemotherapy, and radiotherapy (if not previously received) may all be applied depending on stage. Cure is achievable following second remission.

Nephroblastomatosis

Multiple foci of premalignant tissue, also known as nephrogenic rests, characterize this condition. They may be observed on renal US and CT scan. The condition is associated with Wilms' tumour, but may exist without tumour formation (seen on 1% of routine post-mortem examinations). Close monitoring is required due to risk of subsequent tumour formation.

Other renal tumours in childhood

Mesoblastic nephroma

Occurs in infants and is treated with surgery; chemotherapy is only indicated for incompletely excised cases.

Clear cell sarcoma

A bone metastasizing renal tumour of childhood. It is more aggressive than Wilms' tumour and accounts for about 6% of cases.

Malignant rhabdoid tumour

Rare (<2% renal tumours) and occurs mainly in infants. It is associated with posterior fossa CNS tumours and has an unfavourable outcome.

Bone tumours

These tumours are rare in childhood (5% of all paediatric malignancies).
• Incidence peaks in teenage years, in which they are the 4th most common group of malignancies.
• Majority of cases are osteosarcoma (OS) or Ewing's sarcoma (ES). They are histologically distinct, with different patterns of disease and response to treatment.
• Sarcomas are associated with Li–Fraumeni syndrome (familial mutation of p53), and patients cured of familial retinoblastoma are at a high risk of OS.

Osteosarcoma

Presentation

Localized pain and swelling, pathological fracture, and rarely erythema. Most affect the long bones around the knee (67%) and humerus. The metaphysis is a more common site than mid-shaft. Delay in diagnosis is common.

Metastases

• Seen at diagnosis in 15–25% of cases
• Lungs most common site, followed by bones.

Diagnostic investigations

• Plain X-rays of bony lesion.
• Biopsy (for definitive diagnosis).
• Lactate dehydrogenase and alkaline phosphatase.
• MRI of primary site.
• CT chest.
• Isotope bone scan.

Treatment

Chemotherapy, followed by surgery and then further chemotherapy. The aim is to perform limb-preserving surgery whenever possible.

Prognosis

Adverse outlook is associated with:
• Inability to resect primary tumour.
• Poor response to induction chemotherapy.
• Metastatic disease (especially extrapulmonary disease).

Relapsed osteosarcoma

Most recurrences are isolated pulmonary metastases. Surgical resection can result in long-term survival in 20–30% of patients. The role of chemotherapy for recurrent OS is uncertain. The role of radiotherapy is limited to palliation.

Ewing's sarcoma of bone and soft tissue

ES usually occurs in bone, but may also occur in soft tissues. ES and peripheral PNETs share a common immunophenotype (CD99 or MIC2) and cytogenetic profile (t(11;22) in 85% and t(21;22) in 5–10%). Both tumour categories belong to the Ewing's family of tumours. (*Note:* Peripheral PNET should *not* be confused with CNS PNET tumours.)

Presentation

Localized pain and swelling, and sometimes pathological fracture. The diaphysis of long bones is more commonly affected than metaphysis. The axial skeleton is involved more often than in OS with pelvis the most common site. Metastases to lungs and bone are more common at diagnosis than in OS.

Diagnostic investigations

- Plain X-rays of bony lesion.
- Biopsy (for definitive diagnosis).
- Lactate dehydrogenase and alkaline phosphatase.
- MRI of primary site.
- CT chest.
- Isotope bone scan.
- Bone marrow aspirates and trephines (bilateral).

Treatment

Chemotherapy, followed by surgery and then further chemotherapy. For extremity sites, limb-preserving surgery is the aim whenever possible. Radiotherapy is an effective adjunct, and an alternative to surgery, particularly at axial sites.

Prognosis

Adverse outlook associated with:

- large primaries;
- axial sites;
- poor response to induction chemotherapy;
- metastatic disease.

Bony metastases confer a particularly grave prognosis with <20% long-term survivors.

Relapsed ES

Salvage therapy is rarely successful, and will depend on treatment previously received. Second-line chemotherapy may include combinations involving Etoposide, carboplatin, cyclophosphamide, topotecan and ironotecan. Surgery and radiotherapy may also have a role in treatment.

Rhabdomyosarcoma

Rhabdomyosarcoma (RMS) is the most common soft tissue sarcoma in childhood. It accounts for 6% of all childhood malignancies (commonly aged <10yrs). The majority of cases are sporadic. Most are either embryonal or alveolar (more aggressive) subtypes. Botryoid (good prognosis) and spindle cell types are also recognized. A small number of cases are associated with Li–Fraumeni syndrome.

Presenting features Mass, pain and obstruction of:
- bladder;
- pelvis;
- nasopharynx;
- parameningeal;
- paratestis;
- extremity;
- orbit;
- intrathoracic.

Lymph node involvement is common. Distant metastases are rare.

Diagnosis and staging
- *Imaging of primary site:* CT, or MRI.
- Biopsy for histological molecular and cytogenetic analysis. Alveolar RMS characterized by the presence of t(2;13) or t(1;13).
- CT scan of chest.
- Bone marrow aspirates and trephines.
- Isotope bone scan.
- Lumbar puncture (parameningeal primaries).

Treatment
- Chemotherapy (6–9 courses) with ifosfamide or cyclophosphamide, actinomycin, vincristine, anthracyclines.
- Surgery is reserved for accessible sites (paratesticular, peripheral) after 3–6 courses of chemotherapy.
- Radiotherapy after surgery for residual tumour and alveolar histology.

Prognosis Ranges from <10% survival for bony metastatic disease to >90% for excised paratesticular tumours. Favourable features are:
- Younger age at diagnosis.
- Botryoid or embryonal histology.
- Paratesticular or superficial head and neck sites.
- Absence of nodal involvement or distant metastases.

Off treatment monitoring Imaging of primary tumour site by US or MRI and CXRs to screen for pulmonary metastatic recurrence.

Relapse
- Second-line chemotherapy.
- Radiotherapy may be employed at sites not previously irradiated.
- Outcome for relapse and recurrence is poor.

Germ cell tumours

Germ cell tumours (GCTs) comprise a heterogeneous group of neoplasms, often with mixed histology. They arise from primordial germ cells in gonads or, following aberrant germ cell migration, in midline extragonadal sites, including sacrococcygeal, mediastinal, or CNS sites. GCTs are rare occurring in 3–5 per million children <15yrs of age, with peak incidence seen in children aged <3yrs. 10% of girls with ovarian GCTs are found to have an underlying intersex state.

The *nomenclature* of GCTs is complicated.
- Mature teratoma is benign.
- Immature teratoma may disseminate locally.
- Malignant GCTs:
  - *germinoma* (or seminoma, dysgerminoma, depending on site) is totipotent;
  - *teratoma*, yolk sac tumour (YST), choriocarcinoma (CHC), and embryonal carcinoma (EC) represent more differentiated forms.
- Secreting tumours (YST, CHC, some immature teratomas, and mixed tumours) characterized by secretion of AFP and/or hCG, which may be used for diagnosis, monitoring of treatment response, and detection of recurrence.

Presenting symptoms

Site-dependent. Testicular masses are usually painless. Ovarian tumours present as either painful or painless abdominal mass. Metastases are rarely present at diagnosis (lungs, the commonest site, bone, and bone marrow).

Diagnosis and staging

- Measurement of AFP and β-hCG in serum (and CSF for CNS disease).
- *Imaging of primary:* US, CT, or MRI.
- Biopsy of unresectable tumours (unless unsafe) and/or imaging and markers sufficient to make diagnosis.
- CT scan of chest and abdomen.
- Bone marrow and isotope bone scan to look for metastases.

Treatment of extracranial tumours

- Surgery followed by observation for low risk tumours (e.g. mature/immature teratoma and gonadal stage I).

Note: Testicular tumours should be removed via an inguinal approach. Sacrococcygeal teratomas should be removed together with the coccyx to reduce risk of malignant relapse. Chemotherapy is reserved for intermediate and high risk disease.

Prognosis Survival >90% for malignant extracranial GCTs.

Primary liver tumours

- Hepatoblastoma (HBL) is the commonest primary paediatric hepatic tumour (<1% all cancers), with 2/3 of cases in the first year of life.
- Hepatocellular carcinoma (HCC) an embryonal (undifferentiated) sarcoma of the liver are rare in children.
- Serum AFP levels are raised in >80% HBL.

Treatment

- Chemotherapy including platinum drugs and anthracyclines for HBL.
- Good surgical result is critical for long-term survival. Liver transplant is indicated if local resection not possible.
- Treatment is the similar for HCC, although they are less sensitive to chemotherapy.
- Embryonal sarcoma is usually treated on soft tissue sarcomas protocols.

Prognosis Long-term survival for HBL is >70%, even in presence of lung metastases. Survival for HCC is significantly lower.

Other rare tumours

Up to 5% of malignancies in childhood are very rare. They include:
- Epithelial or adult-type tumours, (e.g. carcinomas and melanoma).
- Embryonal tumours (e.g. rhabdoid tumours).

Malignant melanoma Risk factors include:
- pre-existing conditions;
- giant congenital naevi;
- dysplastic naevus syndrome;
- xeroderma pigmentosum;
- albinism;
- immunosuppressive diseases.

Most cases arise on healthy skin and may be related to sun exposure. Surgery is the mainstay of treatment. Survival around 90% for local disease; 25% for metastatic disease.

Rhabdoid tumours
- Highly aggressive tumours that arise in kidneys or CNS.
- In the CNS, they appear histologically similar to PNETs, but sometimes associated with tumours outside the CNS.
- Treatment includes surgery, chemotherapy, and radiotherapy. Long-term survival is rare.

Phaeochromocytoma
Tumours in the adrenal medulla and sympathetic ganglia are usually sporadic, but may be associated with von Hippel–Lindau disease and multiple endocrine neoplasia types 2a and 2b (see 📖 p.440). They present with endocrine manifestations, (e.g. hypertension, excessive sweating) or a mass. Less than 10% of phaeochromocytomas are malignant.

Investigations Plasma and urine catecholamine levels are usually raised.

Treatment Surgery after α-adrenergic antagonists to control sympathetic symptoms.

Nasopharyngeal carcinoma
The commonest epithelial cancer in children. It is found in teenagers and associated with antibodies to EBV:
- Treatment involves chemotherapy, radiotherapy, and β interferon.
- Overall survival at 5yrs ~70%.

Other carcinomas
These carcinomas are rare.
- *Thyroid* (predominantly the papillary variant and associated with exposure to radiation). May present with asymmetrical nodular goitre (see 📖 pp.420–421).
- Adrenal carcinoma (seen in young adults with occasional occurrences in older children). May present with precocious puberty, inappropriate virilization in females (see 📖 p.480).

Langerhans cell histiocytosis

Langerhans cell histiocytosis (LCH) is a disorder of unknown cause with a wide range of presentations. It is not a malignant condition, but may behave like one in its severest forms. Usually managed by paediatric oncologists.

Langerhans cells are normally found in skin, lymph nodes, and airways. LCH results from monoclonal proliferation and accumulation of histiocytes, with the characteristics of Langerhans cells, in skin, bone, pituitary, CNS, lungs, intestines, spleen, or bone marrow. It may manifest as single- or multisystem disease. Single-system disease is usually confined to bone, occasionally to skin, and seen more in older children. The natural history varies from spontaneous resolution to repeated recurrence, or death.

Note: LCH was previously known as 'histiocytosis X', which was subdivided into eosinophilic granuloma, Letterer–Siwe disease, and Hand–Schüller–Christian disease

Incidence Approximately 1 in 200,000 children affected each year.

Presentation Depends on site of disease, but may include:
• Pain or lump associated with isolated bony disease (most common).
• Skin rash (widespread macular–papular or mimicking seborrhoeic dermatitis of the scalp).
• Discharge from the ear.
• Diabetes insipidus.
• Systemic disturbance (fever, malaise, anorexia, and failure to thrive).

Diagnosis

Biopsy with confirmation of Birbeck granules (or positivite CD1a or S100 immunohistochemistry). Diagnosis can be made without biopsy in the presence of characteristic pituitary/hypothalamic abnormality, where biopsy considered too hazardous, or of lytic bone lesions with clinical features suggesting spontaneous resolution.

Further investigation

Suspected LCH should be fully staged to identify possible multisystem disease. Investigations should include skeletal survey, abdominal ultrasound, early morning urine for osmolality, FBC and film, coagulation studies, and liver enzymes.

Treatment

• Single system LCH, usually involving bone or skin, frequently resolves spontaneously or following biopsy/surgical curettage, but may require topical or intralesional steroids in persistent or recurrent cases.
• Multisystem LCH, seen mainly in young patients (aged <2yrs), requires treatment with steroids and chemotherapy (vinblastine, etoposide, or methotrexate).

Prognosis >80% survive long-term without significant sequelae. Survivors `of multisystem or CNS disease may have lasting disabilities.

Haemophagocytic lymphohistiocytosis

A rare condition that may be 1° (familial haemophagocytic/erythrophagocytic lymphohistiocytosis, FHL or FEL) or 2° to infection (sHLH). Characterized by accumulation of phagocytic mononuclear cells, rather than dendritic or antigen-presenting cells as seen in LCH.

- *Presenting features:* include fever, splenomegaly, and cytopenia (2 out of 3 cell lines—red cells, white cells, and platelets). Neurological symptoms relating to increased CSF cell counts and protein sometimes seen. There may also be lymphadenopathy, skin rash, jaundice and oedema, and hepatic dysfunction.
- *Biochemistry:* shows raised triglycerides and low fibrinogen, sometimes raised serum transaminases and ferritin levels.
- *Other investigations to consider:* include viral, immunological, and genetic testing.

Treatment

Recovery may be spontaneous in sHLH with resolution of infection, but FHL is fatal without treatment. Steroids, etoposide, IT methotrexate may stabilize the disease. Allogeneic BMT is required for cure. Overall survival is ~50%.

Chemotherapy

May be given as adjuvant treatment (following surgery), or neoadjuvant treatment (before surgery). Combinations of drugs used to increase efficacy, reduce development of resistance, and limit single organ toxicity. Maximizing dose intensity (treatment frequency) increases efficacy.

- *Short-term side-effects:* vomiting, myelosuppression, alopecia, and mucositis (inflammation of mucous membranes).
- *Long-term effects:* on organ function (kidneys, gonads, hearing, heart) effects variable and, in general, less than effects of radiotherapy.

Antimetabolites Structural analogues of chemicals found in the intermediate steps in the synthesis of nucleic acids and proteins. They include:

- *6-mercaptopurine (6MP):* 6-thioguanine (6TG), cytarabine (ara-C), fludarabine (used in leukaemia, NHL).
- *methotrexate (MTX)* used in leukaemia, NHL, and OS.

Side-effects include renal toxicity (MTX), myelosuppression, hepatotoxicity, and mucositis.

Anti-tumour antibiotics Originally isolated from bacteria and fungi, they have antibiotic and anti-tumour activity. They include the following:

- *Anthracycline:* daunorubicin, doxorubicin, idarubicin, mitoxantrone, epirubicin used in leukaemia, NHL, HL, neuroblastoma, Wilms', sarcoma. *Side-effects*—myelotoxicity, alopecia, mucositis, cardiotoxicity.
- Bleomycin used in Hodgkin's disease, GCTs. *Side-effects*—include pulmonary toxicity.
- Actinomycin D (dactinomycin) used in Wilms' tumour, soft tissue and ES. *Side-effects*—myelotoxicity (mild), hepatotoxicity.

Epipodophyllotoxins semi-synthetic analogues of podophyllotoxin. They stabilize normally transient DNA–protein complexes by inhibition of topoisomerase I or II:

- *Etoposide (VP16):* inhibits topoisomerase II. Used in leukaemia, NHL, neuroblastoma, sarcoma, GCTs, CNS tumours, palliative chemotherapy (low dose). *Side-effects*—include hypotension, myelotoxicity, alopecia, hepatotoxicity, mucositis, 2° leukaemia.
- Topotecan, ironotecan inhibit topoisomerase I. Used in neuroblastoma, sarcoma, and CNS tumours.

Vinca alkaloids Bind to tubulin, interfering with mitotic spindle:

- Vincristine. Used in leukaemias, NHL, Hodgkin's disease, CNS tumours, Wilms', sarcoma. Side-effects include neurotoxicity.
- Vinblastine. Used in Hodgkin's disease, anaplastic large cell lymphoma. Side-effects include myelotoxicity and mucositis.
- Vinorelbine, new to paediatric practice, causes mild myelosuppression.

Alkylating agents Covalent binding to DNA, to prevent replication and transcription:

- *Cyclophosphamide, ifosfamide:* used in leukaemia, lymphoma, sarcoma, neuroblastoma, high risk Wilms', CNS tumours.
- *Melphalan, busulphan:* used in neuroblastoma, ES.
- Chlorambucil (Hodgkin's disease)
- *Lomustine (CCNU):* used in CNS tumours.

Side-effects—myelosuppression, alopecia, mucositis, tubular nephropathy (ifos), bladder toxicity (cyclo), encephalopathy (ifos), late effects on fertility, 2° leukaemia (CCNU).

Platinum compounds

Permanent cross-linking of DNA and inhibition of DNA synthesis. Cisplatin, carboplatin. Used in sarcoma, neuroblastoma, CNS tumours.

Side-effects—high emetogenicity, nephrotoxicity, ototoxicity, neurotoxicity (mainly cisplatin), myelotoxicity (carboplatin).

Other agents

- Dacarbazine (DTIC) methylates nucleophilic sites. *Side-effects*—mucositis, myelotoxicity, hepatic dysfunction, local pain, 'flu-like' symptoms).
- *Procarbazine:* originally MAOI, but found to be antitumour. Methylates once activated in *vitro. Side-effects*—myelotoxicity, reduced fertility.
- *L-asparaginase:* depletes pool of asparagine, needed by some malignancies, e.g. ALL. *Side-effects*—hypersensitivity, coagulopathy, rarely pancreatitis.
- *Amsacrine:* complex with DNA and topoisomerase II.
- *Hydroxyurea:* analogue of urea; inhibits DNA synthesis.
- *Steroids:* as well as symptom control and reduction of oedema particularly around CNS tumours, have direct anti-tumour effects in haematological malignancies.

Safe administration of chemotherapy

Chemotherapy should only be given by individuals fully trained in the avoidance and management of the complications, working in centres fully equipped and accredited to support chemotherapy.

Route

- *Intravenous:* central venous access is preferred. Risk of extravasation from peripheral access greatest with vinca alkaloids and anthracyclines.
- *IT:* usually for treatment or prophylaxis of CNS disease in leukaemia, *NHL, and some CNS tumours:* safety arrangements for IT' treatment are paramount.

Dosage Usually calculated according to surface area. Intravenous fluid to prevent tumour lysis syndrome (see 📖 p.684) is required with certain drugs (e.g. ifosfamide, cisplatin, methotrexate). Mesna is given with cyclophosphamide and ifosfamide to protect from bladder inflammation.

Monitoring The type and level of monitoring depend on agents used. This may include peripheral blood cell counts, GFR measurement, echocardiogram before and between courses of chemotherapy.

Stem cell transplant

High dose therapy

This involves the delivery of myeloablative doses of chemotherapy and/or radiotherapy, followed by rescue with haemopoietic stem cells. The latter may be autologous (from patient) or allogeneic (from sibling, unrelated donor, or haplo-identical from parent). Indications for use in treatment of childhood malignancy:

- Selected high-risk leukaemia and relapsed ALL (from allogeneic donor).
- High risk solid tumours, including metastatic neuroblastoma, and high risk ES (autologous).

Stem cells are harvested from bone marrow or peripheral blood by leucopheresis following 'mobilization' with granulocyte colony stimulating factor (G-CSF).

Conventional BMT is used for allografts. Peripheral blood stem cell transplants (PBSCT) are favoured for autografts. This offers advantages including less risk of tumour contamination, more rapid engraftment, less severe infections, avoidance of anaesthetic. Conditioning for BMT involves myeloablative radiotherapy or chemotherapy. The aim is to achieve a state of complete remission prior to conditioning. Monoclonal antibodies are used to suppress immune function of donor T-lymphocytes against recipient.

Outcome

Allografts carry greater risk, with approximately 10% procedure-related mortality. Morbidity and mortality from stem cell transplant are due to:

- graft failure;
- infection 2° to profound immune suppression;
- mucositis;
- veno-occlusive disease of the liver.
- multi-organ failure related to the conditioning regimen.

Graft vs host disease (GVHD)

GVHD is a particular risk. It may affect any organ system but commonly skin, liver and the gastro-intestinal system. Ciclosporin A or tacrolimus are given as prophylaxis and steroids, monoclonal antibodies and other immunosuppressants may be employed in treatment.

Radiotherapy

In the use of ionizing radiation to kill cancer cells, dose and fractionation (number of treatments to deliver a total dose) vary according to the nature of the tumour and tolerance of the tissue.

Strategies to increase therapeutic success include:
- *Conformal radiotherapy:* matching beam to 3D shape of target and so sparing surrounding tissue.
- Hyperfractionation and acceleration.
- Targeted radiotherapy with specific isotopes, e.g. I^{131}MIBG for neuroblastoma,
- Radiosurgery (high dose single fraction), brachytherapy (direct application of radionuclides to tumour). Protons (reduced dose to non-target tissues): currently limited availability in paediatrics.

Indications
- Selected cases of Hodgkin's disease, neuroblastoma, Wilms' tumour, soft tissue and ESs, most subgroups of CNS tumours.
- Limited benefit in OS, extracranial GCTs, NHL.
- In leukaemia limited to treatment of CNS and testicular disease and to conditioning for BMT.
- Symptom control in palliative care, e.g. bony metastases, spinal cord compression.

Preparation for radiotherapy
- Planning, by combination of CT and MRI scanning.
- Immobilization using masks/shells, tattoos as markers; sedation or general anaesthesia for youngest children.
- Protection of surrounding tissues, e.g. gonads, using lead shields.
- Play therapists have a central role in this process.

Side-effects
- Acute effects include nausea and vomiting, cutaneous erythema and desquamation, diarrhoea, myelosuppression, pneumonitis, hepatitis. Toxicity is potentiated by actinomycin D or anthracyclines.
- Late effects on growth, CNS, heart, lungs, kidneys, liver (see 🕮 p.688).

Surgery

Surgical interventions for solid tumours include the following.
- *Biopsy only:* chemotherapy and/or radiotherapy may be curative without further surgery, e.g. HL, NHL, RMS, GCTs.
- Resection, primary or following chemotherapy. Completeness of excision influences subsequent adjunctive treatment, e.g. bone tumours, Wilms' tumour, hepatoblastoma, and most CNS tumours.
- Management of the acute abdomen in neutropenic patients.
- Raised ICP and spinal cord compression.
- Tunnelled central venous lines for chemotherapy.

Acute care

All paediatric oncology treatment centres should have clear local guide-lines for supportive management, which should be referred to for details. This section should not be regarded as a substitute for such guidelines. Fever should be treated as an emergency. Immunocompromised children may succumb to overwhelming sepsis within hours. Greatest risk is associated with the nadir white cell count (typically at around 10 days) for most regimens. In the absence of neutropenia, central venous line infection should be considered, particularly if there are symptoms (e.g. rigors) associated with line flushing.

Febrile neutropenia

Fever (temperature >38°C) with neutrophil count $<1.0 \times 10^9$/L, leading to increased risk of bacterial infections. Complicates chemotherapy, spinal radiotherapy, bone marrow disease.

Causes
- Skin or GI bacterial flora.
- Greatest risk from Gram −ve organisms, including *Pseudomonas*.
- Gram-+ve organisms may be associated with central venous catheters.

Examination Include inspection of the skin, mouth, IV line sites, surgical sites, and the perianal area.

Investigation
- FBC and differential count, CRP.
- Culture of blood, urine, stool, swabs of throat, nose, suspicious skin lesions, or central line exit sites.
- CXR/AXR if indicated by symptoms or signs.

Treatment
- Broad spectrum antibiotics should be commenced *without delay* as infection with Gram −ve bacilli △ *may be fatal within hours*.
- Antibiotic choice will vary by institution and local resistance patterns, but must include adequate cover for *Pseudomonas* and Gram-+ve organisms. Include anaerobic cover in the presence of abdominal pain, diarrhoea, or mucositis. Appropriate agents may include:
  - Ceftazidime, ciprofloxacin, meropenem, gentamicin, amikacin, piptazobactam (Gram −ve cover).
  - Vancomycin, teicoplanin (Gram +ve organisms, including coagulase-negative staphylococci).
  - Metronidazole, meropenem (anaerobic cover).
- Antibiotic choice should be reviewed according to results of cultures.

Infection

Viral infections in immunocompromised patients

- *VZV:* if in contact and non-immune, give prophylactic aciclovir or zoster immune globulin. Active chickenpox or shingles should be treated aggressively with IV aciclovir.
- *HSV:* may cause painful oral ulceration; treat early.

Other viruses

- CMV, RSV, and adenovirus may all cause pneumonitis, associated with high morbidity and mortality, especially in BMT patients.

Fungal infections

- Consider in prolonged febrile neutropenia and treat promptly. Mortality remains high, but reduced with newer therapeutic agents.
- Clinical spectrum includes pulmonary aspergillosis, hepatic candidiasis, abscess formation.
- Risk is highest during intensive chemotherapy, such as re-induction for relapsed leukaemia and following BMT.
- Treatment includes fluconazole (limited cover), itraconazole, amphotericin B (liposomal formulation for reduced toxicity), voriconazole, and caspofungin. Prophylaxis is used in high risk treatment regimens.

Pneumocystis pneumonia (PCP)

- *Interstitial pneumonitis:* associated with prolonged immunosuppression; presents with tachypnoea, dry cough, low oxygen saturation readings.
- *Prophylaxis (patients on chemotherapy lasting over 6mths):* co-trimoxazole, monthly pentamidine nebulizers, or dapsone.
- *Treatment:* high dose co-trimoxazole, steroids in severe cases.

Acute care: biochemistry

Tumour lysis syndrome

This involves lysis of malignant cells on starting chemotherapy, releasing intracellular contents, exceeding renal excretory capacity and physiological buffering mechanisms. Abnormalities include:

- Hyperuricaemia.
- Hyperkalaemia.
- Hyperphosphataemia and reciprocal hypocalcaemia.
- Dehydration, leading to risk of acute renal failure.

Mainly seen in ALL, NHL (especially B cell), occasionally AML, rarely solid tumours (e.g. germ cell, neuroblastoma). May occur spontaneously or be precipitated by single dose of steroids or chemotherapy. Risk is increased with high white count, bulky disease, pre-existing renal impairment or infiltration.

Management

Key is prevention and monitoring.

- *Hyperhydration:* e.g. 2.5% or 5% dextrose in 0.45% saline at $3.0L/m^2/$ day 24h before starting treatment, and continued for least 48hr after treatment started. *Avoid added potassium.*
- Ensure good renal output, with diuretic (furosemide) if necessary.
- Allopurinol reduces urate precipitation, use urate oxidase in high risk cases.
- *Hyperkalaemia:* may need treatment with salbutamol, calcium resonium, dextrose/insulin, haemofiltration.
- *Hyperphosphataemia/hypocalcaemia:* increase fluids; haemofiltration in extreme cases; avoid calcium unless symptomatic (tetany, seizures).

Other biochemical disturbances

Hypercalcaemia

Rarely complicates malignancy (usually disseminated), e.g. rhabdomyosarcoma. Manage with hyperhydration (normal saline) and frusemide; bisphosphonates more effective than steroids or calcitonin.

Renal toxicity

Due to chemotherapy or antibiotics.

- Cisplatin (glomerular function, Mg^{2+} loss), ifosfamide (tubular losses of Mg^{2+}, PO_4^{2+}, bicarbonate), high dose methotrexate.
- Amphotericin B (glomerular toxicity and heavy potassium loss), aminoglycosides, vancomycin.

Particular care needed when any of these drugs used in combination.

Acute care: other

The acute abdomen

Possible causes in the oncology patient include the following.

- *Gastric haemorrhage:* $2°$ to gastritis or ulceration. Risk factors include high dose steroids and raised ICP.
- *Pancreatitis:* complicating treatment with steroids or L-asparaginase.
- *Neutropenic enterocolitis or typhlitis (Greek typhlon — caecum):* bacterial invasion (clostridium, pseudomonas) leads to inflammation, full thickness infarction and perforation, sepsis, and bleeding. It is associated with leukaemia. *Symptoms of pain +/− fever may be masked by concomitant steroids* (e.g. in ALL induction). The key to management is early, appropriate antibiotic cover on first suspicion and early involvement of surgeons. Mortality is high.

Haematological support

Blood products should be leucodepleted to reduce viral transmission and incidence of reactions. The latter are treated with antihistamine and/or steroid. Irradiated products should be used to prevent transfusion associated GVHD around the time of stem cell harvesting, following transplant, during treatment with fludarabine, and for patients with Hodgkin's disease.

- *Threshold for blood transfusion:* usually a haemoglobin level of 7 or 8g/dL, but teenagers are often symptomatic at higher levels. (Caution if high concomitant leukaemia, longstanding anaemia, or heart failure).
- *Platelets:* should be maintained above 10×10^9/L if well, 20×10^9/L if febrile or for minor procedure (e.g. LP), 30×10^9/L if brain tumour, and 50×10^9/L after significant bleed or for major surgery. These thresholds should be overridden where there is bleeding.

Nausea and vomiting

Chemotherapy varies in its emetogenicity: oral antimetabolites and vincristine require no prophylaxis; cisplatin and ifosfamide require multiple agents. Aim to prevent severe symptoms.

- *First-line:* domperidone or metoclopramide.
- *Second-line:* ondansetron (5HT antagonist).
- *Dexamethasone:* useful adjunct, but *not in ALL/NHL induction or CNS tumours.*
- *Other agents:* cyclizine useful in children with CNS tumours. In severe cases, nabilone, methotrimeprazine or chlorpromazine can help.

Nutrition and mucositis

Good nutritional status is essential for recovery, but is compromised by the presence of malignancy, direct effects of treatment, and mucositis and infection:

• A dietitian is central to successful nutrition. Support should include making appetizing meals available at all times, calorie supplementation, treatment of mucositis, and use of parenteral nutrition when enteral route inadequate.

• Chemotherapy-induced mucositis leads to oral ulceration, pain, and diarrhoea. Good mouth care (involving basic oral hygiene and antiseptic mouthwashes) helps prevent some infective complications. Prompt treatment with analgesia allows maintenance of oral intake for as long as possible.

Urgent care

Emergency treatment needed for acute complication of tumours, e.g.:
- Leukaemias with high peripheral white blood cell count, leading to hyperviscosity.
- SVC or airway obstruction caused by mediastinal masses.
- Raised ICP.
- Spinal cord compression.

Hyperviscosity
- Risk of sludging of venous blood in cerebral vessels.
- Associated with very high count ALL (WBC >200 × 10^9/L).

Prevention
- Cautious transfusion.
- *Prompt ALL treatment:* hydration, urate oxidase, chemotherapy.
- Leucopheresis may relieve symptoms.

SVC and upper airway obstruction
- May present with dyspnoea, chest discomfort, hoarseness, cough.
- *Findings in SVC obstruction:* plethora, facial swelling, engorgement of veins on upper chest wall, venous dilatation of optic fundi.

Causes
- *SVC obstruction:*
  - upper mediastinal tumours (particularly T cell NHL or ALL);
  - occasionally neuroblastoma.
- *Airway compromise:*
  - thoracic ES;
  - peripheral PNET;
  - rhabdomyosarcoma;
  - malignant GCT.

Management
- Sedation/anaesthesia for diagnostic purposes unsafe in SVC obstruction.
- Empirical treatment based on imaging and non-invasive investigations may need to be used before biopsy confirmation of diagnosis.
- Presence of pleural effusion, common in T-cell NHL, exacerbates symptoms but tap may relieve symptoms and provide diagnosis.

Spinal cord compression
- *Presentation:* back pain; gait, sensory, bladder, and bowel disturbance.
- *Causes:* neuroblastoma, sarcoma, lymphoma, CNS tumours (also infection, osteomyelitis, abscess).
- *Multidisciplinary input vital:* urgent MRI and surgical decompression and biopsy should precede steroids to avoid tumour lysis under anaesthetic. Perform other essential diagnostic procedures (e.g. LP, BM) under same anaesthetic if possible.

Raised intracranial pressure See 📖 p.653. ⚠ *Neurosurgical emergency.* High dose dexamethasone pre-operatively.

Principles of follow-up

Follow-up after completion of treatment is focused on disease recurrence and long-term adverse effects of cancer and its treatment.

Monitoring for disease recurrence

This involves clinical review, combined with imaging or laboratory testing to pick up pre-symptomatic recurrence, which may be amenable to further attempts at curative treatment. For example:

• *CXRs and abdominal US:* Hodgkin's disease.
• *MRI scans:* CNS tumours.
• *Urine VMA and HVA:* neuroblastoma.
• *Serum AFP and hCG:* GCTs.
• *Peripheral blood counts:* leukaemia.

Monitoring for late effects of treatment

This is a growing discipline, since there is now a childhood cancer survivor for every 900 adults. Monitoring is focused on the following.

Late effects of radiotherapy

May occur months or years after treatment has been completed. Sequelae usually progressive and irreversible, and will depend on sites, dose, mode of treatment, and age of patient at time of treatment.

Growth sequelae
• Direct effects on epiphyseal plates.
• Growth hormone deficiency from hypothalamic/pituitary damage.
• Muscle damage and avascular necrosis of bone.

CNS sequelae
• Somnolence and tiredness.
• Hypothalamic and pituitary damage.
• *Intellectual effects:* commonly reduced numeracy and short-term memory.
• Radiation myelitis.
• *Eyes:* cataracts, retinal damage.

Other organ system sequelae
Gonads: infertility/hypogonadism.

'Second' primary malignancies
Risk of 4–6% of occurrence within radiotherapy field. Common second malignancies include solid tumours occurring in the field of radiotherapy, as well as non-melanoma skin cancers. Epithelial tumours predominate.

Late effects of chemotherapy

Sequelae depend on age at the time of exposure, drugs and doses (see 📖 p.678). Well recognized long-term toxicities include:
• Cardiotoxicity following anthracyclines.
• Nephrotoxicity following platinum drugs and alkylating agents.
• Pulmonary fibrosis following bleomycin.

- Impaired fertility following alkylating agents.
- Ototoxicity following antibiotics.
- Second malignancies related to chemotherapy include 2° leukaemia and myelodysplastic syndrome associated with topoisomerase II inhibitors and alkylating agents.

Fertility

- This is affected by gonadotoxic chemotherapy and by radiotherapy fields that impinge on the gonads.
- The younger the patient when treated, the better the prognosis for future fertility.
- More spermatic recovery is seen after chemotherapy than radiotherapy.
- Risk of gonadotrophin deficiency greatest for radiotherapy directed towards suprasellar and nasopharyngeal tumours, but fertility may be preserved with aid of pulsatile gonadotrophin-releasing hormone (GnRH) therapy.

Quality of survival

It is understood that the long-term effects of treatment go beyond the purely physical consequences of treatment and this is an evolving area of clinical research. Cancer survivors (and their family members) are at increased risk of impaired psychosocial wellbeing. Risk is not clearly associated with a specific cancer type or treatment and is likely to be multifactorial in origin. Survivors are also at increased risk for needing special education and, as they enter adulthood, unemployment or underemployment.

Palliative care

Around 30% of children with cancer will die, mostly from progressive disease. Death from complications of treatment is more likely to be swift, with limited opportunity for preparation. Palliative care is the active total care of patients whose disease is no longer curable. It needs to embrace physical, emotional, social, and spiritual needs of children and their families. Chemotherapy, radiotherapy, and surgery may still be used for palliation and control of symptoms.

Breaking bad news

It is extremely important to be honest with an open approach, avoiding false hope. What to tell the child is always difficult; many families tend to be over-protective. This risks loss of their child's trust when the truth can no longer be hidden.

Organization of care

There are few paediatricians specializing in palliative care:
- *Location:* most children die at home, through family preference; some prefer a hospice and a minority the acute hospital ward.
- A multiprofessional approach is required and will vary according to needs and organization of local healthcare.
- The Association for Children with Life threatening or Terminal Conditions (ACT; www.act.org.uk) has played a central role in the development of paediatric palliative care as a specialty in the UK.
- Bereavement support should be considered part of the role of the palliative care team and may be provided by various disciplines within the team, depending on local arrangements.

Symptom control

Anticipated symptoms will depend on the diagnosis. Symptom control measures may be pharmacological or non-pharmacological. Aim to correct the underlying cause, e.g. constipation, infection. Good communication and consideration of psychosocial and spiritual factors will contribute to good control.

Pain
- Oral route is effective for most, until the terminal phase, when SC infusion, often in combination with anti-emetics, sedatives, and anticonvulsants may be preferred. The transdermal route is used for some agents.
- Different agents suit different types of pain, e.g. inflammatory and neuropathic pain, muscle spasm, and raised ICP. Combining different agents is more effective than escalating dose of one.

- World Health Organization (WHO) three step analgesic ladder (see 📖 pp.890, 1018).
  - *Step 1:* non-opioid +/− adjuvants (e.g. paracetamol, NSAID);
  - *Step 2:* weak opioid (e.g. codeine) + non-opioid +/− adjuvants;
  - *Step 3:* strong opioid (e.g. morphine, fentanyl) + non-opioid +/− adjuvants.
- Adjuvants are additional drugs used in pain management. They include:
  - analgesics that relieve pain in specific circumstances, such as gabapentin for neuropathic pain, anti-spasmodics (hyoscine, glycopyrronium), muscle relaxants (diazepam), corticosteroids, bisphosphonates;
  - drugs to control adverse analgesic effects, e.g. laxatives, antiemetics.

Other symptoms
- *Nausea, vomiting:* domperidone, cyclizine (particularly for raised intracranial pressure), methotrimeprazine, haloperidol, ondansetron, metaclopramide.
- *Convulsions, cerebral irritation:* diazepam, midazolam.
- *Spinal cord compression:* dexamethasone, radiotherapy, bladder and bowel management.
- *Terminal restlessness:* midazolam.
- *Dyspnoea:* non-pharmacological measures (position, play therapy, fan), opioids, benzodiazepines, oxygen, steroids.
- *Excess secretions:* hyoscine, glycopyrronium.
- *Anxiety, depression:* diazepam, methotrimeprazine, amitriptyline.
- *Constipation:* anticipate by prescribing laxatives when starting opioids; select least constipating opioids (e.g. fentanyl); may need high enemas.
- *Bowel obstruction:* antispasmodics, stool softeners, rectal preparations to reduce impaction, octreotide to reduce secretions and vomiting.
- *Sweating, from advanced disease fever or drugs:* cimetidine, NSAIDs.
- *Pruritus:* cimetidine if due to disease, antihistamine if opiate induced
- *Haematological* (anaemia, haemorrhage, bruising): transfuse (blood +/− platelets) only for symptomatic improvement and for quality of life; topical tranexamic acid or adrenaline for troublesome mucosal bleeding.

Infectious diseases

Introduction

Infection and infectious disease form a large part of clinical practice in paediatrics and child health. The following list shows the core areas that one should be familiar with.

- The child with fever (📖 pp.696–702).
- Common infections characterized by rash (📖 p.704).
- *Bacteraemia and shock:* see also 📖 Chapter 5 for sepsis and shock (📖 p.70), and 📖 p.714.
- *Mycobacterial infections:* see also 📖 Chapter 9 for TB (📖 p.294), and 📖 p.722.
- *Systemic infections:* see also 📖 Chapter 11 for post-streptococcal glomerulonephritis (📖 pp.374–375), and 📖 p.707.
- *Skin and soft tissues:* see 📖 pp. 718, 826–828.
- Nervous system infection (📖 p.720).
- *Upper and lower respiratory tract infections:* see also 📖 Chapter 9 for the common cold, pharyngitis, bronchitis, bronchiolitis, pertussis, pneumonia, pleural effusion, and empyema (📖 pp.282–293).
- *Cardiovascular system:* see also 📖 Chapters 8 and 5 for endocarditis and myocarditis (📖 pp.242–248).
- *GI system:* see also 📖 Chapter 10 for gastroenteritis and viral hepatitis (📖 pp.338–342, 723).
- *GU system:* see also 📖 Chapter 11 for UTI (📖 p.356).
- *Musculoskeletal:* see 📖 Chapter 20 for osteomyelitis and infective arthritis (📖 pp.738–741).
- *The eye* (📖 pp.146, 914–915).
- *Special hosts:* see also 📖 Chapter 6 for infections in the foetus and newborn (📖 pp.180–183); 📖 Chapter 18 for infections in children with malignancy and transplantation (📖 pp.682–683); and 📖 pp.724–727.
- *Immunizations* (📖 p.728).
- *Tropical diseases* (📖 pp.723, 1026).

The child with fever

In children aged 4wks to 5yrs body temperature should be measured using any one of:
- Electronic thermometer in the axilla.
- Chemical dot thermometer in the axilla.
- Infrared tympanic thermometer.

Fever in babies ≤6mths is rare. Fever >=38.5°C requires further investigation.

Differential diagnosis

The majority of children with fever have a self-limiting viral infection that resolves without any problem. However, in the very young it is particularly important to consider the possibility of an underlying serious infection. When there is no apparent cause of infection, the differential diagnosis of fever includes the following.
- Bacteraemia (see 📖 p.714).
- Respiratory tract infection (see 📖 pp.282–293).
- Meningitis and encephalitis (see 📖 pp.78–79, 720).
- UTI (see 📖 p.356).
- Viral infection (see 📖 pp.704–710).
- Osteomyelitis (see 📖 p.740).
- Bacterial gastroenteritis (see 📖 pp.302, 339).
- Endocarditis (see 📖 p.242).
- Rheumatic fever (see 📖 p.244).
- Malaria (see 📖 p.723).
- Tuberculosis (see 📖 pp.294, 722).
- Post-vaccination fever.

Box 19.1 highlights the signs and symptoms of disease that requires specific medical treatment (see also 📖 pp.698–702).

Box 19.1 Features of illness needing specific treatment

Sepsis including meningococcal sepsis (📖 p.714)
Non-blanching rash (purpuric or petechial lesions is suggestive of meningococcal sepsis) increased HR, respiration rate (RR) for age and capillary refill time ≥2s,

Meningitis including meningococcal meningitis (📖 pp.714, 720)
- *Non-blanching rash:* purpuric or petechial lesions is suggestive of meningococcal disease
- Neck stiffness may not be present in very young
- Bulging fontanelle may or may not be present
- Depressed level of consciousness is a worrying sign
- Seizures

Herpes simplex encephalitis (📖 p.79)
- Focal neurology may or may not be present
- Focal or generalized seizures
- Depressed level of consciousness

Pneumonia (📖 p.290)
- Tachypnoea, nasal flaring, and chest recession
- Chest crackles on auscultation
- Pulse oximeter oxygen desaturation
- May be silent and only detected on CXR

Urinary tract infection (📖 p.356)
- Vomiting, poor feeding, with or without abdominal pain or tenderness
- Lethargy or irritability
- Urinary frequency or dysuria
- Haematuria

Septic arthritis or osteomyelitis (📖 pp.738–741)
- Swelling of limb of joint
- Not using an extremity, non-weight bearing

Kawasaki disease (📖 p.716)
Fever lasting longer than 5 days and at least 4 of the following:
- Bilateral conjunctival injection
- Change in upper respiratory tract mucous membranes with injected pharynx, dry cracked lips, or strawberry tongue
- Change in peripheries with oedema, erythema, or desquamation
- Polymorphous rash
- Cervical lymphadenopathy

Fever: examination and assessment

When assessing a child with a fever a thorough history and examination are required. In the UK the National Institute for Health and Clinical Excellence (NICE) has provided a clinical guideline on 'Feverish illness in children' (see 🔗 www.nice.org.uk/CG047 for updates). The following section is adapted from this guideline. The key priorities are:

- *History:* consider very seriously parent's concerns and perception of a fever in their child. Check for ill contacts, immunization history.
- *Measurements:* make sure that temperature, heart rate, respiratory rate, and capillary refill time are measured as this will determine the order of your priorities (see 📖 Chapter 4, 📖 p.36).
- *Signs and symptoms:* assess the child for the presence or absence of symptoms and signs indicating serious illness.

Boxes 19.2–19.4 summarize the NICE guidelines on features of an illness that are at low-risk of indicating serious illness (green), to intermediate-risk (amber), to high-risk (red).

Box 19.2 Features ('green') indicating low risk of serious illness

- *Colour:* normal colour of skin, lips, and tongue
- *Activity:*
  - responds normally
  - is content and smiles
  - stays awake or awakens quickly if roused
  - strong normal cry
- *Breathing:* normal
- *Hydration:* normal
- *Other:*
  - generally normal
  - no fever at time of examination

Box 19.3 Features ('amber') indicating intermediate risk of serious illness

- *Colour:* pallor reported by parent or carer
- *Activity:*
  - not responding normally and decreased activity
  - prolonged stimulation required to awaken child
- *Breathing:*
  - nasal flaring
  - tachypnoea (>50breaths/min in 6–12-mth-olds; >40breaths/min in >1yr-old)
  - desaturation in air (≤95% in air)
  - chest crackles
- *Hydration:*
  - dry mucous membranes
  - poor feeding
  - reduced urine output
  - capillary refill time >3s
- *Other:*
  - fever ≥5 days
  - swelling of limb or joint
  - non-weight bearing or not using an extremity
  - a new lump >2cm

Box 19.4 Features ('red') indicating high risk of serious illness

- *Colour:* pale, mottled, ashen, or blue
- *Activity:*
  - unresponsive, appears ill, and barely rousable
  - weak high-pitched or continuous cry
- *Breathing:* grunting, severe distress
- *Hydration:* reduced skin turgor
- *Other:*
  - non-blanching rash
  - fever at time of examination
  - bulging fontanelle
  - neck stiffness
  - seizures or focal neurology
  - bile-stained vomiting

Fever: management (green features)

Children with solely *green* features do not need to be admitted to hospital. However, other criteria for admission may include additional factors:
- social and family circumstances;
- parental anxiety, instinct, or concerns;
- child's contact with serious illness;
- child's recent travel abroad to tropical or subtropical areas, or travel to any high-risk areas of endemic infectious disease.

If a child is discharged home, then the parents should be given clear instructions about what to look for and when to call for medical help (Box 19.5).

Box 19.5 Advice to parents of a child with fever managed at home

Urgent problems

Check on your child, even during the night:
- Offer your child regular drinks: if breastfeeding, continue with breast feeds. *Seek medical advice if child stops drinking*
- Look for signs of dehydration, e.g. dry mouth, no tears, sunken fontanelle. *Seek medical advice if present*
- Look for a non-blanching rash. Use a glass tumbler and press it firmly against any rash—if the spots can be seen through the glass and they do not fade, this is a non-blanching rash. *Seek immediate medical advice if present*
- Do *not* sponge your child with water
- If your child has a convulsion *seek medical advice*

Other advice
- Keep your child off school or nursery. This is necessary whilst there is fever; notify them
- If the fever is present for >5 days *seek medical advice*
- If you are not happy with your child's health, or if you have concerns, or if your child gets worse *seek medical advice*

Fever: management (red or amber features)

Children with red/amber features need admission. Those with red features have life-threatening illness and need urgent treatment.

- In hypoxic children or those in shock, follow the emergency care outlined in 🕮 Chapter 5 (🕮 pp.54, 56, 90).
- If there is no apparent source of infection, despite fever, then the investigations should include the following:
  - *Blood*—culture, FBC, CRP, electrolytes;
  - *Urine*—test for UTI;
  - *lumbar puncture*—consider if the clinical assessment dictates and there are no contraindications (see 🕮 p.720);
  - *CXR*—consider if high white blood cell count.

Antibiotics

Immediate treatment

Maximum dose third-generation cephalosporins (cefotaxime or ceftriaxone) should be given to children with fever *and*:

- signs of shock or coma
- signs of meningococcal disease

Consider giving high dose IV aciclovir if suspect herpes simplex encephalitis or disseminated neonatal disease.

Consider giving IV corticosteroid if confirmed bacterial meningitis (but not in infants younger than 3mths

Treatment for suspected bacterial infection

Give third-generation cephalosporin if any of the following are suspected

- *Neisseria meningitidis*
- *Streptococcus pneumoniae*
- *Escherichia coli*
- *Staphylococcus aureus*
- *Haemophilus influenzae* type b

Special cases

Consider choice of antibiotics or route of administration carefully in the following instances:

- *Child <3mths:* add antibiotic against listeria (e.g. ampicillin)
- *Child with decreased level of consciousness:* give parenteral antibiotics.
- *Significant rates of antibiotic resistance:* follow local guidelines

Antipyretics

Fever should be treated if the child is unwell with it:

- Do not use tepid sponging.
- Do not over- or underdress the child.
- Only use paracetamol or ibuprofen if the child is distressed with fever.

Prolonged fever of unknown cause

A fever without apparent cause that has persisted for >21 days is defined as 'prolonged fever of unknown cause'. An explanation is found eventually in the majority of cases. One-third of these will be infectious, and the remaining due to other causes, e.g.:

- *Rheumatological:* juvenile rheumatoid arthritis, systemic lupus eythematosus, rheumatic fever, vasculitis (see 📖 pp.244, 768–776, 780, 788–791); periodic fever syndromes.
- *IBD*(📖 p.332).
- *Malignancy* (📖 p.661).
- *Drug fever.*
- *Factitious illness* (📖 p.999).

Examination and assessment

A thorough history and examination are required. Also consider other factors such as travel, geography, age, and significant exposures. Appropriate investigations include:

- *Blood:* FBC, CRP, ESR, LFTs and renal function tests, albumin.
- *Serology:* CMV, EBV, brucella, and Q fever.
- *Culture:* at least 3 serial adequate volume blood cultures, urine culture, stool culture, and consider need for lumbar puncture and bone marrow culture.
- *Imaging:* of sinuses in the older child and CXR.
- *Bone scan or MRI:* to exclude osteomyelitis.
- *Echocardiography:* to exclude endocarditis.
- *Skin and blood tests:* for TB and *blood test* for HIV after counselling.

Treatment

- *Antibiotics:* these are best avoided until a site of infection has been found. However, in many cases they will have been prescribed already. Remember that antibiotics may be the drug agent causing fever. If the child is critically ill then empiric antibiotics are given.
- *Antipyretics:* these are best avoided during the period of assessment of fever. For example, blood cultures should be taken when the patient is febrile. One can also determine whether there is a specific pattern to the fever.

Common infections characterized by rash

Infections in childhood often have an associated rash. The skin lesion will give some clue to the potential cause (Box 19.6).

> ## Box 19.6 Skin lesions associated with infection
>
> See 📖 p.806 for definitions.
> - *Macules and/or papules:*
>   - *Macules*—red or pink discrete, flat areas that blanch on pressure
>   - *Papules*—small, raised lesions that blanch on pressure
> - *Infections*—measles, rubella, human herpes virus 6, and enterovirus
> - *Purpura and/or petechiae:* red or purple spots that do not blanch on pressure. *Infections*—meningococcal, enterovirus, *Haemophilus influenza,* pneumococcal
> - *Vesicles:* small raised lesions that contain clear fluid. *Infections*—chickenpox, shingles, herpes simplex virus, and hand, foot, and mouth disease
> - *Bullae and pustules:* large raised lesions containing clear fluid or pus. *Infections*—staphylococcal/streptococcal impetigo and scalded skin
> - *Desquamation:* peeling skin, often of the hands and feet. *Infections*—Kawasaki's disease and after scarlet fever (post-streptococcal infection)

An exanthem is a rash that 'bursts forth or blooms' towards the end of incubating an infection. The six classic exanthemata are characteristically:
- widespread, symmetrically distributed on the body;
- red, discrete, or confluent macules or papules.

Box 19.7 gives a summary of the exanthemata. Look at the following sections for more details.

Box 19.7 The six exanthemata

First associated disease: measles virus
- *Incubation:* 8–12 days
- *Duration:* 6–8 days
- *Infectivity:* from 4 days before to 4 days after the rash appears
- *Rash:* maculopapular; starts on the face and spreads
- *Features:* prodromal upper respiratory symptoms and cough, Koplik spots on the oral mucosa rarely seen
- *Treatment:* supportive, contact public health

Second associated disease: group A streptococcus
- *Incubation:* 2–5 days
- *Duration:* 7 days
- *Infectivity:* can become colonized
- *Rash:* fine papular rash on flushed skin, sandpaper texture
- *Features:* sore throat, strawberry tongue, rash, lymphadenopathy
- *Treatment:* penicillin V, consider need for prophylaxis *only* in family where infant less than 1mth of age or multiple family members affected

Third associated disease: rubella
- *Incubation:* 14–21 days
- *Duration:* 2–3 days
- *Infectivity:* from 7 days before to 7 days after the rash
- *Rash:* maculopapular, rapidly spreads and fades
- *Features:* enlarged lymph nodes at the back of the neck and ears
- *Treatment:* supportive

Fourth associated disease: possible coxsackie virus
No longer recognized as a disease entity

Fifth associated disease: parvovirus
- *Incubation:* 4–14 days
- *Duration:* 3–7 days prodrome then rash for 1–4 days; then evanescent rash over 1–3wks followed by arthropathy
- *Infectivity:* no isolation needed for children
- *Rash:* slapped cheek appearance, erythema infectiosum
- *Treatment:* supportive

Sixth associated disease: human herpes virus 6
- *Incubation:* 10 days
- *Duration:* 3–7 days
- *Infectivity:* unclear
- *Rash:* maculopapular
- *Features:* temperature for 3 days then, as the rash appears, the temperature falls rapidly
- *Treatment:* supportive

Exanthem 1: measles

Measles occurs typically in preschool and young children with the peak incidence in late winter and spring.

Signs and symptoms

- *Prodrome:* the 1° infection occurs in the respiratory epithelium of the nasopharynx, and produces fever, coryza, cough, and non-purulent conjunctivitis. Occasionally, a characteristic sign in the mouth is seen opposite the low premolars—'Koplik spots' (which look like grains of sugar on the mucosa). After 2–3 days there is a viraemia with infection of the reticuloendothelial system.
- *Exanthematous phase:* a second viraemia occurs 5–7 days after the initial infection with rash developing some 14 days after initial infection. The maculopapular rash starts on the face and lasts 6–8 days.
- *Infectivity:* 4 days before to 4 days after the onset of rash.
- *Other features:* generalized lymphadenopathy, anorexia, diarrhoea, and fever (may persist 7–10 days). Incubation 7–18 days (av. 10–2 days).

Diagnosis

- *Clinical:* Koplik spots are pathognomonic, but usually seen.
- *Blood film:* leucopenia and lymphopenia.
- *LFTs:* raised transaminases.
- *Oral fluid test:* measles RNA on oral fluid specimen confirms the diagnosis. Serum serology may also be used.

Management

- *Acute treatment:* generally supportive, but could include antibiotics for secondary bacterial infection (e.g. pneumonia, otitis media, tracheitis). Individuals are highly contagious during the viraemia.
- *Prevention:* MMR vaccine at 12–18mths and preschool booster to all children.
- *Vitamin A:* in developing countries vitamin A deficiency and malnutrition lead to a protracted course of illness with severe complications. The rash is dark red and is followed by desquamation and depigmentation. Consider supplements in children older than 6mths.

Complications

Complications commonly occur in young children with almost 20% of cases having at least one additional problem.

- *Acute otitis media* (10%).
- *Lower respiratory tract infection* (LRTI; 5%): bacterial pneumonia, interstitial pneumonia, bronchiolitis, laryngotracheobronchitis.
- *Encephalitis (1 in 5000):* occurs ~8 days after the onset of illness and starts with headache, lethargy, irritability, followed by seizures and coma. Mortality is high and there are neurological sequelae in survivors.
- *Subacute sclerosing panencephalitis* (SSPE, 1/10 000). A rare and fatal neurological disease with progressive intellectual deterioration, ataxia, and seizures about 7yrs after measles infection.

Exanthem 2: group A streptococcus

Scarlet fever is an erythematous rash that may occur with streptococcal pharyngitis. Other patterns of infection caused by group A streptococcus include toxic shock syndrome and necrotizing fasciitis.

Signs and symptoms

- *Prodrome:* infection is spread by respiratory secretions and droplets, or by self-infection from nasal carriage. During the incubation period (2–5 days) the child may have fever, vomiting, and abdominal pain.
- *Exanthematous phase:* 'sandpaper-like' diffuse rash in the neck and chest area (with perioral pallor) spreading to the flexor creases. The pharynx is erythematous and there may be exudative tonsillitis, palatal petechiae, uvular oedema, and strawberry tongue.
- *Other features:* tender anterior cervical lymphadenopathy.

Diagnosis

- *Throat swab:* culture and growth of the organism in a symptomatic individual (note also asymptomatic carriage common)
- *Serum:* antistreptolysin O (ASO) and anti-DNase B titres – one or both may rise in acute infection.

Management

- *Antibiotics:* penicillin V for 10 days. This will prevent the development of rheumatic fever (but not glomerulonephritis) and may reduce the length of illness. Antibiotics should be started within 9 days of acute illness.
- *Isolation:* children should be isolated until 24hr after the start of antibiotics.

Complications

Include peritonsillar abscess, retropharyngeal abscess, acute glomeulonephritis, and rheumatic fever.

Exanthem 3: rubella

Rubella is a mild disease in childhood occurring in winter and spring.

Signs and symptoms
- *Prodrome:* the incubation period is 14–21 days during which time the child may have a mild illness with low-grade fever.
- *Exanthematous phase:* maculopapular rash starting on the face, then spreading to cover the whole body, and lasting up to 5 days.
- *Other features:* suboccipital and post-auricular lymphadenopathy.

Diagnosis
Serology
If there is a risk of a non-immune pregnant woman has been exposed to the child, then the diagnosis should be confirmed by serology.

Management
- Supportive.
- *Prevention:* immunization with MMR (see 📖 p.728).

Complications
Very rarely children may develop arthritis, myocarditis, encephalitis, or thrombocytopenia. (When MMR vaccine uptake is reduced, remember foetal rubella syndrome if a non-immune mother is infected early in pregnancy.)

Exanthem 4: enteroviruses

The majority of infections due to human enteroviruses (coxsackie viruses, echoviruses, and polio viruses) produce non-specific illness. They occur in the summer and autumn months, and occasionally there are characteristic features including the following:
- *Meningoencephalitis:* aseptic meningitis with an associated skin rash, which can present like meningococcal septicaemia (see 📖 p.714).
- *Pleurodynia:* febrile illness with pleuritic chest pain and tender thoracic muscles.
- *Myocarditis.*
- *Hand, foot, and mouth disease:* painful vesicles on the hands, feet, mouth, and tongue.
- *Herpangina:* vesicular and ulcerated lesions on the soft palate and uvula.
- *Polio:* this condition should be eradicated with effective global immunization.

Exanthem 5: parvovirus

Parvovirus B19 induces immune complex formations that deposit in joints and the skin, causing 'erythema infectiosum'. It also infects the erythroblastoid precursors in the bone marrow. The infection occurs in all ages and is more common in the winter and spring.

Signs and symptoms

- *Prodrome:* infection spread by respiratory secretions and droplets. Then low-grade fever, headache, and coryza 7 days after exposure.
- *Exanthematous phase:* a number of days; bright red macules on the face with a 'slapped-cheek' appearance, (also, peri-oral pallor). The rash spreads to the limbs sparing the palms and soles. It is more intense with exposure to sunlight, heat, exercise, and stress.
- *Other features:* other patterns of illness include asymptomatic infection, aplastic crisis, foetal hydrops (from maternal infection).

Diagnosis

- *Clinical:* characteristic rash.
- *Serology:* if the diagnosis is in question titres can be measured.

Management is supportive: antipyretics for fever.

Exanthem 6: human herpes virus 6

Human herpes virus 6 (HHV6) is a benign, self-limiting exanthem commonly infecting children by the age of 2yrs. It is also known as 'roseola infantum' and 'erythema subitum'.

Signs and symptoms

- *Prodrome.* High-spiking fever up to 41°C lasting for up to 4 days. The fever typically stops once the rash appears.
- *Exanthematous phase:* the rose-coloured maculopapular rash appears some days later, beginning on the trunk and spreading peripherally. It lasts for 2–5 days.
- *Other features:* vomiting, diarrhoea, pharyngeal injection without exudates, cervical lymphadenopathy, and febrile convulsions prior to rash (5–10% of cases).

Diagnosis is on clinical grounds. Typical history and there may be associated neutropenia.

Management is supportive: antipyretics for fever.

Complications

The most common complication is febrile convulsion, and HHV6 probably accounts for a third of these in those <1yr of age. Rarely, some children may develop aseptic meningitis, encephalitis, and hepatitis.

Rash: chickenpox and zoster

VZV infection typically occurs between the ages of 1 and 6yrs, with the maximal transmission during winter and spring (📖 p.827).

Signs and symptoms

- *Prodrome:* VZV is spread by respiratory droplets or direct contact with lesions. The infectious period begins 2 days before vesicles appear and ends when the last vesicle crusts over (it is possible to retrieve virus from a crust).
- *Rash:* usually starts on the head and trunk; then the rest of the body. Individual lesions start as red macules, then progress through stages: papule, vesicle, pustule, crusting. Different stages of the rash are seen at the same time and heal completely within 2wks.
- *Other features.* Headache, anorexia, signs of upper respiratory tract infection (i.e. sore throat, cough coryza), fever, and itching.

Diagnosis

- *Clinical.* Characteristic rash, its distribution, and progression.
- *Other.* Serology (VZV IgM), electron microscopy of vesicle fluid.

Management

- *Symptoms:* treatment of fever and itching.
- *School exclusion:* 5 days from *start* of skin eruption
- *Antivirals:* aciclovir is used in severe varicella, encephalitis, pneumonia, babies, and immunosuppressed patients (i.e. steroids, oncology, etc.).
- *VZIG:* Varicella zoster immunoglobulin should also be considered as prophylaxis following contact in at risk individual (see www.hpa.org.uk for guidance).
- *Immunization:* from age 1 not currently part of UK schedule

Complications

2° bacterial infection may occur with invasive group A streptococcus leading to necrotizing fasciitis or toxic shock syndrome. Other rare complications include purpura fulminans, cerebrovascular stroke, and encephalitis. Life-threatening pneumonitis may occur in the young infant and immunosuppressed child.

Herpes zoster (shingles)

A reactivation of latent infection may occur, leading to vesicular lesions in the distribution of a sensory nerve. Rare in childhood, but occurs in the immunosuppressed, or in those who had 1° infection in infancy.

Rash: infectious mononucleosis

Infectious mononucleosis is caused by EBV (90%) and CMV. The source is oropharyngeal secretion. Virus infects B lymphocytes in pharyngeal lymphoid tissue and then spreads to the rest of the lymphoid system.

Signs and symptoms

- *Prodrome:* flu-like illness (headache, low-grade fever, and chills) for 3–5 days. The incubation period is 4–6wks.
- *Features:* exudative pharyngitis; generalized, tender lymphadenopathy; hepatosplenomegaly; widespread erythematous macular rash, especially if inadvertently treated with ampicillin; lethargy.

Diagnosis

- *Classic triad:* lymphocytosis (80–90% of WBC); ≥10% atypical lymphocytes on peripheral blood film; positive serology for EBV.
- *Monospot test:* a low-sensitivity test with false positives occurring in lymphoma and hepatitis.
- *Other.* IgM and IgG are raised early in the disease; raised liver function tests; mild thrombocytopenia. Quantitative PCR in immunosuppressed (not for routine diagnosis).

Management

- *Symptoms:* supportive care
- *Splenomegaly:* patients with splenomegaly should avoid contact sports for 1mth, and adolescents should avoid alcohol.

Complications

- *GI and abdominal:* hepatitis, splenomegaly, and splenic rupture.
- *CNS:* aseptic meningitis, encephalitis, Guillain–Barré syndrome.
- *Post viral tiredness:* is self-limiting, but may take months to resolve.
- *Other.* lymphoma, orchitis, myocarditis, pneumonia.

Lyme disease

- *Cause:* spirochaete *Borrelia burgdorferi* transmitted by tick bite.
- *Age group:* any age.
- *Incubation:* 4–20 days.
- *Rash:* erythematous macule at the site of the tick bite increases in size and forms a painless red lesion called erythema migrans.
- *Early time course (weeks):* the symptoms of fever, headache, myalgia, arthralgia, and lymphadenopathy fluctuate over several weeks.
- *Later time course (months):* dissemination of infection leads to cranial nerve palsies, meningitis, arthritis, or myocarditis.
- *Diagnosis:* the clinical features and serology after 2–4wks.
- *Treatment:* in the young child amoxicillin is used. In the child aged >8yrs use doxycycline. In those with heart or CNS disease use ceftriaxone.

Mumps

Mumps is a viral infection transmitted by respiratory droplets. The virus enters the parotid gland before systemic spread. The peak incidence is in children aged 5–9yrs.

Signs and symptoms

- *Prodrome:* myalgia, anorexia, headache, low-grade fever, and chills. The incubation period is 14–21 days.
- *Features:* 20% of infections are asymptomatic. In 30–40% of cases there is parotitis. In these patients there is often ear pain and tenderness over the gland.
- *Other features:* headache, anorexia, signs of URTI (i.e. sore throat, cough, and coryza), and low-grade fever.

Diagnosis

- *Clinical:* characteristic examination with glandular swelling.
- *Other:* salivary PCR or serology (mumps IgM) in the first week of illness; delayed viral culture of saliva or urine; blood shows lymphocytosis and increased amylase.

Management

- *Symptoms:* supportive care.
- *Immunization:* MMR vaccine confers lifelong immunity.

Complications

- *Meningoencephalitis:* the most common complication and it is usually asymptomatic.
- *Orchitis:* results in testicular swelling, local pain, and later atrophy (see 📖 p.877).
- *Other:* oophoritis, pancreatitis, and myocarditis.

Bacteraemia and shock

Bacterial infection leading to 'sepsis syndrome', and shock is discussed in 📖 Chapter 5 (📖 pp.54, 56–57, 70, 90). The most common cause of bacteraemic shock is *Neisseria meningitidis*, although *Staphylococcus aureus* is in increasing as overall proportion and *Streptococcus pneumoniae* remains an important cause even in the era of routine infant 13 valent conjugate pneumococcal immunization.

Meningococcal septicaemia and shock

Meningococcal disease is rare, but it can be fatal in a previously well child. Unfortunately, at an early stage, the signs and symptoms are non-specific and the child may have features similar to those of a minor viral illness. Meningococcal disease has therefore featured highly in public education; the 'glass test' is used to identify a typical non-blanching purpuric or petechial rash.

Pathogenesis

In the UK, *N. meningitides* serogroup B is the usual cause of illness. (serogroup C is rare since its inclusion in routine vaccination). The trigger and mechanism of invasion are unknown. Once bacteraemia occurs, bacterial autolysis leads to endotoxin release and systemic illness with disseminated intravascular coagulation, capillary leak, and distributive and cardiogenic shock.

Signs and symptoms

- *Non-specific:* fever, malaise, thirst may be the first sign of shock, followed by poor urine output. Pain in proximal muscles, joints, and abdomen is very common.
- *Rash:* initially maculopapular, then petechial or purpuric.
- *CNS:* associated meningitis in 20–30%. Altered conscious level may be due to shock rather than meningitis and respond to initial fluid therapy. Raised ICP is more common in meningitis presentation (e.g. headache, neck pain or stiffness, irritability, and altered conscious level) than sepsis.
- *Respiratory:* features of pneumonia or pulmonary oedema, especially following initial fluid therapy

Diagnosis

Any febrile child who develops a purpuric rash should be considered to have meningococcal septicaemia until proven otherwise.

Management

See 📖 Chapter 5 (📖 p.54). Suspected cases in the community should receive IV benzylpenicillin (IM if no IV access) as an initial single dose:
- Children ≥10yrs, 1g.
- 1–9yr olds, 600mg.
- <1yr, 300mg.

Suspected cases in hospital should receive 80mg/kg/od ceftriaxone (or cefotaxime 50mg/kg/tds. In shock, 20mL/kg fluid volume should be given immediately, consideration given to repeat fluid boluses followed by intubation and ventilation and inotropes following early consultation with paediatric intensive care. Careful attention should be made to correction of electrolyte imbalance, particularly potassium (which is low even in anuric renal failure due to meningoccaemia) and calcium. A management algorithm for health professionals based on the NICE clinical guideline 102 is available at ⌘ www.nice.org.uk/CG102.

Complications
The majority of survivors of meningococcal disease have few or no sequelae. However, there is a significant mortality (2–4%), and morbidity includes loss of digits and limbs due to peripheral vascular disease.

Kawasaki disease

Kawasaki disease is the commonest cause of acquired heart disease in children in the UK. It affects 3.4/100,000 children under 5yrs (boys > girls) and in the UK mortality is 3.7%. It is a systemic vasculitic disease with coronary arteritis leading to coronary artery aneurysms as the most important complication (20–30%). Other complications include coronary thrombosis, myocardial infarction, and dysrrhythmias.

Diagnostic criteria

The diagnosis can be made in children with fever (>38.5°C) present for at least 5 days, without other explanation, in the presence of 4 of the 5 following criteria. Criteria may not be present at the same time (history is important) and misery is a very common feature.

- *Bilateral congestion of the ocular conjunctivae (94%):* non-purulent.
- *Changes of the lips and oral cavity with at least one of the following:* dryness, erythema, fissuring of lips (70%); strawberry tongue (71%); diffuse erythema of oral and pharyngeal mucosa without discrete lesions (70%).
- *Changes of the extremities* with at least one of the following: erythema of palms and soles (80%); indurative oedema (67%); periungual desquamation of fingers and toes (29%).
- Polymorphous exanthem (92%).
- Non-suppurative cervical lymphadenopathy >1.5cm (42%).

Note: The percentage values indicate the proportion of patients manifesting this clinical sign within the first 10 days after onset of fever.

Differential diagnosis

The differential diagnosis for Kawasaki disease includes the following:
- Streptococcal and staphylococcal toxin-mediated diseases
- Adenovirus and other viral infections (enterovirus, measles)
- Drug reactions or Stevens–Johnson syndrome
- Leptospirosis
- *Yersinia* pseudotuberculosis infection
- Rickettsial infection
- Reiter's syndrome
- IBD
- Post-infectious immune complex disease (e.g. post-meningococcaemia)
- Sarcoidosis

Associated features

In addition to the diagnostic criteria of Kawasaki disease, the other features of the condition include the following.
- *Renal:* urethritis with sterile pyuria.
- *Musculoskeletal:* arthralgia and arthritis (35% of patients).

- *CNS:* aseptic meningitis with mild CSF pleocytosis and normal CSF glucose and protein; sensorineural hearing loss (transient high frequency loss or permanent loss).
- *GI:* diarrhoea and vomiting; hydrops of the gall bladder with or without obstructive jaundice.
- *Cardiac:* congestive heart failure, myocarditis, pericardial effusion, arrhythmias, mitral insufficiency, acute myocardial infarction (up to 73%) within 1yr of disease.
- *Coronary aneurysms:* incidence of coronary artery aneurysms varies (15–25% in untreated patients) and resolution varies with age at onset and size and shape of aneurysm.

Investigations

- *Haematology:* leucocytosis with left shift common in acute phase; thrombocytosis peaks in the 3rd to 4th week; normocytic, normochromic anaemia present early and persists until inflammatory process begins to subside; reticulocyte count low.
- *Coagulation:* increased coagulability, platelet turnover, and depleted fibrinolysis.
- *Urine:* mononuclear cells with cytoplasmic inclusions are abundant in the urine early in the disease. These cells are not detected by dipstick methods for 'WBC', which only detect polymorphs.
- *Acute phase reactants:* elevated ESR persists beyond the acute febrile period and gradually returns to normal over 1–2mths. CRP may also be elevated.
- *Biochemistry:* elevated liver transaminases; hypoalbuminaemia.
- *Immunology:* marked activation of circulating monocyte/macrophages; B cell activation elevated immunoglobulin production; T cell lymphopenia.
- *Cardiology:* ECG usually normal, but strain, ischaemia, and/or infarct can be present.
- *Echocardiography:* aneurysms may first be seen from 7–21 days post-onset of fever.

Treatment

- *High dose IV immunoglobulin* is the treatment of choice. 2g/kg over 12hr as a single infusion. Consider repeat dose after 48hr if no deferevescence.
- *Aspirin:* 30—50mg/kg/day (divided qds) reducing to 3–5mg/kg as fever resolves.
- The role of steroids and novel biological therapies is not clear.
- Follow-up is very important for cardiac review.

Skin and soft tissues

Impetigo
- *Cause:* staphylococcal or streptococcal skin infection.
- *Age group:* infants and young children.
- *Features:* erythematous macules (later vesicular/bullous) on the face, neck and hands—often associated with pre-existing skin lesions such as eczema.
- *Infectivity:* nasal carriage is often the source of infection. Auto-inoculation occurs and lesions are infectious until dry.
- *Antibiotics:* topical antimicrobials are often not useful in younger children due to scratching causing further spread of bacteria; if treatment required, use oral antibiotic, taking taste and formulation into account prior to prescription (oral flucloxacillin and erythromycin are often poorly tolerated).

Boils (furuncles)
- *Cause: Staphylococcus aureus.*
- *Age group:* any age.
- *Features:* infection of hair follicles or sweat glands.
- *Infectivity:* nasal carriage is often the source of infection in recurrent boils.
- *Antibiotics:* systemic.

Peri-orbital cellulitis See 📖 p.919
- *Cause:* group A streptococcus, *Staphylococcus aureus*, *Streptococcus pneumoniae*, rarely *Haemophilus influenzae* type b in unimmunized children.
- *Age group:* any age.
- *Features:* fever with unilateral erythema, tenderness, and oedema of the eyelid, often following local trauma to the skin. Complications include local abscess, meningitis, and cavernous sinus thrombosis.
- *Investigations:* if severe (eye movements are not visible or complete ptosis) refer to ENT or ophthalmology and perform cranial CT scan.
- *Antibiotics:* IV ceftriaxone 80 mg/kg/od where eye movements are visible. Add IV metronidazole if eye movements not visible or not improved at 24hr.

Scalded skin syndrome
- *Cause:* exfoliative staphylococcal toxin.
- *Age group:* infants and young children.
- *Features:* fever and malaise with a purulent, crusting, localized infection around the eyes, nose, and mouth. Later diffuse erythema and skin tenderness leading to separation of the epidermis through the granular cell layer. Nikolsky's sign is epidermal separation on light pressure with no subsequent scarring after healing.
- *Antibiotics:* IV flucloxacillin 50mg/kg/qds.

Necrotizing fasciitis
- *Cause:* group A streptococcus, less commonly *Staphylococcus aureus*
- *Age group:* any age.
- *Features:* SC infection of tissue down to fascia and muscle. Symptoms may be due to shock, systemic illness, and severe pain.
- *Antibiotics:* IV, and surgical debridement.

Toxic shock syndrome (TSS)

Cause
- Toxin-producing staphylococci or streptococci
- Multisystem disease due to staphylococcal toxin-1 in 75%

Signs and symptoms
- Systemic illness with high fever
- *GI:* vomiting, watery diarrhoea
- Shock and hypotension, altered conscious level
- *Neuromuscular:* occasional severe myalgia
- *Skin rash:* red mucous membranes and diffuse macular rash; 10 days after infection desquamation of the palms, soles, fingers, and toes

Investigations
- *Haematology:* thrombocytopenia, coagulopathy
- *Biochemistry:* abnormal liver and kidney function

Diagnostic criteria for staphylococcal TSS
- Temperature ≥39°C
- Systolic blood pressure <90mmHg
- Rash (may or may not include desquamation)
- Involvement of three or more of gastrointestinal, musculoskeletal, renal, hepatic, CNS, blood, and mucous membranes

Diagnostic criteria for streptococcal TSS
- Isolation of group A streptococcus
- Hypotension
- Involvement of two or more of coagulopathy, adult respiratory distress syndrome, soft tissue necrosis, rash with desquamation, or renal or hepatic involvement

Treatment
- IV fluids and resuscitation
- Antibiotics against staphylococci and streptococci. Clindamycin often added to flucloxacillin regime due to anti-toxin activity *in vitro*
- IV immunoglobulin

Meningitis

75% of cases of meningitis are believed to occur in those <15yrs of age. Three organisms (*Streptococcus pneumoniae*, *Neisseria meningitides* (mainly group B in the UK) and *Haemophilus influenzae* type b) account for 80% of the cases. *H. influenzae* and meningococcal group C have declined very significantly since the introduction of routine immunization in infancy.

Three important practice points to remember are:

- Infants do not get classical symptoms of meningism with meningitis and there should be an extremely low threshold for doing a lumbar puncture as part of the septic screen in infants with unexplained fever or seizures (see 📖 pp.128, 180).
- Co-existing septicaemia in 20–30% is often the treatment priority to prevent death.
- Do not forget possibility of tuberculous meningitis.

Pathogenesis

The sequence of pathology involves:

- Colonization and invasion of the nasopharyngeal epithelium.
- Invasion of the blood stream.
- Attachment to and invasion of the meninges.
- Induction of inflammation with leak of proteins leading to cerebral oedema.
- Alteration in cerebral blood flow and metabolism.
- Cerebral vasculitis.

Symptoms and signs

In younger children symptoms may be non-specific including fever, poor feeding, lethargy. Rash and seizures may or may not be present. In older children, fever with headache and neck stiffness. Other features include:

- *General:* fever, vomiting, and anorexia.
- *Central:* irritability, disorientation, altered mental state.
- *Seizures:* occur in 30%. Focal seizures suggest localized infarction or subdural collection. Do not assume 'febrile convulsion' in child under 1yr of age or over 1yr of age with additional symptoms.
- *Neck stiffness:* more common in older children.
- *Neurology:* focal cranial nerve signs are more common in children with tuberculous or cryptococcal meningitis.
- *Eyes:* papilloedema is a late sign and not a reliable indicator of raised intracranial pressure. Retinal hemorrhages may be present and may indicate sagittal venous thrombosis or coagulopathy. However, these are rare and in the infant the possibility of non-accidental or inflicted head injury should be considered.

Lumbar puncture

Lumbar puncture is a useful procedure to make the diagnosis of meningitis and identify the organism and it is generally safe. However, patients with bacterial meningitis may have raised ICP so if there is a clinical suspicion of this problem (low heart rate with raised blood pressure, often first sign of which are transient changes seen on cardiac monitors) then the procedure should be deferred. (The cellular and chemical changes of meningitis will remain in the CSF for several days). The contraindications are:

• shock or cardiovascular instability;
• signs of raised intracranial pressure
• focal neurological signs or focal seizures
• infection of the skin at the lumbar puncture site (rare);
• evidence of coagulopathy;
• acute meningococcal disease

Treatment

See 📖 Chapter 5 (📖 p.79). Suspected cases of meningococcal meningitis in the community should receive IV benzylpenicillin (IM if no IV access) as an initial single dose.

• Children ≥10yrs, 1g.
• 1–9yr olds, 600mg.
• <1yr, 300mg.

Suspected cases in hospital should receive 80mg/kg/od ceftriaxone (or cefotaxime 50mg/kg/tds). A management algorithm for health professionals based on the NICE clinical guideline 102 is available at 🕮 www.nice. org.uk/CG102

Steroids

In bacterial meningitis

• Do note use corticosteroids in children younger than 3mths
• There is benefit from the use of dexamethasone and the dosing schedule is 0.15mg/kg qds for 4 days to reduce the severity of neurological sequelae, particularly deafness, after bacterial meningitis (🕮 www.nice.org.uk/CG102).
• If dexamethasone was not given before the first dose of antibiotics, but was indicated, try to give the first dose within 4hr of starting antibiotics, but do not start dexamethasone more than 12 hours after starting antibiotics.

In meningococcal septicemia

• Do not use the meningitic dosing of dexamethasone.
• In children with shock that is not responding to fluids and inotropes, physiological replacement of hydrocortisone ($25mg/m^2$ qds) should be considered after discussion with the intensive care team.

Mycobacteria

Pulmonary tuberculosis

Pulmonary tuberculosis due to *Mycobacterium tuberculosis* (an acid-fast bacillus) is discussed in 📖 Chapter 9 (see 📖 p.294).

Atypical mycobacterial infection could be the cause of the following:

- *Persistent lymphadenopathy:* this infection is diagnosed after histology of
a surgically resected node.
- *Disseminated infection in the immunocompromised patient.*
Mycobacterium avium intracellulare: is an infection often seen in patients
with advanced disease due to HIV.

Tuberculous meningitis (TBM)

TBM is the most feared complication of *M. tuberculosis* infection.

- *Timing:* usually occurs within 12mths of first infection.
- *Age group:* most frequently occurs in those <5yrs of age.
- *Pathology:* the initial pathology is occult haematogenous dissemination
to the cerebral cortex from a 1° site (e.g. gut, lung). This increases
in size until it reaches the meninges and subarachnoid space. A
thick gelatinous exudate is created especially around the brainstem
so that cranial nerves III, IV, and VI are commonly compromised.
Hydrocephalus is common.
- *Clinical course:* the onset is insidious and is characterized by apathy or
disinterest, then intermittent headaches and anorexia. Fever is almost
always present. Vomiting occurs in 50%. Focal neurological signs,
seizures, or severely depressed conscious level may occur.
- *Diagnosis:* 50% will grow *Mycobacteria* from their CSF and the Mantoux
or gamma interferon release assay often positive. 40–90% have CXR
changes of pulmonary disease.
- *Prognosis:* most survive if treated in the early insidious stage. There is
a very high complication rate, especially if the focal neurological signs
are present at the start of therapy.
- *Treatment:* therapy with four antituberculous agents and
corticosteroids is for at least 12mths and should be supervised by
a specialist team.

Tropical infections

Tropical infections may be present in any child returning from the tropics (see 📖 p.1026). A general review in the febrile child should follow the process discussed in the section on 'Acute fever' (see 📖 pp.696–701).

Malaria

- *Agent:* Plasmodium falciparum (also *P. vivax, P. ovale, P. malariae*).
- *Features:* fever (often cyclical, though falciparum is not), diarrhoea, vomiting, flu-like symptoms, jaundice, anaemia, thrombocytopenia.
- *Time course:* onset usually occurs 7–10 days after inoculation, but may occur after a few months in children.
- *Diagnosis:* thick and thin blood film should be examined in all children with fever from infected area without prophylaxis. Repeat daily for 3 samples if there is a high index of suspicion.
- *Treatment:* artesunate is now the first line therapy for *P. falciparum* malaria, although not universally available in the UK. For other forms of malaria consult specialist advice.

Typhoid

- *Agent:* Salmonella typhi or paratyphi.
- *Features:* fever, headache, cough abdominal pain, myalgia followed by GI symptoms a week later. Splenomegaly, bradycardia, and rose-coloured spots on the trunk. Complications include GI perforation, myocarditis, hepatitis, and nephritis.
- *Treatment:* third generation cephalosporin or ciprofloxacin, adjust therapy following antimicrobial sensitivity testing.

Dengue fever

- *Agent:* viral infection spread by mosquitoes.
- *Features:* 1° infection produces a fine erythematous rash, myalgia, arthralgia, and high fever. 2° desquamation follows.
- *Shock:* Dengue shock occurs when a previously infected child has another infection with a different strain.

Viral haemorrhagic fevers

- *Agents:* Lassa, Marburg, Ebola, and other viruses.
- *Features:* highly contagious and often lethal.
- *Management:* if suspected, strict isolation is required and specialist advice needed.

Immunodeficiency disorders

Immunodeficiency may be due to causes that are:
- *Primary*: intrinsic abnormalities.
- *Secondary*: cancer, immunosuppressive agents, HIV infection, splenectomy, nephrotic syndrome, SCD, etc.

Primary immunodeficiency

Caused by defects in the following.

B lymphocytes and antibody production
- *X-linked agammaglobulinaemia:* presents in early childhood with severe bacterial infections
- *Hyper IgM syndrome:* presents with bacterial infection and PCP
- *IgG subclass deficiency:* minor immunodeficiency that may cause recurrent respiratory infection

Tests Immunoglobulin levels and functional vaccine responses as indicated by clinical presentation

T lymphocytes and cellular immunity
Severe combined immunodeficiency (SCID) Presents in first few months. Failure to thrive. Persistent infection due to viruses and fungi

Tests FBC, blood film, lymphocyte subsets and function

Neutrophil defects
Leucocyte adhesion deficiency Presents in infancy with delayed healing of the umbilical cord, chronic skin ulcers, bacterial and fungal infection involving lymph nodes, liver, and lung

Tests Assessment of chemotaxis, neutrophil surface adhesion molecules, and killing (e.g. neutrophil oxidative burst test for chronic granulomatous disease)

Opsonization and other innate immunodeficiencies
Complement deficiency or mannose binding lectin deficiency Rare, but may present with severe meningococcal disease

Tests Complement levels, TOLL receptor pathway assays (second line tests directed by clinical presentation)

Multisystem syndromes
- *Ataxia telangiectasia:* skin, neurological, and immune defects
- *Wiskott–Aldrich syndrome:* eczema, thrombocytopenia, and immunodeficiency
- *DiGeorge syndrome:* hypocalcaemia, branchial arch and heart defects, and immunodeficiency
- *Duncan syndrome:* X-linked lymphoproliferative disease due to prior EBV infection

Tests Chromosomal fragility, genetic polymorphisms

The investigation for these conditions in children with a history of recurrent or severe infection requires a broad screen of tests, which can be directed by the type of infection (e.g. viral, bacterial, fungal).

Treatment

A variety of therapies is required for children with primary immunodeficiency and they should be cared for in designated centres. Therapy includes:

- prophylactic antibiotics;
- supportive care and antibiotics for acute infections;
- replacement immunoglobulins and additional immunization;
- bone marrow transplantation;
- gene therapy (future).

Human immunodeficiency virus

HIV infection in children is a global issue caused mainly by the retrovirus HIV (human immunodeficiency virus) type 1.

Vertical transmission of HIV

See 📖 p.185. Children at risk of acquiring the virus are infants of HIV-positive mothers, although it is now rare because of the success of antenatal preventative measures.

- Infants may become infected during labour and the postnatal period.
- Rate of vertical transmission is 20–40% without suitable management but <1% with effective prophylaxis

Prevention of vertical transmission

- Use of antenatal, perinatal, and postnatal antiretroviral drugs.
- Avoid labour and birth canal contact by elective Caesarean section.
- Avoidance of breastfeeding.

Clinical features

Dormant infection lasts a short period and has few or no clinical features. The later features of paediatric HIV infection are the following.

- *Gastrointestinal:* chronic diarrhoea, failure to thrive.
- *CNS:* delayed development and cerebral palsy
- *Recurrent bacterial and viral infection.*
- *Lymphadenopathy and hepatosplenomegaly.*
- *Opportunistic infections:* Pneumocystis carinii, Candida, herpes virus, Varicella, and atypical mycobacteria.
- *Respiratory distress:* cough, hypoxaemia, bilateral nodular infiltrates on CXR.

Acquired immune deficiency syndrome (AIDS)

Lymphocytic interstitial pneumonitis, *Pneumocystis carinii* (PCP) infection, and *Candida* oesophagitis are 'AIDS defining' in an HIV-positive child; they signify progression to the AIDS phase.

Diagnosis

The diagnosis of HIV infection depends on demonstrating the following:

- *Specific antibody response (anti-HIV antibodies):* infants infected perinatally have an immune response by 4–6mths of age. However, an uninfected infant of a HIV-positive mother can test positive for anti-HIV antibodies for up to 12–18mths.
- *Virus or its components in the blood (PCR):* high specificity tests.

Treatment

- Prophylaxis against PCP.
- Avoidance of live oral polio vaccine and BCG.
- Antiretroviral therapy to suppress viral replication.
- Social, psychological, and family support.

Immunizations

- Immunizations are an important part of child health in the community.
- Immunization should be delayed in the acutely ill child.
- In those where there is a family history of febrile convulsion, advice should be given about control of fever with antipyretics, and when to seek medical assistance.

Schedule

The schedule for vaccinations to be given to an infant growing up in the UK is as follows:

- *BCG:* birth in at-risk groups (e.g. those living in areas of high rate of TB, or those whose parents/grandparents were born in a TB high-prevalence country).
- *Hepatitis B:*
  - birth, 1mth, 2mths in at risk groups;
  - 12, 15, and 18mths in at risk groups.
- *Diphtheria, pertussis, tetanus (DPT):*
  - 2, 3, and 4mths in all infants;
  - booster at 3yrs 4mths to 5yrs old;
  - booster for only diphtheria and tetanus at 13–18-yr-olds.
- *Inactivated polio virus:*
  - 2, 3, and 4mths in all infants.
  - boosters at 3yrs 4mths to 5yrs, and 13–18yrs
- *Haemophilus influenzae type b:* 2, 3, 4, and 12–13mths in all infants.
- *Neiserria meningitidis (meningococcus) C:* 3, 4 and 12–13mths in all infants.
- *Pneumococcal conjugate vaccine:* 2, 4, and 12–13mths in all infants.
- *Measles, mumps, rubella (MMR):*
  - 12–13mths in all infants;
  - booster at 3yrs 4mths to 5yrs.
- *Human papilloma virus (HPV, against cervical cancer):* 3 doses within 6mths in girls 12–13-yr-old.

Live vaccines are contraindicated in children with immunodeficiency. Pertussis immunization is contraindicated in infants who have had a severe local or general reaction to a previous injection. MMR is contraindicated in children allergic to excipients such as gelatin and neomycin.

Table 19.1 Routine childhood immunization programme*

When to immunize	Diseases protected against	Vaccine given
2mths old	Diphtheria, tetanus, pertussis, polio, & *Haemophilus influenzae* type b (Hib)	DTaP/IPV/Hib & pneumococcal conjugate vaccine (PCV)
3mths old	Diphtheria, tetanus, pertussis, polio, & *Haemophilus influenzae* type b (Hib)	DTaP/IPV/Hib, MenC
	Meningitis C (meningococcal group C)	
4mths old	Diphtheria, tetanus, pertussis, polio & *Haemophilus influenzae* type b (Hib)	DTaP/IPV/Hib, MenC, & PVC
	Meningitis C	
	Pneumococcal infection	
Around 12–13mths	*Haemophilus influenzae* type b (Hib) & meningitis C	Hib/MenC
	Measles, mumps, & rubella (German measles)	MMR & PCV
	Pneumococcal infection	
3yrs 4mths to 5yrs old	Diphtheria, tetanus, pertussis, & polio	DTaP/IPV or dTaP/IPV & MMR
	Measles, mumps, & rubella	
12–13yr old girls	Cervical cancer 3 doses	HPV
13–18yrs old	Tetanus, diphtheria, & polio	Td/IPV

* Each vaccination is given as a single injection into the muscle of the thigh or upper arm.
Revised July 2011 ℘ http://www.nhs.uk/Planners/vaccinations/Pages/Vaccinationchecklist.aspx

Bones and joints

Clinical assessment

History

This should focus on the following:

- *Presenting complaint:*
  - *pain*—site, severity, onset, nature, duration/chronicity, exacerbating/relieving factors, rest pain, radiation;
  - if child presents with knee pain, always ask about and examine the hips;
  - *swelling*—site, size, onset, duration, exacerbating/relieving factors;
  - *limp*—refusing to weight bear ± history of trauma or injury;
  - morning stiffness/start-up pain;
  - *deformity*—static/worsening or improving condition.
- *Associated systemic symptoms:*
  - infection (rigors, night sweats, flu-like symptoms);
  - loss of appetite/weight.
- *Antenatal and birth history*—important with congenital conditions.
- Neurodevelopmental milestones (see 🔲 p.557).
- *Past medical history*—previous trauma, surgery, medical illnesses.
- Sports and activities.
- *Drug history*—glucocorticoid usage, allergies.
- *Family history*—hereditary conditions.
- *Neurological screening:*—important in syndromic children.

Examination

Inspection

Observe the child walking and at play (don't forget to watch as they walk into the consulting room).

- *General:*
  - height, weight, proportion (long limbs, short trunk);
  - *skin (scars, lesions, colour, discharge)*—soft tissue (swelling, muscle wasting, contractures), skeletal (alignment, rotation, limb length);
  - *limb*—amelia (absence), hemimelia (absence of distal half), phocomelia (hand/foot attached directly to trunk), syndactyly (fused digits), polydactyly (additional digits);
  - *gait*—antalgic, Trendelenburg, high stepping, short leg, crouch, abnormalities of lower limb/spine (🔲 pp.34, 496).
- *Skeletal alignment:*
  - *Spine*—normally there is a flexible kyphosis of the thoracic spine, a lordosis at the cervical and lumbar spine (not noticeable in neonates). look also for plagiocephaly, torticollis, scoliosis;
  - *lower limb*—check rotational profile, symmetric range of movement, varus/valgus deformity; *always* examine the hips;
  - *feet*—babies have 'flat' feet. The medial longitudinal arch develops during childhood. Look at the shoes!
  - *elbows*—there is a mild valgus deformity when in extension especially in females.

- *Mobility and gait:* toddlers have a wide stepping jerky gait. As the child matures (by the age of 7yrs), the gait becomes more 'adult-like' with the heel strike, stance phase (whole of foot to the ground), push off phase, and arm swing. The cadence decreases and the step length increases.
  - *antalgic (painful) gait*—short stance phase (child does not want to put weight on affected limb);
  - *high stepping gait*—usually due to foot drop (child lifts foot higher off the ground to avoid tripping over);
  - *Trendelenberg gait*—look at pelvis. When weight is loaded on the ipsilateral side, the contralateral hemipelvis tilts downwards (due to weak abductors or neurological, muscular, or hip joint causes in the weight-bearing ipsilateral limb). The upper body is then used to counter-balance;
  - *toe walking*—consider neurological causes (see 📖 pp.34, 496). In boys consider DMD and check creatine kinase (CK).
- *Trendelenburg test:* stand facing the child with your hands out, palms facing upwards. Ask the child to rest their hands (palms down) on your hands. Then ask the child to lift one leg. If the pelvis tilts downwards on the non-weight-bearing side (you will feel the downward pressure on your hand of this side) the test is positive.
- *Gower's sign:* child should be able to independently stand from a sitting position without using their upper limbs. With weak lower limb muscles, the child may 'crawl' hands up thighs in order to stand up, e.g. in muscular dystrophy.
- *Neurodevelopmental assessment:* see 📖 p.557.
- Can the child hop on either foot?
- Can the child climb on to the examination couch?

Feel

Tenderness, warmth, swelling (firmness, fluctuant), leg length discrepancy (true leg length: measure from the anterior superior iliac spine to the medial malleolus), pulses.

Move

- *General:* muscle tone, symmetric full joint range of movement, hyperlaxity/stiffness, contractures (are they fixed or can they be overcome?).
- *Spine:* fixed/correctable deformity?
- *Hip:* Ortolani and Barlow tests (📖 p.748).
- *Knee:* patella instability, anterior drawer/Lachman test (ACL integrity).

The limping child

Exclude trauma and infection before considering other disorders.

Examination

Lower limbs, back, and abdomen need to be examined. Observe the following:

- Limb position of least pain (e.g. in hip septic arthritis, the hip is held in flexion and external rotation).
- Gait (📖 p.34).
- Movement and mobility:
  - ability to weight bear passively and actively;
  - ability to move the joints and limbs freely;
  - palpate for tenderness, heat, and swelling around the joint; palpate the entire length of the extremity, the abdomen, and spine;
  - *leg length difference:* anterior superior iliac spine (ASIS) to medial malleoli. to determine if discrepancy is in femur, or tibia perform galeazzi test (flex knees and hips and examine from the side);
  - *range of movement (ROM):* in individual joint and compare with other side;
  - *neurological and vascular status:* abdominal examination.

Beware of referred pain from joint above or from the abdomen (consider appendicitis, inguinal hernia, UTI with hip pain). Always assess the joint above and below. Hip pathology may present as knee pain.

Investigations

- *Temperature.*
- *Bloods:* FBC, ESR (may be normal), CRP, blood cultures, blood film, rheumatoid factor (RF), antinuclear antibody (ANA), anti-streptolysin (ASO) titre, Lyme titre, HLA-B27.
- *Urine:* dipstick + MSU.
- *X-rays:* antero-posterior (AP), lateral plain X-ray of entire bone involved including joint above and below (e.g. if hip: AP pelvis and frog leg lateral views).
- *US scan:* of muscle and bone.
- *MRI:* very sensitive and specific—good for soft tissues and bone pathology.
- *Three phase bone scan:* when pain not easily localizable; sensitive, but not specific. Radiation exposure.

The limping child: differential diagnosis

Table 20.1 Differential diagnosis according to area of lower limb affected

Back	Hip	Femur	Knee	Foot & ankle
Age 0–5yrs				
Discitis	Developmental dysplasia of hip, transient synovitis, septic arthritis	Osteomyelitis*	Septic arthritis	
Age 5–10yrs				
Discitis	Transient synovitis, Perthes' disease, septic arthritis	Osteomyelitis*	Discoid meniscus, septic arthritis	Kohler's disease, Freiberg's disease, tarsal coalition, verruca
Age 10–15yrs				
Discitis	Slipped upper femoral epiphysis, septic arthritis	Osteomyelitis*	Osgood–Schlatter's disease, osteochondritis dessicans, patellofemoral pain syndrome, chondromalacia patella	Sever's disease, tarsal coalition, verruca, in growing toenails

* Consider with septic joint.

Causes of limp

Tumour
- Neuroblastoma (age 0–5yrs) (📖 p.666).
- Ewing's sarcoma (age 5–15yrs) (📖 p.670).
- Osteosarcoma (age 5–15yrs) (📖 p.670).

Benign tumour
Osteoid osteoma (age 5–15yrs).

Haematological causes (all ages)
- Acute lymphocytic leukaemia (📖 p.656).
- HSP (📖 p.788).
- SCD (📖 p.620).
- Thalassaemia (📖 p.622).

Infection (all ages)
- TB (📖 p.722).
- Malaria (📖 p.723).
- Lyme disease (📖 p.712).
- Viral.

Neurological causes (all ages)
- CP (📖 p.550).
- DMD (📖 p.546).
- Poliomyelitis.
- Hereditary motor sensory neuropathy (📖 p.541).
- Spina bifida (📖 p.170).

Rheumatological causes (all ages) Juvenile idiopathic arthritis (JIA; 📖 p.768).

Trauma (all ages)
- Non-accidental injury (NAI).
- Trauma (open/closed fractures).
- Sprains/contusions.
- Ill-fitting shoes.

Congenital causes (all ages) Congenital limb deficiency/shortening.

Infections: septic arthritis

An infectious arthritis of a synovial joint. The frequency is highest in young children with half of all cases presenting in the first 2yrs. Males > female (2:1).

Pathogenesis

Septic arthritis can develop from osteomyelitis especially in neonates where infection spreads from the metaphysis via transepiphyseal vessels. It may also arise due to haematogenous spread of infection or by direct inoculation.

Aetiology

- *Age <12mths old*: Staphylococcus aureus, Group B streptococcus, Gram –ve bacilli, *Candida albicans*.
- *Age 1–5yrs*: Staph. aureus, Haemophilus influenza (rarely in immunized children), Group A streptococcus (pyogenes), *Streptococcus pneumonia, Kingella kingae, Neisseria gonorrheae* (child abuse).
- *Age 5–12yrs*: Staph. aureus, Group A streptococcus.
- *Age 12–18yrs*: Staph. aureus, Neisseria gonorrhoeae (sexually active).
- Community acquired MRSA (CA-MRSA) is increasing worldwide.

Common joints affected Most (75%) are in lower limb. Knee > hip > ankle. Other 25% are in upper limbs.

Differential diagnosis

This depends on age and joint involved:
- *Hip*: transient synovitis, Perthes, slipped capital femoral epiphysis, psoas abscess, proximal femoral or vertebral osteomyelitis, discitis.
- *Knee*: distal femoral or proximal tibial osteomyelitis. Pain often referred from the hip.
- *General*: cellulitis, pyomyositis, other infectious arthritis (viral, mycoplasmal, mycobacterial, fungal, Lyme disease), sickle cell, haemophilia, trauma, collagen vascular disease, Henoch–Schönlein purpura, reactive arthritis from GI infections or GU infections, streptococcal pharyngitis, viral hepatitis, salmonella, or post-viral (HIV, CMV).
- *>1 joint involved*: pauciarticular arthritis, rheumatic fever, serum sickness, HSP, collagen vascular disease, sickle cell disease, chronic recurrent multifocal osteomyelitis (CRMO).
- *Haemophilia*: increased risk of septic arthritis due to haemarthrosis (predisposes to infection: pneumococci).

Symptoms and signs

Infants characteristically do not appear ill. 50% do not have fever. In the older child—acute onset; decreased range of movements or pseudoparalysis; pain on passive motion; hot, warm, swollen joint; inability to weight bear; systemic symptoms of infection. In <10% of cases more than one joint affected (except gonococcal infections). The clinical picture may be less acute if the child has received antibiotics.

Investigations

- *Blood:* FBC, ESR, CRP, blood cultures; Lyme titres if exposure.
- *X-ray of joint:* usually normal initially (widened joint space suggests an effusion). Subluxation/dislocation, joint space narrowing and erosive changes are later signs.
- *Joint aspiration:* most useful diagnostic investigation. Send aspirate for microscopy and culture. PCR may be useful if already on antibiotics.
- *US:* to detect effusion and guide aspiration.
- *MRI:* if diagnosis in doubt to exclude osteomyelitis, (do not delay treatment while waiting for MRI).
- *CT:* to imaging sternoclavicular and sacroiliac joints. Psoas abscess.
- *Bone scan:* if multiple sites and child too unwell to localize pain.
- *Lumbar puncture:* if a septic joint with *Haemophilus influenzae* (increased incidence of meningitis).

Treatment

- *Medical:* IV antibiotics, *after* aspirate taken, for up to 3wks (until inflammatory markers normalize), followed by oral antibiotics for a total of 4–6wks. Outcome of treatment is time dependent.
- *Surgical:* early referral to orthopaedic team as there is a low threshold for irrigation and debridement of the affected joint (+ drainage of any associated osteomyelitis).
- *Splintage:* In the acute setting a brief period of splintage improves pain and allows inflammation to settle. Splint in position of function.
- *Physiotherapy:* to avoid joint stiffness.

Prognosis

Usually good unless the diagnosis is delayed. Recurrence of disease and development of chronic infection occur in <10%. Long-term follow-up is needed as growth-related sequelae may not become apparent for months or years. Hip joint infection has the worst prognosis for anatomical and functional impairment.

Complications

Chondrolysis, ongoing infection and bone destruction, joint incongruity/stiffness, and growth disturbance. Avascular necrosis of the femoral head can occur.

Infections: osteomyelitis

Infection of bone. The frequency of osteomyelitis is greatest in infants, with 33% of all cases in the first 2yrs, and 50% occurring by 5yrs. Male > female (2:1).

Pathogenesis

Infection usually seen in the metaphyseal region of bones. Most infections are spread via the haematogenous route from a 1° site of entry (e.g. respiratory, GI, ENT, or skin sites). Infection may also occur by direct inoculation (open fractures, penetrating wounds) or local extension from adjacent sites. In the infant, transphyseal vessels are patent and infection may spread to the adjacent joint causing a septic arthritis. In adolescents infection tends to spread through the medullary canal.

Types of osteomyelitis

- Acute.
- Subacute (2–3wks duration).
- *Chronic:* may develop 'sequestrum' (dead bone) and 'involucrum' (new bone).
- Bone abscesses may become surrounded by thick, fibrous tissue and sclerotic bone (Brodie's abscess).

Aetiology

The yield for bacterial growth from synovial fluid and bone aspirate is small; therefore organisms are not always isolated. Staphylococcus aureus is most common in children in all age groups. Other organisms seen include the following:

- *Neonates:* group B streptococcus and Gram –ve enteric bacilli.
- *<2yrs:* Haemophilus influenzae (rare).
- *>2yrs:* Gram +ve cocci, *Pseudomonas aeruginosa*.
- *Adolescents:* Neisseria gonorrhoeae.

Consider salmonella in SCD. Tuberculosis is rare.

Symptoms and signs

- Neonates characteristically do not appear ill and may not have fever.
- Older children have pain, limping, refusal to walk/weight bear, fever, malaise, flu-like symptoms. Overlying bone may be tender (+ warm), with/without swelling. Long bones principally affected: Tibia > femur > humerus.

Differential diagnosis

This includes:

- JIA (📖 p.768).
- Lyme/post-streptococcal arthritis (📖 pp.244, 712).
- Acute leukaemia (📖 p.658).
- Neuroblastoma (📖 p.666).
- Neoplasm (e.g. osteoid osteoma, osteosarcoma, Ewing's sarcoma).
- CRMO.
- LCH.

Investigations
- *Blood:* FBC, ESR, CRP, blood cultures (positive in 50%).
- *X-ray of bone:* early stages may be normal; soft tissue oedema may be visible. Late stages reveal metaphyseal rarefaction. Destructive changes in bone appear after 10 days.
- *US-guided aspiration:* for microscopy and culture.
- *MRI:* soft tissue assessment—bone marrow involvement; abscess formation, joint effusion, subperiosteal extension.
- *Bone scans:* good for acute osteomyelitis; can identify up to 90% of joint involvement (seen as hot spots) and differentiate joint from bone involvement; good for infections of pelvis, proximal femur, and spine.
- Open biopsy may be necessary.
- Consider immunological evaluation if atypical organism.

Treatment
- *Medical:* IV antibiotics for a minimum of 2wks, followed by oral antibiotics for 4wks. Early liaison with microbiologist required.
- *Surgical:* drainage and debridement if there is frank pus on aspiration or a sequestered abscess or collection (not accessible to antibiotics).

Prognosis Usually excellent if treated early. Disease recurrence/progression to chronic infection is seen in <10%.

Complications
- *Systemic:* may include septicaemia.
- *Local:* pathological fracture, sequestration, growth disturbance.

Spinal disorders

General management

History
Pain, onset of deformity, loss of weight, night sweats, family history, disability, other disorders.

Examination
- *Inspection:* asymmetry, scapular prominence, skin lesions (especially midline pits and haemangiomas), *café au lait* spots (associated with neurofibromatosis), foot deformity, leg atrophy.
- *Feel:* spinal tenderness.
- *Move:* forward flexion, hamstring tightness.
- *General:* neurological examination.
- *Investigations:* radiographs, CT, MRI, bone scan.

General spinal disorders

Back pain
Take it seriously! More likely to be caused by significant pathology than in adult (e.g. osteoid osteoma, eosinophilic granuloma). Beware of the following, especially in young children—several weeks of symptoms; night pain; increasing symptoms; abnormal neurology; recent onset of scoliosis; night sweats. Pain may be referred from intra-abdominal or intrathoracic process. Investigate thoroughly, but remember 50% of children experience back pain by 15yrs of age.

Discitis
Inflammation (probably infection) of the disc space:
- *Age group:* any age (infants and children rather than adolescents).
- *Symptoms:* fever; irritability; unwilling to walk; back pain, abdominal pain. Symptoms may be vague.
- *Investigations:* bloods (↑ CRP and ESR); MRI; bone scan.
- *Treatment:* antibiotics (according to local policy), at least until inflammatory markers return to normal.
- *Outcome:* usually do well.

Congenital anomalies
Diastematomyelia: spinal cord is split by a central cartilaginous/bony prominence.
- *Signs:* other abnormalities are common (e.g. scoliosis, clubfoot, cavus foot); cutaneous lesions seen in most children; positive neurology seen in 50%.
- *Management:* consider resection of spur if neurology appears/is progressive.
- Spina bifida.

Regional spinal disorders

Cervical spine: torticollis See 📖 pp.127, 883.

Thoracic spine See Scheuermann's disease (📖 p.744).

Lumbar spine: spondylolysis and spondylolisthesis

- *Definition:* defect of pars interarticularis (spondylolysis). If bilateral and at the same level may result in anterior displacement of one vertebra upon another (spondylolisthesis). Usually due to a stress fracture through a congenitally dysplastic pars.
- *Incidence:* uncommon, associated with spina bifida, metabolic (e.g. osteopetrosis), connective tissue (e.g. Marfan's), hyperextension sports (e.g. gymnastics).
- *Symptoms/signs:* sudden/insidious onset of pain exacerbated by activity. Decreased forward flexion and straight leg raise.
- *Investigations:* X-rays—lateral and oblique spinal views. Look for 'Scotty dog's collar'. Bone scan/SPECT for occult fractures and evidence of healing.
- *Management:* non-operative usually. Rest and change of activities; consider short-term bracing, analgesia, hamstring stretches, and core strengthening. Operative intervention seldom required for stabilization.

Sacral spine: sacral agenesis

- *Definition:* hypoplastic/absent sacrum; most common in infants of diabetic mothers.
- *Signs:* abnormal pelvic ring affecting lower limbs with associated neurology.
- *Management:* tailor towards severity of agenesis and neurology.

Spine: kyphosis

- *Definition*: from Greek Kyphos, a hump. Increased curvature of the spine in the sagittal plane, visible from the side. Normally there is a 20–40° curvature of the thoracic spine.
- *History*: site, age of onset, rate of progression, associated scoliosis/pain/ neurological symptoms, family history.

Examination

Assess:
- *Flexibility*: stand, bend forwards, bend backwards (hyperextension).
- *Ability to lie flat*: associated lumbar lordosis (more prominent with greater severity of kyphosis).
- *Hips for tight hamstrings*: limited straight leg raising.
- Full respiratory (pulmonary function) and neurological examination.

Investigation PA and lateral standing X-rays of entire spine.

Diagnosis

Three major causes are identified by answers to:
- Is it flexible?
- Is it painful?
- When did it start?

Postural kyphosis (most common)

Flexible, usually painless, onset <10yrs old.
- *Other findings*: tall; girls > boys; poor physical development; flat-footed; poor at games.
- *Investigations*: supine hyperextension lateral radiograph confirms complete correction.
- *Treatment*: physiotherapy to improve posture and provide exercises for dorsal spine, education, occasionally brace.
- *Outcome*: corrects spontaneously by end of adolescence.

Congenital kyphosis

Rigid, occasionally painful, onset <10yrs old.
- *Other findings*: severe deformities recognized at birth, associated with congenital spinal abnormality, e.g. spina bifida.
- *Cause*: may be secondary to failure of vertebral formation +/– segmentation during the first trimester.
- *Treatment*: brace, if progression fusion to prevent paraplegia.
- *Outcome*: can progress rapidly and lead to paraplegia.

Scheuermann's disease

- Rigid, aching pain between shoulder blades; onset 10–15yrs (previously normal spine).
- *Incidence*: unknown (up to 7–8% of population in cadaveric studies).
- *Aetiology*: osteochondritis.

Investigations

- *AP and lateral spine X-rays:* >45° kyphosis with >5° anterior wedging at three sequential vertebrae = radiographical definition of Scheuermann's disease.
- May have vertebral body end-plate changes (Schmorl's nodes—vertical herniations of the intervertebral discs into the vertebral end-plate), spondylolysis (30–50%), scoliosis (33%).

Treatment

- *Physiotherapy (extension exercises):* bracing may be considered.
- *Medical:* NSAIDs.
- *Surgical correction:* with severe kyphosis (>70°), the patient is skeletally mature, with severe pain or evidence of cord involvement.

Outcome

Little evidence that patients with kyphosis <70° experience late progression, disabling pain, or neurological compromise.

Spine: scoliosis

Idiopathic scoliosis
- Lateral curvature (>10°) +/− rotation deformity of the spine without an identifiable cause. Description of curvature based on direction of apical convexity. There are 3 types.
- *Infantile (<3yrs old):* left > right side; males > females; associated plagiocephaly (skull flattening), hip dysplasia, and other congenital defects. May be 2° to underlying spinal abnormality.
- *Juvenile (3–10yr olds):* may be 2° to underlying spinal abnormality; high risk of curve progression (70% require treatment with 50% needing brace and 50% surgery).
- *Adolescent:* most common in 11–16-yr-olds. Females > male.

Incidence
- Curves >10°, 2% incidence.
- Curves >30°, 0.2% incidence.
- Right thoracic curves > double major (right thoracic and left lumbar) > left lumbar > right lumbar.

Risk factors
Positive family history; daughters of affected mothers more likely to be affected, Marfans, neurofibromatosis.

Disease progression
Risk factors for curve progression: age <12yrs; skeletal immaturity; female; curve magnitude >20°; spine at greatest risk of curve progression during puberty. Natural history after skeletal maturity is curves < 30° unlikely to progress, if >50° 2/3 will progress. Severe curves (Cobb angle >100°) associated with pulmonary dysfunction, early mortality, pain, poor self-image.

Symptoms
Onset of symptoms, rate of progression, *Is it painful?* (inflammatory or neoplastic.) Ask about respiratory and neurological symptoms.

Signs
- Inspect child standing.
- Describe scoliosis as the side to which the spine is convex (shoulder on convex side is elevated).
- *Inspect:* pelvic height—limb length difference; waistline asymmetry; trunk shift; spinal deformity; rib rotational deformity (rib hump).
- Bend—touch toes. *Is it fixed?*
- *Adam's forward test:* asymmetry of the posterior chest wall on forward bending. If scoliosis disappears: postural (80% of scoliosis).
- Full neurological examination including abdominal reflexes.
- Lower limb examination (other causes of postural scoliosis: unilateral muscle spasm; unequal leg length).

True idiopathic scoliosis
Painless, convex to the right in the thoracic spine, not associated with any neurological changes.

Investigations
- Standing PA and lateral X-rays full spine.
- MRI if pain, neurological changes, rapidly progressive curve, excessive kyphosis, left thoracic/thoracolumbar curves, considering surgery.

Treatment
Based on maturity of patient, magnitude of deformity, and curve progression. The aim is to prevent further progression.

Non-operative
- Close observation (6-monthly X-rays for curves <25°).
- Bracing is controversial. May slow/halt curve progression—the more it's worn, the more effective it is. Consider for children with curves <40°
- Manipulation and casting for young children with more severe curves

Operative
- Anterior/posterior spinal fusion with instrumentation for severe deformities (>45°).
- Posterior instrumentation without fusion
- Vertebral expanding prosthetic titanium rib

Congenital scoliosis

Most common congenital spinal disorder.

Aetiology Abnormal vertebral development in the first trimester.

Associations Can be isolated deformity or associated with other congenital abnormalities: Spinal (40%)> genitourinary (20%) > heart disease (10–15%), also associated with syndromes, e.g. VACTERL (📖 p.848).

Disease progression
Risk of progression dependent on morphology and growth potential of vertebrae. Greatest risk during periods of rapid growth (<2yrs and >10yrs old).

Treatment Early diagnosis; often need surgery.

Scoliosis secondary to neuromuscular disorders
Symptoms and signs
Progresses more rapidly and may continue after maturity; longer curves involving more vertebrae and less likely to have compensatory curves.

Associations
- *Skeletal:* pelvic obliquity, bony deformities, cervical involvement.
- *Pulmonary:* more frequent, ↓ lung function and pneumonia.
- *Neurological:* brainstem, proprioception, Klippel–Feil syndrome.
- *Upper motor neuron disease:* cerebral palsy, spina bifida, spinocerebellar degeneration, syringomyelia, spinal cord tumour/trauma, tethered cord, diastematomyelia.
- *Lower motor neuron disease:* poliomyelitis, spinal muscular atrophy, (myopathic: DMD).
- *Syndromes:* neurofibromatosis, Marfan's.

Hip disorders: developmental dysplasia of the hip

Previously known as 'congenital dislocation of the hip'. Disorder of hip joint development resulting in hip instability/subluxation/dislocation ± acetabular dysplasia.

- *Incidence:* 2:1000 (*but* up to 20:1000 newborn hips are unstable; 90% spontaneously stabilize by 9wks).
- *Risk factors:* family history (1:5), female > male (5:1), Left > right (1.5:1), racial predilection, breech presentation.
- *Aetiology:* capsular laxity (increased type III collagen, maternal oestrogens), decreased intrauterine volume (breech position, first born, oligohydramnios).
- *Associations:* other 'packaging' disorders: torticollis (20%), metatarsus adductus (10%), talipes calcaneovalgus, teratologic dislocation, Down's syndrome.
- *Teratologic dislocation:* a distinct form of hip dislocation associated with neuromuscular syndromes (e.g. myelodysplasia, arthrogryposis, chromosomal abnormalities, lumbosacral agenesis, diastrophic dwarfism). The hip is dislocated *before* birth. It is more difficult to treat.

Disease progression

Capsular laxity + shallow acetabulum → instability/subluxation/dislocation → muscle contracture → progressive acetabular dysplasia with a fibro-fatty substance filling the acetabulum (pulvinar); femoral head becomes hypoplastic.

History Usually uneventful pregnancy; parents may notice delayed walking, painless limp, prone to falls. DDH may be incidental finding.

Examination

All newborn infants should be screened for DDH before discharge and then again at 6wks. High-risk infants are selected for ultrasound screening. Still controversy over selective v universal screening program.

Neonate

- Is hip dislocated? If so, is it reducible? Ortolani's test (O for out). Gently elevate (anteriorly) and **abduct** the dislocated hip to reduce it (clunk of reduction).
- If not dislocated, can I dislocate it (i.e. dislocatable)? Barlow's test. Gently **adduct** and depress (posteriorly) femur; vulnerable hip dislocates.

These 2 provocation manoeuvres become unreliable after age 6–8wks.
- *Infant:* asymmetric gluteal folds, limited abduction, leg length discrepancy. *Galeazzi sign*—flex knees with feet together; +ve sign = affected femur appears short due to dislocated hip joint. (*Note.* Also +ve if femur is congenitally short; –ve with bilateral DDH).

- *Older child:* may walk with limp; positive Trendelenburg test. With bilateral dislocations, the only sign may be an exaggerated lumbar lordosis and limited hip abduction.

Investigations

- *Age <6mths:* hip US (before ossification; operator-dependent).
- *>6mths:* AP pelvis radiograph. A shallow acetabulum with increased acetabular index, and hypoplastic femoral head in superolateral position is demonstrated. Shenton's line broken.

Treatment

Depends on age of child (see Box 20.1). An urgent referral to a paediatric orthopaedic surgeon is needed in order to start treatment as soon as possible. The aim is to achieve and maintain concentric hip reduction to encourage early acetabular development to reduce the risk of future degenerative joint disease.

Box 20.1 Treatment at different ages

Age <6mths
Pavlik harness (maintain hip in flexed position with some hip abduction)

Age 6–18mths
- Manipulation and closed reduction (+/– adductor tenotomy) + hip spica plaster cast
- Open reduction (medial approach if <12mths old; anterior approach if >12mths old) + hip spica plaster cast

Age 18–24mths
- Trial of closed reduction
- Open reduction (anterior approach) +/– pelvic osteotomy + hip spica plaster cast

Age 2–6yrs
- Open reduction (anterior approach) +/– femoral shortening +/– pelvic osteotomy + hip spica plaster cast

---

Complications

- *Early:* inadequate reduction and redislocation.
- *Intermediate:* residual acetabular dysplasia; avascular necrosis.
- *Late:* early osteoarthritic changes.

Prognosis

Any residual acetabular dysplasia may be treated with a pelvic osteotomy as a secondary procedure. Long-term acetabular dysplasia is likely to lead to early degenerative changes in the hip.

Hip disorders: Perthes' disease

Also known as Legg–Calve–Perthes disease. It is due to an *idiopathic* osteonecrosis (avascular necrosis) of the femoral head of unknown aetiology. Incidence: 1:10,000

Risk factors

Boys > girls (4:1); age 4–10yrs. <20% bilateral (usually staged + asymmetric), 10% family history, low birth weight, 4% children with transient synovitis, delayed skeletal maturity.

Aetiology

Unknown, although several risk factors lead to avascular necrosis: trauma, endocrine (e.g. hypothyroidism, renal disease, steroids), metabolic, coagulability (blood dyscrasia, protein C or S deficiency, thrombophilia).

Differential diagnosis

- Multiple epiphyseal dysplasia (📖 p.767).
- Spondyloepiphyseal dysplasia (📖 p.767).
- Hypofibrinolysis.
- Slipped upper femoral epiphysis (SUFE) (📖 p.752).
- Septic arthritis (📖 p.772).
- TB of hip.
- Trauma.
- SCD.

Pathological stages

- *Avascular:* hip appears sclerotic with minimal loss of epiphyseal height
- *Fragmentation:* initially fissures appear in epiphysis, followed by more severe fragmentation and loss of height.
- *Remodelling:* regeneration, new bone formation, and head remodelling
- *Healed:* no avascular bone visible on radiographs

Symptoms Mild/intermittent anterior thigh/groin/referred knee pain with limp; classical 'painless limp'. *Note:* Knee pain: beware hip pathology.

Special signs

- *Look:* proximal thigh atrophy, mild short stature, limp/Trendelenburg/antalgic gait common (see 📖 pp.34, 752).
- *Feel:* effusion (from synovitis), groin/thigh tenderness.
- *Move:* decreased hip range of movement (especially abduction and internal rotation) with muscle spasm.

Investigations
- *AP and lateral pelvic X-rays:* many different classifications, but most useful is lateral pillar classification. The femoral head is divided into thirds. Group A no loss of height of lateral 1/3, B up to 50% loss of height, group C >50% loss of height.
- MRI may help diagnosis especially in the early stages.
- *Technetium 99 bone scan:* decreased uptake in femoral epiphysis due to poor vascular supply.
- Dynamic arthrography to delineate hip joint and plan surgery.

Prognosis
This is a local self-healing disorder. Prognosis depends on bone age and X-ray appearances. Poor prognostic indicators are:
- *Clinical:* heavy child; ↓ range of movement; adduction contracture; flexion into abduction, female and older age at presentation (> 6yrs).
- *Radiological:* Gage's sign; lateral subluxation of femoral head with lateral calcification; whole head involvement; metaphyseal cysts; lateral pillar group C hips.

Treatment is controversial
The aims are to relieve symptoms and signs by eliminating hip irritability and maintaining hip range of movements. This is achieved by:
- Maintaining sphericity of femoral head.
- Containing femoral head in acetabulum whilst remodelling occurs.
- Preventing epiphyseal collapse and secondary osteoarthritis.

Non-operative treatment Observation and activity modification, including bed rest and walking aids. NSAIDs, physiotherapy. Bracing is controversial.

Operative treatment Femoral/pelvic osteotomies to contain femoral head in acetabulum.

Hip disorders: slipped upper femoral epiphysis

Displacement of the upper femoral epiphysis on the metaphysis through the hypertrophic zone of the growth plate. The femoral neck displaces anteriorly and the head remains in the acetabulum.

- *Incidence:* the most common adolescent hip disorder (3:100 000); 25–60% bilateral.
- *Risk factors:* African American, >50% obese (weight >95th percentile), positive family history, puberty, boys (12–16yrs) > girls (10–14yrs).
- *Aetiology:* unknown, but associated with the following:
  - *Endocrine*—hypothyroidism, hypogonadism, renal osteodystrophy;
  - *Mechanical*—retroversion of femoral neck or vertical growth plate;
  - *Other*—Down syndrome, radiotherapy/chemotherapy.

Symptoms and signs

Groin, thigh, or knee pain. Antalgic gait, limited hip flexion and abduction, flexion into external rotation, and thigh atrophy.

Always consider hip pathology in a child presenting with knee pain.

Presentation

Characterized by 2 broad types of children.

- *Obese hypogonadal (low circulating sex hormones):* delayed skeletal maturation bone age.
- *Tall thin, often boys, post growth spurt (younger age in girls):* overabundance of growth hormones.

Diagnostic classification

This is based on duration of symptoms.

- *Preslip:* wide epiphysis; mild discomfort, but normal examination; often seen on contralateral hip.
- *Acute slip:* mild symptoms <3wks, then sudden slippage usually without trauma; pain so severe child unable to weight bear; usually unstable.
- *Acute on chronic:* acute slip on pre-existing chronic slip; usually have previous symptoms (pain, limp, out toe gait) for several months; unable to weight bear; usually unstable.
- *Chronic:* most common type; history for several months; symptoms worsen as slip progresses; child able to walk with mildly antalgic externally rotated gait. Usually stable.
- *Slips may be further sub-classified into stable or unstable (Loder):* in an unstable slip' child unable to weight bear, even with crutches, and cannot do straight leg raise actively. These have increased risk of AVN.

Investigations

- *X-Ray:* AP pelvis and frog lateral hips. Widening of physis, Klein's line intersects lateral capital epiphysis on AP.
- *MRI:* useful in pre-slip diagnosis, and evidence of AVN.
- *Endocrine tests:* if appropriate, e.g. thyroid function.

Treatment

The aim is to prevent further 'slippage' and to minimize complications.

Operative

Usually pin *in situ* (to encourage the proximal femoral epiphysis to close, hence preventing further slippage); usually not reduced as manipulation may increase the incidence of avascular necrosis. Prophylactic pinning of opposite hip is controversial. It is recommended in younger children and those with endocrinopathy.

Complications

- *Chondrolysis (degeneration of the articular cartilage of the hip with narrowed joint space, pain, decreased motion):* associated with more severe slips; occurs more frequently among African American children and females; associated with pins protruding out of the femoral head.
- *Osteonecrosis/avascular necrosis (higher incidence in unstable hips):* due to injury to retinacular vessels (at time of slip or manipulation) or compression from intracapsular haematoma. Commonly leads to degenerative joint disease. Avascular necrosis uncommon in stable slips.

Knee disorders

Anterior knee pain

Common in the growing child and is usually due to overuse. Pain is worse with load-bearing, going downstairs, and prolonged sitting with knee flexed.

Common causes include the following:

- *Osteochondroses:* Osgood–Schlatter's disease (see 📖 p.761).
- *Sinding–Larsen–Johansson disease:* see 📖 p.761.
- *Bipartite patellae:* usually bilateral and a normal variant of ossification. There is a risk of developing an avulsion fracture; thus the child should rest, stop sports, and the knee should be splinted. NSAIDs may help. Once resolved, a gradual return to activities is possible.
- *Patella maltracking:* several causes including dysplasia of the femoral condyles, malalignment of the quadriceps mechanism with relatively weak vastus medialis, genu valgum, tibial torsion, increased laxity. Presents with vague anterior knee pain, instability, +/– episodes of patella dislocation. Treatment is physiotherapy, but some may need surgery.
- *Chondromalacia patellae:* softening of the articular cartilage, which may progress to osteoarthritis (X-rays may be normal) Treatment physio strengthening and stretches.

Genu recurvatum

Congenital hyperextension

- Commonest in breech presentations.
- Associated with arthrogryposis, spina bifida, DDH, talipes equinovarus.
- Severity varies from mild hyperextension to dislocation. Management: look for other abnormalities (e.g. DDH).
- Gentle stretching, serial casting, quadriceps lengthening at 1–3mths if necessary.

Acquired recurvatum

- Physiological 'curved' knee occurring in girls due to joint laxity. May be familial and predispose to sprains or patella instability.
- Consider neurological causes if not bilateral.
- Clinical features include a hyperextended knee, generalized lax joints.
- May be caused by trauma to the proximal anterior tibial physis causing a progressive deformity with growth.

Genu valgum (knock knees)

Defined by position of knees such that, when standing with knees together, the medial malleoli are not touching (therefore it is a frontal plane deformity). Commonly observed between ages 2 and 7yrs.

Causes

Bilateral

- *Physiological:* most common.
- *Metabolic:* renal osteodystrophy, rickets, hypophosphataemia.
- *Skeletal dysplasia:* Kniest's syndrome, congenital dislocation of patella.

- *Haematological:* myelodyplasia.

Unilateral

Asymmetric growth—trauma/infection/tumour/epiphyseal dysplasia to tibia or femur.

Presentation Child is noticed to walk knock-kneed. Establish rate of progression, diet, and family history.

Examination

- *General:* height and body proportions. May be overweight or have dysmorphic features. Full lower limb examination (standing and lying); often accompanied by flat feet (pes planus); measure knee angle and intermalleolar distance.
- *Specific signs.* Tibiofemoral angle assessment. The angle at which the long axis of tibia bisects the long axis of femur can be measured clinically and radiologically. Widened intermalleolar distance (distance between medial malleoli of ankles).

Investigations No X-ray required until >18mths age; then AP and lateral standing full leg length views.

Treatment

- *Non-operative:* mainstay for physiological genu valgum.
- *Operative:* reversible epiphysiodesis (physeal stapling or eight plate) of medial side tibia. If skeletally mature corrective osteotomy

Prognosis 95% physiological valgus resolves with growth achieving normal adult alignment by 7–8yrs.

Genu varum (bowed knees)

Bowing of the knees if patient stands with ankles together. Normally genu varum (15°) at birth progresses to physiological genu valgum by 4–5yrs. Genu varum is common in children <3yrs (especially obese children who start walking <1yrs old)

Causes

- *Physiological: in utero* (curled up) foetal position results in a bowed appearance due to:
  - a tight posterior hip capsule which causes external rotation of the hips;
  - internal tibial torsion.
- *Structural:* osteogenesis imperfecta (📖 p.762).
- *Metabolic:* vitamin D deficiency (nutritional rickets)/resistant rickets, hypophosphataemia (📖 pp.444–445), calcium deficiency.
- *Skeletal dysplasia:* metaphyseal dysplasia, achondroplasia, enchondromatosis (📖 p.766).
- *Local asymmetric growth:* Blount's disease (abnormal growth of medial aspect of proximal tibial epiphysis), osteochondromas, physeal injury (e.g. trauma, infection), dysplasia.

History

Parents notice child is walking bowlegged/in toeing of feet. Establish developmental milestones and rate of progression, family history, diet, social history, etc.

Examination

General examination including height and weight; full lower limb examination including rotational profile, widened intercondylar distance (distance between medial femoral condyles).

Investigations

Weight-bearing AP and lateral lower leg views

Symmetrical physiological bowing, flaring of tibia and femur. Can also measure tibiofemoral angle, metataphyseal–diaphyseal angles.

Treatment

Severe physiological genu varum may be treated by guided growth (reversible epiphysiodesis) using staples or eight plates. Blounts disease may require corrective osteotomes. Refer to orthopaedic paediatric surgeon

Prognosis 95% of cases of physiological varus resolve with age.

Osteochondritis dissecans of the knee

Occurs when an area of subchondral bone becomes avascular and fragments and separates from the underlying bone. May involve the overlying cartilage, leading to mechanical problems (e.g. loose bodies) and joint incongruity. Most commonly involves the lateral aspect of the medial femoral condyle. It may progress to early degenerative osteoarthritis.

- *Risk factors:* adolescents (10–15yrs). Boys > girls. Often secondary to trauma, ischaemia, abnormal epiphyseal ossification.
- *Clinical features:* non-specific knee pain, +/– locking and +/– stiffness. Knee swelling after activities, but no history of acute trauma or injury. May be tender over affected articular cartilage of medial femoral condyle if knee is fully flexed.
- *Disease progression:* the overlying articular cartilage is usually intact in younger children and the bone heals as revascularization occurs. The risk of articular fracture with separation and loose body formation increases with increasing age, larger lesions, and a weight-bearing location.

Investigations

X-rays of knee in AP, lateral, and notch views to assess femoral condyles. MRI may be useful for determining integrity of articular cartilage and defining whether synovial fluid is behind the lesion.

Treatment

Depends on patient age, size, and stability of fragment. Usually a short treatment with rest, anti-inflammatory drugs, and splintage will suffice. However, it may require surgery:

- *Non-operative:* as above, including observation with periodic X-rays and MRIs to assess degree of healing. Bracing and restricted weight-bearing/activities if significant growth remaining.
- *Operative:* adolescent with minimal growth left/loose lesion— arthroscopic assessment with possible debridement and microfracture through subchondral plate to promote revascularization and healing. Fixation of large fragments.

Prognosis Worse with large lesions in lateral femoral condyle in older children.

Note: Osteochondritis dessicans may occur in other major joints including the elbow (capitellum) and less often the lateral condyle of the patella.

Orthopaedic trauma

Trauma is the most common cause of childhood deaths. It is often due to falls especially in the home environment (home> sports > school > road traffic accident).

Road traffic accident is the leading cause of death. NAI should be considered (see 📖 pp.527, 923, 1000).

Fractures

Generally boys > girls with a peak incidence at 12yrs of age, although specific injuries peak at different ages, e.g. NAI at 1yr, femoral fractures at 3yrs, pedestrian vs car at 6yrs, lateral condyle/supracondylar fractures at 7yrs, physeal injury at 11–12yrs. 4% are multiple fractures. Children's fractures usually are more frequent in summer than in winter.

Principles of management

- Stabilize according to resuscitation principles (see 📖 Chapter 4).
- Full history (including nature of injury, left/right handedness) and examination.
- Is the fracture open/closed?
- Is the limb neurovascularly intact? Is there a compartment syndrome?
- Is the associated joint dislocated?
- Splint limb for comfort; analgesia; elevate.
- X-ray affected bone +/– joint above and below.
- Liaise with orthopaedic team.

Complications

Early

- *Neurovascular problems:* e.g. median nerve paraesthesia with distal radius fractures, median/ulnar nerve paraesthesia with supracondylar fractures, radial nerve in humeral shaft fractures, common peroneal nerve with proximal fibula fractures.
- *Compartment syndrome:* especially associated with closed low energy mid-shaft tibia fractures.

Intermediate

- *Joint stiffness:* especially fractures around the elbow.
- *Malunion:* usually well tolerated if malunion is within plane of motion; may be compensated in younger children with remodelling.

Late

- *Overgrowth:* occurs in long bones due to physeal stimulation (from hyperaemia). Femoral fractures in children may overgrow by 1–3cm.
- *Deformity:* if epiphysis is damaged, child may develop progressive deformity several months later. Require long-term follow-up
- *Non-union:* rarely shaft of tibia/ulna.

Common fracture patterns

The most common fracture pattern is a complete fracture of both cortices (e.g. spiral, transverse, oblique, multifragmentary). However, the following fractures are specific to children.

- *Buckle/torus fractures:* children <10yrs. Usually caused by a fall on an outstretched hand (causing compression of one cortex resulting in 'buckle' on the X-ray) resulting in a metaphyseal distal radius fracture. Inherently stable. Treatment immobilize in plaster of Paris/backslab; fracture clinic follow-up within 2–3 days. Remove plaster in 3–4wks and mobilize.
- *Plastic deformation or bend fractures:* traumatic bending/bowing of bone, but insufficient energy to produce a fracture. No fracture seen on X-ray (limb may appear 'bent'). Commonly ulna (look out for radial head dislocation); occasionally fibula. Treat as for torus fracture. If severe bowing or dislocation require manipulation under anaesthetic.
- *Greenstick fractures:* like bending a young twig, the cortex will break on the tension side and bend on the compression side. The energy is insufficient to result in complete bicortical fracture. It may require manipulation under anaesthesia.
- *Salter–Harris fractures (physeal injuries):* 20% of all children's fractures involve the physis (most commonly the distal radius). It is usually extra-articular, but fractures in the proximal femur/humerus, radial neck, distal fibula may be intra-articular.

Some fractures may indicate NAI (📖 pp.527, 1000), e.g. spinal fracture or femoral shaft fracture in the non-ambulant, rib fractures, two separate fractures at different stages of healing. These children should be referred for full investigation.

Osteochondroses

A spectrum of conditions primarily affecting the epiphyses , but may also involve cartilage and bone. Despite the term 'osteochondritis', the condition is not always due to inflammation and may be due to trauma or over-usage, vascular irregularities, or may be a normal variation. The affected devascularized bony region undergoes spontaneous healing with revascularization, resorption, and re-ossification. Symptoms are usually worse with activity and relieved with rest. It is usually a self-limiting condition with clinical outcomes ranging from normal to serious disability. Investigations include radiographs of the affected region, which may demonstrate fragmentation/collapsed sclerotic bone. An MRI scan will confirm the diagnosis. The conditions can be classified anatomically.

'Physeal' (growth plate) osteochondroses

Often require treatment.
- *Madelung deformity (distal radius):* defect in the volar and ulna side of the distal radial physis resulting in a shortened tilted distal radius and a prominent ulna. Occurs in teenage girls and features include pain, decreased range of movement, and abnormal wrist joint. Treated with analgesia and surgery.
- *Scheuermann's disease (vertebra):* see 📖 p.744.
- *Blount disease:* tibial physis.

Articular osteochondroses

Great potential for disability.
- *Freiberg disease:* infarction of the second metatarsal head or epiphysis in teenagers (females > males), presenting with pain on running and dancing. Joint tenderness with decreased range of movement, and pain on tip-toe standing. Managed with change of activities, analgesia, orthotics, intra-articular corticosteroids+/– surgery.
- *Perthes' disease:* see 📖 p.750.
- *Panner's disease (osteonecrosis of the capitellum):* children <10yrs. No history trauma. Mild flexion contracture diffuse synovitis. X-ray shows irregular areas with sclerosis. MRI/CT/USS may aid diagnosis. Treatment NSAIDs, splint, occasionally arthroscopy. Prognosis good.
- *Osteochondritis of capitellum:* occurs in older children. May be due to overloading of the elbow (e.g. overhand throwing/batting) with accentuation of any valgus deformity. Clinical findings include mechanical block +/– flexion contracture, general lateral elbow pain, and swelling. AP X-ray with elbow flexed 45° may demonstrate irregular joint surface. CT/MRI/USS have also been used. Treatment: rest with avoidance of exacerbating factors; anti-inflammatories; arthroscopic removal of loose bodies, drilling, or fixation of unstable lesions.
- *Radial head:* similar to osteochondritis capitellum, except the radial head is affected. Child is prone to developing overgrowth and joint incongruity.

Non-articular osteochondroses

At tendon attachments

- *Osgood–Schlatter's disease (tibial tubercle traction apophysitis):* failure of the tibia tubercle apophysis due to repetitive traction stress from the extensor mechanism in boys (aged 12–14yrs) > girls (aged 10–12yrs). Usually a self-limiting condition with complete resolution through physiological healing (physeal closure) of tibia tubercle within 12–24mths. Presents with painful swelling over a prominent tibial tubercle (usually unilateral), associated with running/jumping. An irregular fragmented tibial tubercle may be seen on X-ray. Treatment includes non-operative (activity modification, rest +/− ice +/− knee brace), physiotherapy (isometric hamstring and quadriceps exercises), medication (NSAIDs), and operative (occasionally excision of separate ossicles may improve symptoms after skeletal maturity).
- *Sinding–Larsen–Johansson syndrome:* related condition arising at distal end of the patella.

At ligament attachments

Adam's disease (medial epicondyle)

Repetitive injury to the elbow following throwing/serving sports (e.g. racquet sports). Results in medial epicondylar fragmentation or avulsion and delayed closure of the growth plate. May have ulnar nerve involvement and point tenderness over the medial epicondyle.

Treated with rest/change of activities, splintage, analgesia (NSAIDs). Gradual return to activities once symptoms have settled. May need surgery to excise loose bodies.

At impact sites

- *Kohler's disease:* infarction of the navicular bone presenting as medial midfoot pain and a limp in young children (males > females) especially with load-bearing sports. Treated with rest from load-bearing sport, in soles/casts. If symptoms are severe, child may need to be non-weight-bearing with gradual return to activities depending on symptoms.
- *Sever's disease:* calcaneal apophysitis. Caused by repeated microfracture (with subsequent inflammation and healing) of the fibrocartilaginous insertion of the tendo-Achilles to the calcaneum during the pubertal growth spurt. Symptoms vary depending on the level of activity and it improves with skeletal maturation. There may be a bony prominence at the tendon insertion due to overgrowth during healing response. Treatment symptomatic NSAIDs, heel cord stretching.

Osteogenesis imperfecta

See also 📖 pp.763, 838. An inherited condition affecting collagen maturation and organization. The incidence is around 1/20 000. Osteogenesis imperfecta (OI) is due to a mutation in type I collagen gene that predisposes
to fracture formation. Following a fracture, initial bone healing is normal,
but there is no subsequent remodelling and the bone heals with deformity.
10% are clinically asymptomatic.

Clinical features

- *Bones:*
  - low birth weight/length for gestational age;
  - short stature;
  - 50% scoliosis.
  - *Joints:* ligamentous laxity resulting in hyperextensible joints.
- Specific signs and X-ray features (see Table 20.2).

Investigations and diagnosis

- Prenatal US scan may detect severe forms in foetus.
- Molecular genetic testing (pre- or postnatal).
- *Biochemistry:* normal/increased alkaline phosphatase (ALP).
- *Skin biopsy:* assess collagen in cultured fibroblasts.
- *Bone biopsy:* histology—increased Haversian canal + osteocyte lacunae
  diameters, increased cell numbers.

Treatment No curative treatment. Aim to prevent and manage fractures with long-term rehabilitation.

Prevention Strategies to decrease fracture frequency include:

- oral calcium supplements;
- bisphosphonates;
- synthetic calcitonin.

Surgical interventions

Intramedullary rods (fixed length/telescoping) to prevent bowing of long
bones, especially for fractures in children >2yrs old. Corrective surgery for
scoliosis deformities >50°.

Prognosis

In severe OI a good predictor of future walking is being able to sit by
10mths. May develop cardiopulmonary or neurological complications.
Usually develop progressive shortening and deformity caused by multiple
fractures, e.g. 'sabre' tibia, 'accordion' femora.

Table 20.2 Osteogenesis imperfecta: Sillence classification

IU fractures	Eyes (sclera)	Bones	X-ray features: thin cortices; osteopenia
Type I Mild; AD (60–80%). Presenile hearing loss in 30–60%, often with aortic valve regurgitation *			
No	Blue	Frequency of recurrent fractures decreases after puberty; diaphyseal > metaphyseal fractures; usually ambulatory	Wormian bones on SXR (occipital)
Type II Perinatal. Lethal (stillborn/death within first year); AD			
Yes	Blue	Relative macrocephaly, large fontanelles, micromelia, triangular facies with beaked nose, bowed limbs, legs abducted 90°	'Beaded' ribs—respiratory insufficiency
Type III Progressive and deforming (most severe non-lethal type) AR			
Yes	White	Pectal deformity, triangular facies, relative macrocephaly, abnormal teeth, easy bruising, severe osteoporosis (fractures), progressive shortening, deformity	'Popcorn' metaphyses, flared lower ribs, vertebral compression
Type IV Moderately severe, AD. Usually able to attain community ambulation skills *			
Yes	White	Bowed long bones, relatively infrequent fractures (frequency decreases after puberty). Moderately short stature	Osteoporotic, metaphyseal flaring, vertebral compression
Type V Moderately deforming; AD			
No	White	Mild/moderate; short stature	IO calcification; hyperplastic calus
Type VI Moderately/severely deforming			
No	White	Short stature, scoliosis	'Fish scale' bone lamellation
Type VII Moderately deforming; AR			
No	White	Short stature; short proximal limbs	

IU, Intrauterine; AD, autosomal dominant; AR, autosomal recessive. * Type A, no teeth involvement; type B, dentinogenesis imperfecta present.

Osteopetrosis

Also known as marble bone disease or Albers–Schönberg disease. This is a rare chromosomal condition defined by failure of osteoclastic bone resorption and hence failure of remodelling.

Classification

- *Malignant/infantile type:* AR. Severe skeletal deformity presenting at birth or shortly after. Poor prognosis. Bone marrow transplantation may help in some cases.
- *Benign type:* AD. Later childhood/adulthood benign presentation. Prone to frequent fractures.

Clinical features

- *Face:* macrocephaly, hydrocephalus, 'abnormal eyes' (optic atrophy, partial oculomotor nerve paralysis), compression of other cranial nerves resulting in deafness, facial nerve palsy.
- *Teeth:* late eruption; early caries, osteomyelitis, and necrosis of mandible.
- *Limbs:* generalized osteosclerosis, fragile bones (due to failure to form lamellated bone in stress areas) with fractures that are difficult to fix and prone to delayed union, dwarfism.
- *Haematological:* encroached marrow cavities leading to anaemia, pancytopenia, spontaneous bleeding/bruises. Spleen (extra medullary haemopoiesis leading to hepatosplenomegaly).
- *Kidneys:* causes distal renal tubular acidosis (type 1 RTA).

Investigations

- *Blood:* pancytopenia and leucoerythroblastic picture (increased primitive cells in blood film). Dry bone marrow tap.
- *X-rays:* dense 'marble' bone (generalized increased density with loss of normal trabecular pattern).
- *Skull:* underdeveloped mastoid air cells and paranasal sinuses.
- *Long bones:* widened ends ('Erlenmeyer flask' proximal humerus/distal femur).
  - *phalanges*—dense transverse band in metaphysis close to epiphyseal line, condensed bone proximal and distal ends of phalanges;
  - *metacarpals*—'bone within a bone' appearance—sclerotic cortex separated from central bone by area of normal calcification;
  - *vertebral bones*—'sandwich/rugger jersey' appearance—relative sclerotic upper and lower plates;
  - *bone scan*—increased uptake in epiphyseal ends of long bones; normal elsewhere.

Treatment

Depends on severity of disease and is mainly supportive. Medical therapy includes glucocorticoids. Bone marrow transplant may help. Treatment of fractures is difficult due to dense bone quality.

Prognosis Malignant type—usually terminal within first 10yrs of life. Benign form—lifespan unaffected.

Cleidocranial dysplasia

Also known as cleidocranial dysostosis. Characterized by deficient ossification of the clavicle (cleido) and bones of skull (cranial). It is a rare congenital autosomal dominant condition.

Clinical features

- *General:* proportionate mild short stature. No mental retardation.
- *Cranium:* large skull, frontal and parietal bossing, delayed imperfect ossification of sutures and fontanelles.
- *Face:* underdeveloped/deficient facial bones leading to prominent forehead, pseudoexophthalmos, and hypertelorism (due to small wide nasal bridge and widely spaced shallow orbits); protruding mandible.
- *Dental:* high arched/cleft palate, late loss of deciduous teeth with slow disordered eruption of secondary teeth (= extra/absent teeth).
- *Ears:* hearing loss +/– frequent ear infections.
- *Upper limb:* mobile drooping shoulders; completely absent/partially absent clavicle (especially lateral part, usually unilateral); recurrent dislocation shoulder/elbow; short middle and distal phalanges; long second metacarpal.
- *Torso:* narrow thorax and pelvis.
- *Spine:* delayed vertebral ossification; scoliosis/lordosis; kyphosis; prominent cervical transverse processes.
- *Lower limbs:* tubular phalanges of feet.

Investigations

- *Skull:* multiple imperfect ossification centres (wormian bones); large open anterior fontanelle; absent/delayed development of sinuses; hypoplastic maxilla.
- *Clavicle:* total absence/partial absence of lateral aspect clavicle (commonest) or bipartite clavicle.
- *Shoulder:* subluxation of humeral heads.
- *Pelvis:* delayed ossification pelvic bones with widened symphysis pubis; coxa vara of hips.
- *Spine:* failure of union of neural arches. Association with syringomelia
- *Renal tract:* association with Wilm's tumour requires imaging kidneys.

Treatment

Usually abnormalities cause little functional disability. Lateral part of clavicle may cause brachial plexus problems (if so, for excision). Recurrent dislocations of the shoulder may require stabilization. Dental anomalies should be treated by maxillofacial surgeons. Coxa vara may require valgus osteotomy.

Prognosis Normal lifespan.

Skeletal dysplasias

This is a heterogeneous group of conditions characterized by abnormal growth of bones. They can be classified according to the region of bone involved or by their genotype (see Table 20.3).

Radial dysplasia

An absent or hypoplastic radius that causes abnormal radial deviation of the hand. This is the most common form of longitudinal upper limb deficiency and is often accompanied by a congenitally absent thumb. Anomalies of other systems may also be associated.

- TAR.
- FA.
- *Holt–Oram syndrome:* AD; cardiac anomalies, and radial dysplasia.
- VACTERL (vertebral anomalies, anal atresia, cardiac malformations, tracheo-oesophageal fistula, renal and limb anomalies).

Management

- Serial castings/splinting.
- Surgery is usually required to place the hand in position to maximize function. If a thumb is absent, pollicization of the index finger could improve function. The index finger is reconstructed and radially positioned to form a functional 'thumb'.

Table 20.3 Classification of skeletal dysplasia

Region	Example of	
	Hypoplasia ('failure of')	Hyperplasia ('excess of')
Epiphysis		
Articular cartilage	Spondyloepiphyseal dysplasia	Dysplasia epiphysealis hemimelica (Trevor's)
Ossification centre	Multiple epiphyseal dysplasia	
Physis		
Proliferating cartilage	Achondroplasia	Marfan's syndrome
Hypertrophic cartilage	Metaphyseal chondrodysplasia (Schmid, McKusick, Jansen)	Enchondromatosis
Type 2 collagen	Diastrophic dysplasia	
Proteoglycan metabolism	Kneist syndrome	
Metaphysis		
Intramembranous bones	Cleidocranial dysostosis	
Formation of primary spongiosa	Hypophosphatasia	
Absorption of primary spongiosa	Osteopetrosis (functionally deficient osteoclasts)	
Diaphysis		
Diaphyseal aclasia		Multiple exostoses fracture
Periosteal bone formation		Engelmann's disease
Endosteal bone formation		Hyperphosphataemia (vitamin D resistant rickets)

Juvenile idiopathic arthritis

JIA is a common chronic childhood disorder (UK prevalence 1/1000; incidence: 1/10 000). It is a diagnosis of exclusion in children <16yrs old with a history of at least 6wks of persistent arthritis. JIA is divided into 7 subsets for research purposes.[1] These are not diagnostic categories, but are useful clinical groups. As a child's symptoms evolve with time (e.g. the appearance of a psoriatic rash), they may change subtype.

Classification of JIA[1]

- *Systemic arthritis:* relative frequency, 10–13%. See 📖 p.772.
- *Oligoarthritis (persistent or extended):* relative frequency, 40%. See 📖 p.773.
- *Polyarthritis (rheumatoid factor +ve):* relative frequency, 3%. See 📖 p.774.
- *Polyarthritis (rheumatoid factor –ve):* relative frequency, 27%. See 📖 p.776.
- *Psoriatic arthritis:* relative frequency, 2–15%. See 📖 p.777.
- *Enthesitis-related arthritis:* relative frequency, 1–7%. See 📖 p.778.
- *Undifferentiated arthritis:* relative frequency, 2–15%.

Differential diagnoses of childhood arthritis

- *Infection:*
  - *bacterial*—septic arthritis; osteomyelitis (📖 pp.738–741);
  - *viral*—rubella; parvovirus B19; infectious mononucleosis (📖 p.711);
  - Lyme, *Brucella*, TB (📖 pp.702, 712, 722).
- *Post-infection:*
  - reactive arthritis;
  - post-streptococcal reactive arthritis;
  - rheumatic fever (📖 p.244).
- *Malignancy:*
  - leukaemia (📖 p.656);
  - neuroblastoma (📖 p.666);
  - 1° bone tumours—benign or malignant;
  - metastatic disease.
- *Orthopaedic:*
  - Perthes and other osteochondritides (📖 p.750);
  - slipped upper femoral epiphysis (📖 p.752);
  - hip dysplasia (📖 p.748);
  - infantile coxa vara;
  - chondromalacia patellae (📖 p.754);
  - irritable hip (📖 pp.734–737).
- *Hypermobility:*
  - *benign hypermobility*—local or generalized;
  - Marfans, Ehlers–Danlos (📖 pp.838, 940);
  - IBD (📖 p.332).

- *Connective tissue disease:*
  - SLE (📖 p.780);
  - juvenile dermatomyositis (📖 p.782);
  - *systemic sclerosis*—limited or progressive (📖 p.786).
- *Metabolic disorders:*
  - gout;
  - mucopolysaccharidoses (📖 p.986).
- *Haematological:*
  - SCD (📖 p.620);
  - other haemoglobinopathies (📖 p.622);
  - haemophilia (📖 p.636).
- *Vasculitis:*
  - HSP (📖 p.788);
  - polyarteritis/microscopic polyangitis
  - Kawasaki disease (📖 p.716);
  - Takayasu arteritis (📖 p.791).
- Immunodeficiency syndromes.
- *Other inflammatory disorders:*
  - sarcoid;
  - chronic recurrent multifocal osteomyelitis (📖 p.740);
  - SAPHO (synovitis, acne, pustulosis, hyperostosis, and osteitis).
- *Idiopathic pain syndromes:*
  - chronic regional pain syndromes;
  - fibromyalgia
  - *'non-organic pain'*—a cry for help (📖 pp.310, 592).

Reference

1 Petty RE, Southwood TR, Manners P, *et al.* (2004). International League of Associations for Rheumatology classification of juvenile idiopathic arthritis: second revision, Edmonton 2001. *J Rheumatol* **31**: 390–2.

Juvenile idiopathic arthritis: clinical principles and management

Before labelling child with diagnosis of JIA it is imperative to exclude the differential diagnoses, the most important of which are sepsis, malignancy, and trauma (see 📖 p.736).

History from carer and child

- Limp, stiffness and loss of function, pain, or malaise.
- Onset usually gradual. Beware of misleading history of trauma as young children frequently fall without significant injury.
- History of non-use, or change in use.
- Child may not complain of pain. Infant may be 'irritable'.
- *Inflammatory symptoms:* worse after rest or inactivity.
- Stiffness is rarely volunteered. Parents sometimes describe child as 'like a little old person in the mornings'. Toddler's behaviour may be perceived as being difficult and uncooperative (e.g. refusing to move in the morning, then running in the afternoon).
- History of associated rash, fever, weight loss.
- History of sore throat, URTI, antecedent infections, and travel.
- Family history of arthritis, psoriasis, colitis, rheumatic fever, or acute iritis.

Examination

- Observe the child before they become self-conscious.
- Watch them playing and walking.
- Examine all the joints and spine for swelling, warmth, pain on movement, or limited movement.
- Measure for leg length inequality and pelvic tilt.
- Examine muscle bulk around affected joints.
- Assess general muscle strength.
- Examine the skin, hair and nails for rashes, psoriasis.
- *General examination:* vital signs, height, weight, and BP.
- Examine mouth and palate for ulcers, dentition; fauces for asymptomatic tonsillitis; heart for murmurs; abdomen for hepatosplenomegaly.

Investigations

- FBC may show mild anaemia and thrombocytosis.
- Neutrophilia suggests sepsis or systemic JIA.
- *Severe anaemia or thrombocytopenia:* consider leukaemia.
- ESR/CRP usually normal or mildly elevated. Very high levels suggest infection or malignancy. High ESR plus thrombocytopenia suggests leukaemia.
- *Infection screen:* throat swab, urinalysis, blood for ASOT, viral serology (CMV, EBV, parvovirus B19, hepatitis) and culture.
- *Rheumatoid factor:* non-specific test, but significant in polyarthritis (>5 joints). Exclusion criterion for oligoarticular JIA.

- *ANA:* non-specific (5% children ANA +ve). In oligoarticular JIA limited prognostic determinant for iritis.
- Muscle enzymes (CK, LDH, aldolase) raised in dermatomyositis, but can be normal. Very high LDH suggests malignancy.
- *Imaging:*
  - *radiographs*—exclude fracture or tumour; *early JIA*—soft tissue swelling, and juxta-articular osteopenia; *later*—joint space narrowing and erosions;
  - *US*—helpful for confirming synovitis and joint effusion;
  - *MRI*—useful for atypical monoarthritis; gadolinium-enhanced MRI is gold standard for diagnosis of synovitis, but does not differentiate from sepsis.
- *Synovial fluid aspirate:* culture for sepsis. Microscopy rarely helpful.

Management

General

- Establish diagnosis and counsel child and parents.
- Start treatment as soon as possible.
- Most children will need regular hospital review to look for presence or reappearance of thickened synovium or effusions.
- *Exercise:* regular, daily aerobic and 'range of motion' exercises.
- *Psychological support for children and carers:* education and support groups (e.g. Arthritis Research Campaign).
- Ask about school performance and support at school.
- Adolescents may need counselling about contraception and alcohol if taking MTX.
- *Amyloidosis:* rare complication of severe disease.

Joints

- Minimize pain and stiffness using NSAIDs:
  - ibuprofen (30–40mg/kg);
  - diclofenac (1.5–2.5mg/kg bd);
  - naproxen (5–15mg/kg bd);
  - piroxicam (5–20mg daily according to weight).
- *Prevent deformity:* regular daily exercises; night splints; intra-articular steroid injections (triamcinolone) may settle inflammation for years.
- *Control disease activity:* MTX oral or SC in resistant cases.
- *Etanercept:* anti- tumour necrosis factor (TNF) if unresponsive to NSAIDs and SC MTX.

Eye screen for uveitis

Must have regular screening, initially 3-monthly, by experienced ophthalmologist. Treat with topical steroids and midriatics. Course is independent of joint disease severity. Potentially blinding.

Growth Measure growth velocity; nutritional status; muscular atrophy.

Dentition Watch for caries.

> Once the diagnosis is established the child should be looked after by a paediatric rheumatologist for specialist drugs and co-ordinating multidisciplinary support.

Systemic arthritis

Multisystem disease is often diagnosed late as joint involvement is often late. Peak age 2–3yrs; 10–20% JIA; equal male:female.

Clinical features

- Fever is essential, typically quotidian up to 39°C, returning to normal between attacks.
- *Rash:* salmon pink, macular/urticarial on chest, trunk, and intertrigones. Present when warm and disappears within minutes.
- Myalgia, arthralgia, and arthritis. Arthritis often appears after first 6mths of illness and can be oligo- or polyarthritis.
- Generalized lymphadenopathy and hepatosplenomegaly.
- Polyserositis with pericarditis, pleuritis, and sterile peritonitis. Silent pericardial effusions (15%). Myocarditis + tachycardia, cardiomegaly, and congestive cardiac failure is rare.
- Growth retardation 2° to disease, steroids, or joint damage.
- *Late complications:* amyloidosis (difficult to treat).
- *MAS:* rare, life-threatening; precipitated by infection or NSAIDs. Haemophagocytic bone marrow with falling WBC, platelets, and ESR, and very high ferritin.

Investigations

- FBC (normocytic or hypochromic anaemia; leucocytosis; thrombocytosis).
- *ESR/CRP can be high:* use to monitor disease during treatment.
- *Hypoalbuminaemia:* multifactorial—poor diet, general ill health with catabolism, possibly proteinuria secondary to renal amyloid.
- ANA and RF usually –ve.
- Viral titres and blood cultures.
- *Malignancy screen:* CXR, US abdomen.
- ECG and echocardiogram.

Management

- NSAIDs for initial management of pain, fever, and serositis. Indomethacin often used for pericarditis.
- Pulsed IV corticosteroids if no improvement after 1wk of NSAIDs.
- Oral steroids at 1mg/kg in divided doses until fever settled and inflammatory markers normal. Taper dose to reduce side-effects. Use alternate day doses and add steroid-sparing agent.
- MTX is used, but is not as effective as in other JIA subsets.
- Intra-articular corticosteroid for flares of single joints.
- *Biological therapy:* anti-TNF and anti-IL6 in resistant cases.

Prognosis

Three groups—monocyclic (11%); recurrent or polycyclic (34%); and persistent (55%). Monocyclic patients do well. More than 33% of the others will have permanent disability with active disease in adult life. Death from infection, MAS, or amylodosis.

Oligoarticular juvenile idiopathic arthritis

- Commonest subtype (previously known as pauciarticular JCA/JRA). 40% of patients.
- *Two subsets are recognized:* persistent and extended. If the number of joints increases to more than 4 within the first 6mths of illness, it is termed extended oligoarticular JIA.
- Children may develop silent, blinding iritis (anterior uvertis). It is usually ANA-positive patients (40–75% of this form of illness) who are at risk of developing iritis.

Clinical features

- Diagnosis of exclusion; rule out infection.
- Milder symptoms than reactive arthritis; no constitutional symptoms.
- Often present with joint swelling or limping rather than pain.
- 2/3 single joint; 1/3 only 2 joints; often asymmetrical; knees, ankles, elbows, wrists common, but any joint possible.
- Careful examination may reveal more extensive disease as the child may be too young to express pain.
- Elbows and knees may lack full extension, but not be painful.
- Affected leg may overgrow; measure leg lengths and check pelvis is level.
- Observe gait for circumduction to compensate for limb overgrowth.

Investigations

- FBC; CRP (usually normal); ANA (prognostic value for uveitis).
- *X-ray:* exclude fracture, tumour; look for overgrowth and damage.

Management

- Regular review to assess joints, eyes, and general growth.
- *NSAIDs for pain and stiffness:* full dose for 8wks (ibuprofen, diclofenac, naproxen, or piroxicam).
- *Intra-articular steroid injections:* may settle inflammation for years.
- If not controlled with oral NSAIDs and intra-articular steroids, MTX oral or SC is used in resistant cases.
- Rarely etanercept (anti-TNF therapy) is needed.
- *Screen for uveitis:* initially 3-monthly, by ophthalmologist.

Disease course and prognosis

- 80% normal at 15yrs. 'Extended' subset have worse prognosis.
- Uveitis is most important extra-articular complication.

Rheumatoid factor-positive polyarthritis

A chronic symmetrical inflammatory polyarthritis (>5 joints) with positive RF on two occasions at least 3mths apart. Typically affects teenage girls, though any age possible. Similar to adult rheumatoid arthritis, but generally a more aggressive disease.

ARA criteria for diagnosis of rheumatoid arthritis[1]

- *Morning stiffness:* >1hr at peak illness
- *Arthritis in at least 3 joints:* witnessed by a physician
- *Hand arthritis:* wrists, MCPs, or PIPs
- Symmetrical arthritis
- Rheumatoid nodules
- Rheumatoid factor-positive
- Erosions on X-ray

All symptoms need to be present for at least 6wks. Four or more criteria need to be fulfilled for diagnosis of rheumatoid arthritis (RA). These are primarily classification criteria (90% sensitivity and specificity).

Clinical features

- History of early morning and immobility stiffness.
- Symmetrical arthritis affecting large and small joints associated with rheumatoid nodules. Wrists and PIPs affected early. Hip involvement can be aggressive and lead to early hip replacement.
- Tenosynovitis common around fingers and ankles.
- *Systemic features:* low grade fever (differential diagnosis systemic JIA); hepatosplenomegaly; lymphadenopathy; serositis (pericarditis and pleurisy).
- *Eyes:* uveitis rare; dry eyes relatively common (10–35%); episcleritis can lead to a painful red eye.

Investigations

- FBC; CRP; LFTs; RF; ANA.
- Renal function and urinalysis.
- X-rays of affected joints and CXR.

Management

- Monitor disease activity and aim for good control of arthritis.
- Regular meticulous assessment for tender and swollen joints, muscle wasting, joint damage, and loss of joint function.
- Monitor growth development and nutritional status.
- *Exercise:* range of joint motion and aerobic activity.
- Psychosocial development can be severely affected and needs addressing.

Treatment

- Start treatment as soon as possible.
- NSAIDs provide relief from pain, stiffness, and swelling.
- All children will need disease-modifying antirheumatic drug (DMARDs): MTX is the least toxic and most well established—orally or SC. Others include hydroxychloroquine, sulfasalazine, azathioprine, ciclosporin, and gold. These have been used in combination with MTX or alone.
- *Steroids:* intra-articular steroids to settle synovitis in individual joints; oral steroids as adjunct to DMARDs; pulsed IV steroids for flare of disease. Aim to minimize total steroid load.
- *Biologic agents:* Anti-TNF agents (etenercept, infliximab, adalimimab) have been shown to reduce joint erosions and may prevent progression to secondary arthritis

Prognosis Most children survive into adulthood though with poor functional outcome because of aggressive, unremitting disease, early erosions, and high incidence of joint replacement. The use of aggressive, early systemic MTX and biological therapies may have improved this outcome.

Reference

1 Arnett FC, Edworthy SM, Bloch DA, *et al.* (1988). The American Rheumatism Association 1987 revised criteria for the classification of rheumatoid arthritis. *Arthritis Rheum* **31**(3): 315–24.

Rheumatoid factor-negative polyarthritis

30% of JIA cases. Previously known as polyarticular onset JCA. Characterized by 5 or more affected joints within first 6mths.

Clinical features

- *Diagnosis of exclusion:* IgM RF-negative 3mths apart.
- *Systemic features:* low grade fever and transient rashes possible, but mild.
- Asymmetrical joint involvement of any joint including jaw, cervical spine, wrists and fingers, and subtalar joints.
- Joint swelling leads to limited mobility and muscle wasting.
- Chronic hyperaemia leads to accelerated bone growth and premature cartilage fusion. Common sites: carpus, subtalar, jaw (micrognathia, dental malocclusion); cervical spine (C3–5 apophyseal joint fusion with instability above and below).
- Tenosynovitis and bursitis around fingers and feet.
- Flexion contractures at elbows, knees, and hips.

Investigations

- *Blood:* FBC, CRP, ANA.
- *X-ray:* affected joints.

Treatments

Start treatment as soon as possible.

- NSAIDs for 8wks in adequate dose, plus intra-articular steroids to target joints.
- Start DMARDs early to try and induce remission with oral or SC MTX (use sulfasalazine or azathioprine if intolerant to MTX; see 📖 p.775).
- *Remission:* continue NSAID for 6mths and DMARD for 1yr.
- *Persistent arthritis:* intra-articular steroids into target joints + combination DMARDs.
- *Etanercept:* anti-TNF therapy if intolerant or unresponsive to MTX.

Prognosis

Heterogeneous group of conditions with variable prognosis. Prognosis has dramatically improved in recent years with the aggressive use of MTX and anti-TNF therapy. However, up to a third will have persistent deformity, disability, and disease activity into adult life.

Psoriatic arthritis

Recently recognized, underdiagnosed subset of JIA; 2–15% of children with JIA; unknown aetiology on a background of strong genetic predisposition (up to 50%).

ILAR criteria for diagnosis of psoriatic arthritis[1]

- Inflammatory arthritis in presence of psoriasis, or inflammatory arthritis with dactylitis or psoriatic nail changes plus a first-degree relative with psoriasis.
- *Exclusions:* RF +ve; HLA-B27 +ve in male >6yrs; any enthesitis-related arthritis or uveitis in first-degree relative; systemic arthritis.

Clinical features

- Arthritis and rash rarely present simultaneously. Rash usually precedes arthritis.
- *Arthritis:* commonest is asymmetrical large joint (knees or ankles). Small joint polyarthritis of fingers and toes (metacarpal phalangeal (MCP), proximal interphalangeal (PIP), and distal interphalangeal (DIP) joints) and dactylitis are also common. Some children have tendonitis or tenosynovitis, especially around the ankles.
- *Skin:* predominantly plaque psoriasis (examine extensor surfaces of elbows and knees, hairline, behind the ears, around the umbilicus, groin, and natal cleft; see 📖 p.810).
- *Nails:* pitting, ridging, onycholysis, subungual hyperkeratosis.
- *Uveitis:* needs regular screening as can potentially blind.
- Psoriasis affects up to 3% of normal population; the association with inflammatory arthritis may be coincidental.

Investigations

- *No specific tests:* need exclusion bloods (see 📖 p.734).
- *Often evidence of chronic inflammation:* raised CRP; thrombocytosis; and low grade normocytic anaemia.

Radiographs

- Periarticular osteopenia and soft tissue swelling.
- Periosteal new bone formation, particularly in dactylitis.

Treatment

Important to diagnosis dactylitis. NSAIDs are the mainstay of treatment. Intra-articular steroid injections often help settle inflammation. Methotrexate and ant-TNF agents are effective for persistent disease.

Prognosis Arthritis can be episodic and continue into adult life. A few patients have a very destructive course with arthritis mutilans.

Reference

1 Petty RE, Southwood TR, Manners P, et al. (2004). *International League of Associations for Rheumatology classification of juvenile idiopathic arthritis*, 2nd revision, Edmonton 2001. *J Rheumatol* 31: 390–2.

Enthesitis-related arthritis

Recently introduced ILAR terminology and category.[1] Previously known as juvenile ankylosing spondylitis or seronegative spondyarthropathy. Characterized by arthritis with enthesitis (inflammation in any tendinous, ligamentous, or muscular insertion on to bone) or arthritis alone or enthesitis alone with 2 of the following features:

• sacroiliac joint tenderness;
• inflammatory spinal pain;
• HLA B27 +ve;
• first degree relative family history of uveitis;
• age of onset 6 >yrs.

Exclude RF +ve; systemic arthritis; psoriasis in patient or first degree relative.

Clinical features

• Commonly adolescent or pre-adolescent boys (M:F, 10:1).
• Oligo- or polyarthritis predominantly in lower limbs.
• Enthesitis especially around the foot (heel pain). Children can present with isolated heel pain many years before spinal symptoms.
• Spinal pain may not be present at onset.
• Progresses to sacroiliac joint tenderness, inflammatory spinal pain, or buttock pain (worse at night plus early morning stiffness).
• Systemic features: low grade fever, weight loss, and fatigue.
• Acute anterior uveitis (10–15%): acutely painful red, photophobic eye—different from uveitis seen with other JIA.
• Associated IBD and reactive arthritis.

Examination

• Examine affected joints: for synovitis, effusions, associated muscle wasting, and range of movement.
• Spine examination: is essential. Test for cervical rotation, thoracic rotation, lateral flexion, and document the Schober test (mark 10cm above and 5cm below the 'dimples of Venus' and note the increase gained by forward flexion). Normal is at least 21cm—varies little with age and gender. Look for loss of normal lumbar lordosis.
• Chest expansion: may be reduced in advanced disease.
• Examine commonly affected enthesitis sites around the heel: Achilles insertion and calcaneum.

Investigations

• FBC (normochromic anaemia, mild leucocytosis, and thrombocytosis).
• If microcytic anaemia think of occult IBD.
• CRP may be raised.
• RF and ANA negative.
• HLA B27 +ve 90%, but also +ve in 8–10% of normal population.

Radiology

X-ray changes lag behind clinical symptoms by up to 10yrs. MRI is the gold standard in adults. Interpretation is difficult in children. Lateral views may show Romanus lesions (small erosions of the corners of the vertebral bodies).

X-rays

- *Affected joints:* soft tissue swelling, periarticular osteopenia, erosions, joint space narrowing, bony ankylosis.
- Heel may show calcaneal spur or fluffy exostoses on Achilles.
- Sacroiliac joints may show erosions, sclerosis, and fusion.
- Thoracolumbar junction may show bony overgrowth syndesmophytes.

Reference

1 Petty RE, Southwood TR, Manners P, *et al.* (2004). International League of Associations for Rheumatology classification of juvenile idiopathic arthritis: 2nd revision, Edmonton 2001. *J Rheumatol* **31**: 390–2.

Systemic lupus erythematosus

Complex, multisystem autoimmune disorder affecting adolescents (rare in younger children; female:male ratio 20:1). Commoner and more severe in Afro-Caribbean, Hispanic, and Far Eastern girls.

The ARA criteria are helpful (90% sensitivity 97% specificity), but less reliable in early disease.[1] One of the 'great mimics' of other conditions.

The revised ARA criteria for the classification of SLE[1]

SLE is diagnosed if 4 of the 11 features present simultaneously or serially:
- Malar rash
- Discoid rash
- Photosensitivity
- Mouth ulcers
- Arthritis (non-erosive)
- *Serositis:* pleurisy or pericarditis
- *Renal disease:* persistent proteinuria >0.5g/24hr or cellular casts
- *Neurological disorder:* psychosis or seizures in absence of known precipitants
- *Haematological abnormality:* haemolytic anaemia or leucopenia <4.0 × 10⁹/L on 2 or more occasions or thrombocytopenia <100 × 10⁹/L
- *Immunological:* raised anti DNA binding antibody, anti-Smith antibody, and/or +ve antiphospholipid antibodies
- Antinuclear antibody

Clinical features

The presenting complaint may affect any organ system.
- *Non-specific constitutional symptoms common:* low grade fever, weight loss, fatigue, anorexia, and lymphadenopathy.
- *Mucocutaneous problems:* hair loss (scarring and non-scarring alopecia); mouth ulcers; photosensitivity (50%); Raynaud's phenomenon (90%); malar 'butterfly' rash over bridge of nose and sparing nasolabial folds; discoid lesions; livido reticularis; urticarial rashes; purpuric rashes; digital vasculitis.
- *Musculoskeletal (90%):* polyarthritis resembling rheumatoid arthritis (non-erosive); tendonitis; arthralgia; myalgia; myositis (5%); aseptic necrosis.
- *Cardiovascular:* pericarditis (silent or rapidly constrictive); myositis, valvulitis with endocarditis (Libman–Sachs).
- *Pulmonary:* pleurisy; pleural effusions; haemoptysis from pulmonary vasculitis; interstitial fibrosis; pneumonitis.
- *Renal:* hypertension; proteinuria; nephritis; nephrotic syndrome; renal failure.
- *Haematological:* anaemia (normochromic normocytic, Coombs +ve haemolytic, renal failure, drug-related); leucopenia and lymphopenia common (80%); thrombocytopenia (20%) chronic, rarely aggressive.

- *Neurological:* migraine (40%); mood disorders (anxiety, depression, emotional liability (70%)); psychoses (rare); seizures (rare); peripheral neuropathies (10%).
- *Careful drug history:* especially tetracyclines for acne (+ve antihistone antibodies).

Investigations

FBC, LFTs; renal function; BP measurement; urinalysis; ANA (99%), dsD-NA (40% , but specific for SLE); RF; coagulation screen; anticardiolipin and antiphospholipid antibodies. ESR may be raised; CRP low unless serositis or infection; C3, C4 low in active disease.

Management: in specialist clinic

- *General:* avoid sun exposure and use sun-screen; treat hypertension; and minimize long-term cardiovascular risks. Use ACE inhibitors for nephroprotection for proteinuria.
- Target and treat aggressively affected organs.
- NSAIDs for musculoskeletal symptoms.
- Hydroxychloroquine for fatigue, rashes, and arthritis.
- Prednisolone and steroid-sparing drugs (azathioprine (AZA), MTX, mycophenolate mofetil (MMF)) for other severe manifestations.
- Prednisolone and cyclophosphamide for active nephritis; then AZA or MMF.
- *Experimental treatments for refractory cases:* rituximab; autologous stem cell replacement.

Prognosis

- Very variable between ethnic groups. Overall 5-yr survival 90% with death from unremitting active disease or immunosuppression.
- Prognosis worse for those with nephritis (60% after 15yrs).
- Bimodal survival curve with long-term increased risk of cardiovascular disease.

Reference

1 Tan EM, Cohen AS, Fries JF, et al. (1982). The 1982 revised criteria for the classification of systemic lupus erythematosus. *Arthritis Rheum* **25**: 1271–7.

Juvenile dermatomyositis

Autoimmune inflammatory disease of skin and muscles. Rare (incidence 2–3 per million) and occurs between ages of 10 and 14yrs. Cause unknown; infectious and environmental triggers are likely.

Diagnostic criteria for juvenile dermatomyositis (JDM)*

Erythematous rash plus two other criteria:
- Symmetrical weakness of proximal muscles
- Periorbital oedema with heliotrope discoloration; scaly rash over MTPs and PIPs (Grottron's papules)
- Elevation of one or more muscles enzymes: CK, AST, LDH, aldolase
- EMG changes of myopathy and denervation
- Muscle biopsy evidence of necrosis and inflammation
- MRI (has largely superseded EMG and muscle biopsy in children)

*Modified from Bohan A, Peter JB. (1975). Polymyositis and dermatomyositis. *N Engl J Med* **292**: 403–7.

Clinical features
- Onset usually insidious, rash may precede muscle weakness.
- *Rash:* periorbital oedema with heliotrope discolouration of upper lids; facial rash includes nasolabial folds (unlike SLE); erythematous maculopapular rash over extensor surfaces of MCP, PIPs, elbows, and knees (Grottron's papules); nail-fold vasculitis.
- *Muscles:* typically symmetrical proximal muscle weakness with fatiguability of arms and legs; truncal weakness (unable to sit from lying); 'Gower's sign' (🕮 p.733); palatal and respiratory muscles affected in severe cases with nasal speech, poor swallowing, decreased lung volume.
- *Arthritis* (60%): 2/3 oligoarthritis; 1/3 polyarthritis.
- *Lung disease* (uncommon): interstitial fibrosis; pulmonary vasculitis.

Diagnosis is usually made by typical rash, proximal muscle weakness, raised muscle enzymes, and typical MRI changes.

Differential diagnosis Infectious myositis (usually viral); overlap with autoimmune disorder (SLE and mixed connective tissue disease (MCTD)); systemic arthritis JIA.

Late complications
- *Calcinosis:* linked with active myositis; occurs in skin, fascia, subcutaneous fat and muscle. Superficial lesions may be painful, erupt, and discharge. Sheets of calcification may prevent movement and usually resolve with time. Tumoural deposits may be surgically removed.
- *Lipodystrophy:* generalized or partial; painless; generalized form associated with insulin resistance, diabetes, liver disease, and short stature.

Investigations

- *Muscle enzymes:* CK; LDH; aldolase; AST; ALT.
- *ANA (6–60%):* may be raised; Myositis-specific antibodies rarely present in children.
- *ESR and CRP:* variable.
- *MRI (STIR or T2 fat suppressed):* diffuse white signal throughout affected muscles.
- *EMG:* low amplitude, short-duration polyphasic potentials with early recruitment, fibrillations, and repetitive discharges.
- Muscle biopsy can show histological evidence of necrosis and inflammation.

Monitoring

- *Regular examination:* muscle strength testing and muscle enzymes.
- Aim to maintain function, normalize muscle enzymes, and limit steroid effects on growth.

Course and treatment The condition may be uniphasic, polyphasic, or continuous. Corticosteroids are the mainstay of treatment. Methotrexate is used in more severe and persistent severe cases as a steroid-sparing drug. Cyclophosphamide is used in some centres for vasculitis. Treat for 18mths after remission induced. Some evidence that aggressive treatment may minimize calcinosis.

Mixed connective tissue disease— overlap syndromes

Combined features of SLE, progressive systemic sclerosis, and dermatomyositis with positive ribonucleoprotein (RNP) antibody.

- Prognosis and management similar to that of SLE , but more benign prognosis because renal and CNS involvement are rare.

Clinical features

- Raynaud's phenomenon (common).
- Swollen hands and fingers (common).
- *Polyarthritis:* symmetrical peripheral.
- *Rashes:* similar to SLE or JDM rash; tight non-elastic skin of hands. See also 📖 p.839.
- Muscle weakness and myositis.
- Restrictive lung disease and pulmonary hypertension (rare).

Differential diagnosis

- Systemic onset JIA (📖 p.768).
- RF-positive polyarticular JIA (📖 p.774).
- SLE (📖 p.780).

Investigations

- Characteristic anti-RNP antibody.
- *Other autoantibodies:* ANA +ve (90%); RF +ve (often).
- *FBC:* leucopenia; thrombocytopenia.
- CXR.
- Renal function.
- *Echocardiogram:* screen for right ventricular hypertrophy secondary to pulmonary hypertension in established disease.

Scleroderma

Hard, tight, inelastic skin and subcutaneous tissue. Female to male ratio is 2:1. Two distinct syndromes.

Localized scleroderma (morphoea, linear scleroderma)

- Lesions confined to the skin are termed morphoea.
- Lesions that involve the underlying tissues, sometimes down to bone, are termed linear scleroderma (LS).
- In both types there is an initial inflammatory phase with single or multiple flesh-coloured or erythematous plaques. These evolve into firm, waxy, yellow-white shiny lesions with violaceous borders.
- Growth of the region under LS is arrested and this can result in severe growth and cosmetic deformities.
- Linear lesions across the forehead to the nose are termed 'en coup de sabre'. These lesions may extend down to the brain and be associated with epilepsy.
- Oligoarthritis (10%) can precede skin changes.
- Oesophageal involvement not infrequent, but no other systemic changes.

Systemic sclerosis (SSC or progressive systemic sclerosis PSS)

- Raynaud's phenomenon is universal (often the presenting symptom); severe attacks can result in digital ischaemia, ulceration, and bony resorption.
- Skin changes follow with oedema and inflammation. Symmetrical involvement of the metacarpal phalangeal (MCP) joint and metatarsal phalangeal (MTP) joints.
- Finger oedema lasts for several weeks and is replaced by taut, waxy, shiny, thickened skin that eventually becomes atrophic. Finger tip skin may crack ('mechanics's hands').
- *Facial involvement:* pinched nose, expressionless façade, and decreased gape.
- Nail folds are ragged with telangiectasia.
- *Joints:* stiff from overlying scleroderma. Occasional oligoarthritis.
- Dysmotility and bowel wall thickening can occur throughout the bowel leading to malabsorption, wasting, bloating, abdominal cramps, diarrhoea, or severe constipation.
- Pulmonary fibrosis and pulmonary hypertension are initially asymptomatic. When more severe they lead to dyspnoea, syncope, and death.
- Myocarditis, pericarditis, and arrhythmias reported.
- Renal disease with crisis used to be commonest cause of death.

Investigations

- FBC, ESR; LFTs, renal function including BP; ANA, anti-centromere, and anti-topoisomerase antibodies.
- CXR; ECG; echocardiogram to screen for pulmonary hypertension.
- LFTs and CT scan if fibrosis or pulmonary hypertension.

Treatment and management

No treatment is consistently effective in slowing or preventing fibrosis and sclerosis in severe progressive cases. MTX, mycophenolate, ciclosporin, and low dose steroids have been used in the inflammatory phase. Steroids and ciclosporin may precipitate scleroderma renal crisis (check for hypertension and treat with ACE inhibitors).

Symptomatic treatment depending on organ involvement:
* *Raynaud's:* hand warmers; double gloves; oral or topical vasodilators; prostacyclin for severe attacks and digital gangrene;
* *GI tract:* avoid NSAIDs. Metoclopramide aids gut motility; proton pump inhibitors for acid secretion; pancreatic supplements.

Prognosis

* *Localized scleroderma:* generally good prognosis. Cosmetic deformities may occur if bone involvement with linear scleroderma.
* *SSC/PSS:* poor prognosis. 5yrs survival 34–73%. Death from pulmonary hypertension and renal crisis.

Henoch–Schönlein purpura

Small vessel vasculitis associated with IgA immune complexes. A triad of arthritis, colicky abdominal pain, and palpable, papular, purpuric rash. Characteristically affects prepubertal boys.

Clinical features

- *Skin rash:* palpable purpura over buttocks and lower legs. Severe skin vasculitis can lead to oedema (dorsum hand, scrotum, and periorbital).
- *Arthritis:* typically short-lived affecting large joints (knees, ankles, or elbows).
- *Gastrointestinal:* colicky abdominal pain (commonest), malaena, haematemesis, intussusception, perforation, appendicitis.
- *Renal:* dipstick haematuria and proteinuria present (50%). Glomerulonephritis and nephrotic syndrome rare.

Investigations

- FBC, renal function, dipstick urinalysis, and full renal investigation with biopsy if evidence of renal involvement (crescentic IgA glomerulonephritis).
- *Skin biopsy rarely necessary:* leucocytoclastic vasculitis.
- Abdominal investigations as per symptoms.

Treatment and prognosis

Most cases have a benign course with complete resolution of symptoms within 6wks. NSAIDs help arthritis symptoms. Corticosteroids for abdominal pain and arthritis may hasten symptom resolution. Test for haematuria because nephritis and nephritic syndrome carry worse prognosis for hypertension and decreased renal function.

Polyarteritis nodosa

Rare, medium-vessel necrotizing vasculitis with aneurysm formation. Male:female ratio 2:1.

Clinical

- Antecedent systemic illness with unexplained fevers, abdominal pains, and arthralgia of up to 1yr.
- Testicular pain in males (often mistaken for torsion).
- Vasculitis or purpuric skin rash.
- *Arthritis (30%) large joints:* exquisite bony tenderness from peripheral vasculitis and periosteal new bone formation.
- *Renal:* hypertension; haematuria, proteinuria; renal failure; intrarenal aneurysms.
- *GI involvement* (50%): abdominal pain; pancreatitis; bowel infarction.
- *CNS:* mononeuritis multiplex; peripheral neuropathy; fits; hemiplegia.

Investigations

- FBC; LFTs may be elevated.
- *Renal function* urinalysis for active sediment.
- MRI; MR angiography to reveal multiple aneurysms.
- *Histology:* panarteritis with fibrinoid necrosis, thrombosis, infarction, weakening of artery walls, and aneurysms. Segmental lesions at bifurcations of small- and medium-vessel walls.

Course and treatment Without treatment may be fatal. Often under recognized and undertreated in children. If treated promptly, with pulsed cyclophosphamide and high dose steroids, prognosis improved.

Wegener's granulomatosis

Triad of **ANCA** positive small vessel vasculitis, respiratory tract granulomata, renal disease. Rare. Usually diagnosed in adolescents (male = female). *Staphylococcus aureus* may have role in pathogenesis since 3 times greater carriage in Wegener's granulomatosis (WG).

Clinical features

- Subacute disease can be present for years. Transformation into systemic disease (malaise, fever, weight loss, vasculitis) occurs.
- *ENT (90%):* nasal crusting, obstruction, and ulceration; serous otitis media; sinusitis. Nasal septum and sinus wall destruction (saddle nose deformity).
- *Pulmonary (80%):* subglottic stenosis (stridor); haemoptysis (25%); lower bronchial obstruction with atelectasis and pneumonia; pulmonary haemorrhage; asymptomatic nodules.
- *Renal (90%):* varies from mild asymptomatic (commoner microscopic haematuria; mild renal impairment) to fulminant diffuse necrotizing crescentic glomerulonephritis and renal failure.
- *Arthritis (50%):* non-erosive polyarthritis; muscle and joint pains common (60%).
- *Skin (40%):* palpable purpura of leucocytoclastic vasculitis; livido reticularis; pyoderma gangrenosum.
- *CNS (30%):* mononeuritis multiplex and sensorimotor peripheral neuropathy.
- *Eye lesions:* episcleritis; uveitis; orbital pseudotumour.

Investigations

- *Blood:*
  - FBC (normocytic, normochromic anaemia, leucocytosis, thrombocytosis). ESR and CRP raised (differential diagnosis: infection);
  - renal screen with BP measurement and urinalysis at each visit. Renal biopsy if active sediment and declining renal function;
  - CANCA (proteinase 3) positive in 90% patients with generalized WG. High specificity.
- *Lungs:*
  - CXR, sputum culture, and cytology; CT lungs; bronchoscopy and biopsy if indicated.
  - CT sinuses +/– nasendoscopy and biopsy.
- *Histology:* necrotizing, giant cell, granulomatous, medium vessel vasculitis in respiratory tract.

Course and treatment

- *Systemic disease:* treated with pulsed IV cyclophosphamide and steroids to induce remission. Remission maintenance with MTX or AZA. Minimize total steroid load. Only stop after min. 12mths disease-free.
- *Subacute and limited disease:* have variable (milder) course; may respond to MTX alone or with low dose steroids. Long-term co-trimoxazole in remission reduces pulmonary infection and relapse rates. 10yr survival 75%; morbidity considerable.

Takayasu's arteritis (pulseless disease)

Rare chronic granulomatous panarteritis affecting aorta and large arteries. Adolescent Asian (Japanese) girls and young women most susceptible.

Clinical features

- *Subclinical prepulseless phase may last years:* anorexia, fatigue, poor growth, unexplained fevers, and episodic arthritis (50%).
- *Pulseless phase:* diagnoses often made incidentally.
  - diminished peripheral pulses and aortic dilatation on CXR or hypertension and renal artery stenosis;
  - dramatic presentation with severe hypertensive encephalopathy and seizures; congestive cardiac failure; aortic valvulitis and aortic regurgitation; pulmonary stenosis;
  - syncope 2° to paroxysmal hypertension or paroxysmal tachycardias with facial flushing headaches, chest pain, dyspnoea, and palpitations. May be triggered by changes in posture or micturition (i.e. baroreceptor hypersensitivity).

Investigations

- FBC (normochromic normocytic anaemia, thrombocytosis); ESR and gamma globulins very elevated even in the prepulseless phase.
- *Imaging:* high resolution carotid US, angiography, or MR angiography show characteristic arterial dilatation, post-stenotic dilatation, aneurysm, thrombosis, and occlusion of the proximal branches of the aorta.

Treatment

- *Manage hypertension:* β-blockers and ACE inhibitors. Avoid vasodilators.
- *Treat vasculitis:* initially high dose steroids (prednisolone 1mg/kg/ day or equivalent) with MTX or AZA as steroid-sparing drugs. Cyclophosphamide for severe or resistant cases.
- *Surgery:* range from angioplasty to bypass grafting.

Prognosis

10yr survival 90%, although the majority (75%) have some impairment of daily living, and 50% are disabled. Prognosis depends on hypertension and aortic incompetence. Successful planned pregnancy is possible.

Adolescent health

Communication

See also 📖 pp.575–576, 1034, 1038. The primary goal of any consultation with an adolescent, regardless of the presenting complaint, is to establish a relationship of trust. This calls for effective and efficient communication. However, achieving this is often difficult and challenging, particularly when faced with a personality who is undergoing rapid psychological and social change, and who does not have an adult's perspective of health issues and society. Young people may be seen by themselves, as well as with their parents. Parents should not be excluded, but it is important to emphasize that the adolescent is the centre of the consultation. Communication of information should be in a manner appropriate for development.

Have a style of communication that is:
- open;
- sensitive;
- empathetic;
- non-judgemental.

A positive regard and respect for any differing values and practices should be exhibited. At all times there must be reassurances about confidentiality.
- Use an open-ended questioning style.
- Avoid medical jargon and inappropriate reassurance of normality.
- Allay fears and anxieties.
- Abstract concepts should be avoided.

The HEADSS protocol (Box 21.1) is a psychosocial history toolkit specifically designed for adolescent health-related consultations.[1]

Box 21.1 The HEADSS protocol*

H   Home life including relationship with parents
E   Education or employment, including financial issues
A   Activities including sports (also note friendships and social relationships, especially close friendships)
A   Affect (mood, particularly whether mood is responsive to situations)
D   Drug use, including cigarettes and alcohol
S   Sex (information on intimate relationships and sexual risk behaviours may be important in both acute and chronic illnesses in adolescents)
S   Suicide, depression, and self-harm
S   Sleep

*Reproduced from Christie D, Viner R. (2005). Adolescent development. Br Med J **330**: 301–4, with kind permission from BMJ (adapted from reference 1).

Reference
1 Goldenring J, Cohen E. (1998). Getting into adolescents HEADSS. *Contemp Pediatr* Jul, 75–80.

Adolescence: overview

Adolescence is the transition period before adulthood. A number of physical and psychological objectives are achieved.

Physical and psychological objectives of adolescence

- Achievement of physical maturation.
- Achievement of sexual maturation.
- Attainment of personal identity.
- Establishment of independence.
- Establishment of autonomy.
- Development of sexual relationships.

Adolescence is therefore filled with major changes that need to be taken into account when caring for adolescents with health-related problems.

Management of adolescents: key areas to consider

Communication issues

Appreciation of adolescent-relevant issues, e.g. sex/drugs/smoking.

Physical examination

- Privacy and personal integrity.
- Pubertal assessment.

Psychosocial issues

- Personal identity.
- Compliance.

Ethical and legal issues

- Consent.
- Competence.
- Confidentiality.

All those working with adolescents need to acquire the appropriate skills to manage and communicate effectively with young people.

Psychological development

Adolescence marks the beginning of the development of more complex thinking processes. These include:

- The ability for abstract thinking (thinking about possibilities).
- The ability to reason from known principles (form own new ideas
- or questions).
- The ability to consider many points of view according to different
- criteria (i.e. compare or debate ideas or opinions).
- The ability to think about the process of thinking.

During adolescence, young people acquire the ability to think systematically about all logical relationships within a problem. The transition from concrete thinking to formal logical conclusions occurs over time. Each adolescent progresses at varying rates in developing his/her ability to think in more complex ways. Some adolescents may be able to apply logical operations to school work long before they are able to apply them to personal dilemmas. When emotional issues arise, they often interfere with an adolescent's ability to think in more complex ways. The ability to consider possibilities, as well as facts, may influence decision-making, in either +ve or −ve ways. The interactions that occur between puberty and psychological development are important, esp. in the context of developing self-esteem and a sense of sexuality and body image.

Social development

Adolescence marks the period of time during which there is a gradual shift in the balance between dependence on others to position of independence. The timing of this process is variable and will depend on the social and cultural environment.

Physical development

Psychological and social changes occur against a background of physical changes of puberty.

Adolescent health problems

The WHO defines adolescence as the period between 10 and 19yrs of age and, in most developed countries, this accounts for 13–15% of the population. In the UK adolescent health problems are increasing. This is thought to be a reflection of poor investment in health care delivery to young people, and also of the increasing proportion of adolescents who are of low socioeconomic status and who belong to ethnic minority groups.

Adolescent mortality

The improvement in mortality rate observed in other age groups over recent decades has not been mirrored in adolescents. The most common cause of death in this age group is traumatic injury (particularly road traffic accidents) and poisoning. Suicide among late teenage males has doubled in the last 3 decades.

Adolescent health problems

The pattern of adolescent illness is distinct. Some of the most common concerns that we see in adolescents are summarized in the Box 21.2.

An increasing trend has been observed in the following adolescent health problems in recent years:

- Substance misuse (📖 p.800).
- Sexual health problems (📖 p.801).
- Mental health problems (see 📖 pp.568, 578–585).
- Obesity (see 📖 p.400).

Box 21.2 Common adolescent-related health problems

- Acne (📖 p.822)
- Chronic illness
  - diabetes mellitus (📖 p.406)
  - cystic fibrosis (📖 p.270)
  - cancer
- Chronic fatigue (📖 p.990)
- Somatic symptom disorders (📖 p.592)
  - chronic pain
  - headache (📖 p.516)
- Constitutional delay in growth and puberty (📖 p.468)
- Substance abuse (📖 p.800)
  - alcohol
  - smoking
  - illicit drugs
  - cannabis
- Psychological problems
  - ADHD (📖 p.600)
  - anxiety disorders (📖 p.584)
  - conduct/behaviour disorders (📖 p.598)
  - depression (📖 p.578)
  - eating disorders—anorexia nervosa (📖 p.594); bulimia nervosa (📖 p.596)
  - school phobia (📖 p.991)
  - stress-related symptoms (📖 p.586)
- Gynaecological disorders
  - oligomenorrhoea/dysmenorrhoea
  - polycystic ovarian syndrome
- Sexual health problems
  - teenage pregnancy (📖 p.801)
  - sexually-transmitted infections (STIs) (📖 p.801)
- Obesity (📖 p.400)
- Sports-related injuries

Substance misuse

Misuse of alcohol, tobacco, and illicit drugs is becoming common amongst adolescents, and causes health problems in this age. Alcohol and tobacco are the most commonly used substances, and are thought to account for 95% of the morbidity and mortality in this age range. Most adolescents who use alcohol or tobacco do not progress to using illicit substances. However, most users of illicit drugs will have used alcohol and tobacco.

- *Alcohol:* in the UK, by 15yrs of age, 40–50% of adolescents will have drunk alcohol. 'Binge' drinking is prevalent in certain societies.
- *Smoking:* smoking rates have not changed in the last 20yrs. In the UK, by 15yrs, 21–26% admit to smoking regularly.
- *Illicit drugs:* cannabis is the most commonly used substance in teenagers in most developed countries. 30% have had experience by 15yrs.

Risk factors for substance misuse

The adolescent and his/her environment

- *Personality traits:* antisocial personality disorder.
- *Behavioural problems:* conduct disorder; depression.
- *Familial factors:* favourable attitudes to substance use; poor or inconsistent parenting practices.
- Early age experience of substance misuse.
- Peer group pressure.
- Poor social environment and relationships.

Signs of substance misuse

- *Non-specific:*
  - emotional changes;
  - personality changes;
  - depression;
  - mood swings;
  - social difficulties;
  - decline in school attendance/performance;
  - behaviour changes;
  - physical changes, e.g. increased fatigue.
- *Signs of drug usage:*
  - pupil constriction;
  - skin changes: venepuncture marks.
- *Withdrawal effects:*
  - agitation/tremor;
  - dilated pupils.

Signs of substance dependence

- Difficulty controlling/limiting substance use.
- Tolerance: the need for greater amounts to achieve same effect.
- Signs and symptoms of withdrawal when substance unavailable.

Sexual health problems

See also 📖 pp.576, 1002. Sexual health is a priority for adolescent care. The median age of first sexual experience in the UK is around 16yrs of age.

Sexual health matters: areas that should raise concern

- Age <13yrs.
- Suspect age or power imbalance in relationships.
- Evidence of bribery and coercion.
- Overt aggression.
- Misuse of substances as a disinhibitor.
- Whether the behaviour places him/her at risk so that he/she is unable to make an informed choice.
- Attempts to secure secrecy made by the sexual partner.
- Whether the sexual partner is known to social services or police.
- Whether the child denies, minimizes, or accepts concerns.

Experience of sex at an early age is often associated with unsafe sex practice. This may be due to lack of knowledge, or access to contraception, being under the influence of drugs, or inability to resist peer pressure. Unsafe sex practices may lead to unwanted pregnancies and STIs.

Adolescent pregnancy

The UK has one of the highest rates of teenage pregnancy in Europe (approx 20–25 per 1000 women aged 15–19yrs). Many such pregnancies occur within marriage. Most unwanted teenage pregnancies occur in the context of poverty, low educational achievement, and adverse social factors (e.g. mental health problems, sexual abuse, and crime). Infants of teenage mothers are at increased risk of being low birth weight (SGA). Prevention of teenage pregnancies is a high priority. Health promotion and sex education are successful in this area.

Sexually transmitted infections

Rates of STIs in UK 16–19yr olds in the UK are increasing. The highest rates of infection occur in Afro-Caribbeans and Africans. 30–40% of sexually active girls in high-risk groups may be infected with *Chlamydia*.

Adolescents: risk factors for STIs

- Avoidance of barrier contraception methods.
- Multiple, sequential, or concurrent partners.
- Mental illness.
- Substance misuse.

Clinical symptoms and signs similar to adults.

Symptoms of Chlamydia in adolescents

- *Males:* asymptomatic (50%); urethritis or discharge.
- *Females:* asymptomatic (70%): confidential screening/testing programmes have been proposed and a national *Chlamydia* programme has been available in the UK since 2006; vaginal discharge (especially early adolescence); pelvic inflammatory disease.

Adolescence and chronic illness

A chronic illness is defined as a condition lasting at least 6mths. The number of young children surviving into young adulthood with a congenital or chronic health problem is increasing. In addition, the prevalence of certain chronic lifelong conditions (e.g. type 1 diabetes) is increasing. It is estimated that 20–30% of young people may have a chronic illness.

Impact on the adolescent

Teenagers with a chronic illness are disadvantaged compared with their healthy peers. Their illness can impact on physical, psychological, emotional, and social development and well-being:

Consequences of chronic illness on adolescent development

Physical

Constitutional delay in growth and pubertal development (📖 p.468).

Psychological
- Poor self-esteem.
- −ve body self-image.
- Sense of alienation.
- Depression.
- Anxiety.
- Behavioural problems.

Social and educational
- Poor school performance.
- Social isolation/integration.

Impact on the family

Chronic illness can adversely impact on the adolescent's family. Parents have to provide additional time for care and support of the teenager with a chronic illness, often with financial consequences. Parents may experience guilt, frustration, and anxiety, and the frequency of mental health problems is increased. Siblings are also disadvantaged, often missing out on parental time and attention. The support of specific agencies and child and adolescent psychology services is often required and may be helpful.

Impact on health professional relationships

Young people are usually more concerned about the 'here and now' issues of adolescence, and less interested in the long-term consequences of their treatment and their behaviour towards it. This often leads to a conflict of priorities between health professionals (and parents) and the adolescent, and may lead to problems with compliance. Improving compliance may be helped by the following:

Treatment discussions
- Should be developmentally and cognitively appropriate.
- Should be alone and in confidence.
- Adopt a non-judgemental approach.
- Explore understanding of illness and treatment. Correct any misunderstanding and educate.
- Identify potential barriers to adherence.
- Avoid medical jargon.
- Encourage treatment 'routine'.

Treatment goals
- Should be relevant to (current) adolescent issues, e.g. appearance, socializing, recreational opportunities.
- Include the adolescent in negotiations.
- Keep goals short-term (weeks–months).
- Use simplest regimen possible.
- Tailor to the adolescent's daily routine.

Treatment application
- Give written instructions.
- Suggest simple reminder strategies, e.g. 'stickies', calendar.
- Enlist support and help from parents, family, peers.

Transition to adult health services

Adolescents requiring ongoing specialist hospital care will eventually need transfer to 'adult' health care services. This transition requires more than a 'simple' transfer of medical records from one service to another. There are many different models of transition of care (e.g. direct paediatric to adult service or indirect via an intermediary 'adolescent' or young adult service). Transition should be carefully planned and the adolescent patient, and their family, should be given plenty of time to consider and prepare. Transition should not take place at a fixed, predetermined age, but rather at a point when the adolescent is ready and has the necessary coping skills to deal with the adult clinic. Personalized transition plans are needed for each patient and careful communication, co-ordination, and organization are required between the paediatric and adult teams.

Dermatology

Assessment of a rash

History
- When did the rash start?
- Where did the rash start?
- Any exacerbating or relieving factors?
- Is it itchy?
- Any contacts with patients with the same rash?
- General drug history?
- Recent medications or skin treatments?
- Past medical history?
- Family history?
- Any recent foreign travel?

Examination
- Undress child and inspect all the skin.
- Describe 1° lesion morphology:
  - *macule*—flat circumscribed lesion <1cm diameter;
  - *papule*—raised palpable circumscribed lesion <1cm diameter;
  - *nodule*—palpable mass >1cm diameter;
  - *plaque-like*—large disc-shaped lesion;
  - *vesicle*—blister containing clear fluid <0.5cm diameter;
  - *bulla*—blister containing clear fluid >0.5cm diameter;
  - *pustule*—visible blister containing pus;
  - *erythematous*—blanching and red;
  - *purpura*—red-purple non-blanching discoloration of the skin due to extravasation of red cells;
  - *petechia*—purpuric lesions <2mm diameter;
  - *telangiectasia*—permanently dilated visible small blood vessels that blanch on pressure;
  - *wheal*—raised, itchy, white papule surrounded by red flare;
  - *scaly*.
- Describe distribution of 1° lesion, e.g. diffusely scattered, linear.
- *Look for and describe:*
  - 2° changes, e.g. excoriation (scratch marks);
  - pigmentation;
  - scarring;
  - atrophy (thinning of the skin);
  - lichenification (skin thickening);
  - sclerosis (induration of skin, often due to increased collagen production);
  - erosion (partial thickness loss of epidermis);
  - ulceration (full thickness loss of epidermis and possibly dermis);
  - crusting (due to dried exudates).
- *Palpate:* may be impalpable, hard, firm, soft, tender, hot. If lesion is red, test if it blanches on pressure.
- *General examination:* taking care to examine nails, scalp, and mouth.

Atopic eczema/dermatitis

The terms atopic eczema and atopic dermatitis are used interchangeably.
- One of the most common skin diseases affecting children, with a prevalence of 5–15% in developed countries.
- The age of onset is less than 6mths in 75%.
- Flare-ups are commonly due to dry skin, irritants, infection, sweating/ heat, emotional stress, and occasionally allergies.

Aetiology
- Genetic susceptibility.
- Impaired epidermal barrier function.
- Immune dysregulation.
- Allergen (food and airborne) sensitization and infection play a lesser role.

Presentation
See Plate 1.
- Acute eczema may be erythematous and weeping.
- Chronic eczema may be lichenified and dry.
- There are often 2° changes of excoriation, post-inflammatory hypo/ hyperpigmentation and infection.
- Infant eczema often affects cheeks, elbows, and knees with crawling.
- Childhood eczema is often flexural; also affects the wrists and ankles.
- Adolescent and adult eczema is also flexural, but may also affect the head and neck, nipples, palms, and soles.

Treatment
- *General measures:* soap avoidance, e.g. soap free bath oil or wash. Limit showers/baths to 5–10min in lukewarm water. Moisturize immediately after showering. Wear loose fitting cotton undergarments. Avoid over heating. Keep finger nails short.
- *Specific measures:* use topical corticosteroids daily until the eczema is clear, then taper off on alternate days for 1wk and then twice weekly before stopping. If the eczema returns resume once daily application until clear and then recommence taper.
  - ointments are generally better than creams;
  - wet dressings improve efficacy and can be done at home;
  - swab suspected infection (viral PCR, immunofluorescence or culture and bacterial cuture);
  - treat promptly with antibiotics or antivirals after this;
  - sedative antihistamines may improve sleep at night for those older than 2yrs.
- In those not improving, review the causes for flare-ups (see ⬚ 'Presentation', above). They may need admission to hospital for intensive wet dressings or referral to a dermatologist for consideration of phototherapy or systemic therapy.
- *For mild eczema:* a mild potency topical corticosteroid ointment, e.g. 1% hydrocortisone, is appropriate daily for anywhere on the body.

- For mild to moderate eczema, a moderate potency topical corticosteroid ointment: e.g. clobetasone butyrate 0.05%, is appropriate and safe for daily use on the face and body, but not the groin.
- For moderate to severe eczema, a potent topical corticosteroid ointment, e.g. mometasone furoate, is appropriate daily for the body, but not the face or groin.

Complications

- Sleep disturbance.
- Emotional upset.
- Family dysfunction.
- Eczema herpeticum (HSV)
- *Staphylococcus aureus* infection
- Growth delay.
- Atopic cataracts.

Prognosis

The natural history tends towards resolution with age. Predicting this is difficult, however, early onset severe disease with associated atopy (hayfever and asthma), and elevated IgE may be associated with a worse prognosis.

Red scaly rashes

Atopic eczema

See 📖 p.808.

Psoriasis

Psoriasis affects 1–2% of the population. One third develops the disease before age 20. It is an immune mediated disorder of T cells. There is a strong genetic component in childhood psoriasis, however, environmental factors such as infection (streptococcal and HIV), stress, smoking (pustular psoriasis) and drugs (beta blockers, calcium channel blockers, thiazides, lithium, interferon and antimalarials) also play a role.

Presentation

See 📖 Plate 2.

- Red, well-demarcated plaques with overlying silvery scale.
- Classically affects elbows, knees, and scalp.
- However, facial (40%) and napkin (25%) psoriasis is a common presentation in children.
- The clinical appearance may be site-modified in the scalp (concretions), genital area (glazed), palms and sole (pustules).
- Variant presentations include guttate (small plaque), annular (ring-like), pustular and erythrodermic (>90% skin affected).
- Common nail signs include pitting, onycholysis (separation of the nail plate from the nail bed) and subungual hyperkeratosis (distal thickening).
- Psoriatic arthropathy may develop (see 📖 p.777).

Treatment

General measures

- Soap avoidance.
- Moisturize immediately after bath/shower.
- Provide emotional support (very important).
- Remove any precipitating triggers.

Specific measures

- Topical steroids
- Topical tar and salicylic acid creams
- Topical calcipotriol (vitamin D derivative)
- Those patients that do not respond to topical therapy and general measures may be referred to a dermatologist for consideration of phototherapy and systemic agents (acitretin, cyclosporin, methotrexate and biologics).

Prognosis May be life-long or spontaneously remit.

Contact dermatitis

Irritant contact dermatitis

In children irritant contact dermatitis due to urine, faeces and friction in the napkin area is common. It spares the folds, favours convexities and there may be 2° *Candida* infection. Frequent nappy changes, drying after bathing and use of a barrier cream may help to prevent this. Hydrocortisone cream in combination with an antifungal cream are the treatment of choice.

Allergic contact dermatitis

Allergic contact dermatitis (delayed type IV hypersensitivity) less common; often occurs in older children. Strong reactions often cause an acute blistering and weeping eczema. Common allergens include nickel (earrings), colophony (sticking plasters), topical medicaments (topical neomycin and preservatives), some henna tattoos, plants (e.g. poison ivy) and rubber. Treatment is allergen withdrawal and topical steroids.

Seborrhoeic dermatitis See 📖 pp.196, 841.

Pityriasis rosea

Self-limiting condition common between ages 1 and 6yrs.

Cause Probably 2° reaction to viral infections.

Presentation

- Distinctive initial truncal (usually) oval, red, scaly 'herald patch' (2–5cm diameter).
- Several days later generalized smaller scaly, yellowish-pink patches develop over trunk and proximal limbs.
- Characteristic 'Christmas tree' distribution common. Patches follow lines parallel to ribs.
- Pruritus, malaise, lymphadenopathy may occur.

Treatment Reassurance. Antipruritics may be required.

Prognosis Resolves after 4–6wks usually, but may persist for several months.

Tinea infections See 📖 p.828.

Papular rashes (1)

Urticaria (hives)

Acute urticaria affects 10% of the population at some time.

Pathophysiology Adverse stimulus → mast cell degranulation → histamine release → localized vasodilatation and ↑ capillary permeability.

Causes

Usually idiopathic or triggered by recent viral infection. Other causes include:
- Allergens (e.g. drugs, foods, inhalants, insect bites).
- Trauma (physical urticarias), e.g. dermographism due to light skin trauma (commonest), pressure, cold, heat, sunlight.

Chronic urticaria (defined as acute urticaria not resolving after 2mths) is idiopathic in >90%, but may be caused by:
- Chronic bacterial, fungal (e.g. oral *Candida*), or parasitic infection.
- Rarely, ingested food dyes.

Presentation

See ☐ Plate 3.
- Rapidly developing erythematous eruption with raised central white wheals and occasionally local purpura.
- Any part of body can be affected and often itchy.
- Lesions last 4–24hr.
- May have associated fever and arthralgia (serum sickness).

Investigation

Apart from good history investigation is usually not necessary. Skin prick testing is rarely helpful. If chronic, consider:
- FBC;
- throat swab (streptococcus);
- urine culture;
- exclude threadworms;
- food and symptom diary.

Treatment

- Oral antihistamines.
- Oral prednisolone, short course if severe.
- Avoid triggering factors, e.g. ingested food dyes and non-steroidal drugs.

Angioedema

Variant of urticaria with significant swelling of subcutaneous tissues, often involves lips, eyelids, genitalia, tongue, or larynx. If severe, may cause acute upper or lower respiratory tract obstruction and may be life-threatening.

Causes As for urticaria. *Hereditary angioedema* is a rare AD condition caused by active C1-esterase inhibitor deficiency.

Investigations and management As for urticaria. If hereditary angioedema is suspected then measure serum C4 complement level initially.

Treatment for severe angioedema
- Give facial oxygen.
- IM 0.1mL/kg adrenaline 1:10 000.
- IM/IV hydrocortisone 12-hourly.
- Nebulized salbutamol.

Prophylaxis
In severe and recurring cases of hereditary angioedema, tranexamic acid or anabolic steroids (e.g. danazole boosts liver production of C1-esterase inhibitor) are effective, but the latter is rarely used in childhood due to its androgenic effects.

Molluscum contagiosum

Common pox virus infection affecting infants and young children.

Presentation

Pink umbilicated (central dimple) papules. Usually affects moist areas, but can occur anywhere. Exacerbated by active eczema or topical steroids.

Treatment

None if uncomplicated as usually spontaneously resolves within a year. If problematic:
- Treat any associated eczema.
- Pinch forcep liquid nitrogen cryotherapy.
- Lesion curettage.
- Application of benzoyl peroxide 5% daily.

Scabies See 📖 p.829

Viral warts See 📖 p.826

Papular rashes (2)

Papular urticaria
Hypersensitivity reaction to insect bites. Itchy small red papules or vesicles evolve into 1–5mm papules +/− surrounding urticaria or surface crusting. Usually on limbs and buttocks. May last for weeks and be exacerbated by new bites elsewhere. Secondary infection common.

Treatment
- Prevent new bites.
- Antipruritics (e.g. oral antihistamines, topical steroids).
- Antibiotics for any 2° infection.

Keratosis pilaris
Common. Any age. Horny plugging of follicles causes asymptomatic rough papular rash +/− erythema. Affects upper outer arms, front of thighs, cheeks.

Treatment Reassurance; emollients, especially urea-based creams.

Papular acrodermatitis (Gianotti–Crosti syndrome)
- Acute, non-itchy, red papules appear over face, limbs, and buttocks.
- Asymptomatic or accompanied by malaise, hepatomegaly, lymphadenopathy.

Causes
- Enteroviruses.
- EBV.
- Adenovirus.
- Mycoplasma.

Treatment Reassurance.

Prognosis Spontaneously resolves after a few weeks.

Vesiculobullous rashes

Erythema multiforme

Cause

Immunologically mediated syndrome. May be idiopathic, but usually precipitated by infection (e.g. mycoplasma, herpes simplex, other viruses) or drugs (e.g. sulfonamides, penicillin).

Presentation

See 📖 Plate 4.
- Crops of characteristic symmetric 'target' lesions develop with pallid or purple centre surrounded by erythematous ring.
- May also be haemorrhagic, red macules or large bullae.
- Lesions last 2–3wks and affect hands, feet, elbows, knees.
- Typically, mucous membrane ulcers occur (buccal, eye, genitalia).

Treatment

If precipitating infection recurs treat early as tends to cause rash again, e.g. topical aciclovir for recurrent HSV.
- Fluid maintenance.
- Analgesic mouthwashes.
- Lip emollient ointment.
- Oral antihistamines.

Prognosis Complete recovery, but may recur.

Stevens–Johnson syndrome/toxic epidermal necrolysis

Severe, and overlapping condition with erythema multiforme except usually drug induced with viral infection rarely implicated.

Presentation

See 📖 Plate 5.
- Widespread blisters/bullae over erythematous, purple macular, or haemorrhagic skin.
- Mucous membranes often affected with haemorrhagic crusting.
- Rubbing may cause skin separation at epidermodermal junction (= positive Nikolsky sign).
- Also possible fever, arthralgia, myalgia, prostration, renal failure, pneumonitis, conjunctivitis, corneal ulceration, blindness.

Treatment

- Supportive, as for severe burns (e.g. hydration, airway protection).
- Identify causative antigen and remove/treat.
- Frequent emollient ointment.
- Specialist eye care.
- 👆 Systemic corticosteroids or immunoglobulin used in first 2–3 days may be helpful if life-threatening.

Prognosis Can be life-threatening. Recovery usually occurs in 3–4wks.

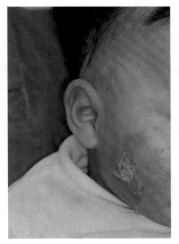

Plate 1 Atopic dermatitis.

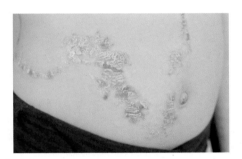

Plate 2 Psoriasis.

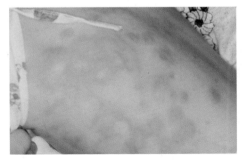

Plate 3 Urticaria.

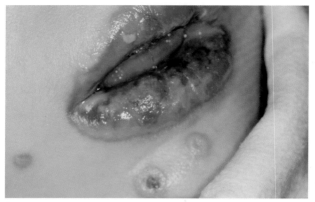

Plate 4 Erythema multiforme.

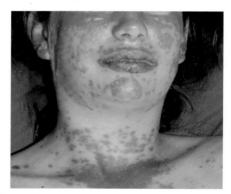

Plate 5 Stevens johnson syndrome.

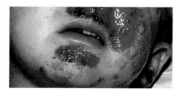

Plate 6 Epidermolysis bullosa.

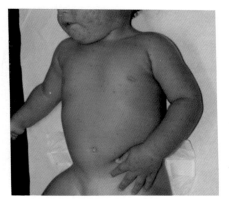

Plate 7 Viral exanthem.

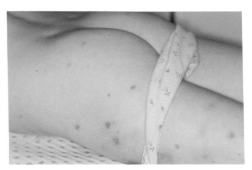

Plate 8 Henoch Schonlein purpura.

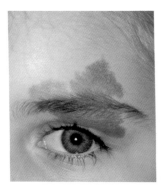

Plate 9 Capillary vascular malformation (port wine stain).

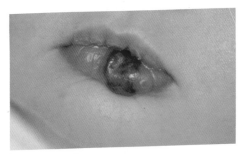

Plate 10 Infantile haemangioma.

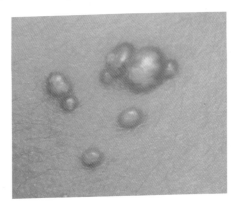

Plate 11 Molluscum contagiosum.

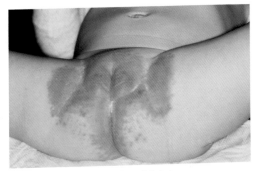

Plate 12 Irritant napkin dermatitis with candidiasis.

Staphylococcal scalded skin syndrome

Exotoxin-mediated epidermolysis 2° to *Staphylococcus aureus* infection (which may be trivial). Occurs in children <5yrs.

Presentation
- Extensive tender erythema with flaccid superficial blisters/bullae ('scalded appearance').
- Erosions and +ve Nikolsky sign.
- Crusting around eyes and mouth, fever.

Treatment
- Supportive treatment and analgesia.
- IV anti-staphylococcal antibiotics.
- Gentle skin care, emollient ointments.

Prognosis Rapid recovery without scarring.

Impetigo

Highly contagious *Staphylococcus aureus* or β-haemolytic streptococcal superficial skin infection. May be 1° or complicate other skin disease (e.g. HSV infection, eczema, scabies). Risk factors include overcrowding and poor hygiene.

Presentation
- Superficial, rapidly spreading initially clear blisters that rapidly develop into straw-coloured 'dirty' looking lesions with yellow crusting.
- Often starts around nose and face; neonates may develop bullous impetigo.
- Risk of staphylococcal scalded skin syndrome or acute glomerulonephritis (streptococcal).

Investigation Skin swabs for bacterial culture and sensitivity.

Treatment
Rapidly resolves if:
- bathe crusts off using antiseptics (contain infectious bacteria);
- antibiotics (e.g. topical mupirocin 2% ointment or oral flucloxacillin);
- treat any predisposing condition.

Eczema herpeticum See 📖 p.826

Traumatic blisters

Caused by friction, burns, or insect bites. Sterile aspiration of blister within 12hr after appearance, and pressure dressing may be curative.

Epidermolysis bullosa See 📖 Plate 6 and 📖 p.840

Other viruses See 📖 pp.826–827

Red blanching (erythematous) rashes

Causes vary with age. Viral causes commonest in younger children. In older children, eczema, psoriasis, and drug reactions (e.g. reaction to ampicillin in glandular fever) predominate.

Viruses (exanthem)

See 📖 pp.704–709. See 📖 Plate 7. Culprits include:
• adenovirus;
• enteroviruses (coxsackie or echovirus);
• EBV;
• influenza;
• parainfluenza;
• human herpes virus 6 (roseola infantum);
• parvovirus b19 (erythema infectiosum);
• rubella;
• measles.

Usually associated with fever and widespread non-specific macular or macular–papular erythematous rash. If child is significantly unwell, lethargic, or peripheral perfusion is reduced, admit and investigate (may be bacterial sepsis). Otherwise, simply reassure and advise symptomatic treatment.

Drug eruptions

Erythematous macular–papular rash commonest (e.g. to penicillins, cephalosporins, anticonvulsants). Drugs may also cause:
• Urticaria (e.g. opiates, NSAIDs, penicillins, cephalosporins).
• Exfoliative dermatitis (e.g. sulphonamides, allopurinol, carbamazepine).
• Erythema multiforme or Stevens–Johnson syndrome/toxic epidermal necrolysis (e.g. anticonvulsants, antibiotics and allopurinol).

Treatment
• Discontinue offending drug, may need prick or patch testing to identify.
• Symptomatic treatment (e.g. antihistamines or emollients for pruritus).

Erysipelas and cellulitis Conditions overlap. Erysipelas is superficial skin infection whereas cellulitis involves deeper subcutaneous tissues. Usually due to *Strep. pyogenes* or *Staph. aureus*; occasionally *Haemophilus influenzae*.

Presentation
• Tender, warm, spreading, sharply marginated erythema +/− oedema.
• May also have ascending red streaks of lymphangitis.
• Regional lymphadenopathy, fever, malaise.
• Deeper infection may co-exist, e.g. osteomyelitis.

Management
• Swab skin and blood culture.
• If erysipelas alone, IV penicillin (erythromycin if penicillin-allergic).
• *Cellulitis:* raise affected part (e.g. limb); combination of IV penicillin and flucloxacillin. Consider cefotaxime instead of penicillin if child aged <5yrs and not immunized against *Haemophilus*.

Erythema marginatum Crops of pink truncal rings (lesions fade rapidly, only to recur) caused by rheumatic fever. No treatment required.

Erythema nodosum

Typically affects older children. Caused by immunological reaction to:
- Tuberculosis.
- Streptococcal infection.
- Mycoplasma infection.
- IBD.
- Sulphonamides.
- Viruses.
- Idiopathic (30%).

Presentation

Multiple discrete, large, red, hot, tender nodules on shins (occasionally thigh and forearms) appear over 10 days. Nodules resolve over 3–6wks, with colour changes similar to fading bruises. Fever, malaise, arthralgia, particularly of knees, may also occur.

Management Investigate for infection. Treat underlying disease; give analgesics.

Sunburn

See also 📖 p.1024. Caused by excessive UV light exposure. Sun avoidance, skin covering, hats, and water-resistant high-factor sunscreens are preventative! Fair-skinned individuals, infants, and those with pre-existing hypopigmented disorders are at particular risk.
- *Presentation:* painful, tender erythema +/– blistering over exposed area. Resolves with skin peeling.
- *Treatment:*
  - Antipyretics;
  - Analgesics;
  - topical calamine lotion;
  - topical corticosteroids if severe.

Intertrigo

- *Cause:*
  - excessive friction between skin surfaces;
  - obesity is a predisposing factor.
- *Presentation:*
  - moist, erythematous eruption typically affecting the groin, axillae, neck, submammary areas;
  - 2° *Candida* infection common.
- *Treatment:*
  - treat inflammation and infection, e.g. topical antibiotic, topical antifungal and low potency topical steroid;
  - improve general hygiene;
  - expose to air.

Kawasaki disease See 📖 p.716

Septicaemia Meningococcal disease, as well as other bacterial pathogens, can present with an erythematous rash (see 📖 p.714).

Pruritus

Is the sensation provoking a desire to scratch? If severe, it leads to excoriation, papules or nodules (localized skin thickening), and lichenification.

Generalized pruritus

Causes

- Skin diseases (see Localized pruritus, p.820).
- Hepatic disease (bile salts).
- Food or drug reaction/allergy (e.g. penicillin).
- Underlying malignancy, particularly lymphoma.
- Chronic renal failure.
- Hypo- or hyperthyroidism.
- Parasites (e.g. scabies).
- Iron deficiency anaemia.

Investigation

In absence of obvious underlying skin disease:
- FBC.
- Blood film.
- CRP/ESR.
- Ferritin.
- LFT.
- U&E and creatinine.
- Glucose.
- TFT.

Treatment

- Treat causative disease.
- Bland topical emollients.
- Emollient bath oils.
- Night-time sedative, e.g. antihistamines.

Localized pruritus

Causes

- Atopic eczema (cheeks, hands, and limb flexures).
- Contact dermatitis.
- Urticaria.
- Insect bites.
- Fungal infection (e.g. tinea capitis).
- Head lice (pediculosis capitis).
- Scabies (finger webs, wrists, groin, buttocks).
- Psoriasis.
- Dermatitis herpetiformis (elbows, shoulders, genitalia, perineum, buttocks).
- Pityriasis rosea.
- Chickenpox.
- Dermatitis artefacta (!).

Investigation In absence of obvious underlying skin disease, investigate as for generalized pruritus.

Treatment As for generalized pruritis.

Pruritus ani
Localized peri-anal itching.

Causes
- Threadworms.
- Anal disease (e.g. anal fissure, haemorrhoids, Crohn's disease).
- Poor hygiene.
- Chronic faecal soiling.
- Chronic diarrhoea.
- Localized skin disease (e.g. candidiasis, psoriasis).
- Contact dermatitis (e.g. to toilet paper).
- Idiopathic.

Investigation Threadworms may be seen during anal inspection or their eggs seen on microscopy of 'sellotape' applied to the anus or skin swab culture.

Treatment
- Treat underlying disease.
- Improve perianal hygiene.
- Mild topical steroid may relieve once infective cause is excluded.

Pruritus vulvae
Localized perivulval itching.

Causes
- Idiopathic.
- Poor hygiene.
- Infection (e.g. candidiasis, trichomoniasis).
- Diabetes mellitus.
- Threadworm.
- Contact dermatitis.
- Localized skin disease (see pruritus ani), e.g. lichen sclerosus.

Treatment As for pruritus ani.

Pustular rashes

Generalized pustulosis is unusual. When the child is <2yrs, immunodeficiency, particularly phagocyte dysfunction, should be excluded. Local causes in older children include:

- acne vulgaris;
- folliculitis;
- impetigo (see 📖 pp.718, 817);
- scabies (see 📖 p.829);
- perioral dermatitis;
- pustular psoriasis (see 📖 p.810).

Acne vulgaris

Acne affects 90–100% of teenagers. However, acne may occur in neonates (spontaneous improvement without treatment occurs), infant (often requires treatment and may imply severe acne in later years) and adult (often women older than 25).

Cause

Excess sebum production, hyperkeratosis of the hair follicle, *Propionibacterium acnes* bacterial proliferation and inflammation of the hair follicle lead to acne.

Hyperandrogenism should be suspected if—acne is severe, sudden and of early onset; if there are other signs of hyperandrogenism including irregular periods, hirsuitism, male or female pattern hair loss and deepening of the voice in women; or there is treatment resistance.

Diet has not yet been proven to impact acne, but a healthy diet and exercise are recommended.

Presentation

Inflammatory (papules, pustules and nodules and cysts) and comedonal (blackheads and whiteheads) acne. There may be hypertrophic and/or atrophic scarring. Acne may affect the face, back, and chest.

Treatment

- *General measures:*
  - use a gentle soap free cleanser daily;
  - use oil free and non-comedogenic make-up.
- *Specific measures:*
  - topical retinoids for comedonal acne, e.g. adapalene, tretinoin;
  - topical antibiotics for inflammatory acne, e.g. clindamycin;
  - topical benzoyl peroxide 2.5–5% for inflammatory acne;
  - oral antibiotics for inflammatory acne, e.g. erythromycin, tetracyclines;
  - oral isotretinoin if severe or unresponsive to above (side-effects: teratogenic, avoid in teenage pregnancy; headaches; myalgia; dry skin/mucous membranes; sun photosensitivity).

Prognosis Resolves, but may persist for years in some cases. Psychological support is important.

Purpuric rashes

Causes

- Viral infections, most commonly enteroviral.
- Septicaemia, most commonly meningococcal (see 📖 p.714).
- Thrombocytopenia, platelet, or clotting disorders.
- Vasculitis, e.g. HSP (see 📖 p.788 and 📖 Plate 8).
- Trauma, including NAI.
- Drug reactions.
- Vasomotor straining, e.g. strenuous coughing or isometric exercise.

Management

If the patient is well and there is an obvious benign cause, reassure as the rash will resolve spontaneously. If cause unclear, initial investigations should include:

- FBC.
- Blood film.
- Clotting studies.
- Blood cultures.
- Check BP, urinalysis, blood U&E and ASOT (if HSP likely).
- If sepsis possible, admit and start IV antibiotics.
- Stop any drug likely to be causative.
- Consider a skin biopsy if diagnosis remains unclear.

Lymphoedema

Diffuse soft tissue oedema due to inadequate lymphatic drainage. May be due to developmental defect, e.g. congenital lymphoedema (isolated or part of Turner's syndrome) or cystic hygroma (which also commonly has a vascular component). Secondary causes include—surgical lymphatic destruction; malignant infiltration; irradiation; recurrent lymphangitis; parasitic infestation (in the tropics—filariasis or elephantiasis).

Presentation

- Pitting firm swelling.
- +/– Hypertrophy of affected limb.
- Lymphangiography may be helpful to identify the area of obstruction.

Treatment

Is often difficult. Limb elevation, pressure garments, or diuretics may be helpful. Give oral penicillin prophylaxis for increased risk of erysipelas.

Blood vessel disorders

Telangiectasia

Telangiectasias are permanently dilated small vessels. Commonest are spider naevi (dilated capillaries radiating from central arteriole). Less than 5 are considered normal. Laser or cautery of central vessel is rarely required. Five or more telangiectasias may be part of:

- Hereditary haemorrhagic telangiectasia (autosomal dominant genetic disorder with telangiectasia on lip, tongue, nasal epithelium, risking recurrent epistaxis +/− GI haemorrhage).
- Ataxia telangiectasia (see 📖 p.724).
- Hereditary benign telangiectasia.

Vascular malformations

Salmon patches Occur on nape of neck, glabella, eyelids and other sites. Often resolve or improve with age (see 📖 p.196).

Port wine stain

Naevus flammeus (see 📖 Plate 9). A capillary vascular malformation evident at birth, which persists with age. Vivid red or purple macule. May affect any site, but face and neck commonest. Involvement of the eyelid may be associated with glaucoma; segmental ophthalmic branch of trigeminal nerve involvement is associated with a risk of Sturge–Weber syndrome (seizures, hemiplegia, mental retardation). Treatment is pulse dye laser.

Klippel–Trenaunay syndrome

A complex venous-lymphatic malformation of the limb associated with limb hypertrophy and varicose veins. Patients may be at increased risk of DVT/pulmonary embolism (PE). Treatment is compression stockings. Lymphatic leakage may be treated with pulse dye laser or CO_2 laser.

Haemangiomas (see 📖 Plate 10)

- There are several types, but the most common by far is the infantile haemangioma (strawberry naevus).
- These occur in 10% of infants. They often present in the first few weeks of life and are more common in females.
- May have a superficial (red colour) and deep (blue colour) component.
- They often undergo a rapid proliferative phase between 4–9mths of age and then slowly involute over years. Complications include ulceration, bleeding and infection.
- If segmental over the face and perineum, they may be associated with PHACES (posterior fossa abnormalities, haemangioma, arterial anomalies, cardiac anomalies, eye abnormalities, sternal cleft or supra-umbilical raphe) and PELVIS (perineal haemangioma, external genital anomalies, lipomyelomeningocele, vesicorenal abnormalities, imperforate anus and skin tags) syndromes respectively.
- Those in the beard area may cause airway obstruction and those in the lumbar midline may be associated with spinal dysraphism. Multiple cutaneous haemangiomas may be associated with internal organ haemangiomas (especially liver and brain).

- Infantile haemangiomas have no risk of Kassabach-Merritt Syndrome (comprises thrombocytopaenia and a consumptive coagulopathy; only occurs in tufted angiomas and kaposiform haemangioendotheliomas).

Treatment

Reassurance and monitoring in most cases is all that is required. However, those in critical or cosmeticially sensitive sites may now be treated with oral propranolol by a dermatologist. Pulse dye laser is a useful treatment for ulceration and residual telangiectasia after involution. Surgical correction may be required to remove the fibrofatty residual after involution of large haemangiomas. Segmental, midline and multiple haemangiomas may need further investigation (see 📖 p.824).

Perniosis (chilblains)

Abnormal reaction to cold with localized, inflammatory, red-blue lesions on extremities (e.g. digits, ears). On rewarming there is pain or itching. Lesions may ulcerate. Resolves spontaneously. Prevented by warm clothing and housing!

Raynaud's syndrome

Episodic artery spasm causes digital ischaemia. The condition is precipitated by cold, finger constriction (e.g. shopping bags), or emotion. Most cases improve with age. Syndrome may be idiopathic (Raynaud's disease) or 2° (Raynaud's phenomenon) to:

- Systemic sclerosis.
- Arterial occlusion (e.g. cervical rib).
- Occlusive arterial disease.

Presentation

Fingers ache, burn, or tingle with colour changes of pallor (ischaemia), blue (cyanosis), and red (reactive hyperaemia).

Treatment

- Treat underlying disease.
- Local warmth.
- Nifedipine.
- Consider sympathethectomy if severe or recurrent.

Skin infection: viral and bacterial

Viral

Warts

Very common. Caused by infection with human papilloma virus. May affect any age, but mainly school-aged children. Warts exists as painless firm papules with rough hyperkeratotic surface. Capillary ends can usually be seen superficially. Typically affect hands, knees, face, and feet. Usually resolve spontaneously within 3yrs.
- Plantar warts (verrucae) may be painful due to pressure-induced in growing.
- Genital or perianal warts (condyloma acuminata) may occur and, although sexual abuse should be considered, causation is commonly innocent.

Treatment

Not usually needed. If painful or embarrassing:
- keratolytic agent (e.g. salicylic acid);
- liquid nitrogen cryotherapy;
- immunotherapy;
- surgical removal.

Molluscum contagiosum

See 🕮 Plate 11 and 🕮 p.813.

Herpes simplex

Most cases due to type I HSV. Type II HSV typically causes genital herpes. Co-infection with active atopic eczema causes eczema herpeticum.

Primary infection

Typically occurs in pre-school children with sore throat, stomatitis, vesicles or ulceration involving mouth, lip, face, and fever. It resolves within 2wks.
- 2° bacterial infection frequently occurs.
- Treat with antipyretics, analgesic mouthwashes, or throat lozenges, topical aciclovir cream. Consider NGT fluids if child becomes dehydrated due to reluctance to swallow. Treat any bacterial 2° infection.

Secondary reactivation

Manifests as initial itch or tingling followed by localized vesicles that then break down. Typically lesions are perioral (cold sore). May be idiopathic, but can be precipitated by illness, immunosuppression, menstruation. Early topical aciclovir cream aborts episode or reduces its severity.

Chickenpox (varicella) (see 📖 p.710)

This is a very contagious infection due to Herpes zoster. Chickenpox with fever, followed by pruritic vesicular eruption over the trunk spreading to face, mouth, and limbs. Lesions evolve at different rates so that macules, papules, vesicles, and pustules will all be present at once. Secondary bacterial skin infection may occur. Illness may cause life-threatening pneumonitis in congenital infection, older teenagers, or immunosuppressed. Infectivity lasts until FINAL vesicle crusts over.

Treatment
- Antipyretics.
- Oral antihistamines.
- Cooling baths.
- Topical calamine lotion.
- IM human-specific *Varicella zoster* immunoglobulin (VZIG) should be given early if risk of severe illness (IV aciclovir in severe illness).

Reactivation (shingles)

Can occur in childhood, particularly when varicella occurs <1yr old. May be severe in immunosuppressed. Presents with localized unilateral pain, itching, or hyperaesthesia, followed by vesicular eruption in the distribution of affected dorsal root ganglia. Treat with oral aciclovir if severe and topical antibiotics if 2° bacterial infection.

Hand, foot, and mouth disease

Infection with coxsackie or enterovirus 71, usually in pre-school children. (*Note:* Completely different infection from foot and mouth disease in animals!) Painful small vesicles (may be linear or oval) affect mouth (stomatitis), palms, and soles, and occasionally nappy area. Lesions spontaneously resolve within 10 days. If uncertain a viral swab can confirm the diagnosis and also exclude potentially more serious HSV/VZV infection.

Treatment Symptomatic.

Bacterial

Impetigo See 📖 pp.718, 817.

Erysipelas/cellulites See 📖 p.818.

Furuncle (boil)
- Confluence of furuncles = a carbuncle.
- Hair follicular abscess (boil) is usually due to *Staphylococcus aureus* infection. Common in post-pubertal males.
- Tender superficial red papule develops into large painful inflamed pustule that ultimately discharges superficially.
- Affects mainly the back, axilla, and buttocks.
- Associated with diabetes mellitus and poor hygiene.
- Recurrent or severe furuncles require surgical drainage, oral flucloxacillin, and daily chlorhexidine baths to decrease *S. aureus* skin colonization.

Fungal skin infections

Dermatophyte infection

Tinea corporis (ringworm)

Annular scaly lesion. Central clearing and sharp edge on trunk, face, or limbs.

Investigation Skin scrapings for microscopy and culture.

Treatment Topical antifungals, e.g. an imidazole cream, terbinafine cream.

Tinea capitus (scalp ringworm)

Red, scaling scalp lesions with hair loss and short hair stumps. May present as tender erythematous patch with pustules (kerion). Investigation as for Tinea corporis. Skin lesions appear fluorescent green under Wood's light.

Investigation Skin scrapings and hair pull for microscopy and culture.

Treatment Topical antifungal shampoo for one week and 6–8wks oral griseofulvin 20mg/kg/day (plus oral steroids if kerion exists).

Tinea pedis (athlete's foot)

Itchy, irritable skin between the toes +/− sole of foot.

Treatment Topical antifungal.

Tinea unguium (onychomycosis)

Nail infection causes discoloured, friable, and deformed nails.

Investigation Microscopy and culture of nail clippings.

Treatment Oral antifungal for 3mths (e.g. terbinafine).

Candida albicans infection

Predisposing factors

- Moist body folds.
- Treatment with broad-spectrum antibiotics.
- Immunosuppression.
- Diabetes mellitus.

Variants include the following:

- Cutaneous candidiasis (e.g. napkin rash; see 📖 Plate 12). Macular erythema, slight scaling, small outlying 'satellite' lesions, in body folds.
- Chronic paronychia.
- Chronic mucocutaneous granulomatous candidiasis (2° to congenital immunodeficiency disorder).

Investigations Skin scrapings for microscopy and culture.

Treatment Oral or topical anti-candidal drugs, e.g. nystatin, fluconazole.

Pityriasis versicolor (Tinea versicolor)

Malassezia infection in post-pubertal children. Asymptomatic hypo/hyperpigmented macules and scaling on trunk/upper limbs.

Treatment Topical imidazole foaming lotion for 3 consecutive nights.

Parasitic skin infections

Scabies

- Caused by *Sarcoptes scabiei* mite.
- Common at all ages.
- Diagnosis is not easy, so look closely for clues. Classically it causes itchy papular rash with visible burrows affecting finger and toe webs, palms, soles, wrists, groin, axillary folds, buttocks (truncal in infants). Excoriation, eczematization, urticaria, or impetigo may develop.
- Diagnosis is confirmed by microscopy of mite removed from burrow (rarely needed).

Treatment

- Treat whole household and close contacts simultaneously with 12hr topical application below the head (in children <2yrs old all body except face) with permethrin cream (5%) or 24hr of malathion liquid (0.5%) washed off and then repeated the next day.
- *Simultaneously*, launder bed linen and underwear in a warm wash.
- Antihistamines or calamine lotion for itch, which may last for 10 days.
- Apply weak topical corticosteroid if scabies nodules are present.

Lice

- Infestation with *Pediculus capitus* (scalp 'nits'), *Pedicularis corporis* (body), or *Phthirus pubis* (pubic area 'crabs').
- Common in all ages.
- Localized pruritis, 2° impetigo or regional lymphadenopathy.
- Lice are difficult to see, but small white eggs (nits) are easily seen attached to hair shafts.

Treatment Daily thorough combing with fine-toothed comb combined with single shampoo with lotions of carbaryl (0.5%) or malathion (0.5%).

Other insects Many biting insects (e.g. fleas, midges, bedbugs, mosquitoes) may cause erythematous macular lesions with central punctum or papular urticaria.

Treatment

- Avoid bites, e.g. treat infested pets.
- Oral antihistamines.
- Topical steroids.
- Antibiotics if there is 2° bacterial infection.

Protozoal skin infections

Cutaneous leishmaniasis

Infection with *Leishmania* spp. Endemic in hot climates (e.g. Mediterranean, South America). Spread by sandflies. Large red-brown papule, nodule, ulcer, or granuloma develops on face after several months incubation. Infection usually resolves within 1yr, but leaves a scar.

Treatment Intralesional or IV antimony compound if severe.

Hair disorders

Hair absence or loss

Alopecia areata

- Commonest cause of hair loss.
- An autoimmune disease.
- Hairless, smooth areas are most often on the scalp. At the margin short remnants of broken hairs are visible ('exclamation marks').
- All of the scalp (alopecia totalis) or the whole body (alopecia universalis) may be involved.
- Hair typically regrows after 6–12mths, but may be recurrent.
- The larger the area of hair loss, the poorer the prognosis.

Traumatic hair loss

May be unintentional (e.g. chronic hair twisting due to ponytail or rubbing of occiput in babies) or intentional (trichotillomania) due to hair pulling, twisting, or cutting as part of habit or 2° to anxiety, chronic social deprivation, or psychological disorder. Characteristically, there is an irregular margin, as well as bizarre patterns without complete hair loss, and broken hairs of different length. Hair re-grows once behaviour is modified.

Scalp infection Tinea capitus, ringworm (see 📖 p.828).

Scarring alopecia

Commonest cause is aplasia cutis. Circumscribed areas of the skin are absent, usually on scalp, which presents at birth with raw, red ulcer that heals with scarring and later absent hair growth. There is a significant incidence of other abnormalities (e.g. trisomies). Irreversible absent localized hair growth will also follow other causes of trauma (e.g. burns, skin disease, trauma).

Congenital diffuse alopecia

A rare autosomal recessive condition. Hair is present in the newborn period, but total hair loss occurs over the next few months and does not regrow. May be associated with other anomalies.

Systemic disease Hair loss can be 2° to hypothyroidism, diabetes mellitus, severe systemic disease, iron or zinc deficiency, chemotherapy.

Management of hair absence or loss

- *History:* include general health, recent illnesses, drug history, family history of alopecia, age of onset.
- *Examination:* pattern of hair loss; scalp and general examination.
- *Investigations:* hair M,C&S; Wood's light (tinea capitis); scalp biopsy.
- Treat any underlying condition.
- Wigs may be helpful.
- Topical steroids may be helpful for alopecia areata.

Excessive hair

Hypertrichosis

Defined as hair growth in areas not normally hairy in either sex.

Causes
- Racial.
- Familial.
- Certain rare syndromes (e.g. Cornelia De Lange syndrome, mucopolysaccharidosis).
- Drugs (e.g. diazoxide, ciclosporin, minoxidil).
- Anorexia nervosa.
- Protein-energy malnutrition.
- Persistence of foetal lanugo hair at birth.

Localized hypertrichosis may be associated with pigmented naevi, spina bifida occulta, inflammatory skin diseases, or topical steroids.

Treatment If required remove or treat underlying cause if possible; hair removal using depilatory creams or waxing.

Hirsutism

Male pattern of hair growth in females.

Causes
- Racial.
- Familial.
- Androgen excess (adrenal hypoplasia or tumour, Cushing's disease, polycystic ovary syndrome).
- Turner's syndrome.
- Drugs (e.g. anticonvulsants, progesterones, anabolic steroids).

Investigate
If there is any suggestion that not racial or familial (e.g. virilization evident).
- FBC.
- Plasma free testosterone.
- Plasma 17-OH progesterone.
- Serum cortisol.
- Urine steroid profile.
- Skull X-ray to detect possible pituitary tumour.

Treatment Treat any underlying disease; reassure if racial or familial; hair removal using depilatory creams or waxing.

Hair diseases

All diseases are rare and include:
- *Menkes kinky hair disease:* wiry wool hair (📖 p.976);
- *Monilethrix:* a rare autosomal dominant condition that causes brittle hair that fails to grow and breaks at 1–2cm;
- *Pili torti:* hair repeatedly twists over 180°, leading to brittle hair that 'flickers' under direct light;
- *Woolly hair syndrome:* wiry woolly Afro-Caribbean-like hair in Caucasians.

Nail disorders

Paronychia

Acute paronychia

Common, particularly in newborns. It presents as acute inflammation and tenderness of nail folds and surrounding skin.

Treatment Topical antiseptics, and, if severe, oral antibiotic, e.g. cephalexin.

Chronic paronychia

Associated with nail dystrophy. It is usually caused by chronic wetness (e.g. thumb sucking, resulting in infection with mixed bacteria and *Candida*).

Treatment Keep nail dry; topical nystatin and antiseptics.

Tinea unguium (onychomycosis) See p.828.

Nail biting

Common habit. Permanent nail damage may occur if nail matrix damaged.

Treatment Gentle dissuasion! Proprietary topical nail solutions that impart a very unpleasant taste may be effective.

Ingrowing toe-nails

Most commonly involves the hallux. A spicule of nail grows into lateral nail fold leading to pain, bacterial paronychia, and granulation tissue.

Treatment
- Local antiseptic.
- Careful trimming of nail spicule.
- Education on correct toe-nail cutting.
- Silver nitrate cauterization of granulation tissue or radical surgery is required when severe.

Subungual haemorrhage

Caused by trauma leading to haemorrhage under nail. Perforation of nail with hot needle is curative and relieves pain immediately.

Nail abnormalities secondary to generalized disease

- Congenital abnormal nails (usually atrophic) may be due to rare inherited conditions, e.g. ectodermal dysplasia.
- *Clubbing:* 2° to chronic pulmonary suppuration, e.g. cystic fibrosis, fibrosing alveolitis, bacterial endocarditis, cyanotic congenital heart disease, malabsorptive states, IBD, hepatic cirrhosis.
- *Onycholysis:* premature separation of nail from nail bed due to psoriasis, trauma, eczema.
- *Koilonychia:* spoon-shaped nails due to chronic iron deficiency anaemia. (Koilonychia is normal in the first few months of life.)
- *Nail pitting:* occurs in psoriasis, eczema, alopecia areata.
- *Beau's line:* transverse groove in nail caused by severe systemic illness.
- *Splinter haemorrhages:* due to bacterial endocarditis, trauma.
- *Yellow nail syndrome:* due to defective lymphatic drainage (also affects the lungs).
- *Nail–patella syndrome:* rare autosomal dominant condition with small rudimentary patella, elbow deformities, reduced or longitudinal split nails. Rarely, chronic glomerulonephritis develops.

Photosensitivity and light eruptions

Photosensitivity

Reactions to sunlight can be precipitated by drugs (e.g. thiazide diuretics, nalidixic acid), soaps, perfumes, plant pollens, plant contact (e.g. giant hogweed plant). Most common is a dermatitis-like reaction, but also it may be erythematous or blistering.

Porphyria

Some forms are photosensitive, e.g. erythropoietic protoporphyria (skin burning, redness, swelling, serous crusting +/− subsequent scarring). Treatment is that of the underlying porphyria together with sun protection (see also 📖 p.819).

Juvenile spring eruption

Red papules and herpetiform vesicles or blisters develop, usually in spring, over light-exposed skin, particularly ear helices. Commoner in boys. Lesions heal without scarring. Topical steroids hasten healing.

Polymorphic light eruption

Itchy, erythematous, papular rash occurring in sun-exposed areas 6–48hr after exposure. Most commonly affects adolescent girls. Treatment is with high factor sun screen.

Actinic prurigo

An uncommon condition precipitated by sunlight. Irritant papules, exudation, and excoriation develop on both exposed and unexposed skin areas. Treatment is with sun protection. Generally resolves after several years.

Xeroderma pigmentosum

A rare autosomal recessive condition in which hypersensitivity to sunlight causes marked erythema followed by dry skin, freckles, hyperpigmentation, atrophy, and scarring. Solar keratosis and skin cancers eventually develop due to the decreased ability to repair DNA damaged by UV radiation.

Pigmentation disorders

Hyperpigmented lesions

Generalized hyperpigmentation (hypermelanosis)

Causes

- Racial.
- Sun.
- ACTH (e.g. hypoadrenalism).
- Chronic renal failure (↑ melanocyte-stimulating hormone (MSH)).
- Malabsorption.
- Drug reaction.

Localized hyperpigmentation (hypermelanosis)

Causes

- Pigmented naevi (see bullet points in *Pigmented naevi*, following).
- Freckles.
- Lentigines.
- *Café au lait* macules.
- Neurofibromatosis (before puberty ≥6 *café au lait* macules >0.5cm diameter, axillary freckles).
- Viral warts.
- Polyostotic fibrous dysplasia (McAS).
- Peutz–Jegher's syndrome (perioral brown macules); post-inflammatory skin disease or trauma.

Pigmented naevi

- *Melanocytic naevus (mole):* developmental anomaly of melanocyte migration. May be brown, black, or pink, macular, papular, hyperkeratotic or smooth, hairy or hairless. Almost universal, commonly on face, neck, or back, appearing after birth throughout childhood, particularly at puberty. *Treatment* usually not required. Surgical removal appropriate for cosmetic reasons, recurrent trauma (e.g. from bra straps), or malignant change (rare in childhood). If congenital, can be extensive—refer to dermatologist/plastic surgeon for treatment and follow-up.
- *Halo naevus:* area of depigmentation around mole due to production of autoimmune antibodies to melanocytes. Usually reassurance alone is needed, but if irregular depigmentation or irregular mole is present refer to a dermatologist.
- *Mongolian blue spot:* macular blue-black lesion present at birth, common in dark-skinned races, particularly over sacrum, buttocks, back, and shoulders. Most fade spontaneously by age 10yrs.
- *Spindle-cell naevus:* benign melanocyte tumour. Red-brown dome-shaped nodule. Treated by simple excision.
- *Malignant melanoma:* rare in childhood. Risk increases with increased sun exposure. Occurs in older children, those with giant congenital pigmented naevi, immunosuppressed, previous chemotherapy, albinism, xeroderma pigmentosum. Change in mole colour, shape, size (unless in proportion to child's growth), ulceration, itch, or haemorrhage requires urgent specialist excision biopsy and histology.

Hypopigmented lesions

Generalized hypomelanosis

Causes
- Hypopituitarism (↓ ACTH and ↓ MSH).
- Oculocutaneous albinism.
- Protein-energy malnutrition.
- Poorly controlled phenylketonuria (phenylalanine acts as a competitive inhibitor of tyrosinases).

Oculocutaneous albinism

An autosomal recessive disorder of melanin synthesis. It presents with hypopigmented skin, blonde hair, pink irises, photophobia, reduced visual acuity, nystagmus.

Treatment Restrict sunlight exposure, e.g. protective high-level sunscreen; ophthalmology referral.

Localized hypomelanosis

- *Vitiligo:* common autoimmune disease (anti-melanocyte antibodies present) resulting in sharply demarcated, often symmetrical white patches. *Treatment* Reassurance. If severe—topical steroids; cosmetics; sun protection; phototherapy. Lesions usually persist.
- *Pityriasis versicolor.* See 📖 p.828.
- *Pityriasis alba:* common in prepubertal children. Represents low grade eczema with post-inflammatory hypopigmentation. Hypopigmented 1–2cm macules +/– fine scale on face or upper body. *Treatment*—topical hydrocortisone 1%, frequent moisturizing. Resolves in 2–3wks.
- *Post-inflammatory depigmentation.*
- *Tuberous sclerosis 'ash leaf' macules:* small oval hypopigmented macules that are more easily seen under Wood's light examination.

Collagen and elastin disorders

Collagen disorders

Ehlers–Danlos syndrome See 📖 p.946.

Comprises a group of several rare genetic (most autosomal dominant) disorders of collagen. In classical EDS the skin is soft, hyperextensible, easily bruised, and heals poorly with thin, atrophic 'cigarette paper' scars. Hypermobile EDS is characterized by soft skin with hypermobility of large and small joints. There is no specific treatment.

Striae (stretch marks)

Result from linear growth exceeding the capacity of new collagen production (e.g. pubertal growth spurt, with glucocorticoids). Linear reddish-purple marks develop. Most commonly occur on lower back and outer thighs. There is no treatment, but the marks slowly fade.

Keloid

An excessive fibrous tissue response to skin trauma. The cause is unknown, but often familial and more common in Afro-Caribbean children. Skin trauma results in well-demarcated raised, smooth, scar that extends beyond original injury.

Treatment Repeated intralesional triamcinolone injections are helpful if given early in keloid development. Radiotherapy also may be helpful if given early or before surgery.

Osteogenesis imperfecta

See 📖 p.762. Group of several rare genetic diseases, mostly autosomal recessive, in which there is inadequate or defective collagen production.

Presentation

Frequent skeletal fractures and multiple deformities; thin skin; defective teeth; hypermobile joints; and blue sclera.

Treatment

There is no specific treatment. Supportive therapy includes use of wheelchairs, orthoses, and analgesics for fractures, etc. Severe forms are lethal in infancy. Less severe forms lead to short stature, multiple or recurrent fractures, and deformities.

Elastin disorders

Cutis laxa

A rare congenital disorder of defective elastin that presents with loose skin folds and easily stretched skin that only slowly returns to original position. It is associated with later hernia, large vessel rupture, and emphysema.

Connective tissue disorders

See 📖 pp.784–787, 789. Skin manifestations of connective tissue disorders include the following:

Systemic lupus erythematosus
Widespread or 'butterfly rash' facial erythema, scalp alopecia, chronic discoid patches, light sensitivity.

Dermatomyositis
Violaceous erythema +/– oedema of face (especially eyelids), upper chest, elbows, knees, knuckles, around nails. Rash may become scaly.

Morphoea
In this idiopathic disorder there is localized sclerosis of the skin. Usually an enlarging large oval plaque of violaceous hue develops which then gradually becomes indurated, smooth, and shiny. Usually resolves spontaneously. Treat severe facial or restrictive linear morphoea with pulsed IV methylprednisolone and oral methotrexate.

Systemic sclerosis
This condition manifests as Raynaud's phenomenon; finger tip ulceration; skin of the face and hands becoming progressively indurated and 'bound down' to underlying tissues; restricted facial movements; beaked nose; mouth puckering; skin atrophy; telangiectasia; pigmentation; calcinosis.

Cutaneous polyarteritis nodosa
Tender nodules (usually lower legs) surrounded by livedo reticularis. Nodules may ulcerate or become necrotic.

Lichen sclerosus et atrophicus
In this idiopathic chronic inflammatory skin disorder localized distinct atrophic changes with associated pallor usually affect genital and perianal regions, almost always in females (the male variety is balanitis xerotica obliterans, which causes phimosis). Pruritus, blistering, or erythema may occur. Treat with emollients, or potent topical steroids if severe.

Miscellaneous skin conditions

Ichthyoses
Inherited group of disorders with underlying abnormal keratinization. The most common variants include:
- ichthyosis vulgaris;
- x-linked recessive ichthyosis;
- lamellar ichthyosis (LI);
- non-bullous congenital ichthyosiform erythroderma (CIE);
- bullous congenital ichthyosiform erythroderma.

Some types present as a 'collodion' baby (LI and CIE most commonly). There may also be eye ectropion and lip eclabium. Otherwise, presents in the first few months of life with dry scaly skin +/- erythema.

Investigation Skin biopsy and histology.

Treatment
Avoid soap and detergents, use bath oils, apply regular urea-containing emollients, or mild keratolytics (e.g. 1% salicylic acid in aqueous cream). If severe, oral retinoids are justified.

Prognosis Most forms improve with age (except X-linked ichthyosis).

Dermatitis herpetiformis
- A rare, chronic autoimmune disease 2° to IgA antibody directed against dermoepidermal junctional antigen.
- Occurs in coeliac disease. Affects ages 6–12yrs.
- Presents as an initial itchy rash of knees, elbows, buttocks, perineum that evolves into blisters.

Treatment Gluten-free diet; oral dapsone. Prognosis is good.

Epidermolysis bullosa
A group of genetically distinct disorders in which the epidermis separates from dermis. Often presents at birth with sloughing of skin (± mucous membranes) following minor skin trauma; blister or bulla formation; exhibits positive Nikolsky's sign. The level of epidermal/dermal cleavage differs between disorders with the more severe form resulting in scarring, finger pseudowebbing, oesophageal strictures, and limb contractions. Nails, hair, teeth may also be affected. Skin biopsy for immunofluorescent mapping determines precise diagnosis.

Treatment
Supportive (e.g. minimal handling, skilled nursing on silk sheets, foam padding, IV fluid/protein/electrolyte replacement as needed, antibiotics for superficial infection, nutritional support, topical paraffin and non-adherent bandaging of blistering areas). Referral to specialized unit is recommended.

Prognosis
Variable and depends on exact disorder. Generally, autosomal recessive forms are more severe, result in scarring, and present at birth. Severe

forms are frequently lethal in newborn period. Prognosis improves with skilled input.

'Adult' seborrhoeic eczema

Affects post-pubertal child. Caused by yeast overgrowth, e.g. *Malassezia ovale*. Presents with erythema with overlying scaling affecting scalp (dandruff), eyebrows, nasolabial folds, cheeks, and joint flexures. Treat with a mild topical steroid/antifungal.

Zinc deficiency

Causes
Dietary deficiency (e.g. breastfed very preterm infants) and *acrodermatitis enteropathica* (rare autosomal recessive defect in zinc absorption).

Presentation
Infants develop demarcated areas of erythema, scaling, and pustules around the mouth, ears, fingers, and toes, anogenital regions; diarrhoea; FTT.

Investigation Low plasma zinc levels.

Treatment Oral zinc supplements restore health.

Ectodermal dysplasia

There are many forms, the commonest is hypohidrotic ectodermal dysplasia (X-linked recessive).

Presentation
Sparse sweat glands, dry skin, sparse hair, thin eyebrows, characteristic facies (prominent frontal ridges in chin, saddle nose, sunken cheeks, thick lips, large ears), and defective peg-shaped teeth. Patients are prone to hyperthermia and heat stroke due to reduced/absent sweating.

Treatment Supportive. Avoid hyperthermia and treat appropriately if it occurs with rehydration and salt replacement. Use dental prosthetics.

Incontinentia pigmenti

In this rare X-linked dominant ectodermal dysplasia girls present in the neonatal period with blistering lesions (cropping circumferentially on the trunk and in a linear distribution on the limbs) that within weeks turn into warty plaques and nodules that resolve to leave streaky hyperpigmentation. Ultimately, the lesions regress by late childhood to leave atrophic, streaky areas of hypopigmentation (often most noticeable on the back of the calves). Associated with dental, eye, musculoskeletal, and neurological abnormalities. No specific treatment available.

Dermatitis artefacta

Caused by self-inflicted skin lesions. Usually affects adolescent girls. Lesions are very variable, but are usually bizarre and sudden in appearance. A helpful clue is that the patient is often inappropriately unconcerned. Occlusive dressing leads to rapid healing. Sympathetic listening is most likely to be helpful. Consider underlying abuse. Psychiatric input may be helpful.

Lichen planus

Cause is unknown. Itchy, flat-topped violaceous papules develop, usually over flexor aspects of wrist and trunk. Papules tend to coalesce into hypertrophic plaque. The nails (pits or ridges) and mouth (white lacy network) are also often involved.

Treatment Topical steroids. Lesions may recur for several years.

Mastocytosis

In this developmental, abnormal collection of skin mast cells, single or multiple macular or nodular lesions urticate when rubbed (Darier's sign). Hyperpigmentation develops after several months. There may be systemic involvement.

Treatment Antihistamines. Lesions and pigmentation resolve.

Paediatric surgery

Symptoms and signs that should cause concern

Neonates and infants

As a paediatrician you will be involved with the surgical care of newborn babies, infants, and older children. It is important that you recognize important symptoms and signs that indicate a surgical emergency.

Neonatal intestinal obstruction

- *Bile-stained vomiting:* the cardinal sign of an intestinal obstruction.
- *Emergency assessment:* check vital signs and commence resuscitation. Pass a 10F NGT if the baby is vomiting.
- *X-ray:* all children with bile-stained vomiting should have an AXR taken.

Radiology

- Dilated bowel loops on the AXR suggest an intestinal obstruction.
- Look for free air to indicate a perforation. In the supine film this will outline the falciform ligament (umbilical vein).
- Be aware of the radiological appearance of a midgut volvulus (see 📖 p.859: prompt diagnosis is essential if the bowel is to be salvaged.

Clinical assessment

- *Anus:* make sure the baby has an anus, especially females.
- *Meconium:* most babies pass meconium within 24hr of birth. Delayed passage of meconium in a baby with abdominal distension could mean Hirschsprung's disease (HSD).
- *Rectal examination:* do not perform a rectal examination, insert a suppository, or perform a rectal washout without seeking advice first because some surgeons use lower GI contrast studies for diagnosis and this may obscure the signs of HSD.

Oesophageal atresia (OA)

- The combination of *polyhydramnios* and a *mucousy baby* is suspicious of OA. See also 📖 p.848.
- Pass a 10F NGT before feeding the baby.
- Babies with OA and a tracheo-oesophageal fistula (TOF) who are ventilated represent a surgical emergency because air escapes down the fistula causing gastric distension that cannot be relieved. These babies are at risk of gastric perforation.

Congenital diaphragmatic hernia (CDH)

Most CDHs are now diagnosed antenatally. Delivery should be arranged in a neonatal surgical centre. At delivery secure IV access so that the baby can be sedated, paralysed, and then intubated. See also 📖 p.852.

- Avoid ventilating the baby with a bag and mask because this distends the stomach.
- If the diagnosis is not made prenatally, suspect CDH in a baby with respiratory distress and apparent dextrocardia.

Intussusception in infants

Suspect intussusception in any infant with gastroenteritis who is not getting better, is unusually miserable, vomits bile or has blood in the stool (see also 📖 p.858. The classical presentation is an infant with:

- intermittent colicky abdominal pain;
- episodic drawing up of the knees;
- passes 'red currant jelly' stool (late sign).

Assessment

- *Resuscitation:* these patients often require large volumes of fluid to restore the circulation.
- Confirm diagnosis by US.
- Do not consider radiological reduction unless you have a surgeon and anaesthetist who are able to operate on the child in the event of perforation or failure.

Incarcerated inguinal hernia

An irreducible swelling in the groin in a baby who is ill and vomiting is probably an incarcerated inguinal hernia. See also 📖 p.868.

- *Resuscitate* the baby.
- *Pass a NGT.*
- *AXR* may clarify the diagnosis by showing an intestinal obstruction and a gas shadow in the bowel trapped in the hernia.
- Transfer to a paediatric surgeon; do not wait overnight.

Older children

Acute appendicitis

Be wary of children with abdominal pain who are taking antibiotics for a presumed sore throat or UTI. The diagnosis may be appendicitis, but the history will be atypical and the abdominal signs are difficult to decipher or absent (see also 📖 p.864).

- *Observe:* admit the child for observation.
- *Urine:* urinalysis is abnormal in 30% of children with acute appendicitis. Resist the temptation to assume the diagnosis is a UTI unless the urine culture is positive.
- *US:* request an US scan if there is clinical doubt.
- *Pelvic appendicitis:* presentation is with diarrhoea and the abdominal signs will be minimal or absent. Exclude a pelvic abscess with US before assuming the diagnosis is gastroenteritis.

Acute scrotal pain

Any boy with acute scrotal pain has a testicular torsion until proven otherwise (see also 📖 p.876).

- Refer all these children to a surgeon.
- The medicolegal consequences of missing a torsion are substantial.

Congenital abnormalities: upper airway

Choanal atresia (CA)

Congenital obstruction of the posterior choana of the nose may be unilateral or bilateral. Babies are obligate nose breathers and bilateral obstruction presents with asphyxia during feeding and sleep. Unilateral obstruction may pass unnoticed. CA may be a presenting feature of the CHARGE association, which is:

- **C**oloboma;
- **H**eart defects;
- **A**tresia of the choanae;
- **R**etardation of growth and development;
- **G**enitourinary abnormalities;
- **E**ar abnormalities and hearing loss.

Diagnosis

- *NGT:* the diagnosis is excluded by passage of a tube down each nostril.
- CT scan will determine whether the obstruction is membranous or bony.

Treatment

- Emergency treatment comprises an oropharyngeal airway and an orogastric tube for feeding.
- Surgery (which is performed through a transnasal approach) restores the patency of the choanae.

Laryngeal atresia

A rare condition that is invariably fatal at birth. The condition is relatively easy to detect using antenatal US because the foetal lungs appear bright and large. The large airways can also be visualized because they are distended with foetal lung fluid. The condition is not amenable to correction (due to lung hypoplasia) and termination of pregnancy should be offered.

Cleft lip and palate

See also 📖 p.191. Approximately 1 baby per 1000 is born with a cleft lip and palate. This may occur sporadically or there may be a family history. A cleft lip is immediately apparent. An isolated cleft palate may not be noticed immediately, but will present with feeding difficulties, particularly nasal regurgitation of milk. A cleft palate will interfere with breastfeeding as it precludes generation of suction. Bottle-feeding may also be difficult unless a squeezable bottle, rather than a rigid bottle, is used.

Management

- *Lip repair:* at around 3mths of age.
- *Palate repair:* at around 6mths of age.
- *Follow-up:* long-term because of problems with speech, dentistry, and hearing.

Pierre–Robin sequence

The Pierre–Robin sequence (Fig. 23.1) is characterized by three features:
- micrognathia;
- glossoptosis;
- cleft palate.

Management
- The large tongue has a tendency to obstruct the airway causing apnoea, particularly during sleep.
- Prone positioning may help, allowing the tongue to fall forward, but occasionally tracheostomy is necessary.
- Endotracheal intubation is often difficult.
- Tube feeding may be necessary.
- The palate is generally repaired between 9 and 18mths of age.
- The airway problems invariably improve with growth.

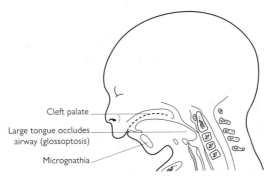

Fig. 23.1 Pierre–Robin sequence.

Congenital abnormalities: tracheo-oesophageal

Tracheo-oesophageal fistula

TOF is usually associated with OA. However, an isolated TOF will present with:
- choking or coughing during feeding;
- abdominal distension;
- recurrent LRTI.

Although symptoms are present from birth the diagnosis is frequently not made until later in childhood. The investigations of choice are a tube injection of X-ray contrast into the oesophagus and bronchoscopy. Treatment is surgical division of the TOF through a neck incision.

Oesophageal atresia and tracheo-oesophageal fistula

See also 🕮 p.844. The incidence of OA and TOF (Fig. 23.2) is 1/3500 live births.
- 75% babies with OA will have a TOF.
- 10% will have isolated OA, which is usually associated with a long gap or defect.
- Rare isolated TOF.
- Rare OA with both upper and lower pouch TOFs.

Maternal polyhydramnios is common, although antenatal diagnosis is rare. Babies present at birth with:
- excess mucus or 'mucousy';
- choking and cyanosis on feeding;
- associated malformations in 50%, usually the VACTERL association (Box 23.1).

> #### Box 23.1 VACTERL association
>
> - Vertebral anomalies (fused vertebrae, hemivertebrae)
> - Anorectal anomalies (imperforate anus)
> - Cardiac anomalies (all types)
> - TOF
> - Renal abnormalities (all types)
> - Limb abnormalities (radial ray anomalies, e.g. hypoplastic thumbs)

Diagnosis
Confirmed or excluded by:
- Passage of a 10F NGT.
- *CXR:* the tube stops in the upper thorax. Air in the stomach indicates a fistula between the trachea and the distal oesophagus (TOF).

Acute management
- The baby should be kept warm and disturbed as little as possible.
- The upper oesophageal pouch should be aspirated regularly by oropharyngeal suction or a Replogle tube.
- Standard IV fluids started.

- Pre-operative antibiotics are not required unless there is evidence of aspiration pneumonia.
- Babies who require mechanical ventilation must be referred urgently for surgery because gas will escape down the TOF and produce progressive gastric distension, which impairs ventilation further, ultimately leading to gastric perforation.

Surgery
- Disconnection of the TOF and anastomosis of upper and lower oesophagus through a right thoracotomy.
- Long gap OA may require a feeding gastrostomy and a cervical oesophagostomy in the neonatal period followed by oesophageal replacement during infancy. Some specialist centres now perform the Foker operation, where prolonged internal 'stretch' makes the remnant of the upper and lower oesophagus 'grow'!
- High-risk babies may have a staged procedure—the TOF is ligated and then the OA repaired a few days later.
- Complications include anastomotic leak, anastomotic stricture, gastro-oesophageal, and recurrent fistula.

Follow-up
- Respiratory morbidity in the early years after OA/TOF repair is relatively high, particularly in the winter months. Consider admitting these children during respiratory infections.
- Obstruction of the oesophagus by food boluses is common in toddlers and young children after OA repair. Usually, it is caused by meat that has not been chewed. Refer for urgent oesophagoscopy.

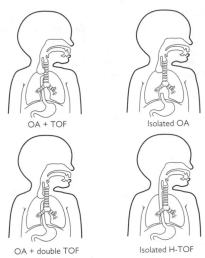

OA + TOF   Isolated OA

OA + double TOF   Isolated H-TOF

Fig. 23.2 Types of OA/TOF.

Congenital abnormalities: oesophagus

Oesophageal stricture

Oesophageal strictures in children may be congenital (5%) or acquired (95%). Strictures may be acquired as a result of reflux oesophagitis, caustic ingestion, or following repair of OA. Congenital oesophageal strictures most commonly affect the middle and distal third of the oesophagus and rarely cause symptoms in the neonatal period. They may be due to:
- membranous diaphragm;
- segmental submucosal fibrosis;
- presence of ectopic tracheobronchial rests.

Presentation
Strictures present with:
- regurgitation of undigested food;
- bolus obstruction;
- failure to thrive.

Diagnosis
- Barium swallow.
- Oesophagoscopy.

Treatment.
- Peptic strictures are an absolute indication for anti-reflux surgery.
- Congenital strictures may respond to dilatation but resection or oesophageal replacement is often necessary.

Caustic ingestion
- *Acute phase:* resuscitate and support with IV fluids and antibiotics.
- *Endoscopy:* to confirm the severity of the burn.
- *Feeding gastrostomy:* in severe strictures.
- *Chronic phase:* serial oesophageal dilatation is performed, but many children require oesophageal replacement.

Congenital abnormalities: lung

Congenital cystic adenomatoid malformation (CAM)

CAM is a congenital malformation of the lung bud characterized by dysplasia of respiratory epithelium. The majority of CAMs are now diagnosed prenatally by US and high-risk cases will be associated with hydrops. Symptomatic CAMs should be resected.

- Large CAMs present at birth with respiratory distress that is managed along conventional lines.
- Small CAMs will be asymptomatic at birth, but may present in early childhood with pulmonary sepsis.

Sequestration

Pulmonary sequestrations are segments of lung parenchyma with an anomalous blood supply from the aorta. There may be an abnormal bronchial connection with the foregut or tracheobronchial tree. The majority are detected prenatally and the management is resection.

- Large sequestrations will present at birth with respiratory distress or with heart failure from high flow through the feeding vessel.
- Sequestrations may present in infancy or childhood with pulmonary sepsis.

Congenital lobar emphysema (CLE)

CLE is an unusual lung bud anomaly characterized by massive air trapping in the emphysematous lobe. This compresses the surrounding normal lung and may result in mediastinal shift.

- CLE presenting with progressive respiratory distress within the first few weeks or months of life nearly always require lobectomy. In the acute phase positive pressure ventilation may produce rapid worsening of the emphysema.
- Lobar emphysema identified on CXR in the absence of symptoms will need close follow-up, and surgery may be avoided.

Congenital abnormalities: chest

Congenital diaphragmatic hernia

See 📖 p.844. The incidence of CDH is 1/2400. The main problem is not the diaphragmatic hernia, but rather the associated pulmonary hypoplasia that is often severe and determines prognosis. The most common type of diaphragmatic defect is posterolateral (Bochdalek) and left-sided, occurring in 90% (see Figs 23.3 and 23.4).

- *Antenatal screening:* most CDHs are identified on antenatal US, but the prognosis for these foetuses is poor (i.e. 20% survive).
- *Birth:* if the diagnosis is not made antenatally and the baby presents at birth, clinical findings may include respiratory distress, scaphoid abdomen, and apparent dextrocardia. The prognosis for survival is ~60%.
- *Coincidental:* ~10% of CDHs are discovered during early childhood, including most anterior (Morgagni) defects. The prognosis is excellent.

Neonatal management

- Initial management consists of sedation, paralysis, endotracheal intubation, and mechanical ventilation with 100% O_2.
- NGT placement and avoid bag–mask–valve ventilation.
- If oxygenation is good and pulmonary hypoplasia is not severe, repair of the diaphragmatic defect is undertaken after a few days either by primary suture or insertion of a prosthetic patch.

Hiatus hernia (HIH)

HIH refers to herniation of the stomach into the chest through the oesophageal hiatus in the diaphragm. The lower oesophageal sphincter also moves and becomes incompetent. Most children with HIH present with gastro-oesophageal reflux (GOR). Two types of hiatus hernia are recognized (Fig. 23.5):

- sliding (common);
- rolling or paraoesophageal (rare).

Management

- Diagnosis is made radiologically by barium meal.
- Treatment comprises management of the GOR, initially medically.
- Surgery is reserved for children who fail to respond to medication, complicated reflux (e.g. peptic strictures), and paraoesophageal hernias (because of the risk of incarceration and infarction of the herniated stomach). Surgery involves repair of the hiatus hernia and a fundoplication to prevent GOR.

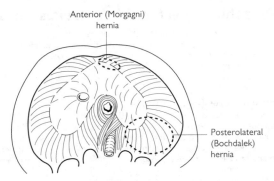

Fig. 23.3 Types of diaphragmatic hernia.

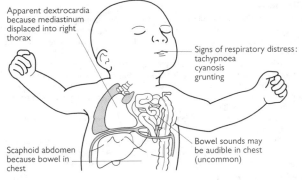

Fig. 23.4 Clinical features of CDH.

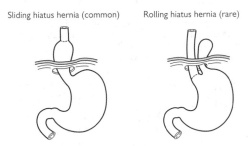

Fig. 23.5 Types of hiatus hernia.

Idiopathic hypertrophic pyloric stenosis

The incidence of idiopathic hypertrophic pyloric stenosis (IHPS) is ~3/1000 live births. Boys are affected more frequently than girls and IHPS is more common in Whites than in dark-skinned races. The pylorus enlarges as a result of hypertrophy of the circular muscle to produce the typical 'tumour'. The cause remains unknown. Familial occurrence is well documented, particularly in girls.

Clinical features (Fig. 23.6)

- *Vomiting*: projectile, starting in the third or fourth week of life. The vomitus is always non-bilious, but it may contain altered blood ('coffee ground') or fresh blood from oesophagitis. Vomiting occurs within an hour of feeding and the baby is immediately hungry. Vomiting may not be projectile in babies who present early (first or second week); they are often misdiagnosed as suffering from GOR.
- *Constipation* is common due to reduced fluid intake.
- *Dehydration, malnutrition, and jaundice* are late signs.
- IHPS is rare beyond 12wks of age.

Diagnosis

- *Test feed*: the baby is allowed to feed from the breast or bottle whilst the examiner palpates the baby's abdomen. This is best conducted with the baby resting on the mother's lap, cradled on her left arm. The examiner sits opposite the mother, on the baby's left. Visible waves of gastric peristalsis may be seen passing across the upper abdomen. The pyloric tumour is usually easiest to feel either early in the feed or after the baby has vomited. 60–90% tumours are palpable. The thickened pylorus is palpable as a firm, 'olive-shaped' mass, just above and to the right of the umbilicus during a 'test feed'.
- *US*: if a tumour cannot be felt, US will usually confirm or exclude the diagnosis.
- *Biochemistry*: the biochemical abnormality of IHPS is a hypochloraemic, hypokalaemic metabolic alkalosis (Fig. 23.7). Assess degree of alkalosis at presentation and monitor correction prior to surgery.

Pre-operative management

- *Rehydrate and correct the alkalosis* before surgery.
- *IV fluids* should be started. 0.45% Saline with 5% dextrose and 20mmol/L potassium chloride at 120mL/kg/day.
- *Feeds*: withhold. The stomach should be emptied with a NGT.
- *Electrolytes and capillary blood pH*: should be checked regularly until they return to normal (usually 24–48h).
- *Blood glucose*: should be monitored.

Surgery

- *Ramstedt's pyloromyotomy*: the treatment of choice (Fig. 23.8). This involves splitting the thickened pyloric muscle. Complications include perforation of the mucosa, which is not serious provided it is recognized and repaired, and wound infection.
- *Oral feeds* are usually withheld overnight. Transient post-operative vomiting is common but invariably settles within 36h. There are no long-term sequelae.

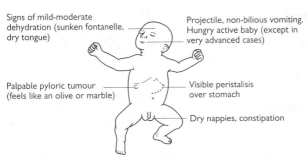

Signs of mild-moderate dehydration (sunken fontanelle, dry tongue)

Projectile, non-bilious vomiting. Hungry active baby (except in very advanced cases)

Palpable pyloric tumour (feels like an olive or marble)

Visible peristalisis over stomach

Dry nappies, constipation

Fig. 23.6 Clinical signs of pyloric stenosis.

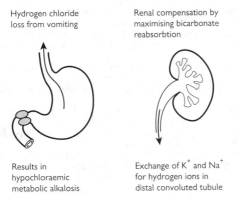

Hydrogen chloride loss from vomiting

Renal compensation by maximising bicarbonate reabsorbtion

Results in hypochloraemic metabolic alkalosis

Exchange of K^+ and Na^+ for hydrogen ions in distal convoluted tubule

Fig. 23.7 Biochemical abnormalities in pyloric stenosis.

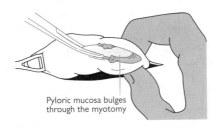

Pyloric mucosa bulges through the myotomy

Fig. 23.8 Ramstedt's operation.

Ingested foreign bodies

See also 📖 pp.51, 857. Swallowed foreign bodies are fairly common in young children. The incident may have been witnessed. Alternatively, the child may present with:

- dribbling;
- regurgitation;
- occasionally cough and stridor.

Diagnosis

Chest X-ray: the majority of ingested foreign bodies are radio-opaque (coins).

Management

- *Oesophageal:* if the foreign body is in the oesophagus it should be removed within 24hr, usually by oesophagoscopy. *Button batteries* in the oesophagus must be retrieved or pushed down into the stomach within a few hours of ingestion. Electrolytic ulceration of the oesophagus occurs rapidly and this may lead to perforation or fistulation into the tracheal or aorta.
- *Below the diaphragm:* if the foreign body is below the diaphragm it will invariably pass spontaneously per rectum and all that is required is reassurance. Serial radiographs are unnecessary. The only proviso is a child who has had previous abdominal surgery in which case adhesions may impede passage of the object:
  - Parents should be asked to examine the child's stools for the foreign body.
  - Colicky abdominal pain and vomiting (i.e. possible signs of intestinal obstruction) warrant review and a repeat X-ray. Provided the child remains asymptomatic, surgery to retrieve the object should be deferred for several months.
  - *Button batteries* below the diaphragm should be treated in exactly the same way as other ingested foreign bodies. The battery will pass spontaneously long before it disintegrates.

Bezoars

Bezoars are FB concretions composed of hair (trichobezoar) or vegetable matter (phytobezoar). The bezoar forms in the stomach and may extend into the small bowel. Bezoars are most commonly seen in young girls who present with:
- weight loss;
- vomiting;
- abdominal pain;
- anaemia.

Diagnosis
- An abdominal mass may be palpable.
- Barium meal or endoscopy will confirm the abnormality.

Surgical treatment
- *Large bezoars:* open surgical removal is necessary.
- *Smaller bezoars:* endoscopic removal.

Midgut malrotation and volvulus

See Fig. 23.9 and 📖 p.845. During the first trimester of intrauterine development the foetal midgut transiently herniates into the umbilical cord. As this reduces, the mesentery normally rotates to bring the caecum to lie in the right iliac fossa and duodenojejunal flexure (DJF) to lie to the left of the midline. The midgut mesentery thus extends diagonally across the back of the abdominal cavity and provides a broad stable pedicle for the SMA to supply the bowel. Malrotation is a failure of this normal rotation that leaves the caecum high in the right upper quadrant and DJF mobile in midline. The result is a narrow base for the midgut mesentery and a narrow mobile pedicle through which the SMA runs. Malrotation is usually asymptomatic and only detected by contrast meal and follow through.

Midgut malrotation

- Midgut malrotation predisposes to midgut volvulus.
- To prevent this complication, surgical correction of a malrotation is advised using Ladd's procedure.
- An incidental appendicectomy is usually performed.

Midgut volvulus

- This is a catastrophic event that occurs without warning.
- The immediate effect is high intestinal obstruction at duodenal level that is rapidly followed by infarction of the entire midgut.

Symptoms

- Bile-stained vomiting.
- Circulatory collapse.
- Tender abdomen.

Diagnosis

- AXR (Fig. 23.10). May appear similar to duodenal atresia with a 'double bubble' and a paucity of gas elsewhere in the abdomen.
- The diagnosis is confirmed by an urgent (even middle of the night) upper GI contrast study.

Surgical treatment

- Immediate laparotomy to untwist the volvulus.
- If the bowel is healthy a Ladd's procedure is performed.
- If bowel viability is doubtful a second look laparotomy may be necessary after 24hr. Frequently, there is massive intestinal necrosis and the child is left with a very short gut in which case long-term IV feeding is required.

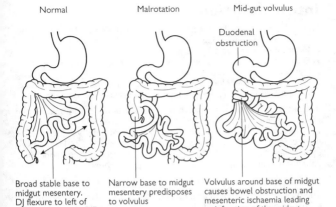

Fig. 23.9 Intestinal rotation and volvulus. RIF, Right iliac fossa; DJF, duodenojejunal flexure.

Normal

Malrotation

Mid-gut volvulus

Duodenal obstruction

Broad stable base to midgut mesentery. DJ flexure to left of midline, caecum in RIF

Narrow base to midgut mesentery predisposes to volvulus

Volvulus around base of midgut causes bowel obstruction and mesenteric ischaemia leading to infarction of the midgut

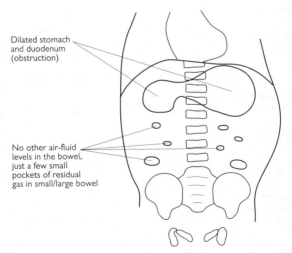

Dilated stomach and duodenum (obstruction)

No other air-fluid levels in the bowel, just a few small pockets of residual gas in small/large bowel

Fig. 23.10 Features of volvulus on AXR.

Intussusception

Intussusception typically affects infants between 6 and 18mths of age. The incidence is 1/500 children. The majority of intussusceptions occur in association with viral gastroenteritis.

- Enlarged Peyer's patch in the ileum acts as the *lead point* that then invaginates into the distal bowel.
- Intussusceptions in older children and adults are more likely to be due to a *pathological lead point*, e.g. a polyp or Meckel's diverticulum.

Intussusception causes a small bowel obstruction. The intussuscepted bowel becomes engorged, which causes rectal bleeding, and eventually gangrenous. Following this, perforation and peritonitis will occur. The most common site for an intussusception is ileocolic (Fig. 23.11) followed by ileo-ileal. Small bowel intussusception may occur as a post-operative complication in infants, typically following nephrectomy.

Presentation

The typical presentation of an intussusception in an infant is as follows:

- Spasms of colic associated with pallor, screaming, and drawing-up legs.
- The child falls asleep between episodes.
- Later, as the intestinal obstruction progresses, bile-stained vomiting develops and rectal bleeding, (i.e. 'red currant jelly stools').
- The child will appear ill, listless, and dehydrated.
- In late cases circulatory shock or peritonitis will be present.

Assessment

- In 30% of cases the intussusception will be palpable as a sausage-shaped abdominal mass.
- Blood may be noted on rectal examination.
- *AXR:* small bowel obstruction and occasionally a soft tissue mass will be visible.
- *US:* confirms the diagnosis by showing a characteristic 'target sign'.

Management

- *Resuscitation:* often large volumes of IV fluid are required to restore perfusion.
- *Antibiotics.*
- *Analgesia.*
- *NGT* passed if the infant is vomiting.
- *Radiological reduction:* provided that there is no evidence of peritonitis, *and facilities for immediate surgery are available*, the treatment of choice is for an expert paediatric radiologist to reduce the intussusception pneumatically by rectal insufflation of air under fluoroscopic control. The risks of this procedure are incomplete reduction and perforation. The latter can be particularly dangerous as a tension pneumoperitoneum develops very rapidly.
- *Laparotomy:* if pneumatic reduction fails, or is contraindicated because of concern about a gangrenous intussusception, laparotomy

is necessary. The distal bowel is gently compressed to reduce the intussusception. If this is not successful then the intussusception is resected. There is a recurrence rate about 10% whether the intussusception is treated radiologically or by surgery. Further recurrence should raise the question of a pathological lead point.

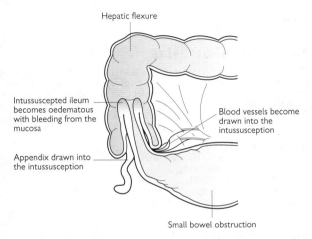

Hepatic flexure

Intussuscepted ileum becomes oedematous with bleeding from the mucosa

Appendix drawn into the intussusception

Blood vessels become drawn into the intussusception

Small bowel obstruction

Fig. 23.11 Ileocolic intussusception.

Duodenal atresia

The incidence of DA is 1/5000 live births.
- One-third of babies with DA have trisomy 21.
- Babies with DA present at birth with bile-stained vomiting.
- AXR shows 'double bubble' sign of gas in stomach and proximal duodenum (Fig. 23.12).
- Surgical treatment consists of side-to-side duodenoduodenostomy. The prognosis is excellent.

Small bowel atresias

The incidence of small bowel atresia is 1/3000 live births. The aetiology is thought to be vascular. The pathology of small bowel atresias varies (depending on how deep in the mesentery the vascular accident occurs) from an atresia in continuity with a mucosal membrane to a widely separated atresia with a V-shaped mesenteric defect and loss of gut (Fig. 23.13). About 10% of atresias are multiple.

Clinical aspects
- *Bile-stained vomiting:* babies present shortly after birth with bile-stained vomiting and abdominal distension.
- *AXR* shows multiple fluid levels (Fig. 23.14).
- *Laparotomy:* end-to-end anastomosis. The prognosis depends on the length of the remaining small bowel.

Meconium ileus

The incidence of MCI is ~1/2500 live births. MCI is associated with cystic fibrosis (CF): 15% of children with CF present with MCI. Lack of pancreatic enzymes results in meconium that is thick and viscous causing an intraluminal obstruction in the terminal ileum. Occasionally the distended obstructed bowel will perforate or result in volvulus *in utero*, so-called 'complicated' MCI. Babies present at birth with intestinal obstruction.

Management
Treatment of MCI involves relieving the intestinal obstruction.
- *Gastrograffin enema:* provided that there is no evidence of intra-uterine perforation the obstruction may be relieved by hypertonic contrast, which draws fluid into the bowel lumen, and the detergent then loosens inspissated meconium.
- *Laparotomy* for unsuccessful enema or complicated MCI.
- *Management of CF* if diagnosed.

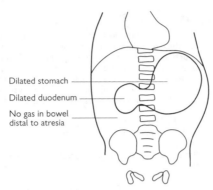

Fig. 23.12 Features of duodenal atresia on AXR.

Atresias in continuity

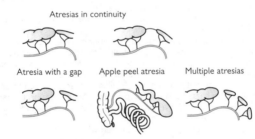

Atresia with a gap   Apple peel atresia   Multiple atresias

Fig. 23.13 Types of small bowel atresia.

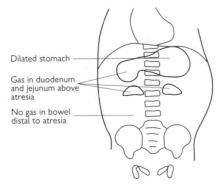

Fig. 23.14 Features of jejunal atresia on AXR.

Acute appendicitis

Acute appendicitis is the commonest abdominal emergency in children, affecting approximately one-sixth of the population. Acute appendicitis begins with obstruction of the lumen of the appendix, often by a faecolith, and this causes vague central abdominal pain. After about 6–12hr an inflammatory process involves the full thickness of the wall of the appendix. After a further 24–36hr the appendix will become gangrenous and perforate. Irritation of the peritoneum results in more severe abdominal pain localized to the right iliac fossa.

- Pain is aggravated by movement.
- Child may prefer to lie still with knees flexed.
- Mild fever is usual.
- Peritoneal irritation results in involuntary spasm in the muscles of the abdominal wall—'guarding'.

Diagnosis

The mortality from appendicitis is virtually zero. However, substantial morbidity is incurred by delayed diagnosis. The diagnosis of appendicitis is clinical and laboratory investigations are generally not helpful.

- The 'classical' symptoms and signs of acute appendicitis are seen in about 60% of cases.
- Of all children admitted to hospital with abdominal pain only about 30% will have acute appendicitis. Not all of these cases are obvious at the initial assessment (probably only 50–70%); if there is any doubt, child should be admitted to hospital for observation.
- Urinalysis is abnormal in about 1/3 children with acute appendicitis: pyuria and even bacteriuria may be present. The temptation to start antibiotics for a presumptive diagnosis of UTI should be avoided unless there are symptoms of dysuria.
- The WCC is normal in 10–20% of children with appendicitis.
- *US:* if there is clinical doubt, US is the investigation of choice. The overall accuracy of US in the diagnosis of acute appendicitis is around 90%.

Mesenteric adenitis

Mesenteric adentitis (MeA) is a condition that mimics acute appendicitis. It is usually the result of an intercurrent viral infection. Children with MeA typically present with:

- fever;
- malaise;
- central abdominal pain.

Diagnosis

- Usually a period of observation is necessary during which time the symptoms remain static or improve rather than progress as would be expected with appendicitis.
- MeA accounts for the majority of children who undergo a normal appendicectomy. After surgery the post-operative course is usually uneventful.

Meckel's diverticulum

Meckel's diverticulm (MD) is:

- A persistence of the embryonic vitelline duct that normally involutes during late foetal development.
- Present in 2% of the population and the majority are asymptomatic.
- A cause of GI bleeding, obstruction, inflammation, and umbilical discharge.

Management

- Rectal bleeding from a MD is painless, fresh, and sufficient to cause a drop in haemoglobin. Sometimes a ^{99m}Tc-pertechnetate isotope scan will identify a MD.
- *Laparotomy:* persistent or recurrent bleeding requires a laparotomy even if the scan is −ve. Diverticulitis or perforation of a MD is clinically indistinguishable from appendicitis.
- Symptomatic MD should be resected.

Gastroschisis

The incidence of gastroschisis is 1/3000 live births, but it is increasing. Most foetuses with gastroschisis are identified on prenatal US and delivery can then be arranged in a regional neonatal surgical centre. The abnormality is immediately apparent at birth as a defect in the abdominal wall to the right of the umbilicus (Fig. 23.15). The bowel is eviscerated and not covered by a sac. As a result of contact with amniotic fluid the bowel is thickened and matted. Associated malformations are uncommon except intestinal atresias (10%).

Management
- Immediate: cover the exposed bowel with Clingfilm™.
- Keep the baby warm and hydrated.
- AXR is unnecessary.
- *Surgery:* the defect requires surgical closure as rapidly as possible. Often this has to be staged using a silo because the abdomen is too small to accommodate the intestine. The silo is reduced serially over a period of 1–2wks and then 2° closure of the defect is performed.
- *Nutrition:* total parenteral nutrition may be required for many weeks because intestinal function is slow to resume after the abdominal wall is closed. However, the long-term outcome is excellent.

Exomphalos (omphalocele)

The incidence of exomphalos is 1/3000 live births (see Fig. 23.15). It is usually identified on prenatal US. It is characterized by:
- Hernia into the base of the umbilical cord—the herniated bowel is covered by a sac (amnion).
- *Exomphalos major:* defect >5cm diameter.
- *Exomphalos minor:* defect <5cm diameter.

Malformations in association with exomphalos are found in 50% of cases:
- *Chromosomal defects:* trisomies 18, 13, 21 and Turner's syndrome.
- Cardiac defects.
- *Syndromes:* BWS.

Surgical treatment
- Closure of the defect in one or more stages.
- The prognosis depends on associated malformations.

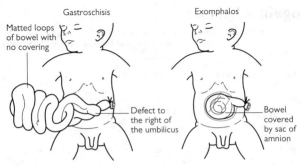

Fig. 23.15 Anterior abdominal wall defects.

Inguinal hernias

Groin hernias in children are almost invariably indirect inguinal hernias. Femoral hernias are rare in children. Inguinal hernias have the following characteristics.

- More common in boys.
- More common on the right side, due to later descent of right testis.
- 15% hernias are bilateral.
- Symptoms are rare.

Clinical care

- A reducible swelling in the groin, often extending into the scrotum (Fig. 23.16).
- Surgical herniotomy. Infants should be repaired within a few weeks of diagnosis because the risk of incarceration is high. The risk of incarceration lessens after the age of 1yr.

Incarcerated hernia

- Incarceration results in an intestinal obstruction.
- There is a 30% risk of testicular infarction due to pressure on the gonadal vessels.
- Treatment of an irreducible inguinal hernia comprises resuscitation of the child and then reduction of the hernia by taxis (i.e. gentle, but sustained pressure is applied to the sac to reduce the contents).
- Most hernias can be reduced safely, although it may be necessary to give the baby morphine first. If the hernia cannot be reduced, emergency surgical exploration is necessary (but this is rare). The use of gallows traction to reduce a hernia is obsolete.
- Provided the hernia is reduced a herniotomy should be performed after 24–48hr to allow for any oedema to settle.

Hydroceles

Infantile hydroceles are common.

- Caused by failure of the processus vaginalis to obliterate after testicular descent through the inguinal canal.
- Clinical signs are a soft swelling around the testis that transilluminates and above which the examiner can get (Fig. 23.16).
- Most resolve by the second year and those that do not should be treated surgically through a short groin incision.
- Check for inguinal hernia.

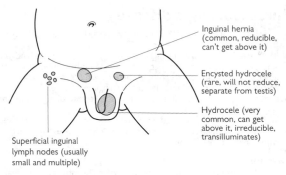

Inguinal hernia
(common, reducible,
can't get above it)

Encysted hydrocele
(rare, will not reduce,
separate from testis)

Hydrocele (very
common, can get
above it, irreducible,
transilluminates)

Superficial inguinal
lymph nodes (usually
small and multiple)

Fig. 23.16 Groin swellings.

Hirschsprung's disease

The incidence of HSD is 1/5000 live births. It may be familial and associated with trisomy 21.

- It is caused by a failure of ganglion cells to migrate into the hindgut.
- This defect leads to an absence of co-ordinated bowel peristalsis and functional intestinal obstruction at the junction ('transition zone') between normal bowel and the distal aganglionic bowel.
- In 80% of cases the transition zone is in the rectum or sigmoid—short segment disease.
- In 20% of cases the entire colon is involved—long segment disease.
- Occasionally, children with short segment disease present in childhood with chronic constipation.

Diagnosis

- Usually presents within the first few days of life with low intestinal obstruction, i.e. failure to pass meconium, abdominal distension, and bile-stained vomiting. 99% of normal newborns pass meconium within 24hr of delivery.
- *AXR:* distal intestinal obstruction.
- *Rectal biopsy:* no ganglion cells in the submucosa.

Surgical treatment

Many surgeons now perform a single stage pull-through in the neonatal period, managing initial intestinal obstruction with rectal washouts, but traditionally a 3-stage procedure is used.

- Defunctioning colostomy, with multiple biopsies to confirm the site of the transition zone.
- Pull-through procedure to bring ganglionic bowel down to the anus.
- Closure of colostomy.

Outcome

- The long-term results are generally satisfactory with approximately 75% of children acquiring normal bowel control, 15–20% partial control, and 5% who never gain control and may end up with a permanent stoma.
- Most important complication of HSD is enterocolitis. A dramatic gastroenteritic illness characterized by abdominal distension, bloody watery diarrhoea, circulatory collapse, and septicaemia. Condition usually associated with *Clostridium difficile* toxin in the stools. Mortality ~10%.

Rectal prolapse

Rectal prolapse refers to a mucosal or full-thickness herniation of rectum through the anal canal.
- Most commonly seen in constipated toddlers squatting and straining.
- Rarely associated with diarrhoea, cystic fibrosis, and coeliac disease.

Management
- Often the prolapse reduces spontaneously after defecation. If not, gentle digital reduction should be performed.
- Constipation should be treated.
- Recurrent prolapse may be managed with submucous injection of 5% phenol in almond oil.
- More complicated surgical procedures are rarely necessary.

Anorectal malformations

The incidence of anorectal malformation is 1/5000 live births. Anorectal malformations comprise part of the VACTERL association (see 📖 p.848). The abnormality should be identified at birth. The baby presents with:
- failure to pass meconium;
- abdominal distension;
- bile-stained vomiting.

Anatomy

The precise anatomy varies but the malformation can be subdivided into high and low/intermediate anomalies in males and females.

Low/intermediate anomalies
- Rectum is present and passes through a normal sphincter complex.
- In boys (Fig. 23.17) there is a tiny fistulous track to the surface of the perineum, often anteriorly on to the scrotum. If meconium is visible on the perineum a local 'cut-back' procedure can be performed to open the fistula back to the rectum in anticipation of normal continence.
- In girls (Fig. 23.18) the rectum usually opens into the back of the introitus as a rectovestibular fistula. This abnormality is termed intermediate because, although normal continence is to be expected, reconstruction involves division of a common wall between rectum and vagina. For this reason treatment involves a 3-stage procedure with defunctioning colostomy, anorectal reconstruction, and then closure of the stoma.
- Vesicoureteric reflux is very common.

High anomalies
- These anomalies are rare in girls but common in boys (Fig. 23.17).
- The sphincter complex is poorly developed and the prospects for continence are mediocre.
- In boys the rectum makes a fistulous connection with the urethra. Treatment involves a defunctioning colostomy within the first 48hr of birth, reconstruction at a few months of age (most commonly involving a posterior sagittal anorectoplasty performed through a midline perineal incision), and then closure of the colostomy.

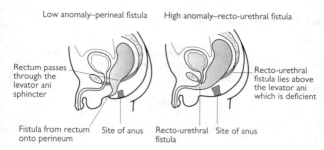

Low anomaly–perineal fistula High anomaly–recto-urethral fistula

Rectum passes through the levator ani sphincter

Recto-urethral fistula lies above the levator ani which is deficient

Fistula from rectum onto perineum Site of anus

Recto-urethral fistula Site of anus

Fig. 23.17 Male anorectal malformations.

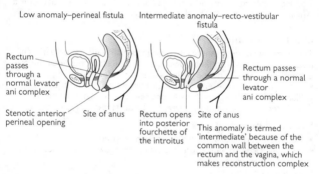

Low anomaly–perineal fistula Intermediate anomaly–recto-vestibular fistula

Rectum passes through a normal levator ani complex

Rectum passes through a normal levator ani complex

Stenotic anterior perineal opening Site of anus

Rectum opens into posterior fourchette of the introitus Site of anus

This anomaly is termed 'intermediate' because of the common wall between the rectum and the vagina, which makes reconstruction complex

Fig. 23.18 Female anorectal malformations.

Umbilical anomalies

Granuloma

The commonest umbilical abnormality seen in infants is an umbilical granuloma (see Fig. 23.19). This is a harmless reaction to the resolving umbilical stump and usually disappears by the 2nd to 3rd week.

Treatment

A persistent granuloma should be cauterized with a silver nitrate stick. Vaseline should be applied round the umbilicus to prevent damage to the surrounding skin and a small dressing placed over the umbilicus to prevent marking of the baby's vest. Multiple applications may be necessary.

⚠ **Caution** A persistent 'granuloma' discharging small bowel contents signifies a patent vitello-intestinal duct (Fig. 23.19). Treatment involves surgical exploration of the umbilicus and excision of the duct with a small segment of ileum. The diagnosis is clinical.

Urachal remnants

These are uncommon anomalies that present in infancy or early childhood. The urachus is an embryonic tubular connection between the bladder and the allantois that normally obliterates before birth.
* *Main symptom:* persistent discharge of urine from the umbilicus.
* *Bladder outlet obstruction* (posterior urethral valves) should be excluded by micturating cystography. Treatment is surgical closure.

Umbilical hernias (Fig. 23.19)

* Common, particularly in Afro-Caribbean children.
* Most will close spontaneously during the first few years of life, regardless of size.
* Complications are rare.
* If the hernia fails to close surgical repair can be performed at around 5yrs of age.

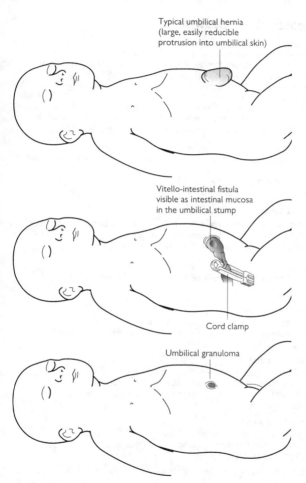

Fig. 23.19 Disorders of the umbilicus.

Testicular torsion

Testicular torsion must be excluded in a child with acute scrotal pain. The peak incidence occurs around 12yrs, but it can occur at any age.

- *Congenital testicular torsion:* rare perinatal event. Newborn infant has a hard, painless scrotal mass. Testis has invariably infarcted and exploration is not necessary, nor is fixation of the opposite testis. The pathology is torsion of the spermatic cord outside the tunica vaginalis.
- *Torsion outside the perinatal period:* the result of an abnormally mobile mesentery of the testis inside the tunica vaginalis. This anomaly is bilateral and allows the gonad to twist on its vascular pedicle.

Presentation

- Sudden onset severe scrotal pain, often associated with nausea and vomiting.
- Tender testis.
- Overlying scrotal skin may be reddened and oedematous.

Treatment

- Immediate scrotal exploration is mandatory to salvage the testis, which should then be fixed to prevent recurrence.
- The contralateral testis should also be fixed.

Differential diagnosis of acute scrotal pain

See also 📖 p.877

Testicular torsion
- Sudden onset pain, swelling, and nausea
- Testis is very tender, and may lie transversely in scrotum
- Scrotal skin may be red

Torted hydatid
- Gradual onset of less severe pain; no nausea
- Focal tenderness at upper pole of testis
- Torted hydatid may be visible through scrotal skin as a pea-sized blue/black swelling

Epididymo-orchitis
- Insidious onset of dysuria and fever
- Usually associated with a urinary tract infection
- Red tender scrotum

Testicular trauma History obvious and there are signs of trauma/haematocele

Idiopathic scrotal oedema
- Child is well
- Scrotal skin is cellulitic but the testes are not tender
- The condition settles spontaneously within a few days

Orchitis and epididymitis

Orchitis

- Orchitis is an uncommon condition in boys that presents with fever and testicular pain.
- Approximately 20% of prepubertal patients with mumps develop orchitis (see 🕮 p.713).
- Diagnosis based on a history of recent mumps or parotitis; mumps orchitis is unilateral in 70% of cases.
- In 30% of cases, contralateral testicular involvement follows a few days later.
- This condition is rare in post-pubertal boys.
- Bacterial orchitis is usually associated with an epididymitis.

Epididymitis

- Usually associated with concomitant orchitis.
- In children epididymo-orchitis is usually associated with a urinary tract infection: infected urine refluxes down the vas.
- Structural abnormality in the renal tract should be excluded.
- Epididymo-orchitis presents with fever, urinary symptoms, and scrotal pain.
- In sexually-active adolescents epididymo-orchitis may be caused by gonorrhoea or *Chlamydia*.
- Epididymo-orchitis should be managed with antibiotics once urine has been sent for culture. Adolescents should be screened for sexually transmitted infection (see 🕮 p.801).

Testicular trauma

A direct blow to the scrotum may rupture a testis. The scrotum is too painful to examine clinically and a gentle US examination should be performed. If the testis is disrupted surgical exploration and repair is necessary to prevent atrophy. If the blow is severe a urethral injury should be suspected and, if necessary, excluded by urethrography.

Undescended testes (cryptorchidism)

The testes descend through the inguinal canals into the scrotum during the first trimester. Cryptorchidism (Fig. 23.20) is seen in 3% of full-term newborn boys and 1% of boys at 1yr. Spontaneous descent may occur in the first 6mths, but is unlikely after this. Cryptorchidism is more common in premature infants.

Clinical aspects

Undescended testes are subdivided into the following.

- *Palpable undescended testes (80%):* usually at the external inguinal ring. These testes can be bought down into the scrotum with an orchidopexy performed through an inguinal incision.
- *Impalpable testes (20%):* intra-abdominal, inside the inguinal canal, or absent. There is risk of malignant degeneration in an intraabdominal testis (1:70, compared with 1:5000 for normal testis). Laparoscopy is the investigation of choice for an impalpable testis. US, CT/MRI are not helpful. If the vas and vessels enter the deep inguinal ring (30%), an inguinal orchidopexy is indicated. If the vas and vessels end blindly at the deep ring (30%), then the testis has torted *in utero* and has resorbed. No further action is necessary. If a testis is seen inside the abdomen then it must be removed or bought down with a two-stage orchidopexy.

When should boys be referred to a surgeon?

- If an undescended testis is noted on routine postnatal check, this should be documented in the medical records.
- Initial follow-up should be with the GP because the majority of these testes will descend during the first 6mths of life.
- If still undescended at 6mths, refer to a paediatric surgeon.

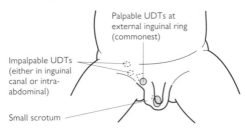

Palpable UDTs at
external inguinal ring
(commonest)

Impalpable UDTs
(either in inguinal
canal or intra-
abdominal)

Small scrotum

Fig. 23.20 Undescended testes (UDT).

Retractile testes

The cremasteric muscle is overactive and the testes retract into the groin. The scrotum is well developed and the parents may notice that the testes are in place when the child is in a warm bath. Examine in a warm environment. The testes can be manipulated into the scrotum and will remain there until the cremasteric reflex is stimulated. Surgery is not necessary.

Hypospadias

Hypospadias affects ~1/350 male births. Characterized by an abnormal position of the external urethral meatus and is classified according to the location of the meatus (penis down to the scrotum; see Fig. 23.21). Severe forms of hypospadias may be associated with chordee—a ventral curvature of the penis. The most common consequences of hypospadias are difficulty urinating while standing and a cosmetic appearance of the penis that differs from that of other boys. Sexual function is not affected unless chordee, which may cause painful erections, is present.

Hypospadias advice

- Make sure you document the diagnosis in the notes.
- Tell the parents *not* to circumcise the child.
- Give the parents a letter stating this advice.
- Refer the child to a paediatric surgeon.

Surgery

Surgical correction involves straightening of any chordee and reconstruction of the urethra to the glans. This may involve tubularizing skin from the prepuce so circumcision is contraindicated. The correction can be completed in one or more operations during early childhood.

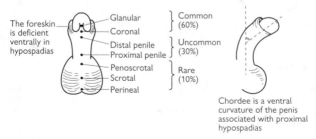

Fig. 23.21 Classification of hypospadias.

Phimosis and paraphimosis

The foreskin develops *in utero* as a protuberance of the penile epidermis, which grows forwards over the glans and adheres to it. The prepuce is normally non-retractable during early childhood. During this period it is very common for parents to notice that the child's prepuce balloons during micturition. It is also very common for boys to complain of intermittent redness and discomfort from the prepuce. This is rarely the result of bacterial or candidal infection, but simply a chemical irritation from urine under the foreskin. These symptoms are self-limiting and resolve during childhood without intervention (i.e. circumcision).

Circumcision

There are few medical indications for circumcision in boys. The majority of non-religious circumcisions performed in the UK are unnecessary (i.e. normal non-retractile foreskins). Genuine indications for circumcision are:

- *Phimosis:* this is almost exclusively caused by balanitis xerotica obliterans (BXO, or lichen sclerosis) which is an uncommon scarring dermatitis characterized by a thickened indurated whitish appearance of the tip of the prepuce. BXO affects 2% of boys by the age of 17yrs and is very rare in those aged <5yrs.
- *Paraphimosis:* the prepuce retracts as the boy gets an erection and becomes stuck behind the glans. The glans becomes swollen and oedematous. The paraphimosis should be reduced under general anaesthesia and circumcision scheduled a few weeks later to prevent recurrence.
- *Recurrent balanitis:* this is rare.

Balanitis/balanoposthitis

Balanoposthitis is acute inflammation of the glans and foreskin associated with a purulent discharge from the preputial orifice. This condition affects 4% of boys, mostly between 2 and 5yrs of age. Recurrent episodes rare.

- *UTI: Staphylococcus aureus* is the most common cause.
- *Treatment:* 5-day course of oral trimethoprim or amoxycillin is appropriate. Topical antibacterials or antifungals are of no value.

Priapism

Priapism is a persistent painful erection. The commonest cause in boys is trauma, usually a fall astride injury to the perineum. Occasionally, priapism is a presenting symptom of acute leukaemia or SCD. Treatment is usually conservative, but may need intervention in SCD (📘 p.621).

Penile trauma

Most penile trauma is iatrogenic as a result of circumcision. Bleeding post-circumcision usually needs exploration under anaesthetic. Clotting should be checked to exclude haemophilia in infants. Entrapment of the foreskin in trouser zips is occasionally seen.

• If the prepuce is caught between the teeth of the zip, then release can be achieved by cutting across the zip and separating the edges.
• This can usually be managed in casualty. Entrapment between the zip slide and the teeth is more complicated because the slider has to be prised off with bone cutters. This is best performed under anaesthetic.

Imperforate hymen

An imperforate hymen usually presents within a few days of life with a lower abdominal mass, sometimes associated with urinary retention. Intrauterine stimulation of the infant's cervical mucous glands by maternal oestrogens causes accumulation of secretions (mucocolpos). The imperforate hymen can be seen bulging through the introitus and treatment consists of incising the hymen. Occasionally, an imperforate hymen is not detected in the newborn period and presents at puberty with 1° amenorrhoea or a painful lower abdominal mass from a haematocolpos. Treatment again comprises incision of the hymen and should be performed under general anaesthesia.

Labial adhesions in infants

Labial adhesions are common in female toddlers. Nappy rash and exposure to urine cause a chronic irritation of the fragile labia which adhere. There is invariably a small opening anteriorly through which urine escapes. Labial adhesions cause no symptoms, but they are a major source of anxiety to parents. Treatment is best deferred until the child is out of nappies. Topical application of oestrogenic cream for 2wks will result in separation of most adhesions but occasionally gentle separation under anaesthetic may be necessary.

Miscellaneous conditions

Tongue-tie

Common and rarely causes symptoms. Tongue-tie does not cause lisp, and is most definitely not responsible for eating problems in an older child. Division of a tongue-tie does not alter the natural history of either condition. Tongue-tie does affect the ability of newborns to breastfeed and division of the lingual frenulum within the first week of life will correct this problem. Bottle feeding is not affected (🕮 p.146).

Dermoid cysts

Common in children (Fig. 23.22). Dermoids are non-tender, mobile subcutaneous cysts filled with keratin, hair follicles, and sebaceous glands. They enlarge slowly and should be treated by excision. Dermoid cysts occur most frequently along lines of embryological fusion, such as lateral corner of the eyebrows (external angular dermoid), midline of the neck, over the bridge of the nose, and suprasternal notch.

Thyroglossal duct cysts (TDC)

Present with midline swelling in the neck, just below the hyoid bone. The swelling rises with tongue protrusion and swallowing. TDCs develop from epithelial remnants left after descent of the developing thyroid from the foramen caecum at the base of the tongue. TDCs gradually enlarge and eventually become infected, which makes excision more difficult. Treatment is surgical removal of the central portion of the hyoid bone along with the cyst and track.

Branchial remnants

Branchial remnants persist from the branchial clefts during embryogenesis of the head and neck. Anomalies of the second branchial cleft are by far the most common. They can be a cyst, a sinus tract, or rarely a fistula.
- *Branchial sinuses:* present as small cutaneous openings along the anterior lower third border of the sternocleidomastoid muscle that discharge mucus (Fig. 23.23). They can communicate with the tonsillar fossa (branchial fistula). Management is excision to prevent infection.
- *Branchial cysts:* uncommon neck swellings along the anterior border of the sternomastoid. The differential includes cystic hygroma, which is more common, and the treatment is surgery.

Cystic hygroma (CH)

A congenital malformation of the lymphatic system. CHs present in early childhood as soft multilocular cystic swellings that often appear after an intercurrent viral infection. CHs are more often found in the neck and axillae, although they can occur anywhere, including inside the abdomen or thorax. Large cervical cystic hygromas may present at birth with airway obstruction. Small CHs require no treatment. Large lesions infiltrate the surrounding tissues making complete surgical excision impossible. Intralesional injection of OK432 (lyophilized product of *Streptococcus pyogenes*) is an alternative to surgery in some cases.

Congenital torticollis

See also 📖 p.127. Within the first weeks of birth a small swelling in the baby's neck is noticed. A sternomastoid tumour is a palpable area of fibrosis in the lower sternomastoid muscle (SM) and is a transient phenomenon that will resolve after a few months. Sometimes there is a history of dystocia. Shortening of the SM results in torticollis with rotation and tilting of the head to the opposite side. Management is conservative in most cases with passive exercises to achieve full neck movements. Hemifacial atrophy and strabismus may develop unless full movement is restored. Occasionally it is necessary to divide the SM, but this is no substitute for physiotherapy.

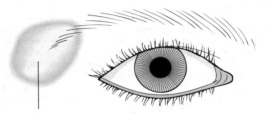

External angular dermoid cyst

Fig. 23.22 External angular dermoid cyst.

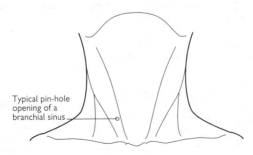

Typical pin-hole opening of a branchial sinus

Fig. 23.23 Branchial sinus.

Perioperative care

Elective children

All children need to have a history and examination:

- The *presenting complaint* should be documented and confirmed.
- Previous medical history, medication, and allergies must be recorded.
- A brief clinical examination should be performed. In the case of undescended testes, hydroceles, and inguinal hernias a mark should be made on the child's thigh to document the side for operation (away from the surgical field to prevent tattooing of the wound).
- If the child is unwell with an intercurrent illness, discuss with the anaesthetist who may decide that the child is unfit for anaesthesia.

Blood tests

These should be kept to a minimum. Children undergoing major surgery should have the following done:

- Haemoglobin checked and blood cross-matched, according to the nature of the operation (usually one unit of blood is sufficient).
- Urea and electrolytes should be checked pre-operatively in children taking diuretics, children in renal failure, and children receiving IV fluids.
- Children at risk of sickle cell disease or thalassaemia should be screened in outpatients before admission.

Fasting prior to elective surgery

This is essential for safe induction of anaesthesia. Recommendations from the Association of Paediatric Anaesthetists are given in Box 23.2.

Box 23.2 Minimum fasting times prior to elective surgery

- *Solid food:* 6hr
- *Formula milk:* 6hr
- *Breast milk:* 4hr
- *Clear fluids (dextrose solution, water):* 2hr

Anaesthetist

The anaesthetist will visit pre-operatively and discuss anaesthesia and post-operative analgesia with the child and parents. In some instances pre-medication may be appropriate.

- IV access will be obtained during induction of anaesthesia and it is sensible to pre-empt this by applying local anaesthetic ointment (e.g. EMLA™) under occlusive dressings to the back of the child's hands or feet, provided a suitable vein is visible.
- Some anaesthetists are happy for children to come down to theatre wearing their pyjamas; others may request a theatre gown.
- Paediatric anaesthetists generally encourage one parent to accompany the child to the anaesthetic room and many will be happy for the parent to remain with the child during induction.

Newborns

Pre-operative resuscitation and preparation are essential if the outcome of surgery is to be successful. Newborns with congenital malformations will be admitted to a neonatal intensive care unit.

Routine preparation

This should include:
- Intramuscular vitamin K.
- FBC to determine the haemoglobin.
- Cross-matching blood. Many laboratories require a sample of maternal blood for typing and this should accompany the baby if the mother is unable or unfit to travel.

Echocardiography

Babies with OA and anorectal malformations should undergo echocardiography before surgery because of the possible cardiac defects in the VATER association.

Renal imaging

Provided the baby passes urine (indicative of functioning nephrons) renal imaging can be arranged electively. Anuria necessitates a renal US scan to exclude renal agenesis.

Intestinal obstruction

Babies will require:
- *IV fluid:* normal maintenance is required. Babies with gastroschisis lose fluid and heat rapidly from the exposed bowel. The baby's abdomen should be wrapped circumferentially in Clingfilm™ (this does not need to be sterile). Regular bolus infusions of 4.5% albumin solution should be given before closure of the defect.
- *NG decompression:* a wide bore NGT is necessary to empty the stomach (8 or 10 French gauge). The NGT should be aspirated every hour and left on free drainage. NG aspirates should be replaced mL for mL with 0.9% saline with 20mmol KCl/L, in addition to maintenance fluids.
- *Biochemistry and acid–base balance:* necessary in babies with prolonged vomiting (e.g. pyloric stenosis).

Consent for surgery

See also 📖 pp.1036–1039.

Consent for surgery: clinical practice

The best person to obtain consent is the surgeon performing the operation

Children

- Whenever possible the procedure should be explained to the child in language that he/she can understand
- Young children are not generally interested in alternative treatments and risk. They are reassured to know that their parents will be with them when they go off to sleep
- Children are interested to know how long the operation will take, how they will feel afterwards, and how long they will get off school

Parents

Informed consent must be sought from the parents. This must include:
- An explanation of the diagnosis and the proposed operation, along with alternative treatments, risks and benefits, and the likely outcomes
- It is prudent to discuss potential complications and provide an estimate of risk. The risk of adverse reactions to general anaesthesia in fit, healthy children is between 1/10,000 and 1/100,000, which is comparable with the risk of injury crossing a road

Emergency

- In an emergency it is justifiable to treat without parental consent
- It must, however, be documented clearly that the child's life is in danger and that attempts have been made to contact the parents
- Ensure that entries in the records are signed, timed, and dated
- Verbal consent from the parents is acceptable in an emergency and this should be recorded on the consent form

Post-operative care: fluids

Day case children

Children admitted for day case surgery will return to the day care ward from the theatre recovery area once they are alert, able to maintain their airway, haemodynamically stable, and comfortable. The presence of a parent in the recovery room is usually beneficial. Oral fluids can be offered in most cases on return to the ward and, if tolerated without nausea, followed by food. Within a few hours most children can be discharged home.

Major surgery

Following major surgery children will return to the ward or intensive care unit. The operation note should include specific instructions regarding antibiotics, catheters, IV fluids, etc.

- *Post-operative IV fluids:* will depend on the nature of the surgery. There is now a general directive to use 0.45% sodium chloride with 5% dextrose or 0.9% sodium chloride for post-operative fluid because the risk of hyponatraemia is minimized. The rate of infusion should be adjusted according to the weight of the child. Potassium chloride 20mmol/L should be added to fluids after the first day.
- *Nasogastric aspirates:* should be replaced mL for mL with 0.9% sodium chloride with 20mmol KCl/L. It is easy to underestimate 'third space losses' (i.e. fluid translocating into the peritoneum, bowel, or chest) after major surgery and this volume of fluid should be added to the maintenance requirements and fluid given to replace continuing losses (e.g. NG aspirates). If the child has cool peripheries and a prolonged capillary refill time the situation will almost always improve after infusion of 20mL/kg of additional fluid (0.45% sodium chloride with 5% dextrose, 0.9% saline, 4.5% albumin, and plasma substitutes are all used in practice).
- *Haemoglobin:* check the haemoglobin on the first post-operative day. Blood transfusion is to be avoided whenever possible and, with the exception of oxygen dependent children, a moderate post-operative anaemia is well tolerated. If transfusion is necessary (i.e. haemoglobin <7.0g/dL) every effort should be made to ensure that the child is only exposed to blood from one donor even if this means that the volume of blood transfused is less than originally calculated. Routine co-administration of diuretics is not necessary in the surgical patient.
- *Biochemistry:* children with high urinary or high stoma losses receiving IV fluids should have blood U&E measured daily. Frequent adjustments to the electrolyte content and rate of infusion may be necessary.
- *Oral fluids:* following abdominal surgery most children will have a paralytic ileus for 36–48hr. After this period, oral intake will resume and IV fluids can be discontinued. If more prolonged IV fluid therapy is necessary consideration should be given to parenteral nutrition.

Nasogastric tubes

NGTs usually inserted to keep the stomach empty. In the pre-operative period this is useful in a child with an intestinal obstruction. A bile-stained aspirate signifies an intestinal obstruction and emptying the stomach will prevent the child from vomiting. Unless otherwise instructed, the NGT should be aspirated every hour and the aspirate replaced intravenously mL for mL with 0.9% saline containing KCl 20mmol/L.

- Common practice to insert a NGT in theatre in a child undergoing abdominal surgery that is likely to result in a paralytic ileus.
- Post-operative management is the same as pre-operative. As the ileus resolves after 24–36hr the volume of the NGT aspirate will decrease and it will become clear. At this stage the NGT can usually be removed and oral fluids resumed. In most cases prescription of the volume of oral fluid is not necessary, but restricting the child to water only for the first 24hr effectively limits the amount they ingest.

Transanastomotic tubes

Following repair of OA in the newborn the surgeon will commonly place a 'transanastomotic tube' (TAT). The purpose of the TAT is to allow early resumption of enteral nutrition.

- Do not attempt to repass a TAT that has been removed inadvertently without seeking advice from the surgeon.
- Perforating an anastomosis is likely to land both you and the baby in trouble!

Newborns and infants

Newborns and infants <44wks post-conception should be transferred to a neonatal or special care baby unit post-operatively. The risk of post-operative apnoea after general anaesthesia is relatively high. Monitoring for a minimum of 24hr post-anaesthetic should include routine nursing observations of:

- temperature;
- pulse;
- respirations;
- pulse oximetry;
- apnoea monitoring.

Post-operative care: analgesia

See also 📖 p.1018.

Analgesia for day cases

Operations are painful and analgesia is essential.

- In many cases, local anaesthetic blocks or wound infiltration will provide complete analgesia for several hours.
- After this simple analgesics, such as paracetamol or ibuprofen are usually all that is required.
- For older children codeine and/or diclofenac may be necessary. A prescription for 2–3 days should be given prior to discharge.

Analgesia for major surgery

After major surgery stronger analgesia is required for a longer period. This applies to neonates, as well as older children.

Continuous epidural infusions of local anaesthetics

There are many advantages to local or regional analgesia and continuous epidural infusions of local anaesthetics (e.g. bupivicaine) work particularly well after major abdominal or thoracic surgery.

- Epidural infusions are not without risk. It is essential that close nursing supervision is maintained (i.e. vital signs and level of the epidural block).
- In many hospitals there is a 'paediatric pain team' who supervise the epidural. If this is not available, close liaison should be maintained with the anaesthetist responsible.
- If the level of anaesthesia seems to be rising to the upper thoracic dermatomes the infusion should be stopped pending advice.
- If the analgesia is inadequate advice should be sought before either removing the epidural catheter or starting opiates.

Continuous IV infusion of morphine

Infusion of morphine or other opiates is another very effective method of post-operative analgesia. For older children, this may be in the form of a patient-controlled analgesia pump with a button the child can press to obtain an increment of analgesic.

- Most hospitals will have guidelines on the use of analgesics for children that should be followed. 'Pain ladders' providing options for analgesics of increasing potency are becoming common.
- It is not acceptable to leave a child in pain and it is simply untrue that administering strong analgesics will mask clinical signs. Peritonitis can be detected reliably in a child who has received morphine.

POST-OPERATIVE CARE: DRAINS AND WOUNDS

Post-operative care: drains and wounds

Chest drain removal

An adult can be asked to suspend respiration in full inspiration before removal of a chest drain. Children will not co-operate with this.

- The best strategy is to remove the drain quickly. Then cover the site with an air-tight transparent dressing (e.g. Tegaderm™).
- The dressing should remain undisturbed for 48hr after which time the wound can be left open.
- Purse-string sutures are painful and not necessary.
- It is not necessary to take a chest radiograph immediately after the drain has been removed provided the child is clinically well.

Wound care

Routine closure of skin wounds in children is by subcuticular suture. The suture runs along below the surface of the wound and provides a neat and water-tight closure. Invariably an absorbable suture is used (e.g. Vicryl™ or PDS™).

- Dressings are a matter for individual preference. If dressings are used it is wise to keep the wound dry until the dressing is removed.
- If no dressing is used, then keep the wound dry for 24–48hr.
- The appearance of clean surgical wounds should improve progressively each day after surgery.
- Parents should be asked to report increasing redness or tenderness so that the wound can be reviewed.

Advice after discharge from hospital

Parents should be given clear simple advice before discharge from hospital regarding analgesia, wound care, and post-operative follow-up. Ideally, written information should also be provided.

- *Following minor day case:* children will generally be back to normal within 24hr. They should be kept off school for 2–3 days and be excused sports activities for 14 days. Routine follow-up of children has now been abandoned by most surgeons. This is, however, a matter of personal preference.
- *Convalescence following major surgery:* specific advice relating to return to school and resumption of sporting activity depends on the operation.

Chapter 24

Special senses

Common presentations

The red eye

Careful evaluation is needed when presentation is acute and there is associated pain, swelling, constant lacrimation, or blurred vision.

Causes
- URTI.
- Viral conjunctivitis.
- Irritant conjunctivitis, e.g. chlorinated swimming pool.
- Bacterial conjunctivitis.
- Stye (infection of eyelash follicle).
- Chalazion (meibomian or tarsal cyst).
- *Other:* corneal laceration/ulcer/keratitis; FB; peri-orbital cellulitis; uveitis.

Differential diagnosis
- *Redness of entire eyelid or swollen eyelid:*
  - peri-orbital cellulitis (📖 p.919);
  - acute ethmoiditis.
- *Associated eye pain or constant eye tearing, blinking:*
  - corneal ulcer;
  - HSV keratitis;
  - eye FB (📖 p.916).
- *Blurred vision:* uveitis (📖 p.915).
- *Infant under age 1mth:* gonorrhoea (📖 p.914).
- *Painless red eye with good vision:* sub-conjunctival haemorrhage
- *Uncomfortable red eye with good vision:*
  - conjunctivitis—viral, bacterial, allergic, or chemical;
  - episcleritis
- *Painful red eye with photophobia:*
  - corneal or sub-tarsal FB;
  - corneal abrasion;
  - corneal ulcer/keratitis;
  - anterior uveitis (iritis);
  - scleritis.
- *Eyelid redness and oedema:*
  - *localized*—stye, meibomian cyst, dacryocystitis (lacrimal sac abscess);
  - *generalized*—pre-septal or orbital cellulitis;
  - acute allergic conjunctivitis;
  - herpes simplex/herpes zoster ophthalmicus.

Ear: pain and discharge

Ear discharge (otorrhoea) may be due to drainage of blood, ear wax, pus, or fluid from the external or middle ear.

- Otitis externa.
- Eczema and other skin irritations.
- Foreign object impaction.
- Otitis media.
- Mastoiditis.
- Perforated eardrum.
- Head injury—CSF leak.

Earache (otalgia) can be a symptom of the conditions noted above. However, it may be the result of pain referred from pathology at another location (referred otalgia):

- Sinusitis
- Parotitis.
- Teeth and jaw (impacted molars, dental caries).
- Acute tonsillitis;.
- Oropharyngeal tumours.

Hearing assessment

A foetus will respond to sound in the latter part of pregnancy (from 3rd trimester). At birth, the baby will react to noise with a marked preference for voices.

Hearing screening

See also 🕮 p.560.

Specific screening questions can be asked when evaluating hearing:
- *Birth*: does baby startle to loud noise?
- *12wks*:
  - Does baby quieten to mother's voice even when mother cannot be seen?
  - Does baby quieten to prolonged loud noise?
  - Does baby settle to a musical toy?
- *5mths*:
  - Does baby smile to familiar voice?
  - Does he/she take turns to vocalize when spoken to?
- *7mths*:
  - Does baby turn to look towards a new sound?
  - Does he/she make tuneful vocalization?
- *9mths*:
  - Does baby recognize own name?
  - Does baby recognize and react to familiar tunes and music?
- *11mths*: Will baby react to calling from out of sight?

The early detection of hearing loss is important. Deafness impairs speech and language development, cognitive development, and socialization. A baby who does not startle when parents come into view may not have heard them approach due to deafness. These children need *urgent* audiological assessment along with children who show absence of appropriate vocalization by age (see bullet points in Hearing screening).

Hearing tests

All health authority areas in the UK have a universal newborn hearing screening (UNHS) programme. UNHS involves otoacoustic emission testing in the first 48hr after birth. In the test a small earpiece is inserted into the ear canal. This delivers a sound that evokes an emission from the ear if the cochlea is normal.

Current hearing screening programmes (Table 24.1)

There is currently some regional variation in the type of tests used.

In line with recommendations once UNHS is in place, universal distraction testing at 7–9mths will be abandoned.

Table 24.1 Hearing screening programmes

Age	Screening test
Birth	Otoacoustic emission. Auditory brainstem-evoked potential. Auditory response cradle test
6–9mths	Distraction test
18mths to 4yrs	Pure tone audiometry (from 3yrs)Speech discrimination test. Impedance audiometry
≥4yrs	Pure tone audiometry

The distraction test

The test is based on the principle that a normal response is observed when sound is presented to an infant, and the infant turns their head to locate the source of the sound. Two testers are required—one presents the sound out of the infant's line of vision, while the other holds the infant's attention in a forward direction. The test involves delivering a frequency—specific stimulus presented at quiet levels (35dB) to the side and slightly behind an infant who is seated on a parent's knee.

Distraction testing requires a behavioural response and is therefore a direct test of hearing sensitivity. The major disadvantages of this test are that an infant must be mature enough to sit erect and head turn, and it is subject to all the common biases found in behavioural testing of hearing. It is therefore unsuitable for neonates, which makes identification of hearing loss before 6mths of age very difficult.

Childhood deafness

Hearing loss or deafness may be congenital or acquired and can be divided into sensorineural (SN) or conductive loss. Hearing loss of up to 20dB tends not to affect development, but a loss of over 40dB will affect speech and language development.

Sensorineural

Inherited/genetic
- Non syndromic.
- *Syndromic:*
  - Ushers syndrome (see Table 24.2);
  - Waardenburg syndrome (see Table 24.2).

Acquired
- *Perinatal:*
  - birth asphyxia;
  - hyperbilirubinemia;
  - congenital infection, e.g. rubella, CMV, syphilis.
- *Postnatal:*
  - drugs, e.g. aminoglycosides;
  - meningitis;
  - head injury;
  - labyrinthitis;
  - acoustic neuroma.

Conductive

External ear abnormalities
Ear canal atresia/stenosis.

Middle ear abnormalities
- Acute otitis media.
- Chronic otitis media (tympanic perforation, cholesteatoma).
- Secretory otitis media.

Table 24.2 Syndromes associated with childhood deafness

Syndrome	Characteristics
Waardenburg	SN deafness + pigmentation anomalies (white for lock)
Klippel–Feil sequence	Deafness (SN or conductive) + short neck with low hair line
Treacher–Collins	Conductive deafness + midface hypoplasia
Pierre–Robin sequence	Conductive deafness + mandibular hypoplasia & cleft soft palate
Alport	SN deafness, pyelonephritis, haematuria, & renal failure
Pendred	SN deafness + hypothyroidism
Usher	SN deafness + retinitis pigmentosa
Jewel–Lang–Nielson	SN deafness + long QT interval on ECG

Disorders of the ear

See also 📖 pp.280–283.

Otitis media

Infection of the middle ear is associated with pain, fever, and irritability. Examination reveals a red and bulging tympanic membrane with loss of normal light reflex. Occasionally there is acute perforation. Causative organisms include:

- Viruses.
- Pneumococcus.
- Group A β haemolytic streptococcus.
- *Haemophilus influenzae*.

Treatment is with broad-spectrum antibiotics (e.g. oral amoxicillin or co-amoxiclav) and analgesia. Decongestants may also help. Complicating mastoiditis (see 📖 p.901) or meningitis are rare. Recurrent ear infections can lead to secretory otitis media.

Secretory otitis media

- This is a middle ear effusion without the symptoms and signs of acute otitis media. It is often the result of recurrent episodes of acute otitis media.
- Duration often last months (chronic secretory otitis media) and the effusions may be serous (thin), mucoid (thick), or purulent.
- Children, although asymptomatic, may be noticeably inattentive, or complain of hearing loss.
- On examination the drum is retracted and does not move easily.
- Fluid effusions may be visible behind the tympanic membrane, which appears opaque. Chronic (>3mths) secretory otitis media, particularly when associated with suspected hearing loss, needs referral to the audiology and otolaryngology (ear, nose, and throat/ENT) teams for further evaluation and possible treatment with myringotomy and insertion of typanostomy ventilation tubes ('grommets').

Otitis externa

- Itching of the external ear canal is common in swimmers and after minor trauma.
- There may be progressive pain and discharge.
- Examination reveals an inflamed ear canal that may be oedematous.
- Treatment is with suction clearance and a combined antibiotic (hydrocortisone 1% + gentamicin 0.3%) and steroid preparation applied topically.

Cholesteatoma

- This is an erosive condition affecting the middle ear and mastoid.
- It may lead to life-threatening intracranial infection.
- Signs include offensive discharge, conductive hearing loss, vertigo, and rarely facial nerve palsy.
- Urgent referral to the ENT team is required for surgery and antibiotics.

Acute mastoiditis

- Uncommon, but may follow an episode of acute otitis media. In the early stage symptoms are indistinguishable from those of acute otitis media, but may evolve to include intense pain, swelling, or tenderness over the mastoid process.
- The latter is due to acute mastoid osteitis and occurs when infection and destruction of the mastoid bony trabeculae has occurred.
- Clinical examination may also reveal outward and downward displacement of the pinna, and swelling of the posterior–superior wall of the external ear canal.
- Purulent discharge may also be present.
- Diagnosis is largely clinical, although CT scan is helpful. Urgent referral to the ENT team is required for IV antibiotic treatment. Mastoidectomy is sometimes indicated.

Foreign body impaction

- Parents may observe a child putting an object in the ear canal, which otherwise may take several days to come to notice.
- On examination with an auroscope, objects that are easily visible (and with a cooperative child) may be extracted using a hook.
- Use of forceps should be avoided as they tend to push the object further down the ear canal and may damage the tympanic membrane.
- Refer to ENT team.

Ear malformations

- Abnormal shape, orientation, or position of the ears should raise suspicions of an underlying congenital or inherited disorder or syndrome.
- Problems with hearing should also be suspected and evaluated.
- Referral to the clinical genetics team is required.

The following conditions are associated with ear malformations.

Low set ear position

- Turner syndrome (📖 p.948).
- Noonan syndrome (📖 p.941).
- Rubenstein–Taybi syndrome.
- Treacher–Collins syndrome (📖 p.950).

Malformed auricles

- CHARGE association (📖 p.950).
- Ehlers–Danlos syndrome (EDS, 📖 p.946).
- Di George syndrome (📖 p.940).
- Down syndrome (📖 p.936).

Common disorders of the nose

Epistaxis
A nose bleed or epistaxis is common in childhood. There is usually no obvious precipitating cause, but it may be associated with minor nasal trauma (direct injury). Rarely an underlying coagulation disorder may be present (e.g. acute lymphoblastic leukaemia or haemophilia). Purulent, bloody nasal discharge should raise suspicions of FB impaction.

Initial management should include sitting with the head tilted forwards and applying firm pressure to the cartilaginous part of the nose with finger and thumb for 10–15min. If simple measures fail to stop bleeding then referral to the ENT team for nasal packing and cauterization under direct visualization. A blood sample for FBC, clotting screen, and blood group testing is warranted in this situation.

Nasal foreign body
- Children may present with a unilateral offensive discharge from the nose.
- Removal of FBs from the nose is more urgent than in the ear as the object may be inhaled.
- Removal may be attempted if the patient is able to cooperate, by having them try to blow their nose.
  - alternatively, attempt removal directly by dislodging with a suitable instrument;
  - an alligator type forceps should be used to remove cloth, cotton, or paper FBs;
  - pebbles, beans, and other hard FBs are more easily grasped using bayonet forceps, or they may be rolled out by getting behind it using an ear curette, single skin hook, or right angle ear hook.
- If these measures are unsuccessful referral to the ENT team is required.

Nasal polyps
Infrequent in childhood. They are associated with allergic rhinitis or cystic fibrosis. Signs include clear watery rhinorrhoea, postnasal drip, and nasal obstruction. Increased snoring intensity may also be a feature. Treatment with topical corticosteroids (e.g. beclometasone) is required.

Nasal malformations
Abnormalities in nasal development may be associated with a number of congenital or inherited conditions. Here are some examples:

Low/depressed nasal bridge
- Achondrogenesis syndromes (📖 p.967).
- Trisomy 21 (📖 p.936).
- Foetal valproate syndrome.
- Mucopolysaccharoidoses (📖 p.968).

Broad/wide nasal bridge
- EDS (📖 p.946).
- Fragile X syndrome (📖 p.943).
- Waardenburg syndrome.

Small nose
- Cornelia de Lange syndrome (📖 p.948).
- Foetal alcohol syndrome (📖 p.951).
- Osteogenesis imperfecta type 2 (📖 p.762).
- Williams syndrome (WS, 📖 p.941).

Hypoplastic nares
- Ectodermal dysplasia (📖 p.841).
- Cleft lip sequence (📖 p.846).

Prominent nose
- Coffin–Lowry.
- Rubenstein–Taybi.
- Smith–Lemli–Opitz.

Choanae atresia
CHARGE association (📖 p.950).

Disorders of mouth and tongue

Gingivostomatitis
Gingivostomatitis refers to inflammation of the oral mucosa and is characterized by the presence of multiple sores and mouth ulcers. The condition is common, particularly among pre-school aged children, and is usually secondary to a viral infection, particularly those that cause common childhood illness such as:
• Herpes simplex (resulting in cold sores and acute herpetic stomatitis).
• Coxsackie viruses (hand, foot, and mouth disease, and herpangina).

Vesicular lesions may erupt on the lips, gums, tongue, and on the hard palate. There is a wide spectrum of clinical features ranging from the mild to the severe, which is often characterized by:
• Pain on eating and drinking.
• High fever.
• Bleeding from gums.
• Extensive ulceration of the tongue, palate, and buccal mucosa.
• Cervical lymphadenopathy.
• Dehydration due to refusal to eat or drink may occur.

Investigation
Usually no specific tests are required for the diagnosis. Nevertheless, blood for coxsackie or herpes virus serology and culture of material obtained from the surface of the sore may identify the viral infection.

Treatment
• Symptomatic (analgesia) and supportive (fluids).
• Good oral hygiene should be maintained with antiseptic mouth washes where tolerated.
• Severe infection may need admission for rehydration with IV fluids and treatment with oral or IV aciclovir.

Macroglossia
Macroglossia is tongue enlargement that leads to functional and cosmetic problems. Although this is a relatively uncommon disorder, it may cause significant morbidity. Macroglossia may be congenital or acquired in origin.

Congenital
• Down syndrome (p.936).
• Beckwith–Wiedemann (p.949).
• Mucopolysaccharidoses (p.968).

Acquired
Congenital hypothyroidism (see p.422).

In infants macroglossia poses early difficulty with feeding and, in the longer term, children may need assistance with speech and language therapy.

Visual development and examination

Normal visual development

- Vision develops rapidly after birth. By 6wks a baby should have eye contact with the mother when feeding and be able to fix and follow a face.
- Early variable angle squints are common and usually resolve as vision improves and binocular function develops.
- Congenital ocular pathology (e.g. dense cataracts) left untreated by 3mths of age will result in permanently poor vision. Since the visual system retains its plasticity over the first 8yrs of life, any ocular abnormality acquired during this period may also disrupt visual development.
- Parental concerns about a baby's vision are usually well founded, so take them seriously.
- Nystagmus, roving eye movements and/or lack of eye contact warrant referral.

Causes of visual impairment in the UK

One in 1000 children have visual acuity worse than 6/18 in the UK, 70% have an additional disability. Children with visual impairment should receive early specialist educational and mobility support.

Causes of visual impairment

Prenatal (50%)
- Genetic/hereditary (e.g. Down, retinal dystrophies, cataract)
- Hypoxia/ischaemia
- Infection/drugs (e.g. CMV, rubella)

Peri/neonatal (30%)
- Hypoxia/ischaemia (e.g. cerebral visual impairment and retinopathy of prematurity)
- Infection
- NAI

Childhood (20%)
- Tumour (e.g. retinoblastoma, craniopharyngioma)
- Raised ICP
- Hypoxia/ischaemia
- Accidental and NAIs
- Specific systemic disorders (e.g. uveitis)

Vision assessment

Early visual development

At birth most babies can fix and follow horizontally. Initially, the eyes move independently and infant may appear to 'squint'. Visual acuity is about 6/200. Retina is well developed, but the fovea is immature. Development of visual acuity is dependent on the production of well-formed images on the retina. A cataract will affect normal development of the optic pathway and visual cortex. Lack of normal development leads to amblyopia.

- *6wks:* both eyes move together and will follow a light source.
- *3mths:* visual acuity is 6/60. A baby should watch their hands and notice toys.
- *6mths:* a baby reaches for toys and passes them from one hand to the other.

Vision screening

Assessment for visual problems should be performed on all children at the newborn examination, the 6–8wks review, and the pre-school (or school-entry) vision check (see 📖 p.908).

Vision assessment

Birth
- *General observation:* eye movements
- *Ophthalmoscopy:*
  - *Red reflex*—dark spots in the red reflex can be due to cataracts, corneal abnormalities, or opacities in the vitreous. The red reflex may be absent with a dense cataract
  - *White reflex*—present with cataracts, retinoblastoma, or retinopathy of prematurity

6–8wks Optokinetics (e.g. nystagmus demonstrated by looking at a moving, striped target)

2yrs Identification of pictures

3yrs Letter matching on the single letter chart, e.g. Sheridan Gardiner chart

5yrs Identification of letters on the Snellen chart

If the following are evident at the age of 6mths, it should arouse suspicions:
- Lack of eye contact/visual inattention
- Random eye movements
- Persistent nystagmus or squint (see 📖 p.910)

Vision screening in the UK

Neonatal examination
- To detect congenital ocular abnormalities, e.g. cataract, corneal opacities, microphthalmia, glaucoma and retinoblastoma.
- Ask about family history of these disorders.
- Use a (bright) ophthalmoscope to examine the eye and red reflex.
- An indistinct red reflex can be caused by cataracts/corneal opacities.
- Retinoblastoma or abnormal retina can cause a white reflex.
- The red reflex may be darker in Asian and Afro-Caribbean babies.
- Refer on if in doubt.

Community screening
- *At 6wks:* GP asks parents about their baby's visual behaviour. Baby should be able to fix and follow a face and large toy. Red reflexes checked with an ophthalmoscope. Squint assessment.
- *At 7–8wks:* health visitor observes visual behaviour. Parents advised of what to look for regarding expected future visual development.
- *At 4–5yrs:* orthoptist checks monocular visual acuity and ocular alignment, children achieving <6/9.5 are referred.

Secondary screening Orthoptic programme for children referred by parents, health visitors and GPs whenever a concern regarding vision or squint is raised.

Eye examination techniques
Visual examination
- *6–8wks:* baby should fix and follow a bright target and your face.
- *4mths:* baby should not squint and should fix and follow toys.
- *6mths:* baby should reach out for toys.
- *2–3yrs:* use picture charts (e.g. Kays pictures).
- *4–5yrs:* use letter charts (e.g. Snellen +/– matching letter card).

Eye movements
- Use a bright toy to attract attention and move in a 'H' shape to assess the action of each muscle.
- Cover test for squint assessment (see Fig. 24.1).

Anterior segment examination
- Use ophthalmoscope set on +20 for a magnified view of the front of the eye, click in the cobalt filter for fluorescein examination.
- Instill anaesthetic drops prior to examination if the child is in pain.
- Check the diameter of the corneas are equal and that the light reflection from each is bright.
- Check the red reflex in both eyes is equally bright.

Posterior segment examination
- Ask the child to look at an interesting target over your shoulder when trying to examine the optic disc.
- Dilating drops are safe to use, but will interfere with neuro-observations for 24hrs: use 1% cyclopentolate (if <1yr old use 0.5%).

a) Pseudosquint: broad epicanthic folds give the appearance of squint, but the corneal reflections are symmetrical

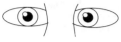

b) Cover test: when a cover is placed over the fixing eye, the squinting eye moves to take up fixation:

Left Esotropia   Left exotropia

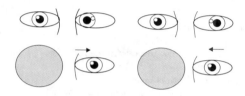

c) Uncover/alternating cover test: the eyes initially appear aligned, but when one eye is covered a latent squint will cause the eye under the cover to deviate. A movement to regain fixation is seen when the cover is removed.

Esophoria   Exophoria

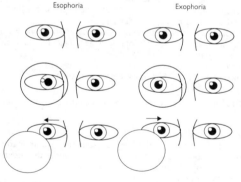

Fig. 24.1 Cover testing.

Squints (strabismus)

Squints are common in childhood. They occur with misalignment of the visual axes of the two eyes so that they appear to point in different directions. If a squint develops in the first 7yrs, it can have a significant impact on visual development.

The causes of squint may be:
• Idiopathic.
• Refractive error.
• Visual loss.
• Ophthalmoplegia (central or peripheral).

Types of squint

There are two main types.

Concomitant (non-paralytic) squint

• Common and usually due to a refractive error in one or both eyes.
• Often convergent.

Non-concomitant (paralytic) squint

• Rare and usually due to cranial (motor) nerve palsy.
• Must exclude an intracranial lesion (e.g. brain tumour).

Describing squints

Squints are described using the following terminology.
• *Convergent:* bad eye turned inwards (cross-eyed appearance)
• *Divergent:* bad eye turned outwards
• *Latent:* a squint that is controlled by subconscious effort and is not always apparent. In certain situations, such as fatigue, the control is lost and the squint will become 'manifest'
• *Pseudosquint:* this arises when wide epicanthic folds give the appearance of a squint, which is excluded on testing

---

Testing squints All squints should be examined using the 'cover test' (see Fig. 24.1).

Management

The aim of treatment is to get the 'weaker' squinting eye 'trained up' in order to prevent amblyopia. Treatments are usually under the supervision of orthoptists in co-operation with ophthalmic surgeons.
• *Correct refractive error:* wear glasses.
• Eye patch wearing on the good eye to 'train' weaker eye.
• Eye muscle exercises.
• Eye (muscle) surgery if large squint and above measures failing.

Note: A child must be seen by an ophthalmologist if squint is:
• Divergent
• Paralytic
• Persistent beyond age of 2mths

Ametropia (refractive disorders)

To see clearly the image must be focused on the retina. In myopia (short/near sight) the image is focused in front of the retina and in hypermetropia (long/far sight) the image is focused behind the retina. Astigmatism results from uneven focusing power at different meridians, causing image distortion. Children are usually born a little long-sighted and the refraction normalizes as the eyes grow. Ametropia may lead to squints and amblyopia. *Quick rule of thumb:* convex lenses (for long sight) magnify; concave lenses (for short sight) minify an image.

Amblyopia

Permanent loss of visual acuity in an eye that has not received clear images in the sensitive period of visual development (up to age 7yrs). Most commonly due to squint, but may also develop with refractive errors and cataracts.

Management

Regular orthoptic monitoring with ongoing correction of the refractive error in the 'lazy'/weaker eye is required.
- *Correct refractive error:* with glasses.
- *Eye patching:* attempt to reverse amblyopia, by covering the better eye to force the 'lazy eye' to work.
- Eye (muscle) surgery.

Visual impairment

Severe visual impairment in 1/1000 births. 50% of severe visual impairment is genetic:
- Identify causes amenable to treatment (e.g. congenital cataracts).
- Use non-visual stimulation (e.g. touch, speech) to aid development.
- Provide a safe environment.

A child is registered blind when the best-corrected vision is less than 3/60. The criterion for partial sight registration is a visual acuity better than 3/60, but less than 6/60.

Causes of visual impairment

Inherited/genetic (50%)
- Trisomy 21 (📖 p.936).
- CHARGE association (📖 p.950).

Congenital
- Cataract (📖 p.916).
- Albinism.
- Retinal dystrophy.
- Retinoblastoma (📖 p.664).
- Congenital infection, e.g. CMV, rubella (📖 p.182).

Antenatal/perinatal (30%)
- Retinopathy of prematurity (📖 pp.188, 920).
- Hypoxic ischaemic encephalopathy (📖 p.172).
- Cerebral damage.
- Optic nerve hypoplasia.

Postnatal (20%)
- Trauma.
- Infection, e.g. ophthalmic herpes simplex.
- *Juvenile idiopathic arthritis:* iritis (📖 pp.768, 915).

Delayed visual maturation

Delayed visual maturation
Babies with delayed visual maturation (DVM) appear blind in the first few months, but their visual behaviour improves with age. There are 3 forms:
- *Isolated DVM:* there is no underlying pathology and there is a rapid and full development of vision between 3–6mths of age. Motor development may also be delayed.
- *DVM associated with cerebral visual impairment:* e.g. infants with cerebral palsy may initially appear blind. The vision usually improves over years, but may be impaired.
- *DVM associated with ocular disease:* congenital ocular disease, e.g. cataracts, and nystagmus can interfere with early visual development. Vision improves over years, but with residual deficit.

Children with DVM should be monitored for general developmental issues. Visual impairment teachers should be involved to help parents to stimulate visual development.

Nystagmus

Nystagmus is an involuntary rhythmic oscillation of one or both eyes (see Table 24.2). The direction of the fast phase, the frequency and amplitude of the nystagmus should be noted. Acquired nystagmus always requires investigation (neuro-imaging and/or electrophysiology). Nystagmus may also occur if there is muscle paralysis or weakness (e.g. secondary to myasthenia gravis) (see 📖 p.544).

Table 24.2 Types and patterns of nystagmus

Type	Pattern/cause
Congenital motor nystagmus	Horizontal jerk
Sensory nystagmus (poor vision)	Usually horizontal jerk
Vestibular nystagmus	Horizontal jerk
Neurological nystagmus	
Gaze paretic	Jerk nystagmus beats towards and worse on lateral gaze
Pendular	High frequency, low amplitude, any direction. Seen in white matter disorders
Upbeat/downbeat	Seen with posterior fossa disorders, e.g. downbeat with Arnold-Chiari malformation
See-saw	One eye elevates while the other depresses,: midline disorders/para-sellar masses
Opsoclonus/ocular flutter	Bursts of high frequency saccades in all directions, e.g. opsoclonus-myoclonus syndrome

Disorders of the eye: infection and inflammatory

Eye infections are common in childhood and largely due to bacterial or viral infections affecting the conjunctiva.

Neonatal conjunctivitis

'Sticky eyes'

Common in the neonatal period starting from the 3rd or 4th day. Swabs are usually negative for significant pathogens. Simple cleaning measures are usually sufficient. Bacterial infection with either *Staphylococcus aureus*, *Pseudomonas aeruginosa*, or streptococcal pathogens can occur. (See also 📖 p.146).

Treatment Topical antibiotic ointment is indicated, e.g. neomycin.

Gonococcal conjunctivitis

Should be suspected if purulent discharge with swelling of the eyelids occurs within the first 48hr of life.

Treatment IV antibiotics required, e.g. cephalosporin.

Chlamydial conjunctivitis

Usually presents at the end of the first week of life. Diagnosis established by specific monoclonal antibody test performed on conjunctival secretions.

Treatment Two-week course of oral erythromycin or topical tetracycline eye ointment is required.

Childhood conjunctivitis

May be due to bacteria (e.g. Gram +ve cocci or *Haemophilus influenzae*), virus (e.g. adenovirus), or to allergic reaction.

Treatment Specific antibiotic eye drops or ointment (e.g. fusidic acid or gentamicin) for 5 days is required.

Allergic conjunctivitis

Acute allergic conjunctivitis can cause rapid onset lid swelling and chemosis (conjunctival oedema). Seasonal/perennial forms present with other features of atopy. Vernal kerato-conjunctivits is a chronic allergic conjunctivitis which is painful and can cause photosensitivity due to corneal involvement. Topical mast cell stabilizers and antihistamines can improve symptoms. Topical steroids are occasionally necessary, but should only be prescribed by a specialist.

Peri-orbital cellulitis See 📖 pp.718, 919

Keratitis

Keratitis is an inflammation or infection of the cornea, which can lead to corneal scarring and requires urgent specialist management. Symptoms include FB sensation, pain, and photophobia with a red eye. It can occur due to viral infection, e.g. HSV or adenovirus in conjunction with skin lesions or conjunctivitis. Bacterial keratitis can occur secondary to corneal exposure in the hospital setting or secondary to contact lens use. Staphylococcal hypersensitivity is a common cause of keratitis in children with blepharitis. Keratitis can also occur as a toxic effect of chemotherapy.

Iritis

Also known as anterior uveitis. Refers to inflammation of the uveal tract structures (i.e. iris, ciliary body, and choroids). It is characterized by symptoms of:
- Ocular pain.
- Photophobia.
- Excessive lacrimation.
- Blurred vision.

Signs include:
- Redness.
- Miosis.
- Keratic precipitates on ophthalmoscopic examination.

Long-term disease may be complicated with the development of cataract, glaucoma, and macular eye degeneration.

Causes of iritis
- *Local infection:* e.g. herpes simplex/zoster.
- Trauma or surgery.
- *Systemic disease:*
  - *Seronegative arthritides*—HLA-B27 positive, ankylosing spondylitis, Reiter's syndrome, psoriatic arthritis (📖 pp.777–779).
  - IBD (📖 p.332).
  - JIA (📖 p.768).
  - Sarcoidosis.
  - Behçet's disease.

Management Referral to the ophthalmologists and treatment with topical steroid drops/ointment and mydriatic agents are required.

Eye foreign body

Small FBs are usually cleared by tear film. Occasionally they may lodge underneath the upper eyelid or become embedded in the cornea causing intense irritation and excessive lacrimation. Examination of the eye to locate and remove the FB should be carried out.

- Instil topical anesthetic drops.
- Perform a visual acuity check (where appropriate) and fundoscopy— examine the anterior chamber and tear film with a bright light (best done with a slit lamp) and examine the conjunctival sacs.
- A loose FB usually adheres to a swab lightly touched to the surface of the conjunctiva, or will be washed out by copious irrigation with saline.
- Referral to the ophthalmology team to exclude any corneal abrasion caused by the FB is usually required.

Cataract

This refers to an opacification of the lens. It may be congenital or acquired.

Causes of cataract

- *Inherited/genetic:*
  - myotonic dystrophy;
  - Walker-Warburg syndrome.
- *Congenital maternal infection:* e.g. rubella, toxoplasmosis (📖 p.182).
- Trauma.
- Radiotherapy.
- *Inflammation:* e.g. chronic iritis.
- Infection.
- *Metabolic syndromes:*
  - galactosaemia(📖 p.967);
  - Wilson's disease (📖 p.976);
  - Lowes';
  - Fabry's (📖 p.968).
- *Other syndromes:* e.g. trisomy 21.
- *Drugs:* e.g. long-term steroid therapy.

Absence of the normal bilateral red reflex, or the presence of a white reflex on ophthalmoscopic examination, should raise suspicion of an underlying cataract and immediate referral to an ophthalmologist is required.

Glaucoma

This condition is associated with raised intraocular pressure; disc cupping, and visual field loss. Primary open angle and secondary closed angle glaucoma are rare in childhood. Congenital glaucoma is also rare and may be due to the abnormal development of the anterior chamber angle. Later-onset glaucoma may result from syndromes that effect eye development. The infant eye, unlike the adult, can enlarge enormously with high intraocular pressures (buphthalmos, 'ox-eye'), developing a hazy cornea and excess lacrimation. The treatment is surgical, but is often unsuccessful. Visual prognosis is poor and often results in blindness.

Orbit and eyelids

Blepharitis and meibomian cyst/chalazion

Blepharitis is a common chronic inflammation of the lid margin, which can result in recurrent styes, meibomian cysts and, occasionally keratitis. The eyelid margins are red and crusty.

Parents should clean their child's lid margins using a flannel soaked in a hand-hot mild baby shampoo solution at bath time. An antibiotic ointment e.g. chloramphenicol can then be applied to the lid margins with a finger-tip. Styes and cysts often respond to this treatment too. If a meibomian cyst persists for months and becomes hard, incision, and curettage under GA may be required.

Congenital eyelid abnormalities

- *Entropion* (in-turned lid) and *ectropion* (out-turned lid) are uncommon in children.
- Lower lid *epiblepharon* can resemble entropion since the lower lashes are in turned due to a fold of skin close to the lid margin. This is seen more commonly in oriental children and resolves as the face grows although repeated corneal abrasion may necessitate surgical correction.
- Congenital *ptosis* due to levator dystrophy can cause unilateral or bilateral ptosis. Neurological causes can be excluded clinically. If the lid covers the visual axis, amblyopia will rapidly ensue.
- Occlusion therapy may be required but, unless the ptosis is severe, surgery is delayed until pre-school age.

Congenital naso-lacrimal duct obstruction

- A common cause of watery and sticky eye(s) in infancy.
- Concurrent conjunctivitis is unusual and the eyes are white despite copious discharge.
- The majority will improve in the first few months of life.
- Advise parents to massage the lacrimal sac (located just inferiorly to the medial canthus) firmly with a finger when the baby is feeding.
- This will express the sac contents into the palpebral fissure where the discharge can be cleaned away with sterile water and a cotton wool pad. It is not necessary to swab the eye or start topical antibiotics if the eye is white.
- Symptoms persisting beyond 12mths warrant referral for consideration of syringe and probing of the tear ducts.

Capillary haemangioma of the lid

- These may be deep and bluish or a superficial 'strawberry' naevus. It can enlarge and cause amblyopia due to ptosis or induced astigmatism in the first years of life.
- Occlusion therapy and spectacle correction are often necessary.
- Oral propranolol is effective at shrinking the lesion and has replaced oral and steroid injections in the management of sight threatening haemangioma.

- Exclusion of a congenital heart defect and intra-cranial haemangioma associated with PHACES syndrome is necessary prior to propranolol therapy.
- *Port wine stains* involving the eyelids may cause glaucoma on the affected side. Ophthalmic referral is required for screening.

Pre-septal, peri-orbital and orbital cellulitis See 🕮 p.718

Pre-septal cellulitis

- This is a bacterial infection involving the eyelids and tissue anterior to the orbital septum.
- The source may be from skin, e.g. an infected insect bite, trauma or meibomian cyst, dacryocystitis (lacrimal sac abscess) or deeper, such as sinusitis.
- Commonest organisms are *Staph. aureus* and B haemolytic *Streptococcus*. Pre-septal cellulitis in a well child can be treated with oral antibiotics.
- Since orbital involvement can develop within in hours, children with severe pre-septal cellulitis secondary to URTI who are systemically unwell should be admitted and started on IV antibiotics (see Orbital cellulitis).

Peri-orbital cellulitis

- Infection of the peri-orbital skin. This is usually due to infection by either *S. aureus* or *H. influenzae* type b (if not immunized).
- May occur s to paranasal or dental abscess in older children. Children are often systemically unwell with fever, erythema, and tenderness over the affected area.
- This requires prompt treatment with a 5–7-day course of IV antibiotics.
- Untreated peri-orbital cellulitis may develop into orbital cellulitis with evolving ocular proptosis, limited ocular movement, and decreased visual acuity.
- May rarely be complicated with intracranial abscess formation, meningitis, or cavernous sinus thrombosis.
- A CT scan of brain should be considered to exclude these complications if suspected.

Orbital cellulitis

- Infective orbital cellulitis arises from bacterial infection of the para-nasal sinuses (consider fungal infection in immunosuppressed children).
- Features include peri-orbital oedema, proptosis, and limited eye movements.
- An ophthalmic emergency, failure to treat adequately will result in visual loss and, potentially, cavernous sinus thrombosis.
- High dose IV second generation cephalosporin (and metronidazole if over 8yrs) without delay.
- Nasal decongestants can be helpful. Children should be co-managed with the ophthalmology and ENT teams.
- CT scanning may detect orbital abscess formation, which requires surgical drainage.

Back of the eye problems

Endophthalmitis

Infection within the eye may be *endogenous* (spread of bacterial or fungal infection from the bloodstream) or *exogenous* (2° to trauma or surgery). Symptoms may vary in severity, but include achy pain, photophobia, floaters, and loss of vision, the eye is usually red and a pus level within the anterior chamber (hypopyon) may be seen. Endophthalmitis requires emergency ophthalmic referral and management with systemic and intra-vitreal agents to prevent blindness.

Retinopathy of prematurity

See also ▢ p.188. This is a fibrovascular proliferative retinal disorder occurring in preterm and low birth weight infants. Its development has been associated with high concentrations of inspired oxygen during the neonatal period. Normal retinal vascularization is not complete until full term. In preterm infants this process is interrupted and, on restarting, may proceed abnormally with aberrant and proliferative new vessel formation.

ROP screening Infants born <31wks gestation, or weighing <1500g are screened from 6wks of age until the retina has vascularized.

Treatment Indirect laser therapy is used in severe cases.

Other medical conditions causing retinopathy

Sickle cell disease

The deformed RBCs in sickle cell disease may cause retinal vascular occlusion or ischaemia. A proliferative retinopathy with new vessel formation, or a non-proliferative retinopathy with scarring and fibrosis may develop. Screening is required with laser photocoagulation for new vessel formation (see also ▢ p.621).

Diabetes mellitus

Diabetic retinopathy is rarely seen in children with type 1 diabetes and not usually before onset of puberty and teenage years (see also ▢ pp.414–415).

Retinitis pigmentosa (RP)

This progressive degenerative disorder of the retina is characterized by typical pigmented retinal appearances. It is an important cause of night blindness, reduced central and peripheral vision, and cataracts. It may occur as an isolated finding or may be part of a systemic disorder.

- *Usher's syndrome:* RP + congenital deafness.
- *Bassen–Kornweig syndrome:* RP + abetalipoproteinaemia, ataxia, and malabsorption.
- *Refsum's disease:* RP + polyneuropathy, deafness, and cerebellar dysfunction (▢ p.972).
- *Kearns–Sayre syndrome:* RP + ophthalmoplegia, cardiac conduction defect (▢ pp.962–963).

Retinal dystrophies

A group of inherited disorders causing rod, cone and/or inner retinal cell dysfunction. Early onset retinal dystrophy may cause blindness in infancy, other forms can cause progressive visual loss during childhood.

Rod dystrophies primarily reduce night and peripheral vision. Cone dystrophies primarily reduce colour vision, central vision, and cause photophobia. Most children are otherwise healthy, but retinal dystrophy can be part of a widespread disorder, e.g. Bardet–Biedl syndrome, Cockayne syndrome, Batten disease, and peroxisomal disorders. Children with early onset SN hearing loss should be referred in order to exclude Usher syndrome. Supportive help with optical and educational aids has been the mainstay of management in the past, but recent success with gene therapy gives us some optimism for future treatment.

Papilloedema/optic disc swelling

There are many causes of optic disc swelling and the term *papilloedema* is reserved for optic disc swelling secondary to raised ICP. Visual acuity is usually good initially, but symptoms such as visual obscurations (momentary loss of vision when leaning over or coughing) and diplopia secondary to bilateral sixth nerve paresis may occur. If left untreated, the papilloedematous nerve will start to become atrophic, initially causing visual field constriction and eventually loss of central and colour vision.

Optic disc drusen are calcific deposits in the optic nerve head that can mimic optic disc swelling. Drusen 'light up' on ultrasonography (performed by an ophthalmologist) and this non-invasive test can prevent unnecessary neurological investigation.

Optic neuritis/neuropathy

Inflammation, infiltration, or compression of the optic nerve cause early loss of central and colour vision. Assessment of optic nerve function should include:
- Visual acuity.
- Visual fields to confrontation (or perimetry if able).
- Colour vision (ask child to compare brightness of red target in one eye to the other).
- Pupil reactions look for a relative afferent papillary defect (Fig. 24.2).
- Visualize the optic disc— it may be swollen or atrophic.

Fig. 24.2 Testing for relative afferent pupillary defect. Left optic neuropathy: both pupils constrict when light is shone in right eye. When the torch is swung over to shine in left eye, both pupils dilate (relative to the previous constriction).

Trauma

Chemical injury (alkali/acids/solvents detergents / irritants)

Start treatment immediately, unless penetrating eye injury is suspected.

- Instill topical anaesthesia (Proxymetacaine 0.5% if available).
- Irrigate with copious saline for 30min.
- Wait 5–10min—ascertain nature of chemical.
- Check pH using litmus paper inside bottom lid.
- Continue irrigation until pH is 7.
- Sweep conjunctival fornices with moistened cotton bud.
- Refer if severe injury and alkali involved otherwise give chloramphenicol ointment tds 2–3 days and SOS appointment.

Corneal abrasion and foreign bodies

Symptoms include sharp, stabbing pain, photophobia, and discomfort on blinking.

- Instill topical anaesthetic to facilitate examination.
- Test visual acuity.
- Examine with ophthalmoscope set on +20 or slit lamp.
- *Instill fluorescein and examine with blue light:* if linear/vertical abrasions are present a sub-tarsal FB is likely.
- Ask the child to look down, but not close the eyes; evert the upper lid using a cotton bud placed on the upper lid crease as a pivot point.
- Use cotton bud to sweep away FB if present.

Large central corneal abrasions should be referred. Central corneal scarring can cause amblyopia to develop in a young child. Otherwise give chloramphenicol ointment tds 1wk with SOS appointment.

Blunt trauma

Blunt trauma is common in older children (especially boys) due to their propensity of throwing things at each other! The child usually complains of achy pain and blurred vision.

- Instill anaesthetic to facilitate examination.
- Check visual acuity.
- *Compare pupil size:* traumatic mydriasis may be seen.
- Examine with ophthalmoscope on +20 for hyphaema (blood in anterior chamber).
- Check red reflex.
- Refer to ophthalmologist if hyphaema/traumatic mydriasis is present.

Penetrating trauma

Suspect penetrating trauma if there is a history of the child falling onto a sharp object (e.g. pencil) or history of high velocity missile, e.g. air gun pellet. The severity of pain and reduction of vision is variable.

- Instill anaesthetic if child is in pain.
- Check visual acuity.
- Examine pupil reactions and look for symmetry.
- Signs of perforation/penetration include:
  - sub-conjunctival haemorrhage;
  - dark pigment on surface or under conjunctiva;
  - distorted pupil and hyphaema.
- Refer immediately, protect eye with hard eye shield and keep nil by mouth.

Inflicted head injury (NAI) See 📖 pp.527, 758, 1000

Severe shaking and shaking/impact injury in infants causes retinal haemorrhages. Haemorrhages are typically multi-layered: *deep retina haemorrhages* (blots and white centered haemorrhages), *superficial retinal haemorrhages* (flame shaped haemorrhages) and *sub-hyaloid haemorrhages* (often associated with a fluid level) occur together. Superficial haemorrhages can disappear within days, but the deeper and sub-hyaloid haemorrhages can take months to resolve. Vitreous traction on the retina may result in perimacular folds in severe cases and papilloedema may be present secondary to sub-dural haemorrhage.

If NAI is considered, a senior ophthalmologist should be requested to document and, if possible, take photographs of the retinal appearance. Often the visual prognosis in such cases is poor, not because of the retinal injury, but because of the associated brain injury.

Genetics

Useful resources

The human genome contains ~25,000 genes, so the few common genetic disorders in this section are a very tiny sample from an enormous range of genetic disorders. Other useful resources for information include the following:

Books

Cassidy SB, Allanson JE (eds) (2010). *Management of genetic syndromes*, 3rd edn. New York: Wiley.

Firth HV, Hurst JA, Hall JG (2005). *Oxford desk reference clinical genetics*. Oxford: Oxford University Press.

Jones KL (2005). *Smith's recognizable patterns of human malformation*. Philadelphia: W.B. Saunders Co Ltd.

Reardon W (2008) *The bedside dysmorphologist. Classic clinical signs in human malformation syndromes and their diagnostic significance*. Oxford: Oxford University Press.

Web-based resources

'Online Mendelian Inheritance in Man' ('OMIM'). Available at: www.ncbi.nlm.nih.gov.

Directory of clinical genetics services in the UK. Available at: www.bshg.org.uk.

Contact a Family (UK). Available at: www.cafamily.org.uk.

Geneclinics. Available at: www.geneclinics.org.

Orphanet. Available at: www.orpha.net.

National Organization for Rare Disorders (US). Available at: www.raredisease.org.

Clinical genetics and genetic counselling

Definition of genetic counselling

'The process by which individuals or relatives at risk for a disorder that may be hereditary are advised of the consequences of the disorder, the probability of transmitting it and the ways in which this may be prevented, avoided or ameliorated.'[1]

Role of the clinical geneticist

Clinical geneticists are doctors with a wide and varied training in medicine and its sub-specialties whose special expertise is in the identification and diagnosis of inherited disorders. Inevitably, these skills lend themselves to the assessment of the child with multiple birth defects but clinical geneticists see patients of all ages and comprising all manner of clinical presentations.

When families come to the genetics clinic, they usually have a number of questions, which may be summarized as follows:

• What is the diagnosis?
• Why did it happen?
• Will it happen again?
• If so, what can be done to ameliorate or prevent it?

The main role of the clinical geneticist is to establish an accurate genetic diagnosis, which is essential in order to:

• Gain an understanding of the condition and possible prognosis.
• Guide optimal management for the child.
• Identify other systems that need surveillance, e.g. hearing or vision.
• Address concerns about events during pregnancy or delivery.
• Enable accurate genetic advice for parents and other family members about the risk of recurrence in future pregnancies.

A basic principle of genetic counselling is that advice is *non-directive*.

Reference

1 Firth HV, Hurst JA, Hall JG. (2005). *Oxford desk reference clinical genetics*. Oxford: Oxford University Press.

When to refer to clinical genetics

A majority of underlying chronic disorders in children are either clearly genetic or have a genetic susceptibility. It is increasingly important for paediatricians to be able to recognize genetic disorders and to know when to enlist the help of a clinical geneticist.

Useful definitions

- *Dysmorphic features:* physical features, particularly unusual facial features, that are not usually found in a child of the same age or ethnic background.
- *Abnormal growth parameters:* height or weight or OFC >98th centile or <2nd centile.

Indications for referral to clinical genetics

- *Congenital anomalies:*
  - multiple congenital anomalies;
  - isolated congenital anomaly in conjunction with dysmorphic features/developmental delay/abnormal growth parameters/a family history.
- *Dysmorphic features:* esp. in conjunction with developmental delay/ learning disability/congenital anomaly/abnormal growth parameters.
- A family history suggestive of a recurrent abnormality.
- *Developmental delay/learning disability:*
  - unexplained severe developmental delay/learning disability;
  - developmental delay/learning disability in conjunction with dysmorphic features/congenital anomaly/abnormal growth parameters/a family history.
- *Multiple problems and no diagnosis:* child with multiple problems and under the care of many specialists with no unifying diagnosis.
- *New diagnosis of a genetic disorder:*
  - enables explanation of the genetic basis of the condition;
  - essential if the diagnosis may have implications for other relatives;
  - important if parents would like advice regarding future pregnancies.
- *Teenager with a genetic disorder:* if a genetic diagnosis was made in infancy/early childhood, refer patient back to clinical genetics in mid-teens so that the young adult understands the genetic basis of their condition and the risks to their own offspring.

Taking a family history

A very important tool in clinical genetics. One of the key skills in taking a family history is drawing a family tree with all relevant symbols (see Fig. 25.1). The approach described here is intended for routine use in a general paediatric setting. A more detailed approach is indicated when assessing a patient with a known or possible genetic disorder.

Drawing a basic family tree

- Start with your patient. Draw a ♂ symbol for a male; ♀ symbol for a female.
- Next add symbols for your patient's parents and siblings. Record basic information only, e.g. age, whether they are in good health, and whether there are any concerns regarding development. If an individual has died, note age and cause of death and annotate the family tree with an oblique stroke through the symbol.
- Ask whether there is any inherited disorder running in the family.
- Ask whether your patient's parents are related (consanguinity increases the chance of an AR disorder). Consanguinity is indicated by drawing a double line on the family tree.
- Ask the key question 'Has anybody else in your family had a similar problem to the patient?' Be aware that some conditions have variable expression, e.g. del 22q11 may present with cleft palate in one member of the family and congenital heart disease in another.
- Extend the family tree upwards to include grandparents and sideways to include aunts, uncles, and cousins. If you have not revealed a familial problem by this stage, do not go further as you are unlikely to have missed an important familial disease with onset in childhood. In the case of a suspected X-linked disorder extend the family tree further on the maternal side (ask a clinical geneticist to help you with this).
- Shade those people in the family tree affected by the disorder. This will help determine whether there is a genetic problem, and, if there is, it will help to suggest the pattern of inheritance.
- For an example of drawing a family tree see Fig. 25.2.

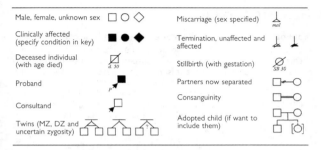

Fig. 25.1 Basic family tree symbols. Taken from Firth HV, Hurst JA, Hall JG (2005). *Oxford Desk Reference of Clinical Genetics*. With permission of Oxford University Press.

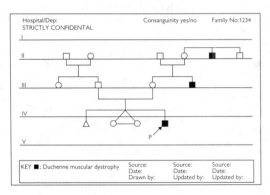

Fig. 25.2 Example of a family tree. Firth HV, Hurst JA, Hall JG (2005). *Oxford Desk Reference of Clinical Genetics*. With permission of Oxford University Press.

Genetic testing

Appropriate situations for genetic testing in a child

- Diagnostic testing in a *child who has features of a genetic disorder*, e.g. chromosome analysis in a child with suspected Down syndrome.
- The child is asymptomatic, but is *at risk for a genetic condition for which preventive or other therapeutic measures are available*, e.g. testing to determine if a child of an affected parent with retinoblastoma (with a known mutation) requires screening by frequent periodic examination under anaesthesia. This is predictive testing and should involve a clinical geneticist.
- The child is *at risk for a genetic condition with paediatric onset for which preventive therapeutic measures are not available*, e.g. SMA type 1. Involve a clinical geneticist. The decision to undertake a genetic test requires a careful balancing of benefit/harm; each case is assessed on its individual merits. Generally, testing is done at parental discretion after careful discussion.

Inappropriate situations for genetic testing in a child

- An asymptomatic child is *at risk for a genetic condition that usually has onset in adult life* for which preventive or effective therapeutic measures are not available, e.g. Huntington's disease.
- Testing for *carrier status*, e.g. siblings of a child with cystic fibrosis. Practice does vary, but we recommend that testing be deferred until the child is old enough to seek testing in their own right, or at least to take part in the discussion about testing. Parents sometimes request testing of young children without having necessarily thought through the difficulties this may lead to later on. We suggest referral to clinical genetics if parents remain keen to perform carrier test.
- Genetic testing of children for the *benefit of another family member* should *not* be performed unless testing is necessary to prevent substantial harm to the family member.

Chromosome tests

Karyotype analysis

A standard chromosome analysis involves a G-banded karyotype viewed by a cytogeneticist using a light microscope. Using this approach, the maximum resolution is ~5–10Mb. One of the major advantages of a chromosome analysis is that it is a genomic survey, i.e. it looks in outline at the whole genome. The normal male karyotype is 46, XY. The normal female karyotype is 46, XX.

Fluorescence *in situ* hybridization (FISH)

Targeted studies are possible at higher resolution using specific FISH probes. Using FISH, it is possible to see the submicroscopic deletions responsible for Williams syndrome (7q) and Angelman syndrome (15q), but only if the clinician specifically requests this.

Molecular kayotyping using microarrays

Microarray analysis is an ever improving technology which enables much higher resolution DNA analysis than is possible with light microscopy. It has recently started to be used in clinical practice and has been especially valuable to clinical geneticists in identifying patients with chromosomal abnormalities previously not diagnosable by standard techniques. However, it is a specialist tool and is not routinely in use in paediatric settings. There are two main types of array:

Targeted arrays

These analyse selected regions of the genome, e.g. known syndromes and sub-telomeric regions.

Genome-wide arrays

These give genome-wide coverage at varying degrees of resolution ranging from 1Mb to 100kb, i.e. 10–100 times greater resolution than conventional light microscopy. It is important to appreciate that at high levels of resolution there is considerable normal variation in the human genome. Copy number variation is routinely identified both in pathological states and as normal family variants. Differentiating between the pathological and non-pathological variation is not within the compass of the non-specialist.

Molecular genetic analysis

The human genome contains ~3,000,000,000 DNA base pairs and ~25,000 genes. In genetic disorders, the pathology may range from a whole extra chromosome, e.g. Down syndrome, to a single DNA base pair alteration, e.g. achondroplasia. Molecular genetic tests are highly specific tests that only reveal information about one very specific gene analysis, generally selected because of a strong clinical diagnosis, e.g. achondroplasia.

• If there is a *commonly occurring mutation*, analysis is simple and comparatively inexpensive, e.g. cystic fibrosis and the CF29 kit tests for the 29 most common mutations in the Caucasian population, and achondroplasia in which two common mutations, G1138A and G1138C in the *FGFR3* gene, account for ~98% of mutations in children with achondroplasia).

• If the *mutation in a family is known*, analysis is usually straightforward and takes ~2–6 weeks for most tests. Such tests, based on information obtained from other family members, should involve a clinical geneticist.

• If the *mutation is unknown*, an entire gene may have to be sequenced. Genetic testing in this situation can be laborious, expensive (often ~£1000), and only a small proportion may be available as diagnostic tests. In the UK, reporting times are being reduced for these tests and now routinely take about 6–8wks, even for a very large challenging gene, e.g. *FBN1* in Marfan syndrome and *TSC1 and TSC2* in tuberous sclerosis. Consult a clinical geneticist about whether genetic testing is appropriate in these circumstances.

Practical issues relating to genetic testing

Counselling the family before testing

Diagnostic testing

Think carefully about the potential impact of the diagnosis you may make with a genetic test. Some genetic conditions are relentlessly progressive and life-limiting, e.g. DMD. Others imply lifelong impairment of a child's ability to learn and communicate, e.g. Angelman syndrome, fragile X syndrome. If you make a genetic diagnosis, it is likely to remain a permanent aspect of that child's life. There may be some treatable elements to the condition, but it is unlikely to be transient or curable. The diagnosis may have implications for other family members. The family should preferably be counselled by a clinical geneticist, before a genetic test is performed. Ensure that the parents understand what you are testing for and why. Explain how long it may take to obtain a result and make careful arrangements for communicating the result.

Predictive testing

The circumstances in which this may be appropriate can be complex and can vary for different disorders. This should be arranged through a clinical geneticist.

Down syndrome

Incidence ~1 in 600–700 live births (incidence increases with advancing maternal age).

Cause

The great majority (~95%) of babies with Down syndrome have trisomy 21, usually due to non-disjunction during maternal oogenesis. ~2% are the result of a Robertsonian translocation. ~2% are mosaic, with a normal cell line as well as the trisomy 21 cell line.

Clinical features

- Usually presents at birth.
- Generalized hypotonia and marked head lag.
- *Facial features:* small low-set ears, up-slanting eyes, prominent epicanthic folds, a flat facial profile, protruding tongue. Later Brushfield's spots apparent in the iris (whitish spots).
- Flat occiput (brachycephaly) and short neck.
- *Typical limb features:* short broad hands (brachydactyly), short incurved little fingers (clinodactyly), single transverse palmar crease, and a wide 'sandal' gap between the first and second toes.
- Mildly short stature.
- Intellectual impairment becomes apparent. IQ scores range from 25 to 70.
- Social skills often exceed other intellectual skills.

Associated conditions

- ~40–50% have congenital heart disease, most commonly atrio-ventricular septal defect (AVSD), ASD, VSD, Fallot tetralogy.
- GI problems include: duodenal atresia, anal atresia, HSD.
- Increased risk of infection.
- Developmental hip dysplasia.
- Eczema.
- *Deafness:* both sensorineural and conductive.
- Cataracts.
- Leukaemia (1%).
- Acquired hypothyroidism.

Diagnosis

If there is clinical suspicion of Down syndrome, a senior paediatrician should discuss their concerns with the parents. The diagnosis is confirmed by a chromosome analysis showing an additional chromosome 21. Most cytogenetics laboratories are able to offer a rapid analysis, e.g. interphase FISH, in order to establish the diagnosis quickly.

Management

- Refer for a detailed cardiac assessment, hip US, and audiology.
- Genetic counselling by a clinical geneticist should be offered. It is not necessary to undertake parental chromosome analysis if the cause is non-disjunctional trisomy 21 or mosaic trisomy 21, but this is very important if the karyotype shows a translocation.
- Putting the parents in contact with a support organization, such as the Down Association, is often helpful (℘ www.downs-syndrome.org.uk and ℘ www.ndss.org).
- Long-term follow-up should ideally be by a multidisciplinary team led by a paediatrician with special expertise, such as a developmental paediatrician, working in a child development centre. Physiotherapy to improve tone and posture is often required.
- Routinely test TFT annually.
- Refer for audiology and ophthalmic assessment 1–2-yearly.
- Almost all children with Down syndrome are now educated in mainstream schools with appropriate educational support.

Prognosis

If deaths from congenital cardiac disease are excluded, life expectancy is well into adult life, although somewhat shortened as almost all develop Alzheimer disease by age 40yrs. Majority of adults can live semi-independently with supervision.

Common chromosomal disorders

Down syndrome See 📖 p.936

Klinefelter syndrome (47, XXY)

- Affects ~1/600–1/800 boys.
- Majority caused by non-disjunction during maternal oogenesis.
- Boys with Klinefelter syndrome enter puberty normally, but by mid-puberty the testes begin to involute and the boys develop hypergonadotrophic hypogonadism with decreased testosterone production (often tall and may develop feminine body build). Testes are small in adult life and men with Klinefelter syndrome are generally infertile (azoospermia). Gynaecomastia develops at puberty in ≥50%. Boys with Klinefelter syndrome typically have an IQ ~15 points lower than their siblings.
- Many boys with Klinefelter syndrome remain undiagnosed throughout childhood, with the diagnosis only coming to light during investigation of infertility.
- Diagnosis is by chromosome analysis.

Patau syndrome (trisomy 13)

- Incidence is ~1/6000 births.
- ~75% caused by non-disjunction during maternal oogenesis; ~20% Robertsonian translocation; ~5% result from mosaicism.
- Trisomy 13 is usually diagnosed by antenatal US scan, since the majority of affected babies have multiple congenital anomalies.
- *Typical malformations include:* holoprosencephaly; SGA; microcephalic; microphthalmia; cleft lip/palate; congenital heart disease (e.g. ASD or VSD); renal anomalies (e.g. fused kidneys); postaxial polydactyly; together with severe/profound mental retardation.
- If there is clinical suspicion of trisomy 13, a senior paediatrician should discuss their concerns with the parents.
- The diagnosis is confirmed by a chromosome analysis (additional chromosome 13). Most cytogenetics laboratories are able to offer a rapid analysis, e.g. interphase FISH, to confirm the diagnosis quickly.

Edwards' syndrome (trisomy 18)

- Incidence is ~1/8000 births.
- Majority caused by non-disjunction during maternal oogenesis.
- Babies with trisomy 18 are usually SGA (mean birth weight 2240g) with an OFC <3rd centile. Other common features include: congenital heart disease, usually VSD +/– valve dysplasia; short sternum; overriding fingers; 'rocker-bottom' feet. There is a strong female excess. Median life expectancy is ~4 days, although some affected babies live for several months.
- If there is clinical suspicion of trisomy 18, a senior paediatrician should discuss their concerns with the parents.
- Initial rapid interphase FISH testing followed by formal chromosome analysis (additional chromosome 18).

Turner syndrome (45, X) See 📖 p.948

Genetic disorders with cardiac features

Many chromosomal disorders and genetic syndromes are characterized by congenital heart disease.

Deletion 22q11 syndrome/velocardiofacial syndrome/Di George syndrome

- Incidence is ~1/4000.
- Caused by a microdeletion on chromosome 22q11.2. Most children have a *de novo* microdeletion, but in ~15% the condition is inherited from an affected parent.
- Apart from cardiac defects, usually involving the aortic arch, features include subtle dysmorphism (wide and prominent nasal bridge, down-slanting eyes, small mouth), parathyroid aplasia/hypoplasia (hypocalcaemia), thymus aplasia (T-cell deficiency). Short stature is common.
- Consider this condition in all children diagnosed with TOF or aortic arch abnormalities, e.g. interrupted aortic arch (~20% will have del(22q11)).
- Also consider in any child with CHD, e.g. VSD, who has hypernasal speech, cleft palate, including submucous cleft palate (may present as nasal regurgitation of milk), hypocalcaemia, asymmetric crying facies, recurrent infections, or learning difficulties, especially speech and language delay.
- Diagnosis will be missed on a routine chromosome analysis; it requires a FISH study.

Marfan syndrome (MFS)

- Incidence ~1/5000 births.
- Variable autosomal dominant multisystem disorder caused by mutation in the *FBN1* gene on chromosome 15q. There is a high new mutation rate (~30%).
- *Features include:* tall and slim body build with long limbs; pectus malformation of the sternum; scoliosis; high narrow palate; long fingers (arachnodactyly); joint laxity. Most affected children are myopic and some may develop lens dislocation (a major diagnostic feature).
- *Cardiac features:* initially, there may be a floppy mitral valve. With time, dilatation of the aortic root (another major diagnostic feature) may occur, leading eventually to ascending aorta aneurysm and aortic dissection. Treatment with *Losartan* has greatly improved the outlook in terms of stabilizing aortic aneurysms.
- If genetic confirmation of the diagnosis is required, this may be possible (in conjunction with a clinical geneticist) by mutation analysis of the *FBN1* gene.

Noonan syndrome (NS)

- Incidence ~1 in 2500 births.
- Autosomal dominant disorder. NS is genetically heterogeneous, with ~50% caused by mutation in the *PTPN11* gene on chromosome 12q. Mutation in several other genes in the RAS/MAP kinase pathway have been reported in other NS cases and in clinically overlapping disorders of cardio-facio-cutaneous syndrome and Costello syndrome.
- *Features:* short stature, typical facial features (hypertelorism, ptosis, ear abnormalities), a broad neck, congenital heart disease (especially pulmonary stenosis), cardiomyopathy, chest malformation with pectus carinatum superiorly and pectus excavatum inferiorly, mild developmental delay, and undescended testes.
- If genetic confirmation of the diagnosis is required, this may be possible (in conjunction with a clinical geneticist) for some children by mutation analysis of the *PTPN11* gene.

Williams syndrome (WS)

- Incidence is 1/7500 live births.
- Caused by a microdeletion on chromosome 7q11 that encompasses the elastin gene.
- Associated cardiac defect is supravalvular aortic stenosis, often with peripheral pulmonary branch stenosis.
- *Facial features include:* peri-orbital fullness; full cheeks; anteverted nares; wide mouth with full lips; small widely spaced teeth. Most have mild mental retardation with strengths in language, but poor visuospatial skills.
- The typical behavioural phenotype is that of over-friendliness, short attention span, and anxiety.
- ~15% of infants have hypercalcaemia.
- Diagnosis is by FISH study for the 7q11 microdeletion
- For further information including growth charts see: ℘ www.williams-syndrome.org/

Genetic testing in cognitive impairment

Amongst children with severe mental retardation, a high proportion will have a genetic cause. This can be elucidated in ~50% of children, with chromosomal disorders being the largest group. Referral to clinical genetics should be considered for all children with unexplained severe global developmental delay/mental retardation.

The referring paediatrician may undertake some basic diagnostic genetic testing, including the following:

- *Chromosome analysis:* investigation with the highest yield for children with unexplained developmental delay. Specific FISH tests for submicroscopic microdeletions, e.g. Williams, 22q11 syndrome, can also be requested.
- *Fragile X analysis:* this is the commonest cause of inherited learning disability, but remains a rare disorder. As it is often difficult to diagnose on clinical grounds, genetic testing should be offered to all children with developmental delay.
- *Creatine kinase in boys:* DMD may present with speech delay and delayed motor milestones and/or global delay.
- *Thyroid function tests:* children born in the UK should have been tested for congenital hypothyroidism on the newborn blood spot screen. If this result was normal (need confirmation), repeat investigation is not required unless there are clinical signs suggestive of hypothyroidism.
- *Amino and organic acids:* inborn errors of metabolism are individually rare, but may present with non-specific features, e.g. developmental delay and/or FTT. Plasma and urine samples should be arranged if there is developmental regression, episodic decompensation, parental consanguinity, a family history, or physical examination findings consistent with a metabolic disorder, e.g. microcephaly, macrocephaly, hepato-splenomegaly. 'Non-specific' abnormalities are more common than true diagnoses.
- *Urine glycosaminoglycans (mucopolysaccharidoses):* consider if developmental regression, glue ear, coarse features, macrocephaly.
- *Ophthalmological opinion:* especially if there is concern regarding vision, eye signs (e.g. nystagmus), neurological signs, microcephaly.
- *Audiology assessment:* especially if there is speech delay or concern regarding hearing.
- *Consider congenital infection:* in children with intrauterine growth retardation, microcephaly, and eye/hearing signs. Requires comparison of maternal booking and current maternal serology. Useful for children up to ~18 months of age.

See ♫ www.phgfoundation.org/pages/work.htm.

Angelman syndrome (AS)

- Incidence ~1/40 000.
- AS is caused by impaired or absent function of the maternally imprinted *UBE3A* gene on chromosome 15q11.13.
- A distinctive neurobehavioural condition with severe developmental delay, profound speech impairment, an ataxic wide-based gait, and a specific behavioural phenotype (excitable personality, hand-flapping, and inappropriately happy affect). Seizures are common.
- The genetics of AS are complex. Refer to a clinical geneticist.

Fragile X syndrome (FRAXA)

- Incidence ~1/5500 males. It is the most common inherited cause of mental retardation.
- Caused by a full expansion (>200 repeats) in the $(CGG)_n$ triplet repeat in the FRAXA gene on chromosome Xq27.3.
- Boys with fragile X syndrome typically have global developmental delay often with gaze avoidance, stereotyped repetitive behaviours such as hand-flapping and resistance to change of routines.
- Up to 50% of girls with a full *FRAXA* expansion will have learning and behavioural difficulties that are similar to, but less severe, than those seen in affected boys.
- Genetic counselling is very complex and there will be genetic implications for relatives. Referral to a clinical geneticist is recommended.

Prader–Willi syndrome See p.949

Rett syndrome

- Affects ~1/10 000 female births.
- Caused by mutation in the *MECP2* gene on Xq28. Girls with Rett syndrome appear normal in the first 6 months of life.
- A severe neurodevelopmental disorder. Almost exclusively affects girls. Presents after age 1yr usually with developmental regression and loss of purposeful hand movements. May develop seizures, scoliosis, erratic breathing with episodes of breath-holding and hyperventilation, and stereotypic hand-wringing.

Smith–Magenis syndrome

- Affects at least 1/25,000 children.
- Usually caused by a *de novo* microdeletion on chromosome 17p11.2.
- Typical features include a broad face with midface hypoplasia, brachydactyly, obesity, developmental delay/learning disability with behavioural disturbance, especially of sleep (night-time waking and daytime somnolence).
- The diagnosis may be missed on a routine chromosome analysis and may require FISH for the 17p11.2 microdeletion.

Williams syndrome See p.941

Genetic disorders with neuromuscular features

The majority of severe neuromuscular disorders affecting infants and children have a genetic basis. In addition to accurate assessment and examination of the child, a detailed family history and examination of parents may sometimes be very helpful in establishing the diagnosis.

Congenital myotonic dystrophy

See also 📖 pp.136–137, 546.

- Caused by a triplet repeat expansion $(CTG)_n$ in the myotonin gene on chromosome 19q. Congenitally affected infants usually have a huge expansion of the triplet repeat with >1000 repeats.
- Occurs in affected babies born to women who also have myotonic dystrophy (an AD disorder with onset usually in adult life), even when mild or undiagnosed.
- Typically, there is polyhydramnios and at delivery the baby is floppy and may require prolonged ventilatory support.
- Diagnosis is usually possible by careful examination of the mother (percussion myotonia) (also enquire if mother sleeps with eyes open) and analysis of a DNA sample from the infant.
- Neonatal mortality is ~20%. Survivors have static or slowly progressive muscle weakness. Many have associated moderate intellectual impairment.

Duchenne muscular dystrophy

See also 📖 p.546.

- *Affects ~1/3500 male births:* DMD is the most common and severe form of childhood muscular dystrophy.
- Caused by mutations (deletions, duplications, and point mutations) in the dystrophin gene on chromosome Xq28.
- Presents with developmental delay, especially late walking and speech delay. In the early phase of the disease, boys have difficulty rising from the floor (Gower's manoeuvre sign where the child climbs up his thighs with his hands to get up off the floor). Later there is early loss of ambulation (mean age ~9 years). Affected boys develop a progressive cardiomyopathy. ~30% of boys with DMD have a mild learning disability that is not progressive.
- Serum CK is grossly elevated, usually >10 times normal levels. Diagnosis is often possible by genetic testing, avoiding the need for muscle biopsy.
- DMD follows X-linked recessive inheritance and expert genetic counselling is an essential part of management.
- Death from cardiorespiratory failure or infection usually occurs in the late teens or early 20s.

Spinal muscular atrophy

See also 📖 p.540.

- An AR disorder caused by bi-allelic mutation in the *SMN* gene on 5q13. ~95% of infants with type 1 SMA are homozygously deleted for exon 7 of the *SMN1* gene.
- In severe cases, babies usually feed normally for the first few weeks with the earliest sign often being of a tiring infant who does not finish his feed. Clinical examination may show fasciculations of the tongue, an important clinical indicator.
- Develop symmetrical proximal muscle weakness as a consequence of degeneration of the anterior horn cells of the spinal cord. Intelligence is unaffected.
- *Several types:*
  - *Type 1 SMA (severe)*—onset in first few months of life. Never able to sit or walk. Usually die from respiratory failure by age 6–12mths.
  - *Type 2 SMA (intermediate)*—onset before age 18mths. Able to sit, but not to walk unaided. Survival into adult life is usual.
  - *Type 3 SMA (mild)*—onset of proximal muscle weakness after age 2yrs. Ability to walk independently initially; survival into adult life.
- Diagnosis can be made by molecular genetic testing.

Genetic disorders with dermatological features

Sometimes it is the cutaneous features that are the key to diagnosis of a genetic disorder (see also 📖 Chapter 22).

Ehlers–Danlos syndrome (EDS)

See 📖 p.838.

- Incidence ~1/5000 births.
- There are numerous types of EDS. Classical EDS is autosomal dominant and caused by mutation in the *COL5A1* and *COL5A2* genes.
- All forms of EDS are characterized by skin fragility, unsightly bruising and scarring, musculoskeletal discomfort, and susceptibility to osteoarthritis. The skin is soft and hyperextensible with easy bruising and thin, atrophic 'cigarette paper' scars, joint hypermobility, varicose veins, and a risk of premature delivery in affected fetuses.
- Hypermobile EDS is a common and usually mild autosomal dominant disorder characterized by soft skin with hypermobility of large and small joints.

Neurofibromatosis type 1

See also 📖 pp.531, 662.

- NF1 has a prevalence of ~1/4000.
- AD condition caused by mutation in the *NF1* gene on 17q11.2.
- For a clinical diagnosis of NF1, the patient should have two or more of the following features:
  - 6 or more *café-au-lait* spots (≥0.5cm in children);
  - 2 or more neurofibromata of any type (dermal neurofibromata are small lumps in the skin that appear in adolescence) or 1 or more plexiform neurofibromata;
  - freckling in the axilla, neck, or groin;
  - optic glioma (tumour in the optic pathway);
  - 2 or more Lisch nodules (benign iris hamartomas);
  - a distinctive bony lesion, e.g. sphenoid wing dysplasia, or dysplasia or thinning of the long bone cortex, e.g. pseudoarthrosis;
  - a first-degree relative with NF1.
- NF1 is a highly variable disorder with a small risk of serious complications, e.g. scoliosis, pressure effects of tumours or malignant change, (e.g. neural crest tumours), hypertension. Regular surveillance, e.g. annual review, is recommended to try and detect these early.

X-linked hypohidrotic ectodermal dysplasia

- The condition follows X-linked recessive inheritance and is caused by mutation in the *EDA-1* gene.
- Boys have reduced/absent sweating that may cause dangerous hyperpyrexia in infancy.
- Carrier females may be mildly affected.

Tuberous sclerosis complex

See also 📖 pp.372, 530.

- Affects ~1/10 000 individuals.
- A highly variable autosomal dominant multisystem disorder caused by mutation in the *TSC1* gene on 9q or the *TSC2* gene on 16p.
- Characterized by hamartomas in the brain, skin, and other organs.
- Commonly presents with infantile spasms. Seizures and mental retardation are often associated.
- Hypomelanotic macules ('ash-leaf' spots) occur in ~95% of affected individuals by the age of 5yrs. A Wood's light (UV) may be needed to visualize these. Angiofibromata occur in later childhood in a butterfly distribution over the nose and cheeks. Other cutaneous features include forehead fibrous plaque, shagreen patches, ungual fibromata, and dental pits.
- 50% of individuals with TSC have normal intelligence, but children who develop infantile spasms and severe epilepsy in the first year of life often have learning disability.
- Thorough clinical evaluation, e.g. cranial MRI, eye exam, renal US, is indicated to make the diagnosis prior to genetic testing.
- Expert genetic advice, with careful evaluation of the parents, is important. ~60% of cases arise as a result of new mutations.
- Genetic testing is possible by mutation analysis of *TSC1* and *TSC2*, but it is helpful to establish a clear clinical diagnosis before embarking on genetic testing.

Incontinentia pigmenti

- Rare X-linked dominant disorder caused by mutation in the *NEMO* gene on Xq28 (~80% carry a common deletion).
- Affected male pregnancies almost invariably miscarry. Girls present in the neonatal period with blistering lesions, cropping circumferentially on the trunk and in a linear distribution on the limbs. Ultimately, lesions regress by late childhood/adult life to leave atrophic streaky areas of pigmentation or hypopigmentation (often most noticeable on the back of the calves). The child remains well and continues to feed. There is often a marked eosinophilia in the blood.
- ~50% have associated abnormalities of dentition, eye (cataracts), or CNS (seizures, microcephaly).
- Genetic testing is possible; ~80% of affected individuals carry a large deletion in the *NEMO* gene.
- No specific treatment available.

Genetic disorders of growth

Assessment of growth plays an important role in deciding whether a child may have an underlying genetic disorder. Measurements <0.4th centile or >99.6th centile nearly always merit further assessment, unless there is a clear explanation. Measurements between the 0.4th and 2nd centiles or 98th and 99.6th need to be interpreted in context and may be clinically significant. If in doubt, discuss with a senior colleague.

Intrauterine growth retardation (IUGR)

Silver–Russell syndrome

- Incidence is unclear (1/3000–100 000 births). Equal sex ratio.
- ~10% of children have maternal UPD7.
- Genetically heterogeneous condition characterized by intrauterine and postnatal growth retardation with short stature and FTT. Typically, babies have disproportionately large head (OFC usually 3rd–25th centile), triangular facies, down-turned mouth, some asymmetry of limbs.
- About 30–50% of cases will show hypomethylation of the paternal chromosome at the IC1 (imprinting centre) on 11p15.5.

Cornelia de Lange syndrome

- Rare; incidence ~1/50,000 live births.
- Intrauterine and postnatal growth impairment, limb anomalies, microcephaly, hirsutism, and distinctive facial features (neat arched eyebrows, short upturned nose, thin lips with down-turned corners of the mouth).
- Approximately 60% of affected children have mutations in the gene *NIPBL* on chromosome 5p13.

Short stature

Turner syndrome

See also 📖 p.469.
- Affects ~1/2500 females.
- Most girls have a single X chromosome (45, X), usually due to non-disjunction.
- As well as short stature, the typical phenotype includes: broad neck; ptosis; wide carrying angle at elbows (cubitas valgus); widely spaced hypoplastic nipples; low posterior hairline, excessive pigmented naevi. Puffiness of the hands and feet is a common neonatal finding.
- Associated abnormalities include: congenital heart disease (15–50%), especially coarctation of the aorta and VSD; structural renal anomalies (~30%), e.g. horseshoe kidney or unilateral renal agenesis; hypoplastic 'streak' ovaries (1° amenorrhoea and infertility).
- The phenotype can be very subtle and is easily missed, and so a chromosome analysis is usually offered to all girls with unexplained short stature.

Tall stature

Marfan syndrome See 📖 p.940.

Obesity

Bardet–Biedl syndrome (BBS)

- Rare condition; incidence in the UK population <1/100 000.
- Genetically heterogeneous with at least 8 genes identified to date. In the majority of families inheritance is autosomal recessive.
- *Features include:* pigmentary retinopathy; postaxial polydactyly; obesity; cognitive impairment; renal defects.

Prader–Willi syndrome (PWS)

- Affects ~1/10 000 individuals.
- Caused by disruption to the paternally derived imprinted domain on 15q11–13.
- Babies are floppy with feeding difficulties and may fail to thrive in infancy. There is rapid weight gain between the ages of 1 and 6yrs.
- Older children have truncal obesity, mild/moderate learning difficulties, and short stature. Typically children have an insatiable appetite with food-foraging and other behavioural problems.
- Diagnosis is by molecular genetic analysis (*SNRPN* methylation assay).

Overgrowth

Beckwith–Wiedemann syndrome

- Incidence ~1/14,000.
- Genetic basis is complex; it is caused by disruption of the imprinted region on chromosome 11p15.
- Usually presents in the perinatal period with macrosomia. Birth weight is usually >97th centile and length is usually > +2SD. Polyhydramnios or preterm delivery commonly occur.
- There may be associated congenital anomalies: exomphalos/umbilical hernia; dysmorphic features (e.g. ear lobe creases, port wine stain, macroglossia (large tongue)); visceromegaly; hemihypertrophy.
- Neonates are at risk for severe hypoglycaemia and should be monitored closely.
- Macrosomia continues through early childhood and then becomes less dramatic with increasing age.
- Some children with BWS are at increased risk for Wilms' tumour.
- In ~50% diagnosis can be confirmed by molecular genetic testing. Uniparental disomy 11p15 analysis requires blood testing of child and *both* parents.

Sotos syndrome

- Incidence ~1/15 000 children.
- Due to mutation or deletion in the *NSD1* gene on chromosome 5q35. Most are isolated *de novo* mutations but familial cases do occur.

Characterized by prenatal overgrowth (birth weight ~4200g in males; ~4000g in females), which persists in childhood, especially through the pre-school years. Final adult height is often in the upper normal range. OFC is also increased and bone age is advanced. Affected children typically have a tall skull with a prominent broad forehead and pointed chin. Developmental delay is almost always present, but varies from mild to severe. Some children have seizures.

Miscellaneous genetic conditions

See Table 25.1

Table 25.1 Miscellaneous genetic conditions

Syndrome	Features	Inheritance	Chromosome	Gene
Achondroplasia	Short limbs, large head, 'trident' hand, flat midface, lumbar lordosis	AD	4p16	FGFR3
Apert	Craniostenosis, beaked nose, cleft palate, severe syndactyly ('mitten hand'), ↓ IQ	AD	10q26	FGFR2
CHARGE (see pp.373, 846)	**C**oloboma, congenital **H**eart disease, choanal **A**tresia, **R**etarded growth (short stature), hypo**G**enitalism, external **E**ar abnormality and deafness	AD (usually de novo)	8q12	CHD7
5p- (Cri du chat)	Hypoplastic larynx (cat-like cry), small stature, microcephaly, micrognathia, low-set ears, hypertelorism, ↓ IQ	Sporadic	5p deletion (5p−)	FGFR2
Crouzon	Craniostenosis, brachycephaly, prominent forehead, proptosis, beaked nose	AD	10q26	TBX5
Holt–Oram	Hypoplastic thumbs ± radius, ASD, VSD	AD	12q	MCPH1-7
Primary AR microcephaly	Sloping forehead, OFC << 0.4th centile (< 4SD), moderate mental retardation	AR	Various	DHCR7
Smith–Lemli–Opitz (SLO)	Ptosis, anteverted nostrils, narrow frontal region, hypospadias, toe syndactyly, ↓ IQ	AR	11q12–13	FGFR3
Thanatophoric dysplasia	Large head, small thorax, short limbs, lethal	Sporadic	4p16	TCOF1
Treacher–Collins	Malar hypoplasia, micrognathia, down-slanting eyes, ear malformations, deafness, lower eyelid coloboma	AD	5q32	PEX1-14
Zellweger	Prominent forehead, large fontanelles, flat facies, hypotonia, stippled epiphyses, nystagmus, hepatomegaly	AR	Various	

Miscellaneous congenital malformations

See Table 25.2

Table 25.2 Miscellaneous congenital malformations

Condition	Features	Cause
Amniotic bands	Congenital facial clefts, limb constrictions, amputations, syndactyly or talipes	Annular amniotic bands
Diabetic embryopathy	Macrosomia, organomegaly (particularly heart and liver), polycythaemia, caudal regression syndrome (sacral and femoral agenesis or hypoplasia), transient hypertrophic cardiomyopathy, neural tube defects	Maternal diabetes mellitus
Fetal compression syndrome	Joint contractions/dislocation, talipes, micrognathia, cleft palate, skull deformity	In utero compression, e.g. maternal pelvic abnormality
Fetal alcohol syndrome	IUGR, hirsutism, microcephaly, mid-face hypoplasia, short palpebral fissures, long smooth philtrum, ↓ IQ, low weight for height.	Excessive maternal alcohol ingestion in pregnancy
Fetal anticonvulsant syndrome	2–3x increase in major malformations, growth retardation, midface hypoplasia, ↓ IQ. Maternal valproate causes a 10x increased incidence of neural tube defects	Maternal anticonvulsant therapy in pregnancy
Goldenhar syndrome	Asymmetric facial hypoplasia, eye coloboma/dermoid, ear hypoplasia, preauricular skin tags, vertebral defects, cardiac defects (Fallot's tetralogy, VSD)	Unknown. Usually sporadic
Klippel–Feil syndrome	Cervical vertebral fusion, low hair line, webbed neck, torticollis, kyphoscoliosis, deafness	Usually sporadic
Moebius syndrome	Immobile face, strabismus, limb defects, syndactyly	Unknown, usually sporadic
Pierre–Robin sequence (see 📖 p.847)	Micrognathia, glossoptosis, cleft palate	Unknown (need to exclude del22q11). Usually sporadic
Potter's sequence	Depressed nasal bridge, crumpled low set ears, talipes equinovarus, joint contractures, lung hypoplasia and respiratory failure. Lethal	Severe oligohydramnios due to renal or urethral abnormalities
VATER association (see 📖 pp.373, 848)	Vertebral defects, Anal atresia, Tracheo-oEsophageal fistula. Renal defects. (VACTERL = additional cardiac and radial limb defects)	Unknown. Usually sporadic

Inherited metabolic disease

General principles

Inherited metabolic disease (IMD) may present at any age and the signs and symptoms may result from:
• Accumulation of substrate that leads to a toxic effect.
• Accumulation of a minor metabolite that in excess is toxic.
• Deficiency of a product of a specific reaction.
• 2° metabolic phenomena.

The commonest error in managing infants and children with IMD is a delay in diagnosis, and therefore a delay in starting treatment. Failure to recognize an IMD may occur because its clinical features are confusing because of:
• Genetic heterogeneity.
• A presenting intercurrent illness.
• similarity with other common, acquired conditions where the differential diagnosis has not been fully explored.

A useful approach is to consider certain 'syndromes' and use this as a framework for investigation (Table 26.1).[1] This approach is widely used and should serve the purpose.

Table 26.1 Differential diagnosis of inherited metabolic syndromes

IMD syndrome	Non-metabolic differential
Neurology (📖 p.956)	*Infections:* enterovirus, herpes
Encephalopathy	*Drug reaction:* CNS depressants, antihistamines, anticonvulsants
Metabolic acidosis (📖 p.958) Lactic acidosis	*Drug reaction:* alcohol, methanol, ethylene glycol, salicylates (see 📖 p.104)
	Deficiency: thiamine
Storage or dysmorphism (📖 p.959)	*Infections:* congenital CMV, congenital toxoplasmosis
	Haematological disorders (see 📖 p.626)
Hepatic (📖 p.960)	*Infections:* hepatitis, enterovirus, infectious mononucleosis
	Drug reaction
	Haematological disorders (see 📖 p.632)
Cardiac (📖 p.962)	*Infections:* enterovirus
	Drug reaction

Reference
1 Clarke JTR (2006). *A clinical guide to inherited metabolic diseases.* Cambridge: Cambridge University Press.

Metabolic syndromes: neurological

There are 7 presentations of IMD with neurological features.

Chronic encephalopathy

Grey matter: developmental delay, psychomotor retardation

Developmental delay is a common problem (see □ pp.557, 562), but the features that warrant investigation for IMD include:

- Global delay affecting all areas of development.
- Progressive course with loss of developmental milestones.
- Objective evidence of neurological dysfunction (e.g. special senses, pyramidal tract, extrapyramidal, cranial nerves).
- Severe behaviours including irritability, impulsiveness, aggressiveness, and hyperactivity.
- Seizures (complex partial or myoclonic) originating early in life that are resistant to usual therapy.

Causes include vitamin B_6 dependency; biotinidase deficiency; neuronal ceroid-lipofuscinosis; GM2 gangliosidosis; cherry-red spot–myoclonus syndrome (sialidosis type I); Leigh disease; Alper's disease; MELAS (mitochondrial encephalopathy–lactic acidosis and stroke-like episodes syndrome).

White matter: gross motor delay, weakness, and incoordination

- *Central involvement only:* Canavan disease; Alexander disease; GM2 gangliosidosis; GM1 gangliosidosis; X-linked adrenoleucodystrophy (ALD); amino acidurias, organic acidurias.
- *Central and peripheral involvement:* metachromatic leucodystrophy (MLD); Krabbe leucodystrophy; peroxisomal disorders.

Chronic encephalopathy with abnormalities outside the CNS

- *Muscle:* mitochondrial myopathy (□ p.971).
- *Hepatosplenomegaly +/– bone:* Gaucher disease, Niemann–Pick disease, mucopolysaccharidosis (MPS) I–IV (Hurler disease, Hunter disease, Sanfilippo disease, Sly disease), GM1 gangliosidosis, sialidosis II, Zellweger.
- *Skin +/– connective tissue:* homocystinuria; Menkes; fucosidosis; multiple sulphatase deficiency; galactosialidosis; prolidase deficiency.

Investigations for chronic encephalopathy

See also □ pp.536–537, 942, 960

- *Clinical:* developmental assessment and neurological examination
- *Imaging:* MRI of head; X-rays of hands, chest, lateral spine
- *Blood:* plasma amino acids; ammonia; lactate
- *Urine:* amino acids, organic acids, and mucopolysaccharide and oligosaccharide screen
- *Electrophysiology:* auditory brainstem reflexes; visual-evoked potentials; somatosensory-evoked potentials; nerve conduction; EMG; EEG

Acute encephalopathy

Deterioration in level of consciousness resulting from IMD:
- may occur in a previously healthy child;
- usually shows no focal features, but ataxia may be present;
- may start with unusual behaviour;
- progresses rapidly, even to the stage of coma.

The likely causes are: hyperammonaemia (urea cycle; 📖 p.964); amino acidopathy (📖 p.965); organic aciduria (📖 p.966); fatty acid oxidation defect (📖 p.970); mitochondrial defect (📖 p.971); hypoglycaemia (📖 p.96).

Stroke

The IMD associated with stroke or stroke-like episodes are:
- Homocystinuria (📖 p.965).
- Fabry disease (📖 p.968).
- *Organic acidopathy:* methylmalonic acidaemia; propionic acidaemia; isovaleric acidaemia; glutaric aciduria I and II (📖 p.966).
- Ornithine transcarbamoylase deficiency (📖 p.964).
- MELAS (📖 p.956)
- Congenital disorder of glycosylation type 1A.
- Familial hemiplegic migraine.

Movement disorder (📖 p.524)

- *Ataxia:* maple syrup urine disease; pyruvate dehydrogenase deficiency; Friedreich ataxia; abetalipoproteinaemia.
- *Choreoathetosis and dystonia:* glutaric aciduria I; Lesch–Nyhan disease; triose phosphate isomerase deficiency.
- *Parkinsonism:* Wilson disease; tyrosine hydroxylase deficiency.

Myopathy

- *Acute intermittent muscle weakness:* hyperkalaemic periodic paralysis; paramyotonia congenita; hypokalaemic periodic paralysis.
- *Progressive muscle weakness:* glycogen storage disease II (GSD, Pompe disease); GSD III.
- *Exercise intolerance with cramps and myoglobinuria:* myophosphorylase deficiency, carnitine palmitoyltransferase II.
- *Myopathy as a manifestation of multisystem disease:* mitochondrial myopathies.

Autonomic dysfunction The causes include: dopamine β-hydroxylase deficiency; neurovisceral porphyrias; Fabry disease; MPS I–III; occipital horn syndrome; mitochondrial neurogastrointestinal encephalomyopathy.

Psychiatric problems

The causes include the following:
- *Child:* MPS II; MPS III; X-linked ALD; Lesch–Nyhan syndrome.
- *Adolescent:* late-onset MLD; late-onset GM2 gangliosidosis; porphyria; Wilson disease; Wolfram syndrome; cerebrotendinous xanthomatosis; urea cycle defect; homocystinuria; adult onset neuronal ceroid lipofuscinosis.

Metabolic syndromes: metabolic acidosis

The emergency care of acid–base problems is discussed on 🕮 p.104. Metabolic acidosis may occur as a result of:
• Abnormal loss of bicarbonate.
• Abnormal accumulation of hydrogen ions in association with a non-volatile organic anion.

These two states can be differentiated by calculating the anion gap (i.e. the difference between plasma [Na^+] and the sum of plasma [Cl^-] and [HCO_3^-]). The normal anion gap is 10–15mmol/L.

Abnormal bicarbonate loss

When metabolic acidosis is due to bicarbonate loss from either the gut or kidney:
• The anion gap is normal.
• Hyperchloraemia is usually present.

To distinguish bicarbonate loss from the gut or from the kidney:
• A history of diarrhoea will distinguish between hyperchloraemia due to GI losses from that due to renal tubular losses.
• Urine net charge (UNC), calculated as [Na^++ K^+] – [Cl^-], is used to estimate urine ammonium (NH_4^+) when there is no accumulated organic acid. A negative UNC implies the presence of adequate or increased urinary ammonium; therefore the acidosis results from abnormal GI loss of bicarbonate. (Note: Urine ammonium is low in renal tubular disorders.)

IMDs associated with RTA include—galactosaemia; hereditary fructose intolerance; hepatorenal tyrosinaemia; cystinosis; glycogen storage disease I; Fanconi–Bickel syndrome; congenital lactic acidosis; Wilson disease; vitamin D dependency; osteopetrosis with RTA; Lowe syndrome.

Accumulation of organic anion

When metabolic acidosis is due to accumulated organic anion:
• It is associated with failure to thrive (🕮 p.308).
• Tachypnoea may be present.
• 2° hypoglycaemia leads to a neurological syndrome (🕮 p.96).
• Organic anion may lead to distinct smell of sweat or urine.
• The anion gap is raised.

The causes include the following:
• *Lactic acidosis:* pyruvate accumulation (e.g. pyruvate dehydrogenase deficiency, pyruvate carboxylase deficiency, multiple carboxylase deficiency); NADH accumulation (e.g. defect of mitochondrial electron chain).
• *Ketoacidosis:* s to IMD (e.g. maple syrup urine disease, organic acido-pathies, glycogen storage disease, disorders of gluconeogenesis; rare p disorders of ketone utilization, e.g. β-ketothiolase deficiency, succinyl-CoA: 3-ketoacid transferase deficiency.
• *Organic aciduria:* a large spectrum of disorders (see 🕮 p.966).

Metabolic syndromes: storage dysmorphism

IMDs associated with significant dysmorphic features

Lysosomal disorders (📖 p.968)
- Mucopolysaccharidoses
- Glycoproteinoses
- Sphingolipidoses

Peroxisomal disorders (📖 p.972)
- Zellweger syndrome
- Rhizomelic chondrodysplasia punctata

Mitochondrial disorders (📖 p.971)

Glutaric aciduria type II (📖 p.966)

Other
- Menkes disease (📖 p.976)
- Homocystinuria (📖 p.965)
- Familial hypercholesterolaemia (📖 p.963)

Lysosomal disorder

The characteristic features of this storage dysmorphic syndrome are:
- coarse facies;
- bone changes (dysostosis multiplex);
- short stature;
- organomegaly (hepatosplenomegaly).

Peroxisomal disorder

The characteristic features of the Zellweger phenotype are:
- psychomotor retardation;
- hypotonia and weakness;
- seizures;
- hepatocellular dysfunction;
- impaired special senses.

Investigations

The initial investigation should include the following.
- *Urine:* mucopolysaccharide and oligosaccharide screen; organic acids.
- *Plasma:* lactate; pyruvate; very long-chain fatty acids; phytanic acid; amino acids; isoelectric focusing of transferrin.

Metabolic syndromes: hepatic syndromes

There are four possible ways in which IMD may present with hepatic involvement.

Jaundice See 📖 pp.130–131, 314–315

Hepatomegaly

See 📖 p.967. The liver enlargement associated with IMD is usually persistent and not tender. The causes include:

- *Glycogen storage disease (GSD) type I:* presents in infancy with hypoglycaemia.
- *GSD type III:* presents in early infancy with failure to thrive, hyperlipidaemia, ketosis during fasting, and deranged liver function.
- *GSD VI:* hepatic phosphorylase deficiency.
- Hereditary tyrosinaemia type I.

Hypoglycaemia See 📖 pp.96–97, 132, 412, 967

Hepatocellular dysfunction See 📖 pp.342–345

IMD with characteristic, severe liver involvement may present at different ages.

- *Infancy:* failure to thrive; mild to severe hyperbilirubinaemia; hypoglycaemia; hyperammonaemia; deranged LFTs; bleeding; oedema; ascites.
- *Children:* presentation with chronic active hepatitis (fatigue, anorexia, hyperbilirubinaemia, tender hepatomegaly), cirrhosis (oedema, gynaecomastia, ascites, clubbing, spider naevi), or neuropsychiatric disease.

Some causes with distinguishing features in infancy

- *Galactosaemia:* hyperbilirubinaemia; haemolytic anaemia; coagulopathy (see 📖 p.967).
- *Hepatorenal tyrosinaemia:* coagulopathy
- *α₁-antitrypsin deficiency:* jaundice; failure to thrive; intracranial and other haemorrhages.
- *Congenital disorders of glycosylation:* failure to thrive; chronic vomiting and diarrhoea; seizures; developmental delay.

Some causes with distinguishing features in childhood

- *GSD type III:* skeletal myopathy (see 📖 p.967).
- *Gaucher disease type III:* massive hepatosplenomegaly; failure to thrive; abdominal protuberance; anaemia; ascites; bleeding diathesis (see 📖 p.969).
- *Niemann–Pick disease, type C:* neurodegeneration; hepatosplenomegaly.
- *Wilson disease:* onset in adolescence with hepatitis, haemolysis, neuropsychiatric disturbance (see 📖 p.976).

Investigation of liver function

Tests of cholestasis
- Bilirubin (conjugated and unconjugated)
- Alkaline phosphatase
- Gamma-glutamyltranspeptidase
- Bile acids (urine)

Blood tests of active liver disease:
- Aspartate aminotransferase
- Alanine aminotransferase

Tests of synthetic function
- Albumin
- Prothrombin and partial thromboplastin time
- Clotting factor levels VII, V
- Ammonium

Specific tests for IMD
- Copper and caeruloplasmin (Wilson disease)
- Alpha-fetoprotein (tyrosinaemia)
- Alpha-1-antitrypsin (PI phenotype, ZZ for deficiency)
- Plasma amino acids
- Urinary organic acids
- Red cell galactose-1-phosphate uridyltransferase (galactosaemia)
- Lysosomal enzymes
- Liver biopsy

Metabolic syndromes: cardiac syndromes

Cardiomyopathy may be the dominant or only clinical problem in a variety of IMDs.

Glycogen metabolism (hypertrophic cardiomyopathy) Pompe disease (GSD II)—presents in early infancy with marked skeletal myopathy, massive cardiomegaly (large QRS, left axis deviation, shortened PR, T-wave inversion).

Fatty acid metabolism (dilated cardiomyopathy)
- *Systemic carnitine deficiency:* presents with skeletal myopathy, hypotonia encephalopathy, hepatic syndrome (hepatomegaly, hypoglycaemia, hepatocellular dysfunction).
- *Long or very long chain acyl-CoA dehydrogenase deficiency:* presents with myopathy, exercise intolerance with myoglobinuria, hypotonia, encephalopathy, hepatic syndrome ± hyperammonaemia.

Organic acidopathy (dilated cardiomyopathy) Propionic acidaemia—intermittent metabolic acidosis; ketosis; hyperammonaemia; neutropenia.

Mitochondrial cardiomyopathy (hypertrophic or dilated)

Sphingolipidoses (hypertrophic cardiomyopathy) Fabry disease— chronic neuritis pain in hands and feet; angiokeratomata; corneal opacities; progressive renal failure; cardiac arrhythmias (intermittent SVT); cerebrovascular disease.

Mucopolysaccharidosis (hypertrophic cardiomyopathy)

Investigation

Initial studies
- *Plasma:* lactate; carnitine (free and total); acylcarnitine profile; ammonium; liver function tests; urea, creatinine, and electrolytes
- *Urine:* organic acids

Suspected fatty acid oxidation defect Fibroblast cultures; enzyme studies

Suspected mitochondrial electron transport defect
- *Plasma:* lactate/pyruvate ratio
- *CSF:* lactate
- *Imaging:* MRI
- *Electrophysiology:* evoked potentials
- *Tissue:* muscle and skin biopsy studies

Suspected lysosomal storage disease
- *Urine:* mucopolysaccharide and oligosaccharide screen, glycolipids
- *Imaging:* skeletal radiology
- *Blood:* lysosomal enzyme studies

Arrhythmias

IMD-related cardiomyopathy may be complicated by arrhythmias including:

- *Heart block:* mitochondrial cytopathy; Fabry disease; carnitine–acylcarnitine translocase (CACT) deficiency; propionic acidaemia.
- *Tachyarrhythmia:* fatty acid oxidation defects; CACT.

Coronary artery disease (CAD)

CAD occurs in Fabry disease, familial hyperlipidaemias, and familial hypercholesterolaemia (FH).

FH affects 1/500 individuals with the following effects.

- *Homozygotes:* severe cholesterolaemia; ischaemic heart disease in infancy or childhood; cholesterol accumulation in the skin (tuberous xanthomas, subcutaneous nodules); and arcus senilis.
- *Heterozygotes:* fatal myocardial infarction in third decade.

Familial hyperlipidaemias causing premature CAD include the following.

- *Type IV:* hyperlipidaemia (increased very low-density lipoproteins).
- *Type IIa, familial hypercholesterolaemia:* hypercholesterolaemia (increased low-density lipoproteins) with tuberous xanthomas, tendinous xanthomas, and arcus senilis.
- *Type IIb:* combined hyperlipidaemia (increased low- and very low-density lipoproteins).
- *Type III, familial dysbetalipoproteinaemia:* β-very low-density lipoproteins with eruptive tuberous xanthoma, planar xanthomas, peripheral vascular disease.

Urea cycle disorders

The urea cycle disorders are a group of conditions in which enzyme defects result in the accumulation of nitrogen in the form of ammonia, which is a highly toxic substance causing irreversible brain damage. Clinical presentation may be in the first few days of life. Hyperammonaemia (usually severe) results in:

• coma;
• convulsions and vomiting.

Clinical confusion with septicaemia is common. In the older child, patients may present with:
• psychomotor retardation;
• growth failure;
• vomiting;
• behavioural abnormalities;
• recurrent cerebellar ataxia and headache.

It is essential to monitor the blood ammonia in any patient with unexplained neurological symptoms.

The urea cycle disorders

• N-acetylglutamate synthetase deficiency (NAGS)
• Carbamyl phosphate synthetase deficiency (CPS)
• Ornithine transcarbamylase deficiency (OTC)
• Argininosuccinic acid synthetase deficiency (citrullinaemia; AS)
• Argininosuccinase acid lyase deficiency (argininosuccinic aciduria; AL/ASA)
• Arginase deficiency (arginaemia; AL/ASA)

All are autosomal recessive except for ornithine transcarbamylase deficiency (X-linked). Individuals with childhood or adult onset disease may have a partial enzyme deficiency

---

Diagnosis
Plasma concentrations of ammonia are elevated, glutamine and alanine (the major nitrogen-carrying amino acids) are usually high, and arginine is low. Specific urea cycle defects can be diagnosed by their characteristic plasma and urine amino acid profiles.

Treatment Management of dietary protein intake with essential amino acids and restriction of protein intake to suppress ammonia formation.

Disorders of amino acid metabolism

Due to defects either in the synthesis of (or the breakdown of) amino acids or in the body's ability to transport amino acids into cells. Most are autosomal recessive. Diagnosis is established by detecting abnormal plasma and urinary amino acid profiles.

Phenylketonuria (PKU)

AR. Occurs in 1/10 000–15 000 live births. In its classical form it is due to a deficiency in phenylalanine hydroxylase. Untreated, brain development is impaired leading to progressive mental retardation and seizures, usually evident by 6–12mths of age. Many children have fair hair and blue eyes. In PKU phenylalanine accumulates and is converted into phenylketones, which are detected in the urine.

- PKU can be managed entirely by a diet low in phenylalanine and high in tyrosine. Adherence to the diet will prevent neurological problems.
- PKU is detected early in a national neonatal biochemical screening programme.

Homocystinuria

Due to deficiency in cystathionine beta-synthase, resulting in increased urinary homocystine and methionine excretion.

Clinical manifestations resemble those of Marfan's syndrome (see 🕮 p.940).

Treatment with high-dose pyridoxine and low-methionine diet, supplemented with cysteine.

Cardinal features of homocystinuria

- *Eyes:* lens subluxation (ectopia lentis); myopia; glaucoma
- *CNS:* seizures; neurodevelopmental delay; behaviour problems
- *Skeleton:* Marfanoid body habitus; high-arched palate; kyphoscoliosis; arachnodactyly
- *Cardiovascular system:* mitral valve prolapse
- *Thromboembolism risk*

Disorders of organic acid metabolism

A large group of disorders characterized by a broad range of clinical symptoms and signs varying in seriousness from trivial to lethal. Includes developmental delay, poor growth, and episodic illnesses with vomiting and metabolic acidosis. Some of these may be precipitated by prolonged fasting or minor viral infection. May be associated with hypoglycaemia and ketosis or ketoacidosis.

- Characterized by urinary excretion of abnormal types and amounts of organic acids.
- Diagnosis by urinary organic acid profile.
- *Treatment:* avoid prolonged fasting, and administer extra carbohydrate during illness.

Examples include the following.

Methylmalonic acidaemia (MMA)

Caused by methylmalonyl-CoA mutase deficiency. Commonly presents in the newborn period with:

- severe metabolic acidosis;
- acute encephalopathy;
- hyperammonaemia;
- neutropenia and thrombocytopenia.

3-hydroxy-3-methyl-CoA (HMG-CoA) lyase deficiency

May present in the newborn period with severe metabolic acidosis, poor feeding and vomiting, lethargy, altered level of consciousness, hypoglycaemia, and hyperammonaemia.

Glutaric aciduria

- GluA type 1 is caused by deficiency of mitochondrial glutaryl-CoA dehydrogenase. The condition presents in infancy with episodes of hypotonia, dystonia, opisthotonus, grimacing, fisting, tongue thrusting, and seizures.
- GluA type II is caused by deficiency of mitochondrial electron transport falvoprotein or dehydrogenase. It may present in the following ways.
  - *Neonatal disease:* with or without dysmorphism (abnormal facies, muscular defects of the abdominal wall, hypospadias in boys, cystic kidneys); hypotonia; hepatomegaly; hypoketotic hypoglycaemia; metabolic acidosis; hyperammonaemia.
  - *Later-onset disease:* episodic metabolic acidosis, failure to thrive, hypoglycaemia, hyperammonaemia, and encephalopathy.

Disorders of carbohydrate metabolism

Autosomal recessive conditions. Often presenting with one or more of the following—episodic hypoglycaemia; lactic acidosis; poor growth and hypotonia; mental retardation/developmental delay; and vomiting; cramps, myoglobinuria, and muscle weakness.

Glycogen storage disease (GSD) Specific enzyme defects preventing mobilization of glucose from glycogen, and resulting in abnormal storage in liver and/or muscle (see Table 26.2).

Table 26.2 GSD types I–V

GSD type	Enzyme defect	Tissue	Key clinical features
I: Von Gierke	Glucose-6-phosphatase	Liver +++	Poor growth Hypoglycaemia Hepatomegaly
II: Pompe	Lysosomal α-glucosidase	Liver ++Muscle +++	Cardiac failure Hypotonia
III: Corri	Glycogen debrancher (amylo-1,6-glucosidase)	Liver ++Muscle +	Poor growth Muscle weakness Hypoglycaemia
IV: Andersen	Glycogen branching (amylo-1,4–1,6 transglucosidase	Liver +++Muscle +	Failure to thrive Liver failure Muscle weakness
V: McArdle	Phosphorylase	Muscle ++	Muscle weakness Cramps

Disorders of fructose metabolism

Hereditary fructose intolerance Fructose-1-phosphate aldolase deficiency. Failure to thrive; hypoglycaemia; metabolic/lactic acidosis; vomiting; GI bleeding.

Galactosaemia

Galactose-1-phosphate uridyltransferase deficiency. Failure to thrive; cataracts; hepatomegaly; jaundice, vomiting and diarrhoea; mental retardation (if untreated). Treatment with galactose-free diet.

Disorders of lipoprotein metabolism

This is a heterogeneous group of disorders resulting in abnormalities of blood lipid profile. May predispose to cardiovascular disease (see 📖 p.963).

Lysosomal storage diseases

See also 📖 p.959. This is a large group of disorders due to defects in lysosomal function.

Mucopolysaccharidoses

A group of IMD caused by deficiency in lysosomal enzymes needed to break down glycosaminoglycans (long chain carbohydrate molecules formerly called mucopolysaccharides). Affects bone, cartilage, tendons, eyes, skin, and connective tissue, leading to accumulation of glycosaminoglycans and progressive cellular and tissue damage.

Clinical features are not apparent at birth, but progress with time as storage of glycosaminoglycans impacts on tissues and organs. Typical features include:

- *Neuropathy:* peripheral/spinal.
- Neurodevelopmental delay; hearing loss (conductive/sensory); hydrocephalus.
- *Visual loss:* corneal clouding/glaucoma/retinal degeneration.
- Coarsening of facial features.
- Short stature/skeletal deformities; joint stiffness.
- Valvular heart disease.

Sphingolipidoses

Clinically the sphingolipidoses show variable severity. They cause progressive peripheral and CNS disease (psychomotor retardation, myoclonus, weakness, and spasticity).

Variants of Gaucher and Niemann–Pick disease that do not affect the nervous system are termed non-neuronopathic.

Sphingolipidoses

- Fabry's disease
- Gangliosidosis
- GM1 gangliosidoses
- GM2 gangliosidoses
- Tay–Sachs disease
- Sandhoff disease
- Gaucher's disease
- Krabbe disease
- Metachromatic leucodystrophy
- Niemann–Pick disease

Fabry's disease

X-linked recessive. Due to a deficiency of alpha galactosidase A, resulting in the accumulation of globotriaosylceramide within blood vessels and other tissues. Clinical features become evident in early childhood and increase in severity with age—anhidrosis; fatigue; skin lesions (angiokeratomas: tiny, painless papules); and burning pain of the extremities. Renal failure, heart disease, and stroke increase with age. Other symptoms include tinnitus, vertigo, nausea, and diarrhoea.

Gaucher's disease

AR. This is the most common lysosomal storage disorder. It is due to deficient activity of beta-glucocerebrosidase and leads to intracellular accumulation of glucosylceramide (glucosylcerebroside) within cells of mononuclear phagocyte origin (producing characteristic 'Gaucher cells').

Gaucher disease is categorized phenotypically into 3 main subtypes:

- *Type I Gaucher disease:* most common form of Gaucher disease—lacks 1° CNS involvement. Wide spectrum of severity, ranging from affected infants to asymptomatic adults. Usually presents in childhood with hepatosplenomegaly, pancytopenia, and bone marrow infiltration. Severe orthopaedic complications, including vertebral compression, avascular necrosis of the femoral head, and pathological fractures of long bones.
- *Type II acute neuronopathic:* acute neuronopathic form of the disorder starts in infancy, and death is often by 2yrs of age. Patients are usually normal at birth, but develop hepatosplenomegaly, developmental regression, and growth arrest within a few months of age.
- *Type III subacute neuronopathic:* subacute form similar to type II Gaucher disease, but has later age of onset and slower progression.

Glycoproteinosis

A heterogeneous group of disorders of glycoprotein storage. A spectrum of phenotypes include neurological deterioration, growth retardation, visceromegaly, and seizures. Also coarse facial features, angiokeratoma corporis diffusum, spasticity, and delayed development.

Types of glycoproteinosis

- Mucolipidosis II (I-cell disease)
- Mucolipidosis III (pseudo-Hurler polydystrophy)
- *Defects in glycoprotein degradation:* aspartylglucosaminuria, fucosidosis, mannosidosis, sialidosis (mucolipidosis I)

Disorders of fatty acid oxidation

Disorders of fatty acid metabolism may be due to deficiency in the acyl dehydrogenase enzyme complex, deficiency in carnitine, or a defect in the carnitine transport process.

- Clinical presentation is with acute encephalopathy with recurrent vomiting, lethargy, drowsiness, and seizures. Hypoglycaemia is usually observed, as well as hepatomegaly and hyperammonaemia.
- Episodes of acute encephalopathy are precipitated by periods of prolonged fasting or by intercurrent illness associated with poor feeding.
- Presentation is usually in the first 2yrs of life.
- Diagnosis depends on a high index of suspicion. A positive family history or a history of previous acute metabolic crisis during trivial intercurrent illness may be present.
- Diagnosis of a specific disorder of fatty acid metabolism is established by demonstrating characteristic abnormalities in urinary organic acid excretion and in plasma acyl carnitine profiles. Abnormalities may not be present when child is well. Molecular genetic testing is also available for some disorders.
- Treatment successfully managed by avoidance of prolonged fasting, high carbohydrate diet, and carnitine supplements. During intercurrent illness, administration of high carbohydrate diet is required.

Medium chain acyl-CoA dehydrogenase deficiency (MCAD)

This is the commonest fatty acid oxidation disorder (1/13 000 births) and is due to mutations in the *MCAD* gene (1p31). Clinical presentation may vary from asymptomatic to fulminant. Newborn screening programs, utilizing neonatal blood spot collection methods, are now in place in many countries for the early detection and management of this condition.

Mitochondrial disorders

Disorders of mitochondrial function result in a wide of clinical problems (see Box 24.1).

Box 24.1 Disorders of mitochondrial function: clinical problems

Common clinical features
- Lactic acidosis
- Muscle weakness/hypotonia
- Poor growth/short stature
- Neurodevelopmental delay
- Seizures

Other recognized features
- *Eyes:* ophthalmoplegia; retinal degeneration
- *Ears:* sensorineural deafness
- *Cardiovascular:* cardiomyopathy; arrhythmias
- *Respiratory:* periodic breathing
- Diabetes mellitus
- Stroke
- Renal tubular dysfunction

- Inheritance may be either autosomal dominant/recessive or X-linked or mitochondrial (i.e. matrilineal), although most arise as *de novo* mutations.
- Diagnosis requires muscle biopsy, with histochemical studies, electron microscopy, and biochemical studies on isolated tissue. Presence of 'ragged-red' fibres in skeletal muscle biopsy is characteristic of disorders presenting with myopathy.

Leigh's syndrome Relapsing acute encephalopathy; lactic acidosis; hypotonia; seizures; +/– cardiomyopathy; +/– hepatic or renal tubular dysfunction.

Pearson's syndrome Failure to thrive; lactic acidosis; sideroblastic anaemia; hypoparathyroidism; diabetes mellitus.

Peroxisomal disorders

Peroxisomes are ubiquitous cellular organelles that function to rid the cell of toxic material. They contain a number of oxidative enzymes and have an important role in the metabolism of fatty acid molecules. Peroxisomal disorders result in abnormalities of lipid metabolism.

Classification of peroxisomal disorders

Disorders of peroxisome development
- Zellweger syndrome
- Neonatal adrenoleucodystrophy
- Infantile Refsum disease
- Hyperpipecolic acidaemia

Defects in peroxisome function
- Rhizomelic chondrodysplasia punctata
- DHAP acyltransferase deficiency
- Acyl-CoA oxidase deficiency
- Bifunctional enzyme deficiency
- X-linked adrenoleucodystrophy*
- Primary hyperoxaluria –Type 1*
- Acatalasaemia*

* Disorders that do not have 'severe peroxisome phenotype'.

Most peroxisomal disorders are associated with 'severe peroxisome phenotype' and share many common features including:
- severe neurodevelopmental delay;
- hypotonia/weakness;
- seizure;
- hepatic dysfunction;
- impaired hearing or vision;
- Sudanophilic leucodystrophy.

Diagnosis is made with liver biopsy and electron microscopy morphological studies. Blood analysis demonstrates characteristic biochemical abnormalities (particularly very-long chained fatty acid, phytanic acid, and bile salt metabolites).

Zellweger syndrome

The classic peroxisomal disorder, due to defect in peroxisome biogenesis. 'Severe peroxisome phenotype' (see 📖 p.959); leads to death within few months of birth.

Infantile Refsum disease

Severe peroxisome phenotype with retinal degeneration, decreased plasma cholesterol, increased plasma phytanate. Survival to early childhood.

Disorders of nucleotide metabolism

A miscellaneous group of disorders characterized by abnormalities in enzymes responsible for metabolism and removal of the purine and pyrimidine components of proteins and amino acids.

Classification of disorders of nucleotide metabolism

Disorders of purine metabolism
- Lesch–Nyhan syndrome
- Gout
- Renal lithiasis (adenine phosphoribosyltransferase (APRT) deficiency)
- Xanthinuria (xanthine oxidase deficiency)

Disorders of pyrimidine metabolism
- Type I and II orotic aciduria
- Ornithine transcarbamylase deficiency

Lesch–Nyhan syndrome

X-linked recessive. Due to a deficiency in hypoxanthine–guanine phosphoribosyltransferase (HPRT) leading to the formation of excessive uric acid.

Children are normal at birth and symptoms and signs develop in the first few months. Classic clinical features include:
- Severe neurodevelopmental impairment.
- Behavioural problems including self-mutilative biting of fingers and lips.
- Spastic CP.
- Choreoathetosis.
- Uric acid urinary/renal stone development.
- Megaloblastic anaemia.
- Short stature.
- Vomiting.

Biochemical analysis demonstrates increased plasma and urinary uric acid levels. Molecular genetic testing for mutations in the *HPRT* gene is available.

Disorders of porphyrin metabolism

The porphyrins are the main precursors of haem, and essential constituents of haemoglobin, myoglobin, the respiratory and P450 liver cytochromes, and of other enzymes (catalases and peroxidases). Deficiency in porphyrin pathway leads to accumulation of precursors, which are toxic to tissues in high concentration. The chemical properties of these precursors determines the site of tissue accumulation, and whether they induce photosensitivity.

The porphyrias (Table 26.3) may be inherited or acquired. They are broadly classified as hepatic porphyrias or erythropoietic porphyrias, based on the site of the overproduction and main accumulation of the porphyrins. They manifest with either skin problems or with neurological complications (or occasionally both) and present either acutely or non-acutely.

- *Hepatic porphyrias:* are characterized by acute neurological attacks manifesting as seizures, neuropathy, behaviour problems/pyschosis, and hallucinations. Muscle (back) pain, vomiting, and abdominal pain are also common. Acute episodes may be triggered by exposure to certain drugs (e.g. alcohol, oral contraceptive agents, and certain antibiotics) and by other chemicals and certain foods. Fasting can also trigger attacks.
- *Erythropoietic porphyrias:* present with skin problems, including light-sensitive blistering rash and increased hair growth.

Spectroscopic and biochemical analysis for abnormalities in porphyrin metabolite profile in urine and stools is required for diagnosis. In nearly all cases of acute porphyria syndromes, urinary porphobilinogen is markedly elevated (except in ALA dehydratase deficiency).

Treatment

Acute porphyria
High carboydrate diet and avoidance of precipitating factors. Haemearginate (early in acute episode). Symptomatic treatment.

Erythropoietic porphyrias
The skin rash that occurs in erythropoietic porphyrias generally requires use of sunscreens and avoidance of bright sunlight. Chloroquine may be used to increase porphyrin secretion.

Table 26.3 Types of porphyria

Porphyria type	Inheritance/site	Enzyme	System involved
Acute porphyrias			
Acute	AR/hep.	ALA-dehydratase	Neurovisceral
Acute/intermittent	AD/hep.	Porphobilinogen deaminase	Neurovisceral
Hereditary coproporphyria	AD/hep.	Coproporphyrinogen oxidase	Neurovisceral + cutaneous
Variegate porphyria	AD/mixed	Protoporphyrinogen oxidase	Neurovisceral + cutaneous
Non-acute porphyrias			
Congenital erythropoietic porphyria	AR/erythro.	Uroporphyrinogen III cosynthase	Cutaneous
Porphyria cutanea tarda	AD/erythro.	Uroporphyrinogen decarboxylase	Cutaneous
Hepatoerythropoietic porphyria	AR/erythro.	Uroporphyrinogen decarboxylase	Cutaneous
Erythropoietic protoporphyria	AD/erythro.	Ferrochetalase	Cutaneous

AR, Autosomal recessive; AD, autosomal dominant; hep., hepatic; erythro., erythropoietic

Disorders of metal metabolism and transport

Wilson disease See 📖 p.346

Autosomal recessive (1/30,000 births); due to mutation in the *ATP7B* gene that encodes for a cell membrane ATP-sensitive copper pump. The condition results in a build-up of intracellular hepatic copper with subsequent hepatic dysfunction, neurological abnormalities, and haemolytic anaemia.

Symptoms and signs

Usually develop from the age of 10yrs onwards (rare <5yrs). Half of patients first present with chronic active hepatitis (which may lead to cirrhosis), and half with neurological symptoms including mood disorder, psychosis, and features consistent with Parkinson's disease. Haemolysis is usually present only in severe cases. Other features seen include renal tubular acidosis, renal stones, and cardiomyopathy.

Diagnosis

- Low plasma concentrations of caeruloplasmin (in 80% of patients). Elevated 24hr urinary copper excretion.
- Ophthalmoscopy to detect Kayser–Fleischer rings (although their absence does not rule out Wilson disease).

Treatment

- Lifelong chelating agents (e.g. D-penicillamine).
- Liver transplantation may be needed in severe disease.

Menkes disease

X-linked recessive. Caused by mutation in the gene encoding Cu^{2+}-transporting ATPase, alpha polypeptide. The disease is characterized by:
- early onset growth retardation;
- peculiar hair development (sparse, steely, or kinky hair);
- focal cerebral and cerebellar degeneration.

The phenotype also includes hypotonia, seizures, microcephaly, and osteoporosis. Predisposition to intracranial haemorrhage is also recognized.

Biochemical analysis reveals low plasma levels of caeruloplasmin and copper.

Haemochromatosis

At least 4 inherited iron-overload disorders have been identified:

- *Classic haemochromatosis (HFE 1):* autosomal recessive affecting 1 in 200 to 1 in 400 of population. Caused by mutation in either *HFE* gene (on 6p21.3) or haemojuvelin gene (*HJV*) (1q21).
- *Juvenile haemochromatosis (HFE 2):* AR.
- *Haemochromatosis type 3 (HFE 3):* AR.
- *Haemochromatosis type 4 (HFE4):* AD.

The clinical features of haemochromatosis are wide ranging and include:

- hepatomegaly;
- Splenomegaly.
- Cirrhosis of the liver.
- Hypermelanotic pigmentation of the skin.
- Heart failure (cardiomyopathy).
- Joint stiffness and arthritis.
- *Involvement of the endocrine glands:* can lead to diabetes mellitus, adrenal insufficiency, gonadal failure, and hypopituitarism.
- Increased susceptibility to certain infections is recognized (e.g. *Salmonella, Klebsiella*).

Primary hepatocellular carcinoma complicating cirrhosis is responsible for about one-third of deaths in affected homozygotes.

Diagnosis Increased serum iron and ferritin levels. Liver biopsy.

Treatment Repeated therapeutic phlebotomy.

Community child health

Introduction

Community child health includes disability, social paediatrics, general paediatrics and health promotion. It involves close working with children's services from education and social care, as well as the primary health care team.

Within a given area a child may have contact with a variety of professionals varying according to the child's needs. Multidisciplinary and multiagency working is essential in order for the child's and family's needs to be effectively met.

Voluntary and charitable organizations

Many different services are available and there is often a close connection between these and statutory agencies particularly for children with disabilities.

- *Homestart:* volunteers offer support in the family's own home to families who have children aged <5yrs.
- *Mencap:* long established national charity for learning disabilities—all ages and causes.
- *Scope:* national charity with focus on CP.
- *National Autistic Society.*
- *Contact a Family:* advice for families with disabled children.

Organizations and structures

The following agencies are responsible for the organization and delivery of child health services in the community.

Primary health care team
- The general practitioner (GP).
- Practice nurses.
- Midwives
- Health visitor and community nursery nurses
- School nurses for mainstream and special schools
- District nurses.

The local authority

The local authority has responsibilities for the administration and delivery of education and social care.
- The Children Act 2004 requires that local authorities have a director for children's services and a lead member responsible for children.
- In the UK, central government is responsible for establishing national policies and guidance and overseeing standards via various means of inspection, but local need determines what services are available.

Education

In the UK there are two levels of services:
- *Central and administrative level (local authority departments):*
  - provide support to schools (includes educational psychology, specialist teachers for learning, behaviour, senses, and educational welfare);
  - responsible for initiation, coordination, and provision of statement of special educational needs according to the 2001 Special Educational Needs and Disability Act.
- *Schools and nurseries:*
  - are directly managed by their governing body;
  - have a special educational needs co-ordinator (SENCO);
  - are allocated some funds to support children with special needs.
  - have access to specialist educational services;
  - are given extra resources as specified in statements of special educational needs for individual children within the school.

Specialist paediatric services
- Include paediatricians in hospital and community
- *Specialist nurses:* e.g., diabetes, epilepsy, asthma)
- *Community paediatric nursing teams:* provide nursing care at home and in other settings for children with complex needs

Health surveillance and promotion

Disease prevention includes the following:[1,2]

- *Primary prevention:* immunizations; accident prevention; dental care.
- *Secondary prevention:* screening for inherited conditions.
- *Tertiary prevention:* reducing impairments and disabilities, e.g. hip dislocation in CP, hypothyroidism and hearing problems in children with Down syndrome.

Primary prevention programmes

These are designed to reduce the number of new cases of disease and disorder presenting within the community.

> ### Examples of primary prevention programmes
>
> - Reducing the incidence of infectious diseases—immunization programme (see 📖 p.728)
> - Reducing the risk of sudden infant death
> - Reducing parental smoking
> - Preventing accidents and poisonings
> - Improving nutrition—breastfeeding promotion
> - Preventing dental disease
> - Promoting child development
> - Preventing child abuse

There is also a range of early intervention programmes designed to promote child development, reduce the risks of child abuse and accidental injury, and improve parents' mental health. Children's centres provide a variety of services to preschool children and their families, and often are a base for different organizations and services.

Primary prevention programmes may be aimed at parents and the family (e.g. poor housing, poverty, illness, disability). Many programmes are also targeted towards at-risk groups (e.g. LBW babies, mothers with postnatal depression, families living in poverty).

There are well established group parenting support programmes on offer which focus on behaviour management particularly. Some are intensively delivered by skilled professionals for at-risk young first time mothers.[3]

Secondary prevention

These programmes reduce the prevalence of disease. The Child Health Promotion Programme in the UK has been the remit of the primary care team, and recent government guidance[2] recommends a much more focused universal approach, with additional services for those with specific needs and risks.

Antenatal screening is a very important component of this, beginning in early pregnancy and is universal at 28wks gestation with an increased focus on those women at higher risk or families requiring extra support or services.(Table 27.1).

Table 27.1 An approach to child health surveillance

Age	Screening procedure
Newborn	General examination with emphasis on eyes, heart, hips
5–8 days old	Blood spot test (hypothyroidism, PKU, CF, metabolic)
up to 4wks	Universal newborn hearing screen
6–8wks old	Examination with emphasis on eyes, heart, hips
By 1yr	Health review
24–30mths	Review and promotion of development
Between 4th and 5th birthdays	Orthoptist assessment of vision to be phased in
School entry	Measurement of height and weight; hearing screening
Primary school	No further screening programme
Secondary school	No universal screening

Other opportunities for health professional contact include immunizations. Early detection of health problems is achieved by:
• Follow-up of babies at risk (e.g. low birth weight, premature).
• Follow-up of children with neurological problems or post-trauma.
• Targeted observation or follow-up of children with a strong family history of genetic disorders, e.g. hearing, vision, dislocated hips, learning difficulties, familial hypercholesterolaemia.
• Detection by parents or health professionals (i.e. neglect).
• Detection by professionals in the course of their work (particularly playgroup, nurseries, and schools, as well as health professionals).

Within each district the preschool programme will vary according to what families need and will be targeted to those who are 'high risk'.

Particular concerns for preschool programmes

- First pregnancies and first time mothers
- Isolated mothers
- Mother with postnatal depression
- Unsupported, young parent living in poverty
- Domestic violence; drug or alcohol abuse
- Parents with learning disability
- Concern about child neglect or abuse
- Infant with difficult feeding, sleeping, or temperament
- Premature baby or child who is disabled
- Refugee families
- Smoking (pregnancy or postnatal)
- Obesity in parents
- Poor attachment and inconsistent care

References

1. Hall DMB, Elliman D (eds) (2004). Health for all children, 4th edn. Oxford: Oxford University Press.
2. Department of Health (2008). The child health promotion programme. London: DoH.
3. Family Nurse Partnership programme (2006). Olds. London: FNP.

Special educational needs

20% of children have special educational needs at some time (see Box 27.1). Only 2% have a statement of special educational needs.

Box 27.1 Reasons for children having problems at school

- Global developmental delay (severe, detected preschool) (📖 p.564)
- General learning difficulties (📖 p.566)
- Specific learning difficulties including dyslexia and dyscalculia (📖 p.988)
- Developmental co-ordination disorder (i.e. dyspraxia) (📖 p.566)
- Behavioural problems (📖 pp.561, 598)
- Asperger's syndrome/high functioning autism (📖 p.602)
- Emotional difficulties (family, bullying, school phobia) (📖 p.991)
- Depression in adolescents (📖 p.578)
- Physical illness (📖 p.802) and disability (📖 p.987)
- Chronic fatigue (📖 p.990)

Statutory assessment of special educational needs (UK)

The Disability Discrimination Act 1995 and amendments legislate for no discriminate against people with disabilities. Schools implemented this Act in 2002. The Special Educational Needs and Disability Act 2001 requires:
- Promotion of the inclusion of such pupils in mainstream schools.
- A graduated response to assessment and help.
- Advice from other professionals including health and education before statutory assessment.

Statutory assessment under the Education Act—UK

The assessment under the Education Act includes advice from:
- Parents and child
- Health: a community pediatrician—'designated medical officer for education'; collates all medical and therapy advice
- Education and educational psychology
- Social services

A provisional statement by the education department is seen by the parents before it is finalized (see 📖 p.987). The annual review is required to ensure that targets and needs have not changed.

Children with disabilities

This includes children with physical and/or learning disabilities. Multi-agency assessments including medical information and a management plan are required. A 'key' worker for these families should be identified in order to minimize disruption and co-ordinate care. Early Support is a national programme that has been developed to facilitate this process, and there is a wide range of information available for families and professionals to access.

Many severely disabled children will also have a statement of special educational needs Each child needs an individual educational plan to identify targets and a means of achieving them, which is regularly reviewed. Other agencies, including therapists and doctors, must ensure that health needs are also met. Therapy advice and targets are given to teachers and school support staff and are incorporated into the child's daily curriculum.

The UK Children's Act stipulates that children with disabilities may require additional services, including social care and respite for the family.

Particular issues for families

- Home adaptations
- *Specialist equipment provision:* standing frames, mobility, feeding, bathing, toileting
- *Augmentative communication:* signing, symbols, speech-aids, speech therapy
- *Financial support:* may be eligible for:
  - Disability Living Allowance (not means tested)
  - Invalid Carer's Allowance (dependent on income)
  - Mobility Allowance (related to level of physical and learning difficulty)
- Learning disabilities and challenging behaviours (common)
- Multiplicity of appointments
- Lack of co-ordination of care

Specific learning difficulties

Dyslexia

Children of normal intelligence who have not learned to read despite exposure to adequate instruction:

- Aetiology uncertain; often family history, M:F 4–8:1.
- Cognitive processes involved include decoding (converting letter strings into sound sequences), encoding (spelling), and linguistic comprehension.
- Diagnosis is educational but a child may have language difficulties and/or co-ordination difficulties.
- If severe, can lead to low self-esteem and school refusal.
- Dyslexia support societies (national and local) are often helpful.
- Specialist advice and support required from education.
- Paediatrician's role is limited to consider the diagnosis and exclude other conditions.

Dyscalculia

A specific learning disability affecting the acquisition of arithmetic skills. Less commonly recognized than dyslexia. Can co-exist with writing difficulties and DCD.

Developmental co-ordination disorder See 🕮 p.568

Previously referred to as dyspraxia or clumsy child syndrome. Defined as marked impairment in the development of motor abilities not explained by mental retardation and not due to a physical disorder. The diagnosis is only made if this impairment interferes with academic achievement or with activities of daily living:

- *Prevalence:* 10% of 8–12-yr-olds; 1–3% of all children. M:F 4:1.
- Presenting features and signs (see Box 27.2).
- Characterized by perceptual difficulties that impede academic progress. For example:
  - poor motor planning;
  - poor visual perceptual skills (discrimination, memory, visual spatial).
- *Clinical assessment:*
  - neurological examination to exclude other conditions (mild CP, muscle disease);
  - overlapping with other conditions including autism and social skills problems;
  - may have additional learning difficulties.
- *Treatment:*
  - physiotherapy;
  - occupational therapy.
- Advice to school as well as parents is vital.

Box 27.2 Presenting features and signs of DCD

Presentation
- Poor motor skills
- Difficulty using cutlery
- Difficulty dressing and riding bike
- Poor attention and organization
- Problems with school progress (reading, copying, maths)
- Behaviour problems (disruptive, low self-esteem)

Signs
- Muscle tone may be low–normal
- Poor balance
- Poor co-ordination
- Excess of overflow movement on effort
- Persistence of primitive reflexes
- Associated sensory difficulties: hypo/hypersensitive to touch, sound, light, taste, smell

Chronic fatigue syndrome

Chronic fatigue syndrome (CFS) is defined as generalized fatigue persisting after routine tests and investigations have failed to identify underlying cause. The fatigue in CFS may be associated with other symptoms:

- Difficulty in concentrating; cognitive dysfunction.
- Disturbed sleep.
- Fatigue (both mental and physical) exacerbated by effort.

The diagnosis should be made as soon as it is clear that the symptoms are causing functional impairment and no alternative explanation has been found (3mths in children).

Investigation

Routine investigations need to be undertaken to rule out plausible alternative causes. Second-line investigations are only undertaken if symptoms/signs or investigations suggest a particular diagnosis.

Investigations for chronic fatigue syndrome

- FBC and film, ESR
- Glucose, biochemistry, CK (muscle), liver function test
- Thyroid tests
- Urine to exclude renal disease
- Screening tests for gluten sensitivity
- Assessment of ferritin levels
- EBV or viral tests only if history indicates recent infection

An assessment of psychological well-being is essential and psychiatric disorders need to be excluded. Psychological morbidities such as anxiety and depression are common and important to recognize.

Management

There is no one single approach for all patients with CFS, but as a minimum the following should be addressed.

Activity management.

Establish baseline level and gradually increase as appropriate. Referral to physiotherapy and occupational therapy to supervise programme and treat symptoms. It is widely assumed that the correct approach is the use of graded activity and CBT, as supported by the literature in adults. However, some patients find it unacceptable to use psychological treatments and have found that any exercise is to be avoided. Parental mental illness, especially depression and anxiety, should be assessed. Treating these presentations may be important in a holistic treatment plan.

Other management

- *Symptomatic treatment* for pain, sleep.
- *Dietary advice* (e.g. poor appetite or weight gain due to immobility).
- *Treatment* for depression and mood disorders—need referral to child psychiatry team.

CFS and education

CFS causes significant disruption to school. The length of absence from school depends on severity and will range from part time attendance to home tuition for many years. Liason with the school is essential in order to formulate a plan for return. Support in school may be needed for mobility or learning, and for some a statement of special educational needs will be required. If the child is too unwell to attend school, home tuition can be organized with support from the paediatrician but the maximum per week is usually a few hours and the child's needs should be monitored closely.

Prognosis

Severe or very severe CFS (house bound or bedridden for 3mths) on rare occasions requires admission to hospital. Some cases the condition may persist for many years. Generally, though, outcome is favourable.[1]

Reference

1 NICE (2007). *NICE guidelines for chronic fatigue*, No. 53. London: NICE.

Absence from school

This may be due to long-term illness (~10%). In many situations the absence from school may be the result of poor provision of extra support in class and/or information and training of the school staff. CFS is an important cause of school absence (see ☐ p.990). Absence due to school refusal has a wide range of contributory factors (see Box 27.3).

Box 27.3 Factors contributing to refusal to go to school

- School phobia
- Anxiety concerning:
  - peers (bullying)
  - teachers
  - difficulties with home life
  - emotional problems
- Poor academic progress whatever reason
- Truancy and antisocial behaviours
- Distressing symptoms such as soiling or wetting

In most cases a thorough medical assessment is needed to ascertain the cause of chronic or recurrent school absence. When it is thought appropriate, home tuition can be provided until the child returns to school.

Constipation and soiling

See also 📖 p.306.
This is a common problem in childhood.[1] Critical periods occur around
the time of infant weaning, toilet training, and starting school. Constipation
may follow a period of dehydration leading to hard stools that become
painful to pass. The child therefore holds on to stool. Secondary soiling
(overflow) is common and leads to anxiety at school that may lead to
school refusal. It is important to review the past medical history for possible underlying reasons and causes of constipation.

Taking the history

Find out when problem first arose. In infants ask about:
• Delay in passage of meconium
• Abdominal distension in early infancy
• Explosive stools

These are possible indicators of underlying HSD or short segment
bowel
   Also ask about:
• Possible precipitants
• Current diet and fluid intake
• Psychological factors
   • coercive or chaotic toilet training
   • fear of toilet
   • parental neglect/discord /illness
   • environmental stressors

Examination and investigations

Examination
• Inspect anus for:
   • fissures
   • infection
   • skin disease—excoriation/fistula
   • dilatation
• Palpate abdomen
• General examination of child including growth: rarely presentation of
   hypothyroidism

Investigations
• AXR (to demonstrate faecal loading)—not routinely needed for
   diagnosis
• Bloods:
   • FBC
   • TFT

Management

Throughout this time parents and child will need considerable support from the nursing team (i.e. health visitor/school nurse/specialist nurse).

Short-term constipation with no soiling

- Soften retained stool, e.g. oral Movicol®, lactulose or docusate.
- Colonic stimulant orally, e.g. oral senna. Continue until bowel pattern regular and then decrease.

Long-term and soiling

- Soften retained stools for at least a week, e.g. lactulose/ docusate/ Movicol®).
- Oral colonic stimulant, e.g. senna, single daily dose until stool passed.
- If no stool passed consider using:
  - oral bowel evacuation preparation;
  - enema;
  - manual evacuation as a last resort (necessary if evidence of impaction).

Maintenance treatment

- Increase dietary fibre and fluid.
- Regular bulk laxative.
- Regular colonic stimulant.
- Persist with medication for at least 6mths.
- Behaviour management may be needed to establish toilet routine.
- Assessment by a clinical psychologist and family therapist if there is a degree of family discord.
- In resistant cases treatment will need to be continued for longer.

Reference

1 NICE (2010). *NICE guidelines constipation in childhood*. No. 99. London: NICE.

Enuresis

Enuresis is the involuntary emptying of the bladder. Although children may 'wet' themselves by day or night, the term enuresis is applied to nocturnal enuresis. When it occurs during the day, while awake, it is known as diurnal enuresis. Nocturnal enuresis is more common.

In order to learn bladder control the young child needs to overcome the infant automatic pattern of voiding. For the young child, conscious awareness of fullness and the ability to postpone voiding by suppressing the urge to void are not perfect. This response is first learned for day-time control. Eventually, bladder control becomes automatic and does not require a conscious act. Night-time bladder control requires that the brain, during sleep, suppress the automatic emptying reflex. Learning bladder control at night occurs gradually, and in some children and families takes much longer than average.

Girls achieve bladder control earlier than boys. Enuresis is defined as the continued wetting in girls beyond the age of 5yrs, and in boys beyond the age of 6yrs.

Enuresis may be primary, with children not having established an appropriate period of adequate bladder control in early childhood, or secondary occurring after a period of established bladder control.

Primary enuresis
- A strong family history.
- Boys more commonly than girls (ratio 2:1).
- 15% of 5-yr-olds, 5% of 10-yr-olds, and 1% of 16-yr-olds have not established total bladder control and will wet the bed once a week or more.
- Majority of cases have no underlying organic cause and it is thought to be due to delayed maturation of bladder control mechanisms.

Secondary enuresis
Needs careful history and investigations because of probable organic cause.

Possible organic causes of secondary enuresis

- *Renal tract:* urinary tract infection
- *Neurological:* spina bifida
- *Endocrine:* diabetes mellitus, diabetes insipidus
- Behavioural problems
- Abuse

Daytime wetting is usually caused by bladder detrusor instability.

History and investigations

History
Assess pattern and types of drink consumed:
- Often limited fluid in the day
- Drink after school and evening
- May have sugary drinks

Voiding habits:
- Infrequent (<4 daily)
- Frequent (>7 daily)
- Dysfunctional/inappropriate place of voiding

Investigations
- Urine testing:
  - culture
  - urinalysis
- US of the renal tract:
  - assess pre- and post-micturition bladder urine residual volume
  - underlying anatomical abnormalities

Treatment

Primary (nocturnal) enuresis
- Encourage regular drinks (water), but restrict in last hour before bed.
- Give drinking/voiding chart.

If primary nocturnal enuresis is associated with arousal from sleep or disturbance, then an enuresis alarm should be considered. This requires careful discussion with families. Compliance is often an issue and the family and child need to be motivated. If enuresis associated with a small bladder, 'bladder training' exercises is first-line approach. Also consider using bladder-stabilizing drugs, e.g. oxybutynin. If nocturnal enuresis and urine output exceeds bladder capacity consider using desmopressin (antidiuretic hormone) and limit fluid intake 1hr before bedtime.

If the problem is resistant to the above treatments, other pathologies need to be considered:
- Urinary outflow obstruction in boys.
- Chronic constipation.
- Neurodevelopmental problems.
- Psychological problems.

Chapter 28

Child protection

Definitions

Child protection The decisive action taken to safeguard children from harm.

Child abuse

This is defined as either:
- Deliberate infliction of harm to a child.
- Failing to prevent harm to a child.

Children may be abused in the family home, in an institutional setting, or, occasionally, by a stranger. Most young people who are abused know their abuser. It is estimated that 1–2 children die each week due to abuse.

Child abuse may be categorized as:
- neglect;
- physical (📖 p.1000);
- sexual (📖 p.1002);
- emotional (📖 p.1003)

Neglect

This is defined as a persistent failure to meet a child's basic physical or psychological needs that is likely to result in serious impairment of the child's health and development. Neglect may occur during pregnancy as a result of maternal substance abuse. Once a child is born it may involve:
- Failing to provide adequate food.
- Failing to protect from physical harm or danger.
- Failure to access appropriate medical care or treatment.
- Failure to ensure adequate supervision

Presentation
- Failure to thrive.
- Consistently unkempt and dirty appearance.
- Repeated failure by carers to prevent accidental injury.
- Lack of social responsiveness and/or developmental delay when there are other concerns about the environment at home.
- Medical advice is not sought, which compromises the health of the child, including if they are in ongoing pain.

Illness fabricated or induced by carers

This is an unusual form of child abuse. It was previously referred to as Munchausen syndrome by proxy (MSbP). The salient feature is that the child is harmed by being presented for medical attention with symptoms or signs that have been falsified by the carer.

- The child is the victim of the abuse and the perpetrator is the person who fabricates the illness.
- Existing mental health difficulties in the perpetrator (child's natural mother in 90% of cases) have been described, but are not essential for the diagnosis.

Presentation

There is a wide spectrum of severity of presentation of harm:

- False medical story.
- Fabrication of signs, e.g. blood on clothing or nappy, or sugar in urine specimen.

The *most serious* presentations include fabrication of illness induced by poisoning or suffocation.

Symptoms

Children may present with one or more of a range of symptoms:

- Seizures, collapse, coma (📖 p.527).
- Apnoea (📖 p.48).
- Vomiting and diarrhoea (📖 pp.300, 302).
- Failure to thrive (📖 p.308).
- Polyuria and polydipsia (📖 p.350).
- Purpura (📖 p.632).
- Recurrent fever (📖 p.702).

Diagnosis

- It is important to realize that the medical profession may potentially harm children because unnecessary investigations are undertaken.
- The diagnosis can be established when the child is separated from the perpetrator and should be considered when other investigations are persistently normal.
- Very careful attention should be paid to the medical history, particularly as to who witnessed events and when they occurred.

Seek an opinion from an experienced colleague, who should arrange a strategy meeting between health-care professionals to decide on what further action is necessary.

Physical abuse

Physical abuse involves any activity that causes physical harm to a child, e.g. hitting, shaking, burning, suffocating. Fabricated illness is also usually included in this category (see 📖 pp.527, 758, 999).

Typical presentations of physical abuse

Any serious or unusual injury with an absent or unsuitable explanation

Bruises
- Symmetrical bruised eyes
- Bruising of soft tissues of the face, especially in small babies. Pre-mobile babies should not get bruises or other injuries
- Bruising of mouth or ears
- Finger marks on legs, arms, or chest (the latter may have associated rib fractures)
- Bruising of different ages
- Linear bruising on buttocks or back
- Distinct patterns of bruising, e.g. handprint marks, implements, kicks
- Uncommon sites for accidents, e.g. stomach, chest, genitalia, neck

Burns or scalds
- Typically with clear outlines or shape of an implement, e.g. cigarette burns, iron
- Soft tissue areas that are unusual, e.g. backs of hands, soles of feet
- Forced immersion, e.g. glove and stocking distribution

Fractures
It is rare for a child <1yr of age to sustain an accidental fracture. Bone disorders, e.g. osteogenesis imperfecta (see 📖 p.762), are rare. Consider the following:
- Long bones (arms/legs) in infants or non-mobile children; ribs
- Multiple fractures in various bones—almost always abuse
- Fractures of different ages

Bite marks
Adult or child bite marks can be determined by forensic dentistry

Scars
Especially if concurrent bruising present

Poisoning
This may be accidental, as a consequence of neglect, or deliberate (as in fabricated illness). An example of deliberate poisoning is salt intoxication, which may prove fatal. This should be considered when severe, recurrent symptoms or signs, such as coma, seizures, or severe GI upset (vomiting or diarrhoea) remain unexplained.

Investigations

Skeletal survey and other imaging

Infants do not localize pain; hence, injuries of differing ages may be missed. X-rays must be carefully planned with the radiology team and the correct views carried out. This may need repeating if inconclusive. Alternatively, consider a radioisotope bone scan.

* *X-rays:* particularly in children aged <18mths and for some older children.
* *Bone scan:* if X-rays inconclusive. Useful for rib fractures but not for metaphyseal or skull fractures.
* *CT or MRI scan of brain:* in infants and young children who present with irritability or coma.

Clotting screen

Perform tests if extensive or unusual bruising, or unexplained cerebral haemorrhage.

* If there is evidence of physical abuse, such as hand marks or marks from implements.
* Should be done if child presents with petechiae or bizarre marks.

Ophthalmology examination by experienced ophthalmologist to look for evidence of retinal haemorrhages. The latter are suggestive of non-accidental head injury (see 📖 p.923).

Sexual abuse

See also □ pp.576, 801.
This involves forcing or enticing a child or young person to take part in sexual activities whether or not the child is aware of what is happening. This may include physical contact, and penetrative or non-penetrative acts. It may also involve non-contact activities, such as looking at or being involved in pornographic or other sexual activities, and includes abuse via the Internet.

Presentation

Children who have been victims of sexual abuse may present in a number of ways, including:
- *Sexually transmitted infections*: gonorrhoea; *Chlamydia*; *Trichomonas vaginalis*.
- Pregnancy.
- Vaginal bleeding in prepubertal girls
- Genital or peri-anal injury with an absent or unsuitable explanation.
- *Behavioural changes*:
  - self-harm;
  - withdrawal;
  - aggression;
  - sexualized behaviour;
  - unexplained deteriorating school performance.
- Disclosure by the child.
- 2° wetting and/or faecal soiling.

Signs

Few signs are diagnostic and there may be no findings in 50–90%.

Acute signs

- *Girls*: acutely—tears in hymen; vaginal bleeding; bruising around genital area; and 'hand' grip marks.
- *Boys*: bruising to genital area; urethral injury; torn frenulum of penis.
- *Anal signs*: anal fissure; gaping anus; swelling of anal margin. *Note*: these signs may disappear rapidly.

Chronic signs

- These signs are more difficult to interpret.
- In girls the following that may be suggestive of previous, repeated penetrative trauma:
  - scar in posterior fourchette;
  - old tear or scar of the hymen;
  - complete absence of tissue at posterior hymen
- *In both sexes*: anal fissure and scars when other causes have been excluded.

Emotional abuse

Persistent, emotional ill-treatment of a child that results in severe impairment in emotional development. This may involve:
- Conveying to children that they are worthless or unloved.
- Imposing age or developmentally inappropriate expectations.
- Causing children to frequently feel frightened and threatened.
- Seeing or hearing the ill-treatment of another as in domestic violence.

This form of abuse often co-exists with other forms of ill treatment.

Presentation

This is almost always gradual and difficult to diagnose. Symptoms are largely behavioural and may include:
- Being excessively clingy.
- Attention-seeking behaviour.
- Overly anxious.
- Overly serious.
- Being anxious to please.

Parental behaviours are a clue to the diagnosis. Any of these must be persistent and severe, and have a major impact on the child in order to reach the threshold for emotional abuse:
- Persistently −ve view of the child.
- Inconsistent and unpredictable responses.
- Expectations that are very inappropriate.
- Induction of a child into bizarre parental beliefs.

Medical involvement in child protection

All health professionals have a role in ensuring that children and families receive the care, support, and services they need in order to promote child health and development. It is likely that health professionals will be the first to have contact with children or families in difficulty. Participation in child protection encompasses a range of activities.

- Recognizing children in need of support or protection, and parents who may need extra help in bringing up their children.
- Contributing to enquiries about a child or family.
- Assessing the needs of children and the capacity of parents to meet their children's needs.
- Planning and providing support for vulnerable children and families.
- Participating in child protection conferences.
- Planning support for children at risk of significant harm.
- Providing therapeutic help to abused or neglected children and parents under stress(usually the remit of the child and adolescent mental health team)
- Contributing to case reviews.

Initial concerns

Where there are concerns about a child, and when there is reasonable belief that a child is at serious risk of immediate harm, doctors should act immediately to protect the interests of the child, and this will almost always involve contacting one of the three statutory bodies with responsibilities in this area:

- Social care.
- Police.
- National Society for the Prevention of Cruelty to Children (NSPCC).

A full report of concerns will be required. The precise action taken should be governed by the procedures set out by the Local Safeguarding Children Boards (see also pp.1005–1010, 1042).

Referrals to other agencies

An experienced/senior member of the medical team must be involved when there are child protection concerns.

Agencies

- *Social care:* lead agency for investigation of child abuse.
- *Police service:* frequently involved in the initial joint investigation or when criminal prosecution is likely.

Referral procedure

- Inform parents unless likely to result in further harm to the child.
- Referral does not need parental permission.
- Specific concerns should be clearly stated.
- Telephone referrals should be confirmed in writing.
- All referrals should be followed up if no acknowledgement is received or action taken.

The child's safety is of equal importance with their medical treatment.

If hospitalization for medical treatment is not indicated they should not be discharged without a clear plan and decision about place of safety and future follow-up. This will be the joint decision and responsibility of the multidisciplinary agencies (medical, social care, and police). The police should be immediately informed if the parents/carers attempt to remove the child from hospital before these decisions are made.

Medical assessment

See also 📖 p.1004. The purpose of the medical assessment is to:
• Assess whether the child has been injured and/or whether there are any other medical or developmental concerns.
• Provide appropriate investigations and treatment for the child.
• Provide an opinion about possible cause.

When assessing a child who may have been the victim of child abuse it is important to inform and involve your senior colleagues at an early stage.

The assessment should be carried out (along with an experienced/senior colleague, if possible) in an environment that provides a sufficient degree of comfort for the child and their parents/carers, as well as sufficient access and lighting for examination. It is good practice to have a nurse or other health professional present at the time of history taking and examination.

History
• A thorough history is required.
• The presenting problem should be documented chronologically, outlining the sequence of events and circumstances leading up to presentation and referral.
• The family history, past medical history (e.g. clotting defects, bone disorders, psychiatric), and social history should be detailed.

Examination
This should include a general examination of all the systems.
• Weight, head circumference, and height should be plotted on a growth chart.
• Neurodevelopmental assessment is appropriate in infants/toddlers.
• External injuries should be recorded in detail, including their location, size/dimensions, and appearance.
• Photographs should be taken (see 📖 p.1007).

Examination of children with suspected sexual abuse should only be undertaken by designated/trained professionals (e.g. the named child protection lead or police-surgeon).

Child protection plan
• Where there are concerns about a child enquires should be made to social care. There is a confidential list of names of children subject to a child protection plan within a local authority area who are believed to be at continuing risk of significant harm. This is maintained by the local authority within the social care department, every local authority is required to hold one.
• A child protection plan is drawn up by professional staff working together with the parents, carers, and the child (where old enough). Children with a child protection plan have a social worker who is responsible for co-ordinating work with the child and the family.

The family must have a clear understanding of the planned outcomes and that they are willing to work to these within a specified time frame.

- A child will be the subject of a child protection plan until it is believed that the child is safe from any future harm. Regular meetings are held with the parents/carers and child to review the work being done and progress made.
- If a child moves out of one area, if they are the subject of a child protection plan, the information must be passed on to the new local authority area.

Consent

This is an important consideration that needs to be taken into account before proceeding with the medical assessment of any child. If the child is deemed to have sufficient understanding to make an informed decision, consent should be obtained from them. This principle is commonly referred to as 'Gillick competency', although now we think in terms of Fraser competency (see 📖 p.1036). Children of sufficient understanding cannot be medically examined without their consent even when an emergency protection order has been made (see 📖 p.1042).

Gillick competency

This is named after the ruling of the House of Lords (Gillick v. West Norfolk and Wisbech Area Health Authority [1985]). It stated that the parental right to determine whether or not a child below the age of 16yrs will or will not have medical treatment terminates if and when the child achieves sufficient understanding and intelligence to enable him to understand fully what is proposed (see also 📖 p.1037). This term has now been replaced by Fraser competency (see 📖 p.1036).

Record keeping

Clear, detailed note keeping is required.

- *Written notes:* full and contemporaneous notes should be kept including comments made by parents and the child. All notes must be signed and dated with the name of the doctor printed underneath an entry.
- *Diagrams:* particularly body maps to illustrate location of injuries.
- *Photographs:* may be helpful, but should be dated and signed or requested from medical photography with parental consent.

Assessment by social care

Social care and the police will undertake an assessment. They will collect the relevant information from all professionals involved. Referrals may result in:

- No further action being taken.
- Provision of support and help for the child and their family.
- A fuller assessment of the needs and circumstances of the child.

Strategy meeting

This is a meeting between professionals from all the relevant agencies (social services, police, education, health) to decide on the next action or steps.

Child protection conference

This will be convened if there are concerns about significant harm. The timing will vary and may be after discharge from hospital as long as the child is in a place of safety. A plan is needed to ensure the child's welfare and safety is addressed. When a child is considered at risk, then following the conference:

- He/she will be the subject of a child protection plan.
- A more comprehensive assessment (core assessment) will be arranged and undertaken.
- A key worker will be appointed.
- A review conference will be arranged within 3mths.

Children not considered at risk have:

- A support plan organized.
- Follow-up between the family and other professionals arranged.

Report writing for child protection conferences

See also 📖 p.1006. Those members of the medical team directly involved in the initial assessment and/or subsequent management of the child should write a medical report. Parents have the right to see reports before a case conference. There are a number of important key points in writing these reports:

- They should distinguish fact from observation and allegation.
- Relevant information should be used from current and past records.
- Medical terms should be explained for the benefit of laypersons.
- Include observations and relevant statements from child and carer.
- State clearly whether the injury is unexplained or does not fit with history.
- State medical opinion only.

Confidentiality and disclosure of medical information

Guidance regarding confidentiality and information disclosure is provided by the UK General Medical Council (GMC). There are various reports from 2004 onwards that can be found on the GMC website (see www.gmc-uk.org/). In addition, there is a useful consultation document that can be downloaded called 'Protecting children and young people: the responsibilities of all doctors' (2011).

- Information can be disclosed without consent in cases of serious crime (including child abuse).
- If information is not disclosed the doctor should be prepared to justify their decision.
- In the absence of consent, confidential medical information about parents or third parties should be shared when relevant and necessary to protect the safety and welfare of the child. The more sensitive this information is, the greater the child's needs must be to justify disclosure.
- Normally permission from parents should be obtained unless it is reasonable to conclude that this would hinder enquiries or place the child at greater risk.

Prevention strategies

Most children referred to social care will be those in need, rather than those requiring protection. Children in need are defined as those whose vulnerability is such that they are unlikely to reach or maintain a satisfactory level of health or development without the provision of support services. The role of social care in prevention is to undertake an initial core assessment and to implement a plan to maximize the child's health and development, including:

• Referral to universal support services, e.g. health visitors, parenting groups, school nurses, nursery placement, home support.
• Referral to specialist services, e.g. mental health (adult or child), paediatrics.

Further reading

Department of Education (2010). *Working Together to Safeguard Children: A guide to inter-agency working to safeguard and promote the welfare of children*. London: DoE. Available at: https://www.education.gov.uk/publications/standard/publicationdetail/page1/DCSF-00305-2010.

NICE (2009). *When to suspect child maltreatment*. NICE guideline CG89. London: NICE. Available at: ℜ http://www.nice.org.uk/CG89

The physical signs of child sexual abuse RCPCH (2008) (see http://www.rcpch.ac.uk/csa where an updated 2012 summary can be downloaded and the hardcopy ordered).

Pharmacology and therapeutics

Prescribing for children

Licensing
Many medicines used in children are not licensed for such use. This does not mean that they should not be used, but that the pharmaceutical company has not sought a license from the regulatory authorities. Hence, many medicines in children are used *off label*, i.e. they are used at a different dose, route, age, or indication than specified within the product license. It is important that medicines are used in children in relation to the scientific evidence available. In certain circumstances this may involve off label use.

Disease states
Certain diseases, e.g. cystic fibrosis, or clinical conditions, e.g. shock, may affect drug metabolism. Both liver and renal failure delay drug elimination, and so require dosage reduction.

Breastfeeding
Most medicines taken by a breastfeeding mother are safe for her infant. Mothers should not be discouraged from breastfeeding because of uncertainty about possible toxic effects. The *British National Formulary (BNF) for children* gives detailed information regarding which medicines to avoid.[1]

Medication errors
Medication errors are a significant problem in children. In particular, *tenfold* errors have been associated with significant mortality and morbidity, especially in the very young. *All health professionals will commit a medication error during their career!* Medication errors include:
- *Incorrect dose:* commonest error and also the type most likely to be associated with a fatality. Knowledge of the child's actual weight and checking of dose calculation is vital, especially on the neonatal unit and with parenteral medicines.
- *Incorrect drug:* second most common type of error and also associated with significant fatalities.
- *Incorrect route:* this is a particular problem with IT drugs. This is a procedure for specialists and great care should be taken when drugs are to be given this way!
- *Other errors:* include incorrect rate of administration, duplicate dosing, and administration of the drug to the wrong patient.

Reference
1 RCPH (2009). *The British National Formulary for Children.* BMJ Publishing Group Ltd, RPS Publishing, RCPCH Publication Ltd. 2009

Adverse drug reactions

One in 10 children in hospital and one in 100 attending outpatients will experience an adverse drug reaction (ADR). 1 in 8 will be severe. ADRs are responsible for almost 2% of children admitted to hospital. ADRs in children can be as varied as in adults. Children, because of growth and development, also suffer specific ADRs. Differences in drug metabolism make certain ADRs a greater problem in children, e.g. valproate hepatotoxicity, or less of a problem, e.g. paracetamol hepatotoxicity following an overdose. The mechanisms of ADRs specifically affecting children are illustrated with examples below.

Mechanisms of ADRs

Impaired drug metabolism

Chloramphenicol, when first used in neonates, led to the development of the grey baby syndrome (vomiting, cyanosis, cardiovascular collapse, and in some cases death). The newborn infant metabolizes chloramphenicol more slowly than adults and so only requires a lower dose of the antibiotic. Reduction in the dosage prevents grey baby syndrome.

Children, particularly neonates, are more likely to have a reduced capacity to metabolize drugs than adults. Therefore, lower doses are usually required.

Altered drug metabolism

Children may have reduced activity of the major hepatic enzymes associated with drug metabolism. To compensate for this, they may use other enzyme pathways. This is thought to be one of the factors contributing to the increased risk of hepatotoxicity in children under the age of 3 years who receive sodium valproate. This risk is raised by the concurrent use of other anticonvulsants which may cause enzyme induction of certain metabolic pathways.

Sodium valproate should not be used as a first-line anticonvulsant in children under the age of 3yrs.

Protein-displacing effect on bilirubin

The use of the sulphonamide sulphisoxazole in ill neonates in the 1950s was associated with the development of fatal kernicterus due to drug displacement of protein bound bilirubin into the blood because of its higher binding affinity to albumin. Ceftriaxone also is highly protein bound and will displace bilirubin in sick neonates.

The protein-displacing effect of medicines should be considered in sick preterm neonates.

Percutaneous absorption Percutaneous toxicity can be a significant problem in the neonatal period due to their higher surface area to weight ratio than that of both children and adults. An example of this is the use of antiseptic agents such as hexachlorophene that have been associated with neurotoxicity.

Drug interactions Ceftriaxone and calcium containing solutions when used together in neonates may result in the precipitation of ceftriaxone—calcium salt in the lungs. This drug interaction can result in fatalities and therefore ceftriaxone should be avoided in neonates.

Ceftriaxone should be avoided in neonates.

Unknown
There are several examples of major ADRs that occur in children for which we do not understand the mechanism. Salicylate given during the presence of a viral illness increases the risk of the development of Reye's syndrome in children of all ages. Since the use of salicylates has been avoided in children the incidence of Reye's syndrome has dramatically reduced. Propofol has minimal toxicity when used to induce general anaesthesia. Used as a sedative in critically ill children, however, it has been associated with the death of over 10 children in the UK alone. The propofol infusion syndrome is thought to be related to the total dose of propofol infused, i.e. high dose or prolonged duration is more likely to cause problems.

Propofol should not be used as a sedative in critically ill children

Suspect ADRs One should always consider the possibility of an ADR being responsible for a child's symptoms. Table 29.1 lists some of the serious ADRs associated with widely used medicines.

Table 29.1 Serious ADRs associated with medicines

Drug	ADR
Corticosteroids	Adrenal insufficiency/sepsis
Cytotoxics	Neutropenia
Carbamazepine	Stevens–Johnson syndrome
NSAIDs (including ibuprofen)	GI haemorrhage
Opiates	Respiratory depression
Sodium valproate	Hepatotoxicity

Preventing ADRs Recognizing which patients are at greater risk of ADRs can help reduce the overall incidence. Health professionals should follow guidelines.

Reporting ADRs Suspected ADRs should be reported to the regulatory authorities. In the UK the yellow card scheme is in operation.

Pharmacokinetics

Pharmacokinetics defines the relationship between the dose of a drug and its concentration in different parts of the body (usually plasma) in relation to time. This relationship is measured and defined numerically. Knowledge of several key terms is needed to understand pharmacokinetic principles.

- *Absorption:* if a drug is given IV, 100% of the dose enters the blood stream. If a drug is given orally, usually only a fraction is absorbed and the term *bioavailability* is used to describe the percentage of the drug administered that reaches the systemic circulation. Absorption is often reduced following oral administration in the neonatal period.

- *Volume of distribution (V):* this is not a physiological volume but rather an apparent volume into which the drug would have to distribute to achieve the measured concentration. Water-soluble drugs, such as gentamicin, have a V that is similar to the extracellular fluid volume. Drugs that are highly bound to plasma proteins have a low V. Children differ from adults because of their body composition (neonates and young children have a higher proportion of body water) and lower plasma protein concentrations.

- *Clearance:* describes the removal of a drug from the body and is defined as the volume (usually of plasma) that is completely cleared of drug in a given time. In adults, clearance is described in relation to volume/time (mL/min). In children, clearance is also described in relation to body weight (mL/min/kg). Clearance is usually reduced in the neonatal period but may actually be higher in infants and young children than in adults.

- *Elimination half-life:* this is the time taken for the concentration of a drug (usually plasma) to fall to half the original value. It is inversely related to clearance. Therefore, 50% of the dose will be eliminated in 1 half-life; 97% of a drug will be eliminated after 5 half-lives. This is also the time required for steady state to be achieved following initial administration of the drug.

Mathematical formulae are available in standard texts that describe the interrelationship between clearance, volume of distribution, and elimination half-life.

Drug metabolism

The major pathways involved in drug metabolism are divided into phase I (oxidation, reduction, hydrolysis, and hydration) and phase II (glucuronidation, sulphation, methylation, and acetylation) reactions. As a general rule, the clearance of drugs in the neonatal period is reduced. For many drugs adult clearance values are reached by the age of 2yrs.

Phase I pathways

The major pathway is oxidation which involves the cytochrome P450 enzymes (CYP). The major CYP enzymes are CYP3A4 and CYP1A2.
* *CYP3A4:* this is responsible for the metabolism of many drugs (e.g. midazolam, ciclosporin, fentanyl, nifedipine). CYP3A4 activity is reduced in the neonatal period and early infancy. Enzyme activity between individuals varies considerably leading to a large range of plasma concentrations after the same dose of an affected drug.
* *CYP1A2:* accounts for 13% of total enzyme activity in the liver. Caffeine and theophylline are metabolized via the CYP1A2 pathway. Enzyme activity is reduced in the neonatal period, but increases rapidly such that by the age of 6 months activity approaches that of older children and adults.

Phase II pathways

Glucuronidation and sulphation are the two major pathways. Glucuronidation is reduced in the neonatal period and there is compensatory sulphation. The development of glucuronidation varies for different drugs. For example, children who are 2yrs old have rates of glucuronidation for morphine similar to those in adults, whilst for paracetamol adult rates of glucuronidation are not reached until puberty.

Pain management

See also 📖 pp.691, 890.

Assessment

Always consider the possibility of a child being in pain, either as a result of their disease or the interventions that are required. Accurate assessment requires an age-appropriate validated pain assessment scale. Self-reporting is the ideal, but the child needs to be ≥3yrs old to be able to do this. Do not use pain scales validated for acute pain to assess chronic pain.

- *Self-report scales:* usually involves the child pointing to a photograph of a child in pain (the Oucher) or a diagram of a child in pain (Bieri Faces Pain Scale or Wong–Baker Faces Pain Scale). The Oucher has been validated in children as young as 3yrs of age, whereas the Bieri Faces Pain Scale has only been validated in children aged ≥6yrs. The Wong–Baker Faces Pain Scale is more reliable in children aged 8–12yrs than in the 3–7-yr age group. The Adolescent Paediatric Pain Tool is for children between the ages of 8 and 17yrs.
- *Behavioural pain scales:* rely on assessment of the child's behaviour. Validated for children aged 1–5yrs. Examples include the Toddler—Preschooler Postoperative Pain Scale (TPPPS) and the CHEOPS. The FLACC has been validated for children aged 2 months–7 years.
- *Neonatal pain scales:* examples include CRIES, NFCS, NIPS, and PIPP. These rely on behavioural observation and, in some, measurements of pulse, BP, and O_2 saturation. It is important to use one that has been validated for the gestation of the infant, e.g. is it valid only in full-term neonates?

Management

It is best to consider pain as being mild, moderate, or severe.

- *Mild pain:* paracetamol is the safest analgesic available and is the first-line drug to be used for mild pain in all ages.
- *Moderate pain:* children who are unresponsive (or unlikely to respond) to paracetamol should receive either a NSAID, such as ibuprofen or diclofenac. Alternatively, codeine or dihydrocodeine can be administered orally.
- *Severe pain:* morphine is the drug of choice. It can be given IV (including patient-controlled analgesia (PCA)), intranasally, or orally.
- *Procedural pain:* for certain painful procedures, e.g. dressing change in burns patients, it may be better to use inhaled entonox. This is an effective and safe analgesic with a short duration of action, which the child can control themselves.

Sedation

There are two main areas where sedation is required—during procedures and whilst receiving paediatric intensive care.

Procedural sedation

There are many sedative agents available. All sedative agents decrease conscious level and, thereby, can have significant toxicity. The choice of sedative agent depends upon local experience and how quickly and for how long sedation is needed. If a child is likely to be difficult to sedate, then consider whether a short-acting general anaesthetic, administered by a paediatric anaesthetist, is safer and kinder to the child.

Prolonged sedation (critical care)

The purpose of sedation in the paediatric intensive care unit (PICU) is to help the child not the health professional. IV midazolam is the drug of choice on admission. Subsequently, once NG feeds are tolerated, chloral hydrate and promethazine have been shown to be more effective than midazolam. Propofol is contraindicated for use in the PICU, with the exception for procedures, in view of the risk of a fatal ADR.

Fever

Fever is a sign of an underlying illness. It is more important to treat the underlying illness than the fever itself. Fever is reduced to make the child more comfortable. The two most used antipyretics (paracetamol and ibuprofen) are also analgesics (see p.701).

Management

Paracetamol is the drug of choice. It is less likely to be associated with a significant ADR than ibuprofen. Ibuprofen is appropriate to use as an antipyretic agent if paracetamol has failed. Although the safest of all NSAIDs, it should not be used in children with gastroenteritis or other GI symptoms.

International health and travel

Child survival: world health

Worldwide, almost 9 million children aged <5yrs still die every year. Child mortality rates vary between world regions, and these differences are large and increasing. Some examples are:
- *1990*. There were 180 deaths per 1000 live births in sub-Saharan Africa, but only 9 per 1000 in industrialized countries—a 20-fold difference.
- *1990–2000*. This 20-fold gap increased to almost a 30-fold difference.

United Nations response

The United Nations set several development goals in September 2000, revised in September 2010:
- *Target:* reduce by two-thirds, between 1990 and 2015, the mortality rate of children under 5yrs.

Since 1990

- The number of children in developing countries who died before they reached the age of 5 dropped from 100 to 72 deaths per 1000 live births between 1990 and 2008.
- The highest rates of child mortality continue to be found in sub-Saharan Africa, where, in 2008, one in seven children died before their fifth birthday.
- Of the 67 countries defined as having high child mortality rates, only 10 are currently on track to meet the Millennium Development Goals target.

World health: childhood illness

Worldwide, half of the deaths in children aged <5yrs are due to:
• pneumonia;
• diarrhoea;
• malaria;
• measles.

Under-nutrition is a major factor contributing to these deaths. Two-thirds could be prevented by interventions already available and feasible today for implementation in low-income countries. In fact, we have the knowledge and instruments to reduce child mortality, but children continue to die because effective interventions are not reaching them. For example, *Haemophilus influenzae* type b vaccine coverage is universally low and, with few exceptions, insecticide-treated net coverage rates in malarial areas are well below 5%.

There are also clear indications in the developed world of health inequalities. Infant mortality rates show an excess associated with social deprivation and ethnic minorities.

The infant mortality rate in England and Wales of 4.7 deaths per 1000 live births in 2009 was the lowest ever recorded in England and Wales and has fallen by 64% since 1978 In sub-Saharan Africa the equivalent rate in children under 1yr was 81 deaths per 1000 live births, 39 in Asia and 19 in Latin America and the Caribbean. In the UK, the rate varies by socioeconomic status, being 69% higher in the 'routine and manual' group compared with the 'managerial and professional group'.

In 2003, data showed also that:
• Excess infant mortality also occurs in children of Asian parents—8.3 per 1000 live births born to mothers whose country of birth was Bangladesh, India, or Pakistan died.
• Babies born to mothers whose country of birth was Pakistan had an infant mortality rate of 10.5 per 1000 live births.
• The factors associated with excess infant mortality include low birth weight, ethnicity, poverty, maternal cigarette smoking, the delivery of health care, and consanguinity.

Taking children on holiday

Parents will often ask advice about taking their child on holiday. Here are some general guidelines to consider in well children. If a child has a chronic illness (e.g. diabetes, cystic fibrosis, CHD), consider whether they will require access to special health needs and provide details of a local expert. Your local specialist should be able to help.

Travel vaccinations

International travel with babies and children has the added dimension of considering the right immunizations long before you go:
- Babies in the UK receive routine immunization (see 📖 p.728).
- Exotic places usually means exotic diseases and therefore the need for immunization. Check with the National Travel Health Network and Centre (at 🖱 www.nathnac.org/pro/index.htm), country by country, in the travel itinerary.
- Babies under the age of 6mths and many immunosuppressed children cannot be given yellow fever injection.
- Babies under the age of 2mths can take antimalarial tablets if the family need to travel to an area requiring prophylaxis. Just as important for very young travellers are the use of a cot mosquito net, and other measures to prevent mosquito and other insect bites.

Flying with babies

Most international travel will require an airline flight. Mothers will not be allowed to fly if they:
- have given birth in the last 48hr;
- had a Caesarean section in the last 10 days.

Families may choose to fly after the baby's 6-wk check. Modern commercial aircraft maintain ambient air pressure equivalent to 8000 ft (2500m) or less, even during flight at altitudes above 13km (43,000 ft). Healthy babies should tolerate this 'altitude' well, although children with respiratory disease may need specialist consideration even if they do not usually require supplementary oxygen at home

Common medical problems encountered on holiday

Sunburn

This problem can be limited by the use of sun suits, hats, high-protection sunscreen, and being disciplined about exposure (see Box 30.1). See also 📖 p.819.

Box 30.1 Advice to parents about avoiding sunburn

It is important to be protected from the sun
- Too much exposure is harmful
- Protection prevents painful sunburn
- Protection reduces the risk of skin cancer in later life
- Some children are sensitive and will develop a rash

Protection entails the following
- Keep infants out of direct sunlight especially in the middle of the day
- Use high-protection, water-resistant sunscreen
- Wear sun suits

If sunburn occurs
- If there is blistering or a rash seek *medical advice* ⚠
- Cool the sunburnt area, but do not let the child get cold

Prickly heat This fine, red rash with tiny pimples is centred around immature sweat glands. It can blister and be uncomfortable.

Diarrhoea

This can be serious in the very young if dehydration occurs (see 📖 p.90). Children returning from abroad should be investigated with stool samples for bacteria, viruses and parasites if the diarrhoea is severe enough to present to hospital or has been present for more than 7 days. This is because some pathogens that require treatment with antimicrobial agents are more common in those returning from abroad (*Giardia lamblia*, *Shigella* and some *Salmonella*). (See NICE guideline).[1]

Reference

1 NICE guideline on 'Diarrhoea and vomiting in children—Diarrhoea and vomiting caused by gastroenteritis: diagnosis, assessment and management in children younger than 5yrs'; M http://www.org.uk/guidance/CG84/NICEGuidance

Illness after international travel

Approximately 3% of people traveling internationally have fever for a short period. Children will require a full assessment of fever as discussed in 📖 Chapter 19 (📖 pp.696–703). When a history of recent travel is known, the additional information needed in your assessment should include:

- review of travel itinerary;
- exposure history;
- duration of fever;
- likely incubation period;
- immunization state;
- use or non-use of antimalarial chemoprophylaxis.

Incubation period

Determining an approximate incubation period is particularly helpful when you are trying to 'rule-out' possible causes of fever. It is also useful to consider causes according to key features. For example, is the fever:

- Non-specific?
- Associated with haemorrhage?
- Associated with central nervous system involvement?
- Associated with respiratory symptoms?
- Associated with exposure to blood?
- Associated with eosinophila?

The following subsection summarizes the likely causes by incubation period and key features. It can be used to guide your history. For example, if fever began more than 21 days after returning from international travel then dengue, rickettsial infections, and viral haemorrhagic fever (e.g. yellow fever, Lassa fever) are excluded, irrespective of the history of exposure. Once the travel exposure and likely duration of symptoms have been identified, your investigations could include:

- Peripheral blood film for malaria.
- FBC and differential WCC.
- LFTs.
- Urinalysis.
- Culture of blood, stool, and urine.
- CXR.
- Specific serology based on the likely incubation period.

📖 Chapter 19 (📖 p.723) discusses some of the infections discussed below.

Causes of fever according to incubation period and key features

Fevers with incubation period <14 days
- *Non-specific fever:*
  - malaria (Plasmodium spp.)—tropics, subtropics, and temperate regions;

- *dengue (virus serotypes 1–4)*—tropics, subtropics;
- *Rickettsial spotted fever*—worldwide;
- *scrub virus*—Asia, Australia;
- *leptospirosis*—tropics;
- *Campylobacter, Salmonella, Shigella*—developed or more commonly developing countries;
- *typhoid fever*—developing countries;
- *East African trypanosomiasis*—sub-Saharan East Africa.
- *Fever with haemorrhage:*
  - meningococcaemia, leptospirosis, bacterial infection, malaria;
  - viral haemorrhagic fever.
- *Fever with CNS involvement:*
  - meningococcal meningitis;
  - bacteria and viral meningitis and encephalitis;
  - malaria, typhoid, and typhus;
  - *rabies*—Africa, Asia, and Latin America;
  - arbovirus encephalitis: worldwide;
  - eosinophilic meningitis;
  - poliomyelitis;
  - East African trypanosomiasis.
- *Fever with respiratory findings:*
  - *influenza*—widespread, seasonal;
  - *legionellosis*—widespread;
  - *acute histoplasmosis*—widespread;
  - *acute coccidioidomycosis*—Americas;
  - *Q fever*—worldwide.

Incubation period 14–55 days
- Malaria.
- Typhoid fever.
- *Hepatitis A:* widespread.
- *Hepatitis E:* widespread.
- Acute schistosomias.
- Amoebic liver abscess.
- Leptospirosis.
- HIV acute seroconversion.
- East African trypanosomiasis.
- Viral haemorrhagic fever.
- Q fever.

Incubation period >55 days
- Malaria
- *Tuberculosis:* worldwide.
- *Hepatitis B and E:* worldwide.
- *Visceral leishmaniasis:* Africa, Asia, S. America, Mediterranean basin.
- Lymphatic filariasis.
- *Schistosomiasis:* tropics.
- Amoebic liver abscess.

Further reading

United Nations millennium goals. Available at: ℘ http://www.un.org/millenniumgoals/pdf/MDG_FS_4_EN.pdf

UNICEF Statistics. Available at: ℘ http://www.unicef.org/sowc2011/pdfs/Table-1-Basic-Indicators_02092011.pdf

Paediatrics, ethics, and the law

Ethics

The development of ethical frameworks has a history as long as medicine itself. Today, ethical traditions can be broadly categorized into three traditions:
- virtue ethics;
- deontology;
- consequentialism.

More recently, principlism has been proposed as a unifying approach.

'Virtue ethics'

Often associated with the tradition of Aristotle and emphasizes the character and moral behaviour of the person or agent. Aristotle proposed nine key virtues: wisdom; prudence; justice; fortitude; courage; liberality; magnificence; magnanimity and temperance.

'Deontology'

Most commonly associated with Immanuel Kant who formulated the concept of the categorical imperative. The tradition emphasizes individual dignity, truth telling, non-maleficence, beneficence, and autonomy. The good will and motive of the individual determine the rightness of the act.

'Consequentialism'

In contrast to deontology, emphasizes that the rightness of an action is determined by its consequences. The tradition is often associated most with the utilitarians such as Jeremy Bentham.

'Principlism'

Traces its origins to the Nuremberg Code (1948), the Declaration of Helsinki (1964), and the Belmont Report (1979) all of which focus on research on human subjects. Beauchamp and Childress have championed moral decision-making in medicine based on principlism emphasizing four moral attributes: autonomy, non-maleficence, beneficence, and justice.

Common law

In England, the United States, Canada, Australia, India, and many other countries the law has mainly developed from judges through case law or precedent, rather than statute or executive action. This system is known as 'common law'. In an idealized form, common law should mean similar cases are decided consistently and that the law will evolve when new circumstances require precedent to be created. Difficulties can present when two or more precedents suggest conflicting courses of action.

We all function within the legal framework of the state in which we live, and we will also have our own personal ethical views and ideas. All of these will have an impact on the way that doctors relate to their patients, colleagues, and everybody else with whom they interact in their professional lives. As a paediatrician you will need to do the following:

• *Identify the legal and ethical problems involving patients that clinicians face most frequently.* When might one anticipate the circumstances in which clinicians may require particular care in deciding a course of action?
• *Identify clearly the clinicians' obligations in each case.* What duties does a clinician have when faced with a moral or ethical problem that affects the care for a patient?
• *Bring expert guidance, wisdom and precedent in complex situations.* What resources can clinicians use to try to resolve legal and ethical problems effectively so that the care of the patient can be continued or altered appropriately?

Recognition of ethical issues in everyday clinical practice

The key areas and issues that arise frequently in paediatric practice are summarized in Box 31.1.

Box 31.1 Key issues in paediatric practice

Consent (📖 pp.1007, 1036)
- Age and Gillick/Fraser competence
- Parental consent or refusal
- Proxy consent
- Refusal of treatment
- Insistence on treatment

Best interests (📖 p.1040)
- Aggressive treatment
- Resuscitation and do-not-resuscitate orders
- Refusal of treatment by doctors
- Cultural factors (e.g. circumcision, blood transfusion in Jehovah's Witness)

Confidentiality (📖 p.1038)
- The doctor–patient relationship (📖 p.1035)
- Rights of minors with or without competence (📖 p.1036)
- Rights of the child versus the family
- Rights of parents

Neonatal and paediatric intensive care (📖 p.1040)
- Resuscitation
- Withholding and withdrawing treatment and end-of-life decisions

Child protection (📖 p.1042)
- Duties of the doctor and breaching confidentiality
- Conflicts of interest: general practitioner's duties to the family

Clinical case study

During clinical practice, as a postgraduate trainee or an undergraduate medical student, there are many opportunities to consider some of the common ethical and legal issues at the core of paediatrics and child health. In order to help with consolidating this aspect of your learning we suggest that you undertake this clinical case study. First, identify a case that has caused you to think. There are then 4 steps. In the first two you note your initial thoughts. Step 3 is completed after a case discussion conference with your team and other learners. Step 4 is for your reflection. Write down a summary of each step—it will help to clarify your thoughts and you shouldn't need more than 250 words for each of the sections in Box 31.2.

Box 31.2 Steps in a clinical case study

Step 1. Clinical vignette
Describe the key issues in your patient or scenario:
- The medical facts?
- Contextual factors?
- The patient's capacity?
- The child's preferences?
- Surrogate decision makers?
- Competing interests?

Step 2. Medical, ethical, and legal issues
- What problems are posed by the case or scenario?
- What options were there for resolution?

Step 3. Clinical goal-setting and decision-making
After you have had an opportunity to discuss steps 1 and 2 in a group:
- Write down what you discussed in the group
- Was there an answer or resolution to the problem?
- How was this achieved and what options or interventions were considered?

Step 4. Implementation and evaluation
- How was the matter dealt with?
- Comment on whether the plan of action worked
- In retrospect, do you think the problem could have been avoided or improved, etc.?

The doctor–child relationship

Involving children in decision-making about their own care presents some problems. The law in England is not clear and relies on the clinician exercising clinical judgment. In general, consider:
- *Doctors should act in partnership with children whenever possible.*
- *The Children Act (1989)* states that children's views should be heard.
- *The United Nations Convention on the Rights of the Child* indicates that clinicians should give 'due weight to the views of the child according to age and maturity'.

The Children Act 1989

The legal framework within which action takes place to safeguard children. The key principles of this act include:
- The welfare of the child is paramount.
- Children are best brought up in their own home and agencies should seek to work in partnership with parents.
- The social services authority has a duty to investigate the circumstances of individual children where there are reasonable grounds to believe that the child is at risk of suffering or suffers 'significant hardship'.

Note the following:
- 'Harm' is defined as ill-treatment (i.e. all forms of abuse) or impairment of health or development.
- 'Significant' is not defined in the Act, but means considerable, noteworthy, or important.

The Children Act 1989 was added to in The Children Act 2004 which gave legal underpinning to 'Every Child Matters: Change for Children' (2004) and meant that from April 2006, education and social care services for children have been brought together under a director of children's services in each local authority.

Closely linked to the Children Act are:
- Protection of Children Act 1999.
- Safeguarding Vulnerable Groups Act 2006.
- The Children and Young Person Act 2008.

The Human Rights Act 1998

Public authorities must act consistently with the European Convention on Human Rights. Most relevant are the following.
- *Article 2:* The right to life.
- *Article 8:* The right to respect for private and family life.
- *Article 5:* The right to liberty and security of person.
- *Article 3:* That no one shall be subjected to torture or inhuman or degrading treatment or punishment.

Parental responsibility

This is defined as 'all the rights, duties, powers, responsibilities, and author-ity which by law a parent has in relation to the child and his property'.

Parental responsibility (PResp) is allocated as follows.

- PResp is automatically given to the mother.
- *The father has PResp if:*
  - he and mother were married at the child's birth;
  - unmarried, but name registered on birth certificate (after December 2003);
  - unmarried and entered into a PResp agreement with the mother;
  - unmarried and obtained a court order for PResp;
  - unmarried and obtained a Residence Order.
  - In addition unmarried fathers can acquire PResp by marrying the child's mother.
  - Parents cannot lose PResp unless the child is freed for adoption (or awarded to local authority as part of EPO or care order).

The doctor–parent relationship

Most professionals do not have any difficulty with the idea that compe-tent adult patients should be involved in their treatment. In the case of children, their parents are the proxy decision-makers. In this regard, the following must be considered.

- *All doctors have a duty to act in the best interests of their patients.* In the UK the General Medical Council requires this standard from medical practitioners.
- *Parents have the right to make decisions about a procedure on behalf of their child.*
- *Parents do not have the right to insist on a doctor doing something that they do not consider to be in the child's best interest.* Given this responsibility, there will be times when a doctor may be forced to act against the parents in the interests of a child.

Assent and consent

In the USA, the term 'assent' in a child is used to distinguish valid 'consent' from a competent adult. The American Academy of Pediatrics suggests that assent should include at least the following elements:

- *Helping the patient achieve a developmentally appropriate awareness:* of the nature of his or her condition.
- *Telling the patient what to expect:* with tests and treatment.
- *Making a clinical assessment of the patient's understanding of the situation:* the factors influencing how he or she is responding (including whether there is inappropriate pressure to accept testing or therapy).
- *Soliciting an expression of the patient's willingness to accept the proposed care:* do not solicit a patient's view without intending to weigh it seriously. Where the patient will have to receive medical care in spite of his/her objection, tell the patient that fact. Do not deceive them.

The American Academy of Pediatrics suggests that clinicians seek the assent of the school-age patient as well as informed permission of the parent for procedures such as:

- *Venepuncture* for diagnostic study in a 9-yr-old;
- *Orthopaedic surgery device* for scoliosis in an 11-yr-old.

With regard to consent, the clinician must present information in a manner suited to the child's developmental level. Parents should be able to assist, but in some cases they may be too close to the situation to assess the child's state accurately. Other professionals can provide important insight into a particular child's developmental level and comprehension of the information presented. In the process of consent, the child's situation influences each of these elements:

- Nature and the purpose of the therapy.
- Risk and consequences of therapy, and of not having therapy.
- Benefits and the probability that therapy will be successful.
- Feasible alternatives.

Consent

In the UK, consent must be sufficiently informed and freely given by the designated person who is competent to do so. (See also 📖 p.1037).

- The adolescent if aged >16yrs.
- The adolescent if aged <16yrs and judged to be competent.
- Parents.
- Individual or local authority with parental responsibility.
- A court.

Competence

Defining whether an adolescent demonstrates competence can be difficult and may depend on the nature of the procedure, as well as the child. The adolescent must possess qualities associated with self-determination and self-identity, appropriate cognitive abilities, and the ability to rationalize and reason hypothetically. Understanding, intelligence, and experience are also important qualities that may determine competence.

Criteria for establishing competence

The patient must:

- Demonstrate an understanding of the nature, purpose, and necessity of the proposed therapy.
- Demonstrate and understanding of the benefits, risks, and potential consequences of not having the treatment.
- Understand that this information applies to him/her.
- Retain and use that information to make decision.
- Ensure their decision is made without being pressurized.

Assessing competence is the legal responsibility of the patient's doctor or other designated health care professional. A patient's refusal to co-operate with competence assessment should not be regarded as demonstrating incompetence. In England, Wales, and Northern Ireland adolescents aged 16–18yrs can consent to treatment, but cannot refuse treatment that is otherwise intended to prevent their serious harm or death. Adolescents aged less than 16yrs may legally consent to treatment if they fulfill the criteria for competence. In Scotland, all children and adolescents may consent to treatment irrespective of age, so long as they are deemed competent to do so.

Confidentiality and disclosure

When should you tell the whole truth? What if you make a mistake? What do you say to the team? What will you say to the family? Will you disclose your error? Will you say you are sorry? How will you handle this in terms of your personal feelings? How will you feel about yourself? These are questions we all have to think about—whatever our level of seniority and whatever field of practice. The General Medical Council provides guiding principles and responsibilities of the doctor in these situations. It should be remembered that deception or flawed disclosure may take many forms, e.g. presenting 'just the facts', or saying 'there's always hope', or thinking that 'you can't tell a patient everything', or omission, or evasion.

Confidentiality in regard to patients

In adolescent practice, the issue of confidentiality arises when the young person presents for certain types of advice or treatment (e.g. contraception, abortion, STIs, substance misuse, mental health issues, and family problems).

- The duty of confidentiality owed to a person under 16 is the same as that owed to any other person.
- It is not absolute and may be breached where there is risk to the health, safety, or welfare of the young person or others.
- Disclosure should only take place after consulting the young person.
- The personal beliefs of a practitioner should not prejudice the care offered to a young person.

Objections to disclosure of information should be respected, although in certain situations disclosure may be required by law for the purposes of protecting the adolescent or others from significant harm.

Breach of confidentiality and disclosure of information

It may be proven legal to breach confidentiality in the following situations:

- *Incompetent individual:* any situation in which there is a risk of harm to the adolescent or to others.
- *Competent individual:*
- history of current or past sexual abuse;
- history of current or recent suicidal thoughts or self-harm behaviour;
- homicidal intentions;
- where serious harm to the individual is likely to occur.

The patient should always be informed that the information will be disclosed and the reason why. Attempts should be made to encourage the patient to agree to disclosure. Legal guidance from professional bodies or from medico-legal services may need to be sought.

Confidentiality and disclosure of medical information to other agencies

Improving children's well-being is dependent on agencies being able to share relevant information about them. The general rule is to seek consent to share information unless you believe it is contrary to the child's welfare. It is the parents (or whoever has parental responsibility) who can give consent.

In UK law, the parental right to determine whether a child <16yrs has medical treatment terminates if and when the child achieves sufficient understanding and intelligence to understand fully what is proposed. In practice, a young person <16yrs of age can consent to treatment, but if they refuse it, parents may override their decision. This is termed Fraser or Gillick competence (📖 p.1007). Whether an adolescent is Fraser competent depends on the complexity of their medical needs as well as their emotional maturity and intellect.

Disclosing personal information and medical information about a child to other professionals (teachers, social worker, police, other health professionals) is not a problem if consent is given but should be proportionate.

• Judgement needs to be exercised and very personal medical information should only be shared if relevant and necessary to promote the child's well-being.
• Medical and other sensitive information about parents needs their permission to divulge. Only share relevant facts when needed.
• If consent is not given then it can be justified if:
• there are very good reasons to do so (see 📖 Chapter 28); *or*
• it is in the public interest.
• Whatever decision is made this must be in keeping with the Data Protection Act, the Human Rights Act, and the common law duty of confidence and also guidance from the General Medical Council (UK).

Withholding or withdrawing treatment in children

There are medical situations where the treatments used to try to keep a child alive will neither restore them to health, nor provide them any other meaningful benefit. In these circumstances treatments such as mechanical ventilation, heart pumps, etc., may no longer be in the child's best interests.

Ethical framework

- *Duty of care and the partnership of care:* our duty as part of the health care team is to comfort and to cherish our patient, the child, and to prevent them experiencing pain and suffering. We undertake this in partnership with the child's parents or carers.
- *Legal duty:* all health care professionals are bound to fulfill their duty within the framework of the law. Any practice or treatment given with the intention of causing death is unlawful.
- *Respect for children's rights:* our treatments for children should have 'their best interests' as a 1° consideration.

Double effect

It is recognized in English and Scottish law that, e.g. increasing doses of analgesia, necessary for the control of pain or distress, may shorten life. We use opiates for the benefit of the child during life and we do not use them to cause or hasten death, but this may be a consequence—the double effect. The principle has four frequently cited conditions:

- The action must be either morally good or neutral.
- The bad effect must not be the means by which the doctor achieves the good.
- The intention of the doctor must be the good effect.
- The good effect must be equivalent or greater than the bad.

Euthanasia

Withholding or withdrawal of treatments, such as ventilation often does not lead to death. It should be clear that active measures to shorten life are not appropriate or legal and that palliative care is to be continued.

Process of decision-making

Making a decision about withholding or withdrawing life-sustaining treatment requires time. It is advisable that the whole team is involved, and enough information and evidence about the child's condition is available. The decision to withhold or withdraw life-sustaining therapy should always go hand in hand with planning palliative care needs.

- *Process:* while decisions are being made the child's life should be safeguarded in the best way possible.
- *Responsibility:* the clinical team carries the corporate moral responsibility for decision-making. The senior member of the team is the consultant in charge of the child's care and should lead the decision-making

process: s/he bears the final responsibility for the chosen course of action.

- *Family and parents:* the final decision about withdrawal of treatment is made with the consent of the parents. Good communication is essential, as is building a relationship based on trust.
- *Second opinions:* it is good practice to consider this option. Other consultants working within the team may have advice. However, additional input from experts in another hospital may be required. This is particularly useful in unusual circumstances where there is uncertainty about prognosis and the child's likely future impairments.
- *Legal input:* with time, effective communication, and support, the decision-making process in most cases can be brought to a resolution. There are instances where hospital legal advisers and court involvement are required, especially where there is disagreement between parents or parents and the medical team involved about the right way to proceed.

Professional framework

See also 🕮 pp.198–199. The Ethics Advisory Committee of the Royal College of Paediatrics and Child Health (RCPCH) identified five situations where it may be ethical and legal to consider withholding or withdrawal of life-sustaining treatment. These are summarized in the Box 31.3.

Where there is disagreement, or where there is uncertainty over the degree of future impairment, the RCPCH advises that the child's life should always be safeguarded until these issues are resolved.

Box 31.3 Ethics Advisory Committee of the RCPCH recommendations

See 'Withholding or withdrawing treatment in children', May 2004, 🔗 www.bapm.org/publications/document/guidelines/Withholding&withdrawing_treatment.pdf

- *Brain death:* mechanical ventilation in such circumstances, where specific criteria are met, is futile and the withdrawal of ICU treatment is appropriate
- *Permanent vegetative state:* this state, which has specific diagnostic criteria, follows brain insults such as trauma and hypoxia. It may be appropriate to withdraw or withhold life-sustaining treatment
- *No chance:* the child has such severe disease that life-sustaining treatment simply delays death without significant alleviation of suffering. Treatment to sustain life is inappropriate
- *No purpose:* the child may be able to survive with treatment, but the degree of physical or mental impairment will be so great that it is unreasonable to expect them to bear it
- *Unbearable:* the child or family feel that, in the face of progressive and irreversible illness, further treatment is more than can be borne. They wish to have a particular treatment withdrawn or to refuse further treatment irrespective of the medical opinion that it may be of some benefit

Good ethical and legal practice in suspected child abuse

A full account of the reporting of child abuse is given in 📖 Chapter 28 (📖 pp.998–1010). The crucial issue for doctors is the safety of the child and this overrides considerations such as confidentiality.

- *Reporting:* as soon as abuse is suspected it is important to share this information with other clinicians and social services and police.
- *Parents and carers* have parental responsibility for their children. Share your concerns and course of action with them as far as is safe for the child.

Criminal proceedings

- Crown prosecution service decides whether to bring a criminal case.
- Burden of proof needed is 'beyond all reasonable doubt'.
- No hearsay evidence is permissible.
- Magistrates Court or Crown Court.

Civil proceedings

- Burden of proof needed is 'on balance of probability'.
- Magistrates Court, County Court, or High Court.
- Divorce and other civil matters included as well as child abuse.

Court orders (Children Act 1989)

Police Protection Order

- *Application:* by the police in case of emergency.
- *Duration:* maximum 72hr.
- Child removed to suitable accommodation or prevention of removal from a current location of safety (e.g. hospital ward).

Emergency Protection Order

- *Duration:* 8 days, but can be extended for a period of 7 days on one occasion only.
- *Application:* by anyone but usually by social services.

Child Assessment Order

- Implemented when parents are uncooperative. In practice little used and not if there are grounds for an emergency protection order.
- *Duration:* 7 days.
- *Application:* by an authorized person, usually the local authority.

Interim Care Order

- *Duration:* maximum 8wks.
- *Application:* by the local authority usually (or NSPCC).
- Gives parental responsibility to the local authority (i.e. social services).

Supervision orders

- *Duration:* 12mths in the first instance.
- *Application:* by social services or NSPCC.

Note: The courts have powers to authorize or prohibit medical examination of a child at the time the order is made or during the course of the order.

Serious case reviews

Following 'Working Together to Safeguard Children 2006' serious case reviews are commissioned in cases where a child dies or sustains serious injuries, and abuse or neglect is known or suspected to be a factor. They were previously referred to as 'Part 8 reviews' as defined in section 8 of 'Working Together to Safeguard Children' (Department of Health, 1999).[1]

The purpose of serious case reviews is to:
- Establish lessons to be learnt about the way in which local professionals and organisations work together to safeguard and promote the welfare of children.
- Identify what those lessons are, how they will be acted on, and what is expected to change as a result.
- Improve inter-agency working and better safeguard and promote the welfare of children.

Reference

Department of Health (1999). *Working Together to Safeguard Children: a guide to inter-agency working to safeguard and promote the welfare of children.* London: HMSO.

Legal aspects of international adoption

The Adoption and Children Act 2002 and the Family Procedure (Adoption) Rules 2005 have comprehensively reformed the law on adoption. A new process called 'placement' has replaced the process of 'freeing for adoption'. The following notes cover some basic information for UK citizens wishing to bring an adopted child from another country.

- In general anyone over 21 can legally adopt a child.
- The UK does not have a statutory upper age limit, but each local authority has the power to determine if a prospective adoptive parent is above its acceptable age limit.
- Married couples must adopt 'jointly', unless one partner cannot be found, is incapable of making an application, or if a separation is likely to be permanent.
- Unmarried couples may not adopt 'jointly', although one partner in that couple may adopt.

UK requirements for adoption

It is a criminal offence if a parent adopts a child overseas with the intention of bringing the child to the UK without having been approved.

- A person must be approved for adoption by their local social services department before a child can be identified.
- A detailed 'home study' will be conducted by local social services or an 'approved adoption society'. A list of approved societies can be obtained from the British Association for Adoption and Fostering (📎 www.baaf.org.uk).
- A medical clearance and full police background check are also required.
- Once the approval for adoption has been granted, the prospective parent(s) should then contact the following departments for advice: the UK Border Agency—Inter-country adoption and immigration rules (📎 www.bia.homeoffice.gov.uk/sitecontent/documents/residency/intercountryadoption.pdf)
- The prospective parent(s) must also apply to the nearest British Embassy or Consulate to obtain clearance for the child to enter the UK. The Home Office Immigration service has an information package (RON117) that explains the procedures.

The UK has now ratified the Hague Convention on Protection of Children and Co-operation in respect of Intercountry Adoption 1993. This means that, in many cases, provided an adoption order is obtained in the child's country of origin, it will not be necessary for the applicant to obtain an order in the UK as well. However, where the child's country of origin has not ratified the Hague Convention, the procedures are more stringent. Applications for adoption in the UK are still necessary and may be transferred to the High Court.

Medical care

There is now a growing literature on the medical problems encountered by some internationally adopted children, albeit in predominantly US journals.

It should be remembered that many internationally adopted children have come from institutions in countries with many endemic diseases. In the USA, international adopted children have been reported to have the following conditions identified on arrival:

- Hepatitis B.
- Intestinal parasites.
- Tuberculosis.
- Congenital syphilis.
- Anaemia
- Lead poisoning.
- Deficient immunization.
- Emotional and behavioural problems.
- Unsuspected medical problems.
- Developmental delay.
- Microcephaly.

In some instances, parents now consult an expert in adoption-medicine to review the information given by the adoption agency. The American Academy of Pediatrics has recommendations on pre-adoption review and screening on arrival. The pre-adoption review will include the following:

- The specialist should be able to advise on the medical summary, the risk of foetal alcohol syndrome, and explain the meaning of Russian diagnoses, such as 'perinatal encephalopathy', 'hypertensive–hydrocephalic syndrome', and 'pyramidal insufficiency'.
- Assessment of growth and development charts, and any photographs and videos.

Once the child has arrived, it is advisable to document the adequacy of immunity gained from any immunizations. In addition to considering and testing for the diseases noted above, the child will require testing for the following infections on arrival and 4–6mths later.

- Hepatitis B.
- Hepatitis C.
- HIV (note that very few internationally adopted children arrive with this infection).

Last, the adoptive parents should consider long-term developmental follow-up.

Index

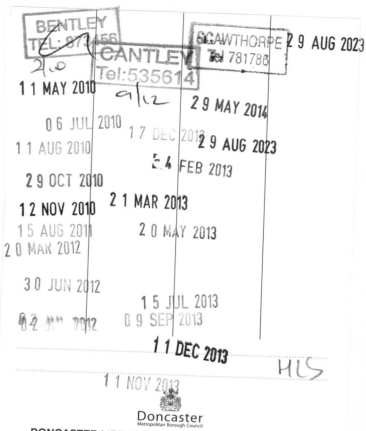

'My God! Ella, you're pregnant!' he breathed, clearly shocked.

'Well, I'm glad to see that all those years of training weren't wasted,' she retorted acidly.

'So, who's the father? I hadn't heard you'd got married.'

For a moment Ella didn't know whether to laugh or cry, but ended up determined to do neither.

'You *stupid* man!' she exclaimed shrilly as all those months of wondering and hurting finally boiled over. 'I'm not married. I have never been married and I have no intention of ever getting married. Furthermore, whether you believe it or not, you are the only man I've ever slept with, but to save you wasting money on DNA testing I'll tell you here and now that I won't be asking you for a single penny to raise this child. At least you'll go away from here secure in the knowledge that I have no intention of using the baby to destroy your marriage.'

Josie Metcalfe lives in Cornwall now, with her long-suffering husband, four children and two horses, but as an army brat, frequently on the move, books became her only friends that came with her wherever she went. Now that she writes them herself she is making new friends, and hates saying goodbye at the end of a book—but there are always more characters in her head, clamouring for attention until she can't wait to tell their stories.

Recent titles by the same author:

THE ITALIAN EFFECT
COMING HOME TO DANIEL
THREE LITTLE WORDS